P9-BZX-620

3 1611 00326 7769

Institutional Review Board
Management and Function
Second Edition

GOVERNORS STATE UNIVERSITY
UNIVERSITY PARK
IL 60466

Elizabeth A. Bankert, MA

Dartmouth College

Robert J. Amdur, MD

University of Florida College of Medicine

JONES AND BARTLETT PUBLISHERS

Sudbury, Massachusetts

BOSTON   TORONTO   LONDON   SINGAPORE

R
852.5
.A46
2006

World Headquarters
Jones and Bartlett Publishers
40 Tall Pine Drive
Sudbury, MA 01776
978-443-5000
info@jbpub.com
www.jbpub.com

Jones and Bartlett Publishers Canada
6339 Ormindale Way
Mississauga, Ontario L5V 1J2
Canada

Jones and Bartlett Publishers International
Barb House, Barb Mews
London W6 7PA
United Kingdom

Jones and Bartlett books and products are available through most bookstores and online booksellers. To contact Jones and Bartlett Publishers directly, call 800-832-0034, fax 978-443-8000, or visit our website, www.jbpub.com.
Substantial discounts on bulk quantities of Jones and Bartlett publications are available to corporations, professional associations, and other qualified organizations. For details and specific discount information, contact the special sales department at Jones and Bartlett via the above contact information or send an e-mail to specialsales@jbpub.com.

Copyright © 2006 by Jones and Bartlett Publishers, Inc.
Cover Image: © Photos.com

All rights reserved. No part of the material protected by this copyright notice may be reproduced or utilized in any form, electronic or mechanical, including photocopying, recording, or any information storage or retrieval system, without written permission from the copyright owner.

Production Credits
Acquisitions Editor: Kevin Sullivan
Associate Editor: Amy Sibley
Editorial Assistant: Katilyn Crowley
Production Editor: Susan Schultz
Marketing Manager: Emily Ekle
Manufacturing and Inventory Coordinator: Amy Bacus
Text Design: Anne Spencer
Cover Design: Kristin E. Ohlin
Composition: Graphic World
Printing and Binding: Courier Corporation
Cover Printing: Courier Corporation

Library of Congress Cataloging-in-Publication Data

Institutional review board : management and function / [edited by]
    Elizabeth A. Bankert, Robert J. Amdur. — 2nd ed.
      p. ; cm.
    Rev. ed. of: Institutional review board / Robert J. Amdur, Elizabeth
A. Bankert. c2002.
    Includes index.
    ISBN 0-7637-3049-1 (case bound)
    1. Institutional review boards (Medicine)—Management.
    I. Bankert, Elizabeth A. II. Amdur, Robert J. III. Amdur, Robert J.
Institutional review board.
    [DNLM: 1. Ethics Committees, Research—organization & adminis-
tration. 2. Ethics, Medical.   W 20.5 I6173 2006]
    R852.5.A46 2006
    616'.027—dc22
                                            2005018289

Printed in the United States of America
09 08 07 06 05   10 9 8 7 6 5 4 3 2 1

Contents

vi

FOREWORD

Jesse's Intent

Paul Gelsinger

Born on June 18, 1981, Jesse Gelsinger was a real character in a lot of ways. Not having picked out a name for him prior to his birth, we decided to name him Jesse three days later. When considering a middle name, we pondered James, but decided that just Jesse was enough for this kid. His infancy was pretty normal. With a brother 13 months his senior, he was not overly spoiled. He crawled and walked at the appropriate ages. When he started talking, it quickly became obvious that this was one kid who would speak his mind and crack everybody up at the same time. He nursed until he was nearly two years old. It wasn't until Jesse was about two years and eight months old that his metabolic disorder reared its ugly head.

Jesse had always been a very picky eater. Since weaning, he would more and more refuse to eat meat and dairy products, focusing instead on potatoes and cereals. After the birth of his sister in late January 1984 and following a mild cold in early March 1984, Jesse's behavior became very erratic over a brief period of time. Because his mother had previously experienced schizophrenic behavior, I was very concerned that Jesse was exhibiting signs of psychoses. His speech was very belligerent—as if possessed. My wife, Pattie, and I took him to see our family doctor. Thinking that Jesse was anemic because of his poor diet and lethargy, the doctor put Jesse on a high protein diet. That was the worst thing for Jesse. Forcing him to eat peanut butter sandwiches, bacon, and to drink milk over the next two days overwhelmed Jesse's system.

On a Saturday in mid-March 1984, Jesse awoke, parked himself in front of the television to watch cartoons, and promptly fell back asleep. When we were unable to rouse him we became alarmed. His mother called the doctor and insisted that we be allowed to take Jesse to Children's Hospital, just across the Delaware River from our home. Upon arrival at the hospital, Jesse was admitted to the emergency room in what they called a "first-stage coma." He responded to stimuli but would not awaken. After several tests indicated high blood ammonia, the doctor told us that Jesse most probably had Reye's syndrome, which upset us very much. Several hours later they told us that other tests indicated that this was not Reye's, and that they would need to run more tests to determine what was wrong with Jesse.

Within a week we had the diagnosis of ornithine transcarbamylase deficiency syndrome (OTC). OTC, we were told, was a very rare metabolic disorder. Jesse's form of the disorder was considered mild and could be controlled by medication and diet.

And so, after eleven days in the hospital, Jesse came home. We hawked everything he ate and made certain he took his medications. From there on Jesse progressed fairly normally, although he remained small for his age. It wasn't until he was ten that he needed to be hospitalized again. Following a weekend of too much protein intake, Jesse's system was unable to rid itself of the ammonia buildup fast enough and he again slipped into a coma. His specialist scrambled to understand how to get him well again, not ever actually having had to treat hyperammonemia. Within five days, Jesse was again well enough to go home, having suffered no apparent neurological damage.

As Jesse entered his teenage years, he resisted taking his medications. He felt that he could control his disorder and only took his meds when he didn't feel well. His mother and I had divorced in 1989, two years after our move to Tucson, Arizona. Jesse was under my care. At age sixteen, Jesse was taking nearly fifty pills a day to control his illness.

Note: This chapter presents an edited transcript of the keynote talk given by Mr. Gelsinger at the meeting of the Applied Research Ethics National Association (ARENA) in San Diego, CA on October 31, 2000.

My new wife, Mickie, and I kept careful watch over Jesse, but as he grew older we expected him to take better care of himself. With six children between us, we had much to consider. Jesse was being seen at a state-funded metabolic clinic in Tucson twice a year to monitor his development and, while not always compliant, he was progressing into adulthood.

In September 1998, Jesse and I were made aware by his specialist of a clinical trial being done at a renowned medical facility in Philadelphia. They were working on what he described as gene therapy for Jesse's disorder. We were instantly interested, but Jesse was told that he could not participate until age eighteen. That fall, Jesse was stressing his metabolism as he had never done before. He had acquired a part-time job and an off-road motorcycle, so I saw him only now and then. As a senior in high school, Jesse had a very busy schedule. Unknown to me at the time, he was having symptoms of his disorder but was trying to hide them. He didn't want restrictions placed on him. I knew that he took his medications inconsistently because I rarely had to order them. I spoke with him every other week about his need to take better care of himself. It took his nearly dying to wake him up.

On December 22, 1998, I arrived home in mid-afternoon to find Jesse curled up on the couch. A close friend was with him. Jesse was very frightened. He was vomiting uncontrollably and could not hold down his medications. After about five minutes with him, I determined that I could not manage his recovery. I convinced his pediatrician and specialist that Jesse needed to be hospitalized and placed on intravenous fluids. With his ammonia levels at six times normal, Jesse was in trouble. After no significant changes in his condition by December 24th, the hospital let Jesse go home for Christmas. Listless all day, Jesse crashed Christmas night and was admitted to intensive care, where they discovered hypoglycemia—seriously low blood sugar. His specialist was certain that it was due to one of his medications, l-arginine, and discontinued it. He also decided that Jesse's primary medication, sodium benzoate, was not effective enough and ordered that a newer, better medication be provided.

While awaiting his new medication, Jesse recovered well enough to be placed in a regular room at the hospital, but his ammonia levels refused to drop. I was staying in the hospital at Jesse's side day and night. Two days after Christmas, on a Sunday afternoon, Jesse and I had a conversation about how he was doing. I described to Jesse how it seemed that he was stuck up a tree, not knowing whether he was going to climb down or fall out. I went home to be with the rest of my family and sleep in my own bed for one night. Jesse called me at about 11:00 p.m. and said, "Dad, I fell out of the tree." He was again vomiting uncontrollably. I rushed back to the hospital and spent a heart-rending two days trying to help my son through his crisis. On Monday, I discovered that the insurance company was balking at paying for Jesse's new medications and that they had not been shipped. I told the pharmacist to purchase the new medications ($3,300 for one month's supply) with my credit card and that I would deal with the insurance company later. The insurance company relented at that point, authorized the medications, and they were ordered on Tuesday. By Tuesday afternoon, December 29th, Jesse was so listless that I grew very alarmed that he would not get well.

At 5:00 p.m., Jesse's vomiting returned and he became incoherent. I moved into the hall to get help. There I found his pediatrician examining his chart. I summoned him to Jesse's room and, while he called in the intensive care doctor, I called my wife and told her to come immediately. Jesse's aunt and grandmother arrived for a visit only to find Jesse in crisis. Mickie arrived and together we held Jesse while they prepared a bed for him in intensive care. The intensive care doctor, seeing Jesse's deteriorating condition and believing Jesse mentally impaired, inquired if life support would be appropriate. It was then that I realized that these people had not known Jesse well, and I explained that the loss of mental faculties that they were seeing was not Jesse's normal state at all. Jesse developed tremors and began to vomit. Suddenly he just stopped. I whispered to Mickie, "He's still breathing, isn't he?" I asked Jesse's pediatrician to check him. After placing his stethoscope on Jesse's chest for a few moments, he told the nurse to call a code blue. We were whisked from the room while they intubated and manually ventilated Jesse and took him to intensive care. We were distraught, believing Jesse to be near death. After fifteen minutes, they indicated that they were getting him under control and that his heart never stopped.

For two days, Jesse lingered in an induced coma to allow the ventilator to control his breathing. He weighed in at only ninety-seven pounds, down from his healthy weight of one hundred twenty pounds. His old medication only partially lowered his ammonia level.

On Thursday morning, Jesse's new medications arrived. Through a gastrointestinal feed, the doctors gave Jesse a special nutritional formula containing his new medications. Within twenty-four hours, Jesse's ammonia levels started falling. We waited at his side as he began to regain consciousness. His first conscious act was to motion us to change the television station. We knew then that Jesse was back.

Within a day, Jesse was out of intensive care, his ammonia levels normal, something he had never known his entire life. He was ordering and eating food like a teenager—again something he had never experienced. We were ecstatic. When his specialist came to see him, I shook his hand and told him that he had a medical miracle on his hands. One week after nearly dying, Jesse was back in school full time with a newfound zeal for life.

By early February 1999, Jesse had recovered enough strength to consider returning to work, but he came down with a serious case of influenza. Because illness often triggered Jesse's metabolic disorder, I stayed home to keep an eye on his condition. Jesse was kind enough to pass the bug on to me. It was the sickest I'd been in twenty years: a fever for six days and fatigue for four weeks. Jesse recovered within a week and was back in school. I had him tested twice while he was ill and his ammonia level was only slightly elevated. The new medications were working wonderfully.

Near the end of February, Jesse returned to his part-time job as a courtesy clerk at a supermarket three miles from our home. On Saturday the 27th, he called me at 11:00 p.m. for a ride home. I picked him up in my work van, and on the way home we had a fateful conversation. I had been asking Jesse to find out if his job would offer him medical insurance once he graduated from school in May. Being a typical teenager, he had done nothing. I told him in no uncertain terms that he needed medical insurance if he didn't intend to continue his education. At the time, we believed that Jesse would not be covered under our insurance once he left school.

Jesse rarely raged at his illness, but this time he flung a half-full bottle of soda against my windshield while cursing his disorder. In anger, I gave him a backhand punch to the shoulder and chastised him. Only two blocks from home, Jesse flung open the door and told me he was jumping out. I said, "Whoa! Wait until I stop." As I was coming to a stop, he gave me a look like he was jumping and went out the door. All I could envision was Jesse falling under the van and my running him over. Sure enough, even though I had nearly stopped, he fell. As I stopped, I could hear him screaming that I was on his arm. Now, my van is a work van loaded with tools and weighing six thousand pounds. Thinking "Oh, God, no!" I threw the van into park and raced around in back to find Jesse's right arm and elbow pinned under my right rear tire. Making certain that his body was clear; I rolled the van forward off his arm.

The kid was crying in agony. As I cradled him in my arms, I cried, "You idiot! What were you thinking?" and then, "Jesse, I'm sorry." He begged me not to move him, and I knew he would need an ambulance. His arm was a red mess from wrist to upper arm with the elbow area gouged out. The tire print was evident on the underside of his arm.

As I began to think about seeking help, a woman who had witnessed what happened while driving from the other direction asked if she could help. I told her to please call 911 and she drove off to do so. A neighbor, hearing the commotion, came out and offered his help. Another passerby offered me his cell phone and I called my wife. Within minutes the paramedics arrived, strapped Jesse to a gurney, and whisked him off to the hospital. After the police informed me that I had done no wrong, that I could not control his actions, it was all I could do to drive the one block home. I had been there to help Jesse through his near-death experience in December and through a serious bout with the flu only to nearly end his life in an accident.

Shaking and emotional, Mickie drove me to the hospital. Jesse was okay; he hadn't even broken his arm! He had suffered extensive road rash and a serious wound to his elbow, but he recovered full use of his arm following two days in the hospital and a month of physical therapy. I was an emotional wreck for a week following the accident. This kid was something else. His sister told him that if he caused me to have a heart attack she was going to kill him. A month later I got word from our insurance company regarding Jesse's status if he did not continue his education. He was covered until age twenty-five as long as he remained our dependent. I joked with him that I had run him over for nothing. He was proud of his war wound from dad. God, what a relief to see this kid bounce back again.

In early April 1999, Jesse again had an appointment at the metabolic clinic. While there, the subject of gene therapy and the clinical trial at Philadelphia came up again. Jesse and I were both still very interested. I informed the doctor that we were already planning a trip to New Jersey in late June, that Jesse would be eighteen at that time, and to let those running the clinical trial know we were interested. I received a letter from the clinical trial people in late April firming things up. By late May, our visit was set. We would fly in on June 18th and he would be tested on the 22nd. Jesse was none too happy about flying in on the 18th; that was his birthday and he wanted to party with his friends. A few days later he told me it was okay to fly on his birthday. I told him that it was a good thing, since I had already bought the tickets for all six of us a month earlier.

So on Friday, June 18, 1999, Jesse, his three siblings, PJ (19), Mary (15), and Anne (14), and Mickie and I boarded a plane to take us down a path we never imagined. We had a party for Jesse that night at my brother's house. We had a reunion with ten of my fifteen siblings and extended families that Sunday. It was great to see everyone. The kids got to meet cousins they hadn't seen in twelve years. Jesse's cousins nicknamed him Captain Kirk because of the way he struck the volleyball with a two-handed chop. This was turning into a great vacation.

We hung out on Monday, and on Tuesday, June 22nd, we all headed over to Philly to meet with the clinical trial people. We arrived a few minutes late because of a wrong turn on the expressway only to discover that they weren't ready for us. The nurse in charge rounded up the doctor who was the principal investigator, and after a lengthy wait we were all ushered into a hospital room to go over consent forms and discuss the procedures that Jesse would undergo. The doctor described the technique that would be used. Jesse would be sedated and two catheters would be placed into his liver; one in the hepatic artery at the inlet to the liver to inject the viral vector and another to monitor the blood exiting the liver to assure that the vector was all being absorbed by the liver. He explained the dangers associated with this and that Jesse would need to remain immobile for about eight hours after the infusion to minimize the risk of a clot breaking free from the infusion site. The doctor also explained that Jesse would experience flu-like symptoms for a few days. He briefly explained that there was a remote possibility of his contracting hepatitis. When I questioned him on this, he explained that hepatitis was just an inflammation of the liver and that the liver was a remarkable organ, the only organ in the body with the ability to regenerate itself. In reading the consent form, I noticed the possibility of a liver transplant being required if the hepatitis progressed. The hepatitis seemed such a remote possibility and the need for transplant even more remote that no more alarms went off in my head.

The doctor proceeded to the next phase and what appeared the most dangerous aspect of the testing. A needle biopsy was to be performed of Jesse's liver one week after the infusion. Numbers explaining the risks of uncontrolled side effects were included. There was a one in ten thousand chance that Jesse could die from the biopsy! I said to

Jesse that he needed to read and understand what he was getting into, that this was serious stuff. The risks seemed very remote, but also very real. Still, one in ten thousand weren't bad odds in my mind. There would be no benefit to Jesse, the doctor explained. Even if the genes worked, the effect would be transient because the body's immune system would attack and kill the virus over a four- to six-week period.

After our forty-five minute conversation with the doctor ended, Jesse consented to undergo the five-hour N15 ammonia study to determine his level of enzyme efficiency. Many vials of blood were taken before Jesse drank a small vial of N15 ammonia. This special isotope of ammonia would then show up in Jesse's blood and urine. The rate at which it was processed out of the body would determine Jesse's efficiency. Going into this study, we were aware that Jesse's efficiency was only six percent of that of a normal person. After waiting with Jesse for two hours, we all decided to head out to Pat's Steaks for lunch and tour South Street for a few hours. On our return to the hospital, Jesse was finished and ready to go.

It was now mid-afternoon and we decided to see the Betsy Ross house and Independence Mall. After we checked out the Liberty Bell, the kids wanted to see the Rocky statue, so we headed over to the Art Museum. Four of us, Jesse, PJ, Mary, and I, raced up the steps Rocky-style (we had watched the movie the night before). Finding only Rocky's footsteps, we learned that the statue had been moved to the Spectrum. So we headed over to Pattison Avenue. A Phillies game was about to start, so I stayed in our rented Durango while the kids had their pictures taken by Mickie. It was a fun time for everyone, especially Jesse. He was starting to feel good about what he was doing. This was his thing and he had a chance to help.

The following day, we toured New York City. Everybody got to pick a place to visit. Jesse chose FAO Schwarz toy store where he bought four pro-wrestling action figures. We all had a great day, finishing with the Empire State Building and the Staten Island Ferry.

Four weeks later, back in Tucson, we received a letter addressed to Mr. Paul Gelsinger and Jesse. It was from another of the principal investigators of the clinical trial, a world-renowned OTC expert, confirming Jesse's six percent efficiency of OTC and stating that they would like to have Jesse in their study. I presented the letter to Jesse and asked him if he still wanted to do this. He hesitated only a moment, then said yes. This same doctor called about a week later to follow up his letter and spoke to Jesse briefly. Jesse told him that he would need to call back and talk to me and explain everything. Jesse was deferring to me to understand this and the doctor was well aware of that.

When I spoke to the OTC expert, we discussed a number of things. Because they had forgotten to include the graph showing Jesse's N15 results, he faxed it to us. I asked if Jesse was the least efficient patient in the study. The doctor explained that he was, and steered the conversation to the results they had experienced to date. He explained that the treatment had worked temporarily in mice, even preventing death in mice exposed to a lethal injection of ammonia. He then explained that the most recent patient had shown a 50% increase in her ability to excrete ammonia following gene therapy. My reaction was to say, "Wow! This really works! So, with Jesse at six percent efficiency, you may be able to show exactly how well this works." His response was that there was hope, and that it would be for these kids. He explained that there were another 25 liver disorders that could be treated with the same technique and that, overall, these disorders affected about one in every 500 people. I did some quick math and figured that's 500,000 people in the U.S.A. alone, 12 million worldwide. I dropped my guard. This doctor and I never discussed the dangerous side of this work. When I presented to Jesse what the OTC specialist had to say, he knew the right thing to do. He signed on to help everybody and, hopefully, himself in the long run. The plan was for him to be the last patient tested. The procedure was tentatively scheduled for mid-October.

By late July 1999, Jesse had a new focus in his life, but he also had other priorities. He had just gotten a tattoo on the back of his right calf. Of course, he didn't discuss it with me first and had used the money he owed me to get it done. I had just bought him a used street motorcycle as a graduation present and he was getting his driver's license. It was great to see him grinning ear to ear as he drove off on his bike for the first time. We saw little of Jesse over the next two weeks. If he wasn't working, he was out riding with his buddy, Gar, or spending the night at a friend's house. He was still living at home and paying $35 a week for rent and $15 a week to pay for the bike insurance that we had fronted for him. This kid was really living and we were so proud of him.

In mid-August, we heard from the clinical trial people that they were having trouble scheduling their next patient and were wondering if Jesse would be available in September. I explained that I would have to check with him. He okayed it and arranged to take an unpaid leave of absence. Most communications with the hospital staff were done via e-mail at this point. The finalized date of admission would be September 9, 1999. I wanted to go with Jesse, but being self-employed and not seeing any great danger, I scheduled to fly in for what I had perceived as the most dangerous aspect of the testing, the liver biopsy. I would fly in on the 18th and return with Jesse on the 21st.

As September 9th approached, we all became more and more focused on Jesse's trip. Mickie bought him some new clothes. Jesse assembled his pro wrestling, Sylvester Stallone, and Adam Sandler videos, and I worked like a dog to get as much done as possible in preparation for my own departure. So with one bag filled with videos and another with clothing, Jesse and I headed off to the airport early on Thursday the 9th. He was both apprehensive and excited. He had to change planes in Phoenix and hail a cab to the hospital once he arrived in Philly. Jesse had never been away from Tucson on his own prior to this trip. Words cannot express how proud I was of this kid. Just eighteen, he was going off to help the world. When we reached his gate, I gave him a big hug. I looked him in the eye and told him he was my hero. As I drove off to work, I thought of him and what he was doing. I started considering how to get him some recognition. Little did I know what effect this kid was going to have.

Jesse called us that night using his phone card. He was well, but had a little mix-up with the cabbie about which hospital to take him to. The cabbie was cool about it though, he said. Reminded him of a scary version of James Earl Jones. Jesse was to have more N15 testing the following day and again on Sunday before the actual gene infusion on Monday, September 13. Saturday was an off day and he would be able to leave the hospital. Two of my brothers had arranged to visit with Jess, and that had put me at ease about not going. Jess had a blast with his uncle and cousins on Saturday and a good visit with his other uncle and aunt on Sunday. Mickie and I spoke with Jesse every day. His spirits were good. He grew apprehensive on Sunday evening. The doctor had put him on intravenous medications because his ammonia was elevated. I reasoned with him that these guys knew what they were doing, that they knew more about OTC than anybody on the planet. I didn't talk with the doctors; it was late.

I received a call from the principal investigator on Monday, just after they infused Jesse. He explained that everything went well and that Jesse would return to his room in a few hours. I discussed the infusion and how the vector did its job. He didn't like the word invade when I explained what I thought the virus did to the liver cells. He explained that if they could affect about one percent of Jesse's cells, they would get the results they desired. Mickie and I spoke with Jesse later that evening. He had the expected fever and was not feeling well. I told Jesse to hang in there, that I loved him. He responded, "I love you too, Dad." Mickie got the same kind of goodbye. Little did we know it was our last.

I awoke very early Tuesday morning and went to work. I received a mid-morning call from the doctor, asking if Jesse had a history of jaundice. I told him not since he was first born. He explained that Jesse was jaundiced and a bit disoriented. I said, "That's a liver function, isn't it?" He replied that it was and that they would keep me posted. I was alarmed and worried. My ex-wife, Pattie, happened to call about 20 minutes later, and I told her what was going on. She reminded me that Jesse had jaundice for three weeks at birth. I called the hospital back with that information and got somebody who was apparently typing every word I said. That seemed very unusual to me. I didn't hear from the doctors again until mid-afternoon. The other principal investigator, the OTC expert, called and said Jesse's condition was worsening, that his blood ammonia was rising, and that he was in trouble. When I asked if I should get on a plane, he said to wait, that they were running another test. He called back an hour and a half later. Jesse's ammonia had doubled to 250 micromoles per deciliter. I told him I would be there in the morning.

It's a very helpless feeling, knowing your kid is in serious trouble while you are a continent away. My plane was delayed out of Tucson, but got into Philly at 8:00 a.m. Arriving at the hospital at 8:30 a.m., I immediately went to find Jesse. As I entered through the double doors into surgical intensive care, I noted a lot of activity in the first room I passed. I waited at the nurses' station for perhaps a minute before announcing who I was. Immediately, both principal investigators approached me and asked to talk to me in a private conference room. They explained that Jesse was on a ventilator and in a coma, that his ammonia had peaked at 393 micromoles per deciliter (that's at least ten times a normal reading, but only slightly above the highest reading Jesse had ever had), and that they were just completing dialysis and had his level down under 70. They explained that he was having a blood-clotting problem and that, because he was breathing above the ventilator and hyperventilating, his blood ph was too high. They wanted to induce a deeper coma to allow the ventilator to breathe for him.

I gave my okay and went in to see my son. After dressing in scrubs, gloves, and a mask because of the isolation requirement, I tried to see if I could rouse my boy. Not a twitch, nothing. I was very worried, especially when the neurologist expressed her concern at the way his eyes were downcast. Not a good sign, she said. When the intensivist told me that the clotting problem was going to be a real battle, I grew even more concerned. I called and talked to my wife, crying and afraid for Jesse. It was at least as bad as the previous December, only this time they had been in his liver. I would keep her posted.

They got Jesse's breathing under control and his blood ph returned to normal. The clotting disorder was described as improving, and the OTC expert returned to Washington, D.C. by mid-afternoon. I started relaxing, believing Jesse's condition to be improving. My brother and his wife arrived at the hospital around 5:30 p.m. and we went out to dinner. When I returned, I found Jesse in a different intensive care ward. As I sat watching his monitors, I noted his oxygen content dropping. The nurse saw me noticing and asked me to wait outside, explaining that the doctors were returning to examine Jesse. At 10:30 p.m. the doctor explained to me that Jesse's lungs were failing, that they were unable to oxygenate his blood even on 100% oxygen. I said, "Whoa. Don't you have some sort of artificial lung?" He thought about it for a moment and said yes, that he would need to call in the specialist to see if Jesse was a candidate. I told him to get on it. I called my wife and told her to get on a plane immediately.

At 1:00 a.m., the specialist and the principal investigator indicated that Jesse had about a 10% chance of survival on his own, and a 50% chance with the artificial lung, the ECMO unit. Hooking up the unit would involve inserting a large catheter into the jugular to get a large enough blood supply. I said, "Fifty percent is better than 10. Let's do it." It seemed like forever for them to even get the ECMO unit ready. Jesse's oxygen level was crashing.

At 3:00 a.m., as they were about to hook Jesse up, the specialist rushed into the waiting room to tell me that Jesse was in crisis and rushed back to work on him. The next few hours were really tough. I didn't know anything. Anguish, despair, every emotion imaginable went through me. At 5:00 a.m., the specialist came to see me and said they had the ECMO working, but that they had a major leak, that the doctor literally had his finger on the leak. I quipped that I was a bit of a plumber—maybe that's what they needed. He returned to work on Jesse and I began to worry for my wife. Hurricane Floyd had made landfall in North Carolina at 3:00 a.m. and was heading toward Philly.

At 7:00 a.m., I entered through the disabled double doors into the intensive care area and, after noting four people still working on Jesse and another half dozen observing, approached the nurses' station to get them to see if my wife would get in okay. They agreed to check and asked if I would like a chaplain. I'm a pretty tough guy, but it was time for spiritual help. At first they sent a young woman who I think was Jewish. I guess she felt a bit out of place because I am Christian, and another chaplain—a Christian man a few years younger than me—was called in to help me. At this point, I was trying to contact my family—my mother especially—to get emotional support. A hospital staffer was very helpful in that respect.

By mid-morning, six of my siblings and their spouses had arrived. Mickie's plane got in just before they closed the airport, and she arrived by taxi at the hospital in the pouring rain. We weren't able to see Jesse until after noon. The OTC expert was stuck on a train disabled by the hurricane. The two doctors on site described Jesse's condition as very grave; whatever reaction his body was having would have to subside before he could recover. His lungs were severely damaged, and if he survived it would be a very lengthy recovery. They had needed to use more than ten units of blood in hooking him up.

When we finally got to see Jesse, he was bloated beyond recognition. The only way to be sure it was Jesse was the scar from his battle with dad and the tattoo on his right calf. My siblings were shaken to the core. Mickie touched him gently and lovingly. Our hearts were nearly breaking.

Because the hurricane was closing in and threatening to close bridges, my siblings left by late afternoon. My sister and her husband stayed to take us to dinner and drive us to our hotel. Exhausted, I slept for an hour. Then I arose, compelled to return to see Jesse. After leaving Mickie a note, I walked the half-mile back to the hospital in a light rain. Hurricane Floyd had skirted Philly and was heading out to sea. I found Jesse's condition no better. I noted blood in his urine. I thought, "How can anybody survive this?!" I said a quiet goodbye to Jesse and returned to the hotel at about 11:30 p.m. I found Mickie preparing to join me. I described Jesse's condition as unchanged and returned to bed. Mickie went out walking for a couple of hours.

In the morning, we arrived at 8:00 a.m. at Jesse's room. A new nurse indicated that the doctors wished to speak to us in an hour or so about why they should continue with their efforts. We went to have breakfast at the hospital cafeteria. I told Mickie we should be prepared for a funeral. She wanted to believe Jesse would get well.

The principal investigators were with Jesse when we returned. They told us that Jesse had suffered irreparable brain damage and that his vital organs were all shutting down. They wanted to shut off life support. They left us alone for a few minutes, and we collapsed into each other. When they returned, I told them that I wanted to bring my family in and have a brief service for Jesse prior to ending his life. Then I told them that they would be doing a complete autopsy to determine why Jesse had died, that this should not have happened.

While waiting for my siblings, rushes of anger toward the doctors swept over me. Then I said to myself, "No, they couldn't have seen this." I went so far as to tell the OTC expert that I didn't blame them, that I would never file a lawsuit. Little did I know what they really knew.

Seven of my siblings and their spouses and one of my nieces were present for the brief ceremony for Jesse—more for us, at this point. I had all the monitors shut off in his room. Leaning over Jesse, I turned and declared to everyone present that Jesse was a hero. After the chaplain's final prayer, I signaled the doctors. The specialist clamped off Jesse's blood flow to the ECMO machine and shut off the ventilator. After the longest minute of my life, the principal investigator stepped in and I removed my hand from Jesse's chest. After listening with a stethoscope for a moment he said, "Goodbye, Jesse. We'll figure this out." Not a dry eye all around. This kid died about as pure as it gets. I was humbled beyond words. My kid had just shown me what it was really all about. I still feel that way.

I supported these doctors for months, believing that their intent was nearly as pure as Jesse's. They had promised to tell me everything. Even after the media started exposing the flaws in their work, I continued to support them. I discovered that federal oversight was woefully inadequate, that many researchers were not reporting adverse reactions, and that the FDA was being influenced into inaction by industry. I decided to attend the Recombinant DNA Advisory Committee meeting in December where all the experts were to discuss my son's death. It wasn't until that three-day meeting that I discovered that there was never any efficacy shown in humans. I had believed this procedure was working based on my conversations with the OTC expert, and that is why I defended them and their institution for so long. These men could not go in front of their peers at the RAC meeting in Bethesda and say this was working.

There is so much more to Jesse's story. Please remember Jesse's intent when you review studies or when you make policy. You are professionals and you know the issues. I ask—and life itself demands—that you take the time and energy to review each protocol as if you were going to enroll your own child. Please use Jesse's experience to give you the strength to say no or the courage to ask more questions.

If researchers, industry, and those in government apply Jesse's intent—not for recognition, not for money, but only to help—then they will get all they want and more. They'll get it right.

PREFACE

Thank you to all of the readers who communicated their appreciation for the first edition of this book. We convey that gratitude to the authors, as it certainly was a collaborative effort. The book has traveled far and wide and has been used as a resource for institutional review boards (IRBs) across the country.

We started the first edition of this book at the ARENA/PRIM&R meeting in San Diego in October of 2000. Since that time, the volume and complexity of research has increased tremendously. When the publisher approached us to produce a second edition we knew the timing was right. As many of the core issues that remain the same, we hope the second edition will provide continuity; however, we have also made efforts to reorganize and improve the educational value of the book as follows:

- **Revisions and updates:** The majority of the chapters from the first edition return in the second edition. All chapters were revised as needed to include new information, improve readability, and to update references.

- **Deletions and reorganization:** We removed and/or reorganized a few chapters, both to reduce redundancy and to maintain a manageable length. Several chapters were combined; for example, since OHRP provided new guidance related to oral histories we combined the *Oral History* chapter with the *Qualitative Social Science* chapter.

- **New chapters:** The second edition contains seven new chapters: *Institutional Review Board Closure of Study Files* (7-6), *HIPAA and Research* (8-1), *Vulnerability in Research* (9-1), *Research in Public Schools* (9-2), *Phase I Clinical Trials in Healthy Adults* (9-3), *When are Research Risks Reasonable in Relationship to Anticipated Benefits?* (10-1), and *Internet Research: A Brief Guide for IRBs* (10-2).

The IRB is still the backbone of our country's system for protecting human research subjects. Individuals who work with the IRB still feel passionately about finding a way to conduct research according to the highest ethical standards. We cannot predict the challenges that lie ahead but it is certain that we will always need practical advice from people with experience and insight. The authors of this book have worked hard to make it an important contribution to the IRB mission. It is in this spirit that we present the second edition of *Institutional Review Board: Management and Function*.

Elizabeth A. Bankert and Robert J. Amdur

CONTRIBUTING AUTHORS

Robert Amdur, MD
Professor of Radiation Oncology
University of Florida College of Medicine
Gainesville FL

Natalie M. Bachir, MD
PGY-3, Internal Medicine
Duke University Hospital
Durham NC

Elizabeth A. Bankert, MA
Director
Committee for the Protection of Human Subjects
Dartmouth College
Hanover NH

Deborah Barnard, MS, CIP
Assistant Director
Quality Assurance and Education
Partners Human Research Committee
Boston MA

C. J. Biddle, CRNA, PhD
Professor
Graduate Program in Anesthesia
Virginia Commonwealth University
Richmond VA

Michael B. Blayney, PhD
Director
Environmental Health and Safety
Dartmouth College
Hanover NH

Alan J. Bliss
PhD candidate
Department of History
University of Florida
Gainesville FL

David Borasky, CIP
Associate Director
Office of International Research Ethics
Family Health International
Research Triangle Park NC

Angela J. Bowen, MD
President
Western International Review Board
Olympia WA

Joseph S. Brown, PhD
Associate Professor
Psychology
University of Nebraska at Omaha
Omaha NE

Sherry Bye
Retired

Denise Niles Canales
President and CEO
API, Inc.
Lexington KY

Timothy C. Callahan, PhD
Associate VP for Academics and Research
Bastyr University
Kenmore WA

Rebecca Carson Rogers, MA
Assistant Director
Institutional Review Board
Dartmouth College
Hanover NH

Gary L. Chadwick, PharmD, MPH, CIP
Associate Provost and Director
Office for Human Subject Protection
Professor of Community and Preventive Health
    and Medical Humanities
University of Rochester
Rochester NY

Sanford Chodosh, MD
Wayland MA

Jeffrey M. Cohen, PhD, CIP
President
HRP Associates, Inc.
Training and Consulting in Human Research Protections
New York NY

Jeffrey A. Cooper, MD, MMM
Deputy Director
Association for the Accreditation of Human Research
    Protection Program, Inc. (R)
Washington DC

Amy Davis, JD, MPH
ARENA Director
Public Responsibility in Medicine and Research
(PRIM&R)
Boston MA

Susan J. Delano, CIP
Deputy Managing Director
Research Foundation for Mental Hygiene, Inc.
Menands NY

Christina A. Di Tomasso, BS
Manager
Office of Clinical Investigation
Children's Hospital Boston
Boston MA

James M. DuBois, PhD, DSc
Associate Professor
PhD Program Director
Center for Health Care Ethics
Saint Louis University
St. Louis MO

Anne Dyson, MPH
IRB Administrator
Office of Clinical Investigation
Children's Hospital Boston
Boston MA

Marianne M. Elliott, MS, CIP
Department of Navy
Human Research Protection Program
US Navy
Washington DC

Kevin J. Epperson, BGS, RRT
IRB Administrator
Office of Regulatory Affairs
University of Nebraska Medical Center
Omaha NE

Richard B. Ferrell, MD
Associate Professor
Psychiatry
Dartmouth Hitchcock Medical Center
Lebanon NH

Susan S. Fish, PharmD, MPH
Associate Director, Office of Clinical Research
Director, Human Subjects Protection
Boston University Medical Center
Boston MA

Ann Barry Flood, PhD
Professor of Community and Family Medicine
    and Sociology
Director of Policy Studies
Chair, PhD Program and the NRSA Postdoctoral Program
Center for the Evaluative Clinical Sciences
    at Dartmouth
Dartmouth Medical School
Hanover NH

David G. Forster, JD, MA, CIP
Assistant Vice President, Office of Compliance
Auxiliary Faculty, Medical History and Ethics
Western IRB and University of Washington
Olympia WA

William L. Freeman, MD, MPH, CIP
Director of Tribal Community Health Programs
Human Protections Administrator
Northwest Indian College
Bellingham WA

Dean R. Gallant, AB
Director, Science Center and Executive Officer
Committee on the Use of Human Subjects in Research
Harvard University
Cambridge MA

Bruce Gordon, MD
Associate Professor
Pediatric Hematology/Oncology
    and Stem Cell Transplantation
University of Nebraska Medical Center
Omaha NE

Ronald M. Green, PhD
The Eunice and Julian Cohen Professor for
    the Study of Ethics and Human Values
Chair, Department of Religion and Director
    of Ethics Institute
Dartmouth College
Hanover NH

Dale E. Hammerschmidt, MD, FACP
Associate Professor of Medicine
Coordinator for Research Ethics
    and Human Subjects Protection,
Department of Medicine, University of Minnesota
Editor-in-Chief, Journal of Laboratory and Clinical Medicine
Minneapolis MN

Karen Hansen, BA
Director, Institutional Review Office
Fred Hutchinson Cancer Research Center
Seattle WA

Erica J. Heath, MBA, CIP
President
Independent Review Consulting
San Anselmo CA

Todd F. Heatherton, PhD
Professor
Psychological and Brain Sciences
Dartmouth College
Hanover NH

Sallyann Henry, PhD
President
Professional Testing Corporation
New York NY

Rachel Hepp, BS, CIP
Clinical Research Coordinator II
Cancer Center Protocol Office
Massachusetts General Hospital
Boston MA

Lorna C. Hicks, MS
Director, Program for the Protection of Human Subjects
    in Non-medical Research
Duke University
Durham NC

Jay G. Hull, PhD
Professor
Psychological and Brain Sciences
Dartmouth College
Hanover NH

Kevin M. Hunt, MED, CHFP
Director of Revenue Management
Concord Hospital
Concord NH

John M. Isidor, JD
CEO
Schulman Associates Institutional Review Board, Inc.
Cincinnati OH

Sandra P. Kaltman, RN, BSN, JD
Attorney
Cincinnati OH

Sayaka Kanade
Northern Plains Tribal Epidemiology Center
Aberdeen Area Tribal Chairmen's Health Board
Rapid City SD

Thomas G. Keens, MD, CIP
Chair, Committee on Clinical Investigations (IRB)
Childrens Hospital Los Angeles
Professor of Pediatrics, Physiology, and Biophysics,
Keck School of Medicine of the University
    of Southern California
Los Angeles CA

Sarah Khan
Medical IRB 2
Office for the Protection of Research Subjects
University of California, Los Angeles
Los Angeles CA

Felix A. Khin-Maung-Gyi, MBA, CIP
CEO, Founder
Chesapeake Research Review, Inc.
Columbia MD

Susan Z. Kornetsky, MPH, CIP
Director
Clinical Research Compliance
Children's Hospital Boston
Boston MA

Gail Kotulak, BS
IRB Administrator
University of Nebraska Medical Center
Omaha NE

Christopher J. Kratochvil, MD
Vice-Chair, IRB
Assistant Professor of Psychiatry
University of Nebraska Medical Center
Omaha NE

Rachel Krebs, BS, CIP
Administrative Director
Office for Human Research Participant Protection
Boston College
Chestnut Hill MA

Judi Kuhl, BS, CIP
Professional Associate II
Office of Research Integrity
University of Kentucky
Lexington KY

Eric Larsen, MD
Medical Director
Maine Children's Cancer Program
Scarborough ME

Robert J. Levine, MD
Professor of Medicine and Lecturer in Pharmacology
School of Medicine
Yale University
Woodbridge CT

Sally L. Mann, MS
IRB Administrator
Office of Regulatory Affairs
University of Nebraska Medical Center
Omaha NE

Peter Marshall, BA, CIP
Human Subjects Protection Scientist
AMDEX Corporation
Office of Research Protections
U.S. Army Medical Research and Materiel Command
Silver Spring MD

J. Allen McCutchan, MD
Professor of Medicine
UCSD School of Medicine—Division of Infectious
    Diseases UCSD Antiviral Research Center
San Diego CA

Helen McGough, MA
Director
Human Subjects Division
University of Washington
Seattle WA

Linda Medwar, BS
Senior IRB Coordinator
Children's Hospital Boston
Boston MA

Matthew Miller, MD, MPH, ScD
Associate Director
Health Policy and Management
Harvard Injury Control Research Center
Harvard School of Public Health
Brookline MA

Paul B. Miller, MA, MPhil, JD
PhD candidate
Department of Philosophy
University of Toronto
Toronto ON Canada

Lawrence H. "Doc" Muhlbaier, PhD
Assistant Professor
Biostatistics and Bioinformatics
Duke University Medical Center
Durham NC

Daniel K. Nelson, MS, CIP
Associate Professor and Director
Human Research Studies, School of Medicine
The University of North Carolina at Chapel Hill
Chapel Hill NC

Robert "Skip" Nelson, MD, PhD
Associate Professor of Anesthesiology and Critical Care
Department of Anesthesiology and Critical Care
University of Pennsylvania School of Medicine
The Children's Hospital of Philadelphia
Philadelphia PA

Susan Nicholson, JD
Attorney
Ropes and Gray
Boston MA

J. Michael Oakes, PhD
Division of Epidemiology
University of Minnesota
Minneapolis MN

Gwenn S. F. Oki, MPH
Director, Research Subjects Protection
City of Hope National Medical Center and
the Beckman Research Institute
Duarte CA

Elisabeth A. Smith Parrott, BA, BS
Research Officer
Committee on the Use of Human Subjects
Harvard University
Cambridge MA

Lucille Pearson, CIP
Retired

Steven Peckman, MFA
Associate Director for Administration and Planning
Institute for Stem Cell Biology and Medicine
University of California, Los Angeles
Los Angeles CA

Robin Levin Penslar, JD
Senior Legal Researcher
Ogilvy Renault Barristers & Solicitors
Toronto ON Canada

Ernest D. Prentice, PhD
Professor, Genetics, Cell Biology and Anatomy
Co-chair, IRB
Associate Vice-chancellor for Academic Affairs,
    Regulatory Compliance
University of Nebraska Medical Center
Omaha NE

Tom Puglisi, PhD
Deputy Chief Officer
Office of Research Oversight
Department of Veterans Affairs
Washington DC

Joan Rachlin, JD, MPH
Executive Director
Public Responsibility in Medicine and Research
Boston MA

Francine C. Romero, PhD, MPH
Northern Plains Tribal Epidemiology Center
Aberdeen Area Tribal Chairmen's Health Board
Rapid City SD

Michele Russell-Einhorn, JD
Director of the Office for the Protection of
    Research Subjects
Dana Farber Cancer Institute
Boston MA

Patricia M. Scannell
422 North Hanley Road
St. Louis MO

Toby L. Schonfeld, PhD
Assistant Professor
Department of Preventive and Societal Medicine
University of Nebraska Medical Center
Omaha NE

Kathy Schulz, CIP
Human Research Compliance Officer
Clinical Research Office
San Francisco VA Medical Center
San Francisco CA

Ada Sue Selwitz, MA
Director
Office of Research Integrity
University of Kentucky
Lexington KY

Laurie B. Slone, PhD
Research Associate
Department of Psychiatry
Dartmouth College
Hanover NH
National Center for PTSD, VA MC (116-D)
White River Junction VT

Marjorie A. Speers, PhD
Executive Director
Association for the Accreditation of Human
Research Protection Programs, Inc. (R)
Washington DC

Mark E. Sobel, MD, PhD
Executive Officer, American Society for Investigative
Pathology
9650 Rockville Pike
Bethesda MD

Elizabeth Stanton, JD
Risk Management Director
Risk Management
Dartmouth-Hitchcock Medical Center
Lebanon NH

Jennifer J. Tickle, PhD
Assistant Professor of Psychology
St. Mary's College of Maryland
St. Mary's City MD

Jan L. Trott
Director
Office of Research Affairs
Maine Medical Center Research Institute
Scarborough ME

Pamela Wright, MA
HRPP Coordinator
Albany VA
Albany NY

Harold Y. Vanderpool, PhD, ThM
Professor, History and Philosophy of Medicine
Institute for the Medical Humanities Department of
Preventive Medicine and Community Health
University of Texas
Galveston TX

Daniel R. Vasgird, PhD, CIP
Director, Research Compliance Services and Research
Integrity Officer
University of Nebraska-Lincoln
Office of Research and Graduate Studies
Lincoln NE

Celia S. Walker
Retired
Fort Collins CO

Cynthia S. Way, CIP, CCRP
Manager, Regulatory Support
Covance Clinical Research Unit, Inc.
Madison WI

Charles Weijer, MD, PhD, FRCPC
Canada Research Chair (Tier I)
Associate Professor
Department of Philosophy
Talbot College
The University of Western Ontario
London ON Canada

Matthew D. Whalen, PhD
Co-founder and Chief Development Officer
Chesapeake Research Review, Inc.
Columbia MD

Mark R. Yessian, PhD
Director of Regional Operations
Office of Evaluation and Inspections
Office of Inspector General
U.S. Department of Health and Human Services
Washington DC

John A. Zaia, MD
Chair of IRB and Director
Virology
City of Hope National Medical Center
Duarte CA

ACKNOWLEDGMENTS

We are grateful to The Dartmouth Committee for the Protection of Human Subjects for being exceptionally dedicated and a continued source of inspiration. We also acknowledge the important role that the Committee's office staff plays in making it possible for our IRB to function effectively. Thank you to Priscilla Grover, Ann O'Hara, Tracy Ostler, Courtney Rogers, and Rebecca Carson Rogers. And finally, there is Nancy Wray, whose mentorship and encouragement brought this project to fruition.

Elizabeth A. Bankert
Robert J. Amdur

PART 1

Background and Overview Topics

An Ethics Primer for Institutional Review Boards

Harold Y. Vanderpool

INTRODUCTION

Institutional review board (IRB) members and administrators are regularly reminded that ethics is a critical component of the review and approval of research protocols. Ethics training for researchers and IRB members and administrators is required at the federal level. In addition, advisory committees tell us that ethical reasoning is imperative for the protection of human subjects. The Advisory Committee on Human Radiation Experiments, for example, discovered "serious deficiencies" in our present system of protection. To correct these deficiencies, the committee declared that efforts must be "undertaken on a national scale to ensure the *centrality of ethics* in the conduct of scientists whose research involves human subjects."[1(pp.817–818)]

Some IRBs can call on the expertise of someone who can describe the nature and content of research ethics in clear, practical, and useful terms. However, many IRB members and administrators remain puzzled and uncertain about how to use ethical analysis. Given two notable barriers, this puzzlement is not surprising. Before discussing what ethics is and how and why ethical analysis is necessary for the protection of human subjects, we need to know why ethics has been—and remains—so often neglected.

Barriers to Understanding and Using Ethics

Ethics and Regulations

The first barrier to the use of research ethics is erected by two unsuspecting sources. It is created by the two most important documents that IRBs are commissioned to follow: The Code of Federal Regulations Title 45 Part 46: Protection of Human Subjects (CFR)[2] and *The Belmont Report*[3] (*Belmont*). This assertion is so surprising—and important—that it needs to be carefully explained.

That these critically important documents constitute a barrier to ethical analysis is surprising and disturbing because they were composed for the protection of human subjects and are, in fact, necessary for such protection. Although they share this common goal, their means for accomplishing the goal of protecting research participants are exceedingly different. The problem over ethics occurs because the relationship between the means of protection in the CFR on the one hand and *Belmont* on the other is not mentioned or specified in either document. The CFR hardly mentions ethics, not to speak of the functions of ethics in protecting human research subjects. At the same time, *Belmont* details ethical principles and applications without specifying how they relate to interpreting and applying federal regulatory rules. IRBs need to be aware of this fundamental flaw in our two most important federal documents, and they need to know how to correct this flaw. This chapter indicates how the right hand of the CFR relates to the left hand of *Belmont's* ethics.

The CFR contains bureaucratic rules that IRBs must follow. Many IRBs follow these rules in rote fashion with little attention to ethics. Many CFR rules pertain to organizational and enforcement matters—the necessity and structure of IRBs, the documentation of informed consent, record keeping, and so on. Other rules detail the "general requirements" of informed consent,[2[Sec.111(a)(4), 116]] factors related to risk/probability of benefit determinations,[2[Sec.111(a)(1)(2)]] and a few sentences about the "equitable selection" of research subjects.[2[Sec. 111(a)(3)]] To apply this last set of rules requires ethical awareness and analysis, but the CFR is virtually silent about the value, not to speak of the necessity, of using ethics.

> **1.** The crucial section in the main body of the CFR that lists what IRBs should use—law, institutional regulations, and standards of professional practice—to "ascertain the acceptability of proposed research"[2[Sec. 107(a)]] does not even mention ethics or ethical reasoning.

2. The CFR mentions ethical standards or principles only twice—both times in its later subparts B[2(Sec.202)] and D[2[Sec.407(b)(1)(ii)]] without any elaboration about what these terms call for.

3. The place where a "statement of ethical principles" is mentioned in the main body of the CFR[2[Sec.103(b)(1)]] pertains to an institution's assurance of compliance agreement. Such a statement is considered optional, and no directions are given as to how any adopted code or ethical statement should be used.

4. The importance of using *Belmont's* three ethical principles (respect for persons, beneficence, and justice) and their respective applications to research (informed consent, risk/benefit assessment, and selection of subjects) is not discussed in the CFR.

These points lead to a disturbing conclusion. Insofar as IRBs follow and focus exclusively on the CFR for research protections (the main, possibly exclusive focus of many IRBs),[1(pp.697,707–709,817)] they may either neglect ethics altogether or relegate ethical concerns to the periphery of protocol review.

Let us now turn to the main ethical problem arising from *Belmont*. *Belmont* was produced by the National Commission for Protection of Human Subjects of Behavioral and Biomedical Research and was published in *The Federal Register* in 1979. *Belmont* was adopted as an authoritative policy statement by the U.S. Department of Health, Education, and Welfare (now called the Department of Health and Human Services), the National Institutes of Health, and the Office for Protection from Research Risks, now called the Office of Human Research Protections.

Does *Belmont* fill the ethical void in the CFR? Assuming the *Belmont* is studied and understood, it can do this, but it fills the void indirectly, not clearly or explicitly.

1. In spite of its official status, the degree to which *Belmont* is actually read, understood, and used by IRBs remains an open question.

2. Importantly, *Belmont's* exclusive focus is that moral awareness and reasoning are imperative for strengthening and assuring human subject protection. *Belmont's* stated purposes are first to demonstrate to researchers, subjects, IRBs, and interested citizens that ethical issues are "inherent in research involving human subjects." Second, and especially important for IRBs, *Belmont* provides an analytical framework composed of principles and their applications that will help resolve ethical problems arising from research.

3. *Belmont* also asserts that its principles will enable IRB members and others to formulate, criticize, and interpret the regulatory rules of research found in the Nuremberg Code, the Declaration of Helsinki, and the CFR. Unfortunately, *Belmont* never describes or gives examples of how existing regulatory rules can be criticized, interpreted, revised, or supplemented.

4. In short, *Belmont* offers no explicit guidance that will enable IRBs to do what they are precisely responsible for doing as they work with the rules of the CFR.

To summarize these points about the first major barrier to the use of ethics in protecting human subjects: The CFR neglects ethics, and *Belmont* does not discuss how its ethical principles and applications relate to interpreting and applying the CFR's rules.

Esoteric Language of Ethics

The second barrier to clarity about how to use ethics in IRB deliberations pertains to befuddlement and confusion over ethics itself. Ethics as a discipline of inquiry is readily associated with terminology, assumptions, arguments, and distinctions that seem esoteric and impractical to those who have not studied philosophical ethics. The esoteric nature of ethics reflects the fact that this discipline is explored primarily in elective college courses, graduate schools, and various types of intensive short courses for medical and other professionals. Because traditions of ethical reasoning are very rarely studied in high schools or the earlier years of public and private education and are not the subject of required courses in college or most professional training programs, the esoteric jargon and concepts of ethics are often not translated into ordinary language and commonly understood categories.

Clarity About Ethical Analysis

A responsible ethical analysis of any proposed action or course of action does not need to be identified with or surrounded by technical and esoteric jargon. Ethical analysis and decision making involves making judgments that are based on accurate facts, common experience, and coherent and convincing reasons. Ethical judgments or judgment calls pertain to what individuals and groups ought to do and how they/we ought to behave. Ethics focus on what is right or wrong (or something in between) and on what is good and virtuous or reprehensible.

All of us indulge in ethical thinking and argumentation even if we do not recognize it as ethical reasoning in a formal or academic sense. We use common and shared patterns of reasoning and experience to arrive at what we take to be an acceptable (moral) or unacceptable (immoral) course of action. At times, even extensive and thoughtful ethical analysis will not uncover some clearly "correct" answer to a moral problem. Given the complexities of human life, some problems appear to have equally strong arguments for and against two or more possible solutions—problems that are rightly called *moral dilemmas*. At other times, a clearly correct answer cannot be discovered or agreed on, but a more or less responsible ethical judgment call can be made. This responsible search for the best possible answer should be distinguished from irresponsible skepticism or laziness.

Ethics as a discipline of reasoning dwells on and wrestles with the many moral beliefs and patterns of thinking that persons in every culture use to make moral assessments and decisions. Over time, ethicists have identified and categorized types of principles and arguments, which they examine to discover which principles and arguments are the most believable and convincing. Disciplined and fully responsible ethical reasoning includes identifying, making explicit, and/or becoming aware of the types and relative strengths of the moral assumptions that we may take for granted. Do we assume that the probable consequences of some action determine its morality? Is this consequentialist assumption sufficient for determining what is moral, or do other assumptions such as freedom of choice (moral autonomy) regardless of the consequences carry more moral weight? When we appeal to consequences, what do we have in mind—increased pleasure, happiness, or some other valued good such as greater knowledge about the natural world?

Ethical reasoning includes the following factors:

1. Identifying a problem that appears to be morally questionable or troubling

2. Accurately understanding the facts and circumstances pertaining to the problem

3. Identifying common and shared values (including the three principles in *Belmont*) that pertain to the problem

4. Identifying and using tried and true moral arguments

5. Making a considered moral judgment (finding an ethical solution) by relating the moral values, arguments, and pertinent examples to the problem in question

A reasonable and responsible ethical solution to some issue should be viewed as the most convincing answer that an informed and well-meaning group of persons can discover. In the process, the group upholds commonly accepted ethical principles and strives to arrive at a sensible and rationally defensible decision.

Because ethical analysis commissions us to make *judgments* based on thoughtful analysis and deliberation, this analysis contrasts with simply *asserting* that something is right or wrong, regardless of the frequency or strength of such assertions.[4(pp.1–4)] As a form of reasoned discourse based on knowledge and common experience, ethical analysis comes to a halt—sometimes to a screeching halt—when someone in a group asserts that some action is right or wrong based on a personal opinion or the authority of a family member, famous person, or hallowed book or tradition. Such authorities may indeed be wellsprings of moral guidance and insight, but to serve as wellsprings, they must be shown to be relevant and convincing before they can carry ethical weight.

Belmont and the Ethics of Research

These brief points enable us to understand what research ethics is. The ethics of research should be defined as the application of the steps and modes of ethical reasoning to the problems and situations arising from research involving human beings.

Belmont is a succinct and compact summary of research ethics that many, if not most, IRB members are unlikely to characterize as easy reading. This is not surprising; *Belmont* traverses a middle road between the somewhat technical (and unquestionably cryptic and compact) concepts and distinctions in its section entitled "Basic Ethical Principles" and its more easily grasped

(but still distinction filled) discussions under the title "Applications." Both sections, especially the first, are like the tips of icebergs that rest on extensive philosophic tradition, the National Commission's deliberations that were predicated on scholarly essays by philosophers and bioethicists, and examples drawn from a number of the reports the National Commission had completed before it completed and published *Belmont*.

Nevertheless, *Belmont* discusses ethics in clear, jargon-free terms. It identifies only three of a number of ethical principles because these three principles (beneficence, respect for persons, and justice) are especially applicable to research. Other commonly recognized ethical principles such as the moral duties of gratitude, fidelity (faithfulness to others), promise keeping, and veracity (truth telling) are also applicable to research, but in less comprehensive ways.

The three principles accented in *Belmont* are set forth as duties that encompass a number of moral concerns and can be readily grasped by persons of varied backgrounds. With respect to the encompassing nature of its principles, *Belmont* includes the far-reaching principle of nonmaleficence (the duty of not harming others) under its principle of beneficence.[5(pp.189–193)] *Belmont* also includes the duty of protecting vulnerable persons from harm (a dimension of nonmaleficence) under its principle of respect for persons.

With respect to how its principles are generally understandable, *Belmont's* principle of respect for persons, for example, can be understood as crediting human beings of all ages with dignity and worth for a variety of reasons. To the chagrin of many bioethicists, *Belmont's* principle of respect for persons is not merely, nor neatly, drawn from philosophic arguments that speak of the necessity of respecting human autonomy, that is, respecting persons as individuals who are credited with the right to make their own unforced decisions.[6(pp.2–4)] Instead, the principle of respect for persons in *Belmont* represents a basic moral standard that makes sense to persons with different backgrounds and training. This principle reflects the U.S. Constitution's emphasis on the rights of self-determination and privacy. It emphasizes the sacredness and value of human life in religious traditions as well as basic human dignity in everyday life. It also reflects the moral arguments advanced by philosophers, such as Immanuel Kant, who based morality on the freedom of the will, and John Stuart Mill, who defended the liberty of free choice.[7] This last point enables us to understand how *Belmont's* ethical principles should be understood. They are presented as "an easily grasped set of moral standards" for persons with diverse backgrounds and training.[8(p.181)] As "the common coin of moral discourse,"[9(p.333)] these principles constitute condensations or essential elements of morality derived from and generally acceptable within human culture. They are also, as *Belmont* accents, "particularly relevant" to research with human subjects. The sections that follow indicate how these principles and guidelines can and should be used to interpret, apply, and reformulate the rules in the CFR previously indicated. These essential tasks pertaining to the use of ethics by IRBs are not discussed in either the CFR or *Belmont*.

Although the ethical framework of *Belmont* is easily understood, the document itself is intellectually challenging. Members of IRBs should not be discouraged if they do not fully grasp *Belmont's* many messages the first time they read—even carefully read—this historic document. Each time it is studied or discussed, its richness and usefulness are more fully grasped. *Belmont* needs to be discussed, dissected, and reflected on. Should, for example, its three principles be equally and fully upheld, or can they be "balanced" off of one another in some instances? *Belmont* never indicates whether all of its principles must be upheld for each research protocol (such that fully informed consent is never compromised) or whether one principle (such as respect for a subject's autonomy) can at times be outweighed when another principle (such as beneficence in the form of a favorable benefit-over-harm ratio) appears to warrant protocol approval. This lack of clarity has led to extensive scholarly debate over how *Belmont's* principles should be understood and applied. See, for example, the essays by Veatch, Jonsen, and Ackerman in *The Ethics of Research Involving Human Subjects.*[4(pp.33–104)]

Ways to Think About and Use Ethics to Review Research Protocols

The topics that follow display how members of IRBs and researchers can use ethics to protect research subjects/participants. The headings suggest a practical method that can be used to explore some important component of research ethics. The ethical components in these headings represent examples only, not the range, of ethical concerns addressed in *Belmont*. Although an extensive body of literature on research ethics exists, this chapter focuses on *Belmont* as a primary source of ethical insight.

Learning Suggestion: Dwell on Belmont's Applications

Research Ethics Topic: The Moral Autonomy of Individuals Clearly and repeatedly, *Belmont* says that its ethical principles lead to or serve as justifications for its applications. This implies that its principles are primary, while its applications are secondary and inferior because they are derived from its principles. This is deceiving for two reasons. First, both the principles and applications are referred to and viewed as ethical "requirements" and "obligations," which means that they are morally equal, even though the principles are general and the applications are more specific. Second, and of greater practical importance at critical points, *Belmont's* human subject protections are far greater in the applications than in the principles.

As a historical footnote, it is highly unlikely that the members of the National Commission first determined what their ethical principles should be and then deduced ethically required applications from these principles. They had already published four reports (on research involving prisoners [1976], children [1977], disclosure of information [1977], and IRBs [1978]) filled with applications related to the ethical obligations of informed consent, of protecting vulnerable subjects, and so on.

The commissioners apparently chose their three principles because of their reciprocal connections with and support of their applications.

This is illustrated by the way the moral autonomy of each individual is understood under the principle of respect for persons in comparison with the way the autonomy of persons is depicted in *Belmont's* applications. To honor the principle of respect for persons, *Belmont* says that researchers must "give weight" to autonomous persons' considered opinions and choices. This conveys the message that researchers can decide when the subject is to be treated as a free and self-determining agent. This contrasts with *Belmont's* applications, which hold that the subject's choice is free and final. For example, prospective subjects must be granted "the opportunity to choose what shall or shall not happen to them." In addition, they must be given all of the information that a "reasonable volunteer" would need to know to decide "whether they wish to participate" in the research.

The practical implications of this example are clear. Members of IRBs can profit from *Belmont's* principles, but the ethical strength, specificity, and applicability of the report's research ethics are primarily found in its applications.

Learning Suggestion: Uphold the Duty to Supplement CFR's Rules

Research Ethics Topic: Protecting the Voluntarism of Research Subjects and Other Dimensions of Informed Consent It is critical for IRB members and investigators to make a fundamental distinction between codified rules and ethical analysis. In its second paragraph, *Belmont* says that the rules found in the Nuremberg Code, the Helsinki Declaration, and the CFR (all of which are specified in its first endnote) "are often inadequate." In addition, they "come into conflict" and "are frequently difficult to interpret or apply." Because *Belmont* never indicates why this is true and what should be done about it, let us explore how ethical analysis exposes the inadequacy and incompleteness of a number of the CFR's rules.

Consider, for example, the rules pertaining to the voluntarism of research subjects, which are given in two places. The introductory paragraph in CFR 46.116 says that investigators should seek consent under circumstances "that minimize the possibility of coercion or undue influence." In 46.116 (a) and 46.116 (a) (8), the CFR holds that one of the "basic elements of informed consent" is "a statement that participation is voluntary." Members of IRBs are very familiar with the boilerplate language in consent forms. These reflect how the rules of the CFR are registered verbatim in most of these forms: "taking part in this study is voluntary. . . . You may withdraw from the study at any time without penalty or loss of any benefits to which you are otherwise entitled."[1(p.708)]

Whether research subjects are indeed approached, recruited, and treated as volunteers is hardly captured by this rote listing of rules in consent forms. Fortunately, *Belmont* contains an excellent discussion of the meaning and ingredients of voluntarism when it summarizes some of the conditions voluntarism requires. *Belmont* says that undue influence occurs "through an offer of an excessive, unwarranted, inappropriate, or improper reward or other overture in order to obtain compliance." It also argues that "unjustifiable pressures" occur when "persons in positions of authority . . . urge a course of action for a subject." This includes manipulating a prospective subject's choice by using the "influence of a close relative." *Belmont's* discussion calls ethical reasoning and judgment making into play because "it is impossible to state precisely where justifiable persuasion ends and undue influence begins." In global terms, IRBs should determine how undue influence (and coercion) should be avoided when they review specific protocols.

When IRBs explore and discuss these issues, they are using ethical reasoning to protect human subjects with the recognition that regulatory rules only touch the hem of the ethical garment. If recruitment strategies are not outlined in the protocol under review, the primary reviewer from the IRB must explore what strategies will be used. This can be done in nonconfrontational ways by asking, for example, "Would you briefly describe how you plan to recruit your research subjects?" Furthermore, IRB members need to be ever alert to the possibility that some subjects are unlikely to receive medical treatment and/or free medical treatment if they do not become enrolled. At times, this requires an awareness of stated or unstated departmental policies that may have the effect of unduly pressuring patients to enlist in research. This wrestling over issues pertaining to the voluntarism of research subjects supplements the CFR's cryptic references about minimizing coercion or undue influence and its rule that subjects should be told that their participation is voluntary.

These concerns about the voluntarism of research subjects can be extended to the other elements of informed consent registered in the rules of the CFR. As we learned from the analytical framework of *Belmont* previously depicted, informed consent involves adequate information, comprehension, and voluntariness. The first paragraph of CFR 46.116 briefly mentions these three areas of concern, but they are inadequately emphasized. This is true because all the "basic elements of informed consent" in the CFR[2[Sec.116(a)(1)–(8)]] and all of the CFR's "additional elements of informed consent"[2[Sec.116(b)(1)–(6)]] deal with only one of *Belmont's* categories: information. This directly encourages IRBs and investigators to equate the basic elements of consent with rules pertaining to the information subjects should receive in consent forms. This links informed consent to information on consent forms, rather than to a process of responsible and ongoing communication between investigators and prospective research subjects.

As a historical footnote, the language and categories pertaining to the "basic elements of informed consent" in the CFR reflect the precise wording of the DHEW/Public Health Service/National Institutes of Health Yellow Book. The book, entitled *The Institutional Guide to DHEW Policy on Protection of Human Subjects*, was published in 1971. Unfortunately, those who revised the CFR kept the language and categories of the Yellow Book instead of revising the CFR so that it conforms with the basic elements of informed consent in *Belmont*. *Belmont* has more comprehensive and protective categories of information, comprehension, and voluntariness. To be ethically responsible, IRBs need to recognize this important flaw in the CFR, and they need to deal with the informed consent of research subjects in terms of *Belmont's* ethically responsible principles and applications.

Learning Suggestion: Recognize the Open Endedness of Some CFR Definitions

Research Ethics Topic: Definition of "Minimal Risk" in Research with Children The CFR defines minimal risk as "the probability and magnitude of harm or discomfort . . . not greater . . . than those ordinarily encountered in daily life or during the performance of routine physical or psychological examinations or tests."[Sec.102(i)] This definition is evoked at crucial places in the CFR with respect to the permissibility of expedited review,[2[Sec.110(b)(i)]] research involving prisoners,[2[Sec.306(a)(2)(A)]] and research involving assenting children and/or the permission of their parents or guardians.[2(Sec.404)]

To be ethically responsible, IRBs should recognize that this definition is subject to wide-ranging interpretations that must be made explicit as protocols are analyzed. In research involving children, for example, this minimal risk definition has been taken to mean everything from gently scraping the inside of a child's mouth with a wooden spatula to remove surface cells to taking fluid from a child's middle ear via a needle passed through the ear drum.[10(pp. 343,349–356)] Although none would quarrel with the first procedure, the ethical permissibility of the second—even if it is "routine" for children with certain types of ear problems—depends on whose perspective is determining risk and harm.

Should minimal risk be determined by the researcher, IRB members, the parents, and/or prospective child subjects? The subjective nature of this key regulatory concept is not noted in the CFR, but it has become the subject of intense debate in the literature involving research with children.[10(pp.349–356)] Informed by the section in *Belmont* entitled "The Systematic Assessment of Risks and Benefits," IRBs need to make discriminating judgments about the variables that pertain to this definition. This includes the medical problems children have, the probable responses and feelings of the children, and the benefits they are likely to receive. To refer to the language of *Belmont*, IRBs need to recognize that a number of the definitions and rules in the CFR are "frequently difficult to interpret and apply."

Learning Suggestion: Think in Terms of Problems

Research Ethics Topic: Payments to Research Participants In keeping with the suggestions made in the section on clarity about ethical analysis, IRBs employ ethical analysis when they identify morally troubling or debatable problems on the basis of a factually accurate understanding of the problem. They identify ethical principles that bear on the problem and then use moral arguments to discover a sensible and defensible solution to the problem. In many or most instances, the problem will encompass more than one ethical principle and its respective applications. Sound ethical judgments will arise from an open and informed discussion that takes all of these factors into consideration.

Consider, for example, the increasingly prevalent practice of paying persons who participate in research. Few, if any, IRBs believe that modest, compensatory payments for transportation, parking, and time commitments by research participants in low-risk protocols pose an ethical problem. However, sizable "salaries" offered to participants who are being asked to participate in invasive protocols (protocols, for example, that require a number of muscle biopsies over the course of several weeks) are another matter. Why? First, these types of protocols can quite easily become coercive for poorer and needy patients—the unemployed, students in need of funds, and so on. Payments of $350 to $600 for six 2-hour clinical experiments can constitute offers that such populations of prospective subjects find difficult to refuse.

Related to this worry about coercion is the concern that such protocols are unlikely to secure an equitable representation from the general population of prospective subjects.[2][Sec.111(a)(3)] This single reference to equitable selection in the CFR is much more completely and thoughtfully discussed in the "Selection of Subjects" section found under *Belmont's* applications. *Belmont* holds that "the principle of justice gives rise to moral requirements that there be fair *procedures* and *outcomes* in the selection of research subjects." It further argues that "unjust social patterns" contribute to an unjust distribution of the burdens and benefits of research because economically or socially disadvantaged persons are "easy to manipulate as a result of their illness or socioeconomic condition."

These points about coercion, manipulation, and injustice should be taken seriously by IRBs that review invasive or risky protocols with payment scales that are likely to attract needy subjects. These studies are highly unlikely to attract wealthier participants who may, in fact, be the ones who will receive the greatest benefits from the research that is being conducted.

This example demonstrates how problems or possible problems that were never addressed in *Belmont* continue to surface and how their being resolved requires thoughtful ethical scrutiny and analysis based on several ethical principles and arguments.

Taken together, all of the topics and examples in this section illustrate how research subjects are not adequately—much less fully—protected without responsible ethical analysis on the part of IRBs

Conclusion

Members of IRBs and investigators are faced with the challenge of overcoming the strong and long-standing barriers that block or discourage the use of ethical analysis in the review and submission of research protocols. What ethical analysis entails has been clearly and sensibly described. The topics and examples discussed in this chapter demonstrate that to protect the rights and well-being of human beings who enroll in research the rules of the CFR must be supplemented and interpreted by the ethical principles and applications of *Belmont*. To protect human subjects, responsible ethical analysis and decision making by IRBs are inescapable imperatives, not expendable luxuries.

References

1. Advisory Committee on Human Radiation Experiments. *The Human Radiation Experiments: Final Report.* New York: Oxford University Press; 1996. http://tis.eh.doe.gov/ohre/roadmap/achre/report.html (DOE 061-000-00-848-9)

2. Code of Federal Regulations. Title 45A—Department of Health and Human Services; Part 46—Protection of Human Subjects, 1 October, 1997. Access date 18 April, 2001. http://www4.law.cornell.edu/cfr/45p46.htm

3. National Commission for the Protection of Human Subjects of Biomedical and Behavioral Research. *The Belmont Report: Ethical Principles and Guidelines for the Protection of Human Subjects of Research.* (DHEW [OS] 78-0013 and [OS] 78-0014.4). Washington, DC: U.S. Government Printing Office; 18 April, 1979. Access date 22 March, 2001. http://ohsr.od.nih.gov/mpa/belmont.php3

4. Vanderpool HY. Introduction and overview: Ethics, historical case studies, and the research enterprise. In: Vanderpool HY (ed.). *The Ethics of Research Involving Human Subjects: Facing the 21st Century.* Frederick, MD: University Publishing Group; 1996:1–4.

5. Beauchamp TL, Childress JF. *Principles of Biomedical Ethics,* 4th ed. New York: Oxford University Press; 1994.

6. Churchill LR. Disrespect for autonomy: Why the Belmont Report needs revision. Paper presented at "Belmont Revisited," a conference held at the University of Virginia, 16–19 April, 1999.

7. Vanderpool HY. Unfulfilled promise: How the Belmont Report can amend the Code of Federal Regulations Title 45 Part 46—Protection of Human Subjects. In: National Bioethics Advisory Commission (ed). *Ethical and Policy Issues in Research Involving Human Participants,* Vol. II. Commissioned Papers and Staff Analysis. August 2001. http://bioethics.gov/human/overvol2.html

8. Beauchamp TL. Principalism and its alleged competitors. *Kennedy Inst Ethics J* 5:181–198, 1995.

9. Jonsen AR. *The Birth of Bioethics.* New York: Oxford University Press; 1998:333.

10. Bartholome WG. Ethical issues in pediatric research. In: Vanderpool HY (ed.). *The Ethics of Research Involving Human Subjects: Facing the 21st Century.* Frederick, MD: University Publishing Group; 1996:339–370.

Reflections of an Outsider

Mark R. Yessian

INTRODUCTION

I am an outsider because of my job. My role in the Office of the Inspector General is to evaluate how well programs and mandates of the U.S. Department of Health and Human Services are being carried out. I am concerned. After many years of evaluating the protections provided to human subjects participating in clinical research, I have found that even with the good work of so many committed members of institutional review boards (IRBs) there are signs that the long-established system of protections is being undermined. This development could threaten not only human subjects, but also the field of clinical research itself.

This commentary begins by quickly reviewing the studies that we have conducted that serve as the basis for my reflections and by outlining the dynamics of change that are altering the clinical research landscape so profoundly. These observations provide the context for the three suggestions I offer to IRB members.

Six Years of Intensive Review (1996–2001)

During this period, we have visited at least 25 to 30 IRBs of all kinds, talked with representatives of over 100 IRBs, and immersed ourselves in the literature on IRBs. In addition, we have examined records of all kinds and reviewed all of the relevant data that we could get our hands on. On the basis of this inquiry, we have produced eight reports, testified at three congressional hearings, and given presentations at 40 to 50 professional meetings. Our style has been not only just to issue reports, but also to engage the issues with those heavily involved in the work of protecting human subjects. This interaction has deepened our insights and further reinforces the suggestions that I offer in this commentary.

One might say that our involvement in this field began by accident. In a study addressing investigational medical devices, we discovered disturbing inadequacies concerning IRB oversight. These concerned matters such as the implantation of a device in three times the number of human subjects specified in the IRB-approved research protocol. In another instance, a research effort was initiated without the changes the IRB called for in the informed consent document, and another research project was continued even though the IRB suspended it. It was these findings that led us to conduct a more intensive and enduring review of the overall system of human-subject protections.

Reports on IRBs

In June 1998, we issued a series of reports on IRBs. The reports, which received considerable national attention, warned that the effectiveness of IRBs was in jeopardy. The reports elaborated that IRBs review too much, too quickly, with too little expertise. They conduct minimal continuing review of approved research, face conflicts that threaten their independence, provide little training to investigators or IRB board members, and devote little emphasis to evaluation of their performance. These findings and our accompanying recommendations struck some in the clinical research field as being alarmist, but they raised awareness among researchers, administrators of academic health centers, and public policy makers. A short time later, the federal Office for Protection from Research Risks, which had conducted only one site visit to an IRB in the 11 months preceding the issuance of our report, became much more proactive. The Office for Protection from Research Risks generated much controversy itself by terminating ederally funded research at some institutions because of failures in their protection of human subjects.

Congressional Inquiries

Two years later, in response to congressional inquiries, we issued a follow-up report documenting the minimal progress made at the federal level in carrying out our recommendations. This report served as the basis of a congressional hearing. In June 2000, we issued two additional reports drawing attention to many disturbing human-subject recruitment practices, particularly for industry-sponsored clinical trials. These involved the use of financial incentives to investigators, physicians targeting of their own patients as potential subjects, the use of referral fees, and misleading advertisements.[1]

In September 2001, we issued a report that addresses the significant growth of clinical drug trials conducted in foreign countries and raises concern about the adequacy of the oversight conducted to assure human-subject protection in those trials. After this report, the Office of Public Health and Science in the U.S. Department of Human Services issued a Federal Register notice seeking comment on proposed criteria for determinations of equivalent protections of human services.

A Changed Research Environment

During the 1970s and early 1980s, when federal IRB regulations were formulated, the clinical research environment was much different than it is now. Most research involving human subjects took place with government support in university teaching hospitals with established research-related controls and an underlying culture of professional norms. Trials typically were conducted by a single investigator at a single institution and involved a small cohort of subjects. IRBs had manageable workloads and functioned in an environment where, in the wake of the Tuskegee experiments and other noted abuses, there was heightened awareness of the risks that research could pose for human subjects.

The environment at the beginning of the 21st century is vastly different. It is characterized by the increased commercialism of research, the proliferation of multisite trials across the nation and, indeed, around the globe, and a significant expansion of research in many new areas such as gene therapy and xenotransplantation. The heightened cost and pressures make it difficult for IRB members to volunteer their time or to raise questions that could slow down the research process and thereby jeopardize funding for an institution and/or investigator. Not least of all, a rise in patient consumerism has led many potential subjects themselves to worry less about the risks of research than about their rights to gain access to research trials.

In this dramatically altered environment, significant changes must be made in the way that protections are afforded. In my view, there is too little recognition of that. Clearly, IRBs alone cannot do it all. Sponsors, investigators, and government agencies themselves must also assume ongoing responsibilities for ensuring adequate protections. Recently, a number of promising federal initiatives have been taken. Nevertheless, IRBs still have a basic responsibility. IRBs are the only ones in the research process that exist solely to protect human subjects. How best to do that in an environment full of obstacles is a challenge to which all IRB members and others concerned about human-subject protections must devote some attention.

Suggestions

Amid so much change, complexity, and turbulence, it is essential for IRB members to keep an eye on the big picture and to consider their role with some perspective. It is in that context that I offer three suggestions. Each points to a direction of thought and action that can help make IRBs most relevant in these difficult times.

Sustain a Capacity for Independent Review in Substance and in Appearance

I lead with this procedural suggestion deliberately. If the IRBs are not independent of the research enterprise and all of the parties and interests associated with it, then they will be hard pressed to do the job expected of them. Perhaps I have an institutional bias here because as a representative of the Inspector General's office I am expected to conduct oversight in an independent manner, separate from the particular interests of programs and their advocates. Our credibility rests on that independence—so, too, I would argue, does that of IRBs. Their job is to ensure the adequacy of protections, even if doing so slows the research process or adversely affects the immediate interests of an institution, sponsor, or investigator. This does not mean that they should oppose those interests or be unmindful of the abiding societal interest in research, any more than we (in our evaluations) should oppose the interest of a program or fail to be cognizant of its social purposes. However, in both cases, our core responsibility requires the capacity and will to act independently. Otherwise our work is likely to be compromised.

This emphasis on independence, I recognize, disturbs many in the IRB community. I have spoken enough with IRB members to know that many (perhaps most) regard their role as a collegial one. They volunteer their time to help fellow investigators ensure that their research plans are in accord with federal and institutional expectations. They speak in terms of a community of interest and an enlightened sense of professionalism rather than an independent role that functions more like that of a gatekeeper or watchdog. They emphasize the importance of trust.

These are important considerations. Certainly, we do not want to establish an adversarial culture that emphasizes confrontation and ignores the importance of professional ethics and sense of responsibility. However, it is important to recognize that changes have occurred not only in the research environment but also in our society since the 1970s. We live in an age of increased commercialism and consumerism, where the body politic is not inclined to grant as much discretion to professionals. This is a society where public accountability and disclosure, in all sectors, are increasingly emphasized. Whether we like it or not, we must acknowledge and deal with these realities. Thus, what actions can be taken to sustain a capacity for independent review? Here are three actions that I suggest.

Ensure that the IRB functions with as much organizational independence as possible. For IRBs that are part of an institution, ensure that they are not part of an organizational unit responsible for bringing in research funds. For independent IRBs, ensure that equity owners do not participate in the review process. In themselves, such measures will not guarantee sufficient independence any more than the lack of them necessarily means that IRBs are not functioning independently. However, they reinforce the significance of independent review and public perception of it.

Achieve broad representation on IRBs. IRBs, particularly those in academic health centers and hospitals, are too narrowly focused in their membership. Federal law requires only that they include one noninstitutional and one nonscientific member. Often this requirement is met simply by including a single member who meets both criteria. This deprives the IRB of a valuable counterbalance to pressures that threaten its independence. I would suggest that IRB independence be nourished in important ways by ensuring that its membership includes ample representation from nonscientific members and from scientists who are not part of the institution at which the research is occurring. Again, this is in contrast to established norms of collegial review, but better fits the modern environment.

Foster public accountability. IRBs, too, must be accountable to the broader public, not just to an institution, sponsor, or government funder. Public support for clinical research rests in large part on confidence that that research is conducted in ways that protect human subjects. IRBs can foster such confidence by making their activities as transparent as possible. This is difficult given the proprietary nature of much of the research they now review. I suggest that IRBs determine the steps that they can take that would contribute to a more open atmosphere yet are consistent with the reality that certain information must be kept confidential. One element that could help in this regard is to conduct independent, publicly disclosed evaluations of IRB performance regularly.

Strengthen Continuing Review
I recall that when I was first informed about IRBs, an IRB member at an academic health center pulled me aside and counseled me that the job of IRBs is to ensure human subject protections up front, not to serve as an ongoing watchdog. Like so many of his colleagues that we would later meet, he emphasized that the system is based largely on trust, and that any movement toward policing would undermine the credibility that IRBs have developed. Many of the reactions to our first set of reports reiterated that we were pushing IRBs toward an oversight role that was inappropriate.

Nevertheless, as vital as trust is to the effective protection of human subjects, the IRB as a review body must function on the basis of "trust, but verify." This necessity is not just a reflection of the current age but, in fact, has been part of the IRB mandate from the very beginning. It was reinforced to me by one of the leading figures who served on the national commission that developed the current system of human-subject protections in the 1970s. In fact, one of the reports of that commission clearly envisioned an active role for IRBs. For instance, it indicated that IRBs may interview human subjects about their research experience or require that investigators provide subjects with a form with which they may report their research experiences to the IRB.

Ironically, the significance of the IRB's initial review of research applications may be decreasing as that of continuing review may be increasing. In the current research environment, where so much research involves sponsor-initiated multisite protocols, the realistic opportunities for IRBs to influence the research design are diminished. Many observers add that the IRB does not have or should not be expected to have the scientific expertise to review many of these designs. In contrast, the continuing review role could become more important as an ongoing check that initial plans and expectations are being met. After all, one of the central notions justifying IRBs in the first place was that they could provide a local presence based on a familiarity with the investigators and with local conditions and norms.

For the skeptical, I would ask that if the IRBs do not assume responsibility for identifying deviations from research plans that threaten human-subject protections (such as those concerning investigational medical devices that I noted at the outset of this commentary), then who should? If IRBs excuse themselves from this oversight role because it violates a tradition of trust and appears too much like policing, or for whatever reason, their inaction could diminish their relevance to human-subject protections. For, surely, some party must play an active part in such monitoring. IRBs, I would submit, are the ones in the best position to play that role and carry it out in a way that is still respectful of the professionalism that must be part of the research enterprise.

The continuing review role can encompass much more than ensuring that protocols stay on track. Among the key questions that IRBs should address during the course of a trial are the following:

1. How is the human-subject recruitment process working? Is it undermining informed consent? Is it jeopardizing patient confidentiality? Is it fostering the equitable selection of subjects?

2. How is the informed consent process actually working? Is it functioning in a way that fosters human-subject understanding?

3. How is the continuing safety of subjects being ensured? Are reportable adverse events in fact being reported? If so, are they being adequately analyzed and addressed to protect subjects?

These, I recognize, are large questions that overburdened IRBs are hard pressed to address in a concerted way. However, neither can they ignore them. IRBs must play an ongoing role in raising and addressing such questions and stimulating sufficient attention to them by all of those connected with clinical research.

Serve as an Ambassador for Human-Subject Protections
This, I suggest, is a more important role than is generally recognized. When there are disclosures of human subjects being harmed unnecessarily, there tends to be widespread outrage and a call for corrective action. However, in a more fundamental way, it seems to me that there is more ongoing societal support (reflected in the actions of

elected officials) for the research itself than for ensuring human-subject protections. We are all vitally interested in the search for cures to diseases and seek rapid access to the benefits of effective therapies. In subtle ways, this can translate into more substantial political support for reducing burdens on the research process rather than on conducting reviews to ensure adequate human-subject protections. The latter can readily be demonized as bureaucratic red tape that impedes scientific progress.

This is an ongoing tension that cannot be avoided altogether. IRBs (and the federal officials establishing rules for IRBs) must be attentive to the need to make the review process as efficient as possible so that it does not unnecessarily delay the research process. Nevertheless, any IRB worth its salt will encounter instances in which it must confront powerful research interests and take a stand in support of its consumer protection responsibilities.

IRBs are the players in the research process who have the most singular and focused responsibility to protect human subjects. However, if the other parties—sponsors, investigators, government agencies—do not internalize such protective responsibilities in their own spheres as well, then IRBs cannot succeed. IRB members should speak out regularly, reminding all of the key parties of their obligations in protecting subjects and of how ongoing societal support for the research depends on carrying out those obligations effectively.

This kind of outreach can be particularly important if it involves drawing attention to troubling developments that warrant greater attention by the research community as a whole. In this context, IRBs—individually and collectively—can provide valuable early warning signals of emerging concerns and help generate greater examination of them. Such concerns include the following:

1. The questionable human-subject oversight for many foreign trials that increasingly serves as a basis for new drug applications
2. The disturbing financial incentives sometimes given to investigators for recruiting human subjects
3. The possible erosion in many settings of meaningful informed consent
4. The uncertainty about how fully sponsors monitor their trials for adherence to human-subject requirements

IRBs should exert more public leadership on these and other such issues. They have a long-established credibility in speaking for human subjects and ought not let their overflowing agendas obscure for them the gains that can be achieved from speaking out more extensively. The issues are too important to be left only to ethicists, academics, and advocacy organizations or for that matter to oversight bodies such as the Office of the Inspector General.

Acknowledgment

The author thanks Aimee Golbitz, Steven Keenan, and China Eng for their comments on an earlier version of this chapter. The views expressed in this article are those of the author and do not necessarily represent those of the U.S. Department of Health and Human Services or the Office of the Inspector General.

Reference

1. Office of Inspector General. Recruiting human subjects: Pressures in industry-sponsored clinical research (OEI-01-97-00195), June 2000. Access date: 12 April 2001. http://www.hhs.gov/oig/oei/reports/a459.pdf

A Unified Human-Research Protection Program

Sanford Chodosh

INTRODUCTION

This chapter is intended to relate my personal perspective on the development of systems to protect subjects studied in research while still advocating the advancement of scientific knowledge. I have had the unusual opportunity to observe and participate in this process over the past 45 years. This included involvement with institutional review boards (IRBs) and proactive involvement in the development of Public Responsibility in Medicine and Research for over 30 years. When I began my career as a clinical investigator before 1960, investigators almost universally developed their own protocols, and the majority was based at academic institutions. The IRB did not exist, and the consent process was primitive at best. When I was asked to become a member of our Human Studies Committee in the late 1960s, the system had minimal guidelines and little institutional support.

Since those early years, much has changed in terms of where and by whom human research is conducted. Institutionally based IRBs are no longer the only game in town. In addition, the progressive increase in research funds, the numbers and complexity of protocols, and the burden of regulatory requirements have all compromised the ability of the IRB to properly carry out its responsibility to protect human research subjects. There is a sense that IRBs have become so involved with the workload of properly reviewing protocols and complying with regulatory details that providing systems that actually protect human subjects has slipped from the IRB's primary function to a secondary role.

From the perspective of past experience, it is important to review why such protection programs are necessary. What current problems exist that need to be resolved so that meaningful and effective systems can be established to truly protect those individuals studied in research? When studying humans in research, a basic tenet is to respect the dignity of such individuals and to minimize the possibility of harm. *The Belmont Report* restated the basic ethical principles that should guide our interactions with all humans, whether in the context of research or everyday living. Unfortunately, the history of research has become marked with terrible examples of how these basic ethical principles have been ignored. Although the majority of scientists have followed these principles, the exceptions created a need for legal measures designed to avoid future problems. These steps were not taken in the Western world until long after the World War II Nazi experiments became

known. The assumption was that, in a civilized society, scientists abided by ethical standards that would not permit such atrocities. This was true in the majority of cases. In the academic world, most risky research was biomedical, and clinician–investigators understood the principle to do no harm to their patients that they carried over to how they dealt with their research subjects. In those early years, additional assurance came from the oversight by clinical service chiefs, who provided guidance to the investigators in their departments. This oversight became more tenuous as clinical services grew in size and complexity and research generated more and more of the operating funds of services and institutions.

After Tuskegee and other ethical failures in research, the public and the scientific community realized that a better means of protecting subjects in research needed to be implemented. These misadventures led to distrust by the public of the ethical behavior of those responsible for the conduct of research. Federal agencies that had initially recommended simple peer review of research now promulgated regulations requiring a stricter review of protocols and developed an assurance process in which institutions receiving federal funds promised to comply with the new rules. Most of these assurances also promised coverage of nonfederally funded human research. IRBs were established wherever federal funds were received or research involving investigational drugs and devices was carried out. Institutions depended on their IRBs to provide a mantle of ethical credibility to the conduct of their research. The IRB was clearly identified as the central focus of an institution's program for the protection of human subjects. As research increased in volume and complexity and as regulatory demands increased, IRBs found themselves inundated with work. However, increased resources did not always follow. The IRB's primary role in protecting human subjects often became secondary to meeting regulatory requirements. The institution's need to meet the conditions of their assurances and continue the income and prestige of the institution's research program became the primary IRB function.

IRBs also had less time and resources to devote to their vital role to investigators in the protection of human research subjects. Institution-based scientists were assumed to be qualified to do research because of their staff appointments. Investigators felt the pressure to do productive research in terms of their academic advancement and funding. Some investigators and institution officials began to view the IRB as an adversary that obstructed research opportunities. Often, IRBs became wary of making mistakes in judgment for which they and their institutions could be held accountable. Delays in approving protocols reinforced the sense that the IRB worked against the best interests of the institution and investigators. Conversely, because most research was funded by federal agencies or under federal regulations, lack of compliance could result in funding cutbacks. If the IRB did not promptly review and approve protocols, their forwarding to be considered for approval by funding agencies would be delayed. While trying to meet these conflicting demands, IRB members often lost the respect of their peers and superiors. In addition, service on the IRB frequently meant less time for teaching, research, and practice with little recognition for performing a difficult job.

New problems arose in the 1980s. Federal and foundation research support increased progressively, leading to more investigators and investigations. Budgetary pressures caused institutions to expect more from their clinicians and teachers. Concomitantly, there was a huge increase in industry-sponsored research in both drugs and devices. Congress now pressed the Food and Drug Administration (FDA) to expedite the approval of investigational products, and industry was allowed to help fund the FDA so that they could comply. Industry, realizing the financial rewards of obtaining earlier approval for marketing, pressed investigators to complete studies as rapidly as possible. Academic institutions could not supply the numbers of subjects fast enough to meet this demand. Institution-based IRBs were also viewed as being too slow or too demanding of changes to their multicenter designed protocols. The FDA allowed industry to develop a noninstitutional-based source of subjects—namely, practicing physicians—to meet their requirements. Research increasingly took place in foreign countries. A new industry developed to provide IRB approval for these multicenter protocols for these geographically diverse practitioner–investigators. These new central and independent review boards supplied the "peer" review for the practicing clinician who was not affiliated with an institution. With 60% to 70% of pharmaceutical

research being accomplished in this setting, large central and independent IRBs, as well as the incorporation of practicing clinicians into business units to facilitate managing more protocols, developed. This new paradigm resulted in a different set of relationships than existed when the institution, IRB, and investigator were all part of a single organization. Because the noninstitutional IRB is usually geographically separate from the investigator, IRB members are unlikely to know these sponsor selected investigators personally. These practitioners often do not answer to a professional peer organization other than their state licensure agency. The sponsor, rather than the investigator, usually submits the protocol and consent form to these noninstitutional IRBs.

These revolutionary changes have increased the speed with which new drugs and devices have been approved. However, there are questions concerning the protection of the subjects in this new system. Although there may be conflicts of interest in academia, they are not as obviously financial as they can be in the noninstitutional setting. The inducement to enter as many subjects as possible is overtly evident because the funds often go directly to the investigator rather than to an institution that can control the investigator's income.

The logistical needs for review by IRBs of multicenter and cooperative studies have not been limited to industry-sponsored research. Increasing numbers of National Institutes of Health (NIH), Veterans Administration, and oncology studies require access to numbers of subjects rarely available at a single site. Besides the requirement for significant numbers of subjects for scientific validity, it is often important to include subjects from diverse geographic or demographic populations. The use of multiple centers may be the only way of recruiting sufficient numbers of subjects to study diseases that occur infrequently. Obviously, the protocols used for multicenter or cooperative studies must be scientifically uniform or the data cannot be combined. Central review of such protocols can be more scientifically rigorous and timelier. However, the issue of the responsibility for the protection of subjects must also be considered, and local review is more likely to take into account special circumstances that could influence the risk/benefit assessment. Currently, how the investigator relates in the setting of central review is not always clearly defined, and the chain of responsibility for protecting the individual subject may also be vague. Guidelines need to be developed that more clearly define the responsibilities of the various components in these circumstances so that the best elements of central and local review are preserved.

IRBs, whether they are institutionally based, central, or independent, face problems that can undermine the ethical standards that are essential to scientific investigations and that protect subjects from risks when benefits are not honestly expected. The common problems are (1) the lack of efficient methods or resources to oversee/monitor ongoing approved studies; (2) pressures by the organization, sponsors, and investigators to approve studies for financial or prestige reasons; and, similarly, (3) pressure to look sideways at the questionable scientific values of a study versus the financial benefits. Additional problems primarily affect institution-based IRBs. There is much evidence that institutions often supply inadequate financial and leadership support. IRB chairs and members often are not given appropriate recognition for their service. With increasing pressures to bring in income from managed-care practice and research, IRB work is often not counted as valued time and effort. Large institutions with very large research programs require very efficient management to accomplish their responsibilities. Institutions that do only a small volume of research often lack the workload to justify the administrative expertise and may not have the capability for appropriate scientific review. A possible solution would be to use an independent IRB or join with other small institutions to support an IRB that would have appropriate resources.

What is clear is that IRBs cannot be expected to continue to be the prime element in the protection of humans studied in research. That responsibility must be broadened to stress the role of the governance of the organization in setting high ethical standards and to emphasize the critical role that the investigator and the research team must play. These three components of the human-research protection program (HRPP) can no longer be adversarial, but must operate as a single entity whose basic value is the ethical treatment of all individuals studied in research. Even when all of the components of an HRPP are not institutionally based, there should be a clear plan for how the HRPP will function to integrate the various aspects required for the protection of subjects, regardless of where the various components are physically located. Multicenter and cooperative studies must designate to whom the responsibility for the subjects' protection will be assigned.

An integrated HRPP must establish policies and procedures to support the role played by each component. The investigator is the key element in the responsible conduct of the research and for the protection of the subjects recruited into studies. The investigator and the research team are perfectly positioned to accept this responsibility. This team must be sufficiently knowledgeable to implement the scientific aspects of the investigation in an ethical manner. It is likely that measures of competency for the research team will become accepted practice.

Whatever measures are implemented, the intent to do the right thing must remain the driving ethical principle. The governance of the HRPP must establish and maintain high ethical standards that are clearly disseminated to the IRB, investigators, and the community they serve. There should be appropriate support of the IRB and investigators so that their responsibilities can be carried out appropriately and expeditiously. Meaningful conflict-of-interest policies must be established and implemented for all components of the HRPP. Visible recognition of the contribution made by IRB members and staff helps to promote respect for the IRB function and for the organization's commitment to ethical research.

Adequate functioning of the IRB requires the support of a trained staff with access to needed resources. The governance should select an IRB chair who can be a leader with stature and credibility in the organization. Chairs should not be rotated on a short-term basis, as stability of IRB functions is more likely to be maintained when there is continuity of leadership. IRB members should be selected with the understanding that this is an important organizational function and should be given the same recognition as research, teaching, or clinical activities.

I am hopeful that the evolution of the system to protect humans studied in research will again become the organization's primary goal by returning to simple humane and ethical principles. There is a need to refocus the primary effort to strengthening the front line of this endeavor, namely, the investigator/subject interface. Any actual or perceived conflicts of interest cannot be allowed to interfere with the protective role of the HRPP. Although the system has a great need to evolve to correct the past problems in research involving humans, we must nevertheless always return to the basic ethical principles in dealing with our fellow human beings. Simply stated, "Do unto others as you would have others do unto you."

A Shared Responsibility for Protecting Human Subjects

Steven Peckman

INTRODUCTION

This chapter addresses the importance of the shared responsibility for creating an institutional culture of respect and trust in the protection of the rights and welfare of human research subjects. It outlines the separate responsibilities of the institution, as represented through the institutional official, investigators, and the institutional review board (IRB) in promoting an ethical and safe research environment. The chapter also highlights the collective responsibility for building the culture of respect and trust through education and support.

A Culture of Respect for the Mission of the IRB

An IRB is defined as "an administrative body" composed of scientists and nonscientists "established to protect the rights and welfare of human research subjects recruited to participate in research activities conducted under the auspices of the institution with which it is affiliated."[1(Chap.IA)] The IRB conducts a prospective review of proposed research and monitors continuing research in order to safeguard the rights and welfare of the participants. Although the IRB is responsible for the review and approval of proposed research, the institutional official is responsible for all parties engaged in the review or conduct of research under the auspices of the institution. Thus, the institutional official should have the "legal authority to act and speak for the institution, and should be someone who can ensure that the institution will effectively fulfill its research oversight function."[1(Chap.IB)]

The requirement that each federally funded institution engaged in human experimentation must constitute a local IRB encourages the institution to promote an environment that supports the highest ethical standards for the review and conduct of its research. Moore[2(p.375)] highlighted the importance of "the intellectual and ethical climate of the institution. Such a climate is difficult to regulate or standardize, at times even to recognize or describe. Yet it is more important than any other single consideration in protecting the willing patient from unwise, inexpert, or ill-advised therapeutic innovation." Moore's 1969 comments on the importance of institutional culture remain largely true today. Most importantly, the imprimatur of the institution makes the local IRB an agent of the highest ethical standards embraced by the institution itself, rather than a foreign agent of the government or an adversary of research, and creates a community that supports such standards.

The research institution is uniquely situated to create a culture in which ethics are valued and the importance of IRB review is honored. Levine[3(p.342)] noted that "to function most effectively, the IRB must not only be, but also must be perceived to be, an agent of its own institution." To achieve Levine's goal, it is incumbent on the institutional official to use his or her moral and academic authority to require the highest ethical conduct from the faculty and staff. The institution should develop and implement local policies and procedures that reflect the ethical principles of *The Belmont Report*[4] and the federal regulations to create an internal standard of acceptable behavior. Institutional policies and procedures translate into a demonstration of philosophical and practical support for the autonomy and authority of the IRB while facilitating a fair, timely, and collegial review of proposed research. An institutional ethos that highlights the importance of ethical principles will also insist on well-conceived and properly executed research. The requirement should be evident in written institutional policies, the actions and communications of institutional officials, and the IRB. Research that is designed or conducted so poorly as to be unethical or invalid exposes subjects and the institution to unnecessary risk. The institutional standard for well-conceived and properly conducted research minimizes the potential for conflicts between the IRB and the research community, facilitates local review, and assures the protection of the rights and welfare of the human subjects.

Investigators will perceive such internal standards as an expression of a communal commitment to ethical behavior rather than as an intrusion into academic research by a colonizing federal authority. The IRB is thus perceived by the research community as an expression of its own commitment to human subjects' protection and the expression of an institutional mandate and policy, rather than an alien and disembodied review process. As noted by the National Commission for the Protection of Human Subjects in Biomedical and Behavioral Research, such an environment demystifies the review process and builds the trust of the research community and the public.[5]

The institution underscores the importance of ethical conduct by convening IRBs with a respected membership that reflects the highest level of scientific expertise and community participation and support. An IRB that has the respect of the research community is better able to fulfill its principal charge as outlined by the National Commission: education of the research community.

> The commission believed that the rights of subjects should be protected by local review committees operating pursuant to federal regulations and located in institutions where research involving human subjects is conducted. Compared with the possible alternatives of a regional or national review process, local committees have the advantage of greater familiarity with the actual conditions surrounding the conduct of research. Such committees can work closely with investigators to assure that the rights and welfare of human subjects are protected and, at the same time, that the application of policies is fair to the investigators. They can contribute to the education of the research community and the public regarding the ethical conduct of research. The committees can become resource centers for information concerning ethical standards and federal requirements and can communicate with federal officials and with other local committees about matters of common concerns.[5]

The institutional official recognizes that the board can only carry out its regulatory, educational, and ethical functions when there are sufficient resources and high-level support staff to communicate effectively with the research community and to ensure adequate protections of subjects through oversight, including continuing review and monitoring of approved research.

The Belmont Circle

Human research is based on trust. The biomedical and social/behavioral investigator must build a relationship of trust with the subject in order to obtain information that will help answer a scientific question. All parties are entrusted with the responsibility to ensure the rights and welfare of research participants through IRB review and compliance with the federal regulations. This means that they are *allowed* to perform human research only after demonstrating an understanding of the responsibility by obtaining an IRB approval. Therefore, human-subjects research is a *privilege* and not a *right*. A federal court determined that human research is not a right, such as the right of intellectual inquiry embodied in academic freedom.

Rather, it is a privilege given by the institution to individuals who have assured their willingness to work within the federal guidelines and state law.[6]

The National Commission outlined three ethical principles in *The Belmont Report* to guide research with human subjects and ensure the maintenance of a culture of trust: respect for persons/autonomy, beneficence, and justice.[4] The ethical principles of *The Belmont Report* and the federal regulations are applied through the creation of an institutional culture that honors and demonstrates respect for human subjects through the process of IRB review of research protocols, as well as the conduct of research by investigators and support by institutional officials.

Successful IRB review balances the interests of three distinct but interrelated social and political entities: scientists, society, and the individual human subject. The IRB, however, does not balance these interests alone. The IRB functions in a dynamic relationship with federal agencies, research sponsors, institutions hosting research, investigators, and the public. The dynamic relationship balances the competing interests of all parties and facilitates the continued conduct of human research in an ethical and collegial environment. Ultimately, an effective system of protections is a collective responsibility that requires a collaborative effort. When all parties acknowledge their shared ethical responsibilities at both the local and national level and a balance of interests is met, they create a culture of trust. This allows for their effective collaboration with the public and research subjects.

The creation of a supportive institutional culture is based on the ability of all parties to apply the concepts of trust embraced by *The Belmont Report* and the federal regulations through successful working relationships with their colleagues. In other words, to apply the *Belmont* principles to human research subjects effectively, they must first share a common goal: the application of these same principles, not in a hierarchical way but in a circular fashion, to interactions with IRBs, support staff, investigators, sponsors, and federal agencies. This is called the Belmont circle (Figure 1.4.1). A circle is created that links all parties equally, and each party demonstrates

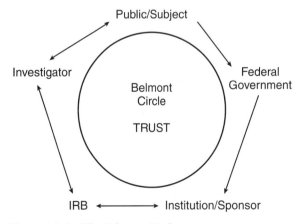

Figure 1.4.1 The Belmont Circle

dedication, both individually and collectively, through education and cooperation, to upholding human dignity through the application of the letter and spirit of the National Commission's report. Using various ethical codes and regulations, they create an environment that ensures the protection of human subjects as well as the advancement of science. The collaboration must exist in a culture of trust, complete openness, and honesty. By upholding the highest ethical principles and standards, they build public support for the pursuit of greater knowledge in a safe research environment.

The Three Levels of Accountability or Compliance

The circle of trust remains whole only when all responsible entities within the institution dedicate themselves to upholding the federal assurance and the concepts within *The Belmont Report*. The responsibility of ensuring accountability or compliance for human research is often placed solely on the shoulders of the IRB and the IRB administrator. The creation of a successful local human-subject protection system, however, is predicated on the interlinking relationship of the three institutional levels of responsibility as outlined in the regulations and guidelines: institution, investigator, and IRB.[1(Chap.ID)]

Each party—investigator, IRB, and institutional official—holds the responsibility for ensuring respect and collegiality in the IRB review process. We should understand the role that each of the participants is expected to play in order to ensure accountability.

The federal regulations embody a self-regulating system that depends on the honesty and integrity of the participants, namely, the institutions, the researchers, and the IRBs. The efficacy of the system is predicated on the ability of the institutions, IRBs, and investigators to work together in a supportive environment of mutual trust toward a common goal: the safe and ethical conduct of research. The systems will not work unless the three levels of accountability reflect and enhance each other. History has shown that a breakdown in any level of compliance will weaken the protection of human subjects, erode the public's trust in scientific research, and result in a demand for broader and stronger regulation and oversight.

Institutional Accountability

Active institutional support is the foundation for a successful, ethical human-research program. The institutional official is responsible for upholding the assurance and is accountable for the actions of investigators and the IRB. Institutional noncompliance is defined as a systemic failure of the institution to implement practices and procedures contained in the institution's assurance. The institution must ensure that (1) the IRB is properly constituted and functions in accordance with the regulations, (2) the IRB receives appropriate institutional support and adequate staffing, and (3) the investigators meet their obligations to the IRB.[7(Sec.103)] Systemic failure to abide by the terms and conditions of an institution's assurance may result in withdrawal of approval of the assurance.[1] Such an action could effectively result in the suspension of all human research at the institution and the requirement that each investigator apply directly to the Department of Health and Human Services/Office for Human Research Protections for the review and approval of each protocol.

The institution ensures that the IRB retains the ultimate authority for the approval of research with human subjects and has the authority to approve, to require modification of, and to disapprove proposed human research.[7(Sec.109)] The IRB also has the authority to suspend or revoke its approval of ongoing research.[7(Sec.113)] It is, therefore, the institution's obligation and responsibility to support IRB decisions made within the course and scope of its charge. Institutional support, however, does not absolve the IRB from the responsibility of working collegially with investigators, nor does it make the IRB the federal police. Rather, it requires that the board serve as an educational resource for the local research community. The Advisory Committee on Human Radiation Experiments highlighted the importance of education: "The historical record makes clear that the rights and interests of research subjects cannot be protected if researchers fail to appreciate sufficiently the moral aspects of human subject research and the value of institutional oversight."[8] The institutional official, therefore, should set the highest ethical standards for the research community and insist on an institutional culture that demonstrates support for the charge of the IRB, namely respect for human dignity.

The institution, therefore, is uniquely situated to take responsibility for various aspects of human research, such as the following:

1. It should create an institutional culture that promotes and upholds the highest ethical standards in the conduct of human research.

2. It should educate and mentor the research community and provide sufficient resources and staff to support the educational mandate of the IRB.

3. It should create an IRB with sufficient scientific expertise and community representation to assess proposed research projects.

4. It should involve all interested parties in the review process, emphasizing open communication and interaction with the community (the source of potential research subjects).

5. It should oversee research.

6. It should be aware of local resources and standards that may impact proposed research.

Investigator Accountability

Investigators are required to submit research for prospective IRB review. They must comply with all IRB conditions of approval, institutional policy, and federal and state regulations and laws. The Office for Human Research Protections (OHRP) noted that the most common lapses in compliance include (1) unreported changes in the protocol, (2) misuse or nonuse of the informed consent document, and (3) failure to submit protocols to the IRB in a timely fashion.

"Occasionally, an investigator will either avoid or ignore the IRB. Such cases present a more serious challenge to the systems of human subject protection. Regardless of intent, investigators initiating unapproved research involving human subjects place those subjects as well as the institution at an unacceptable risk."[1(Chap.ID)]

IRB Accountability

The IRB must ensure that all appropriate review procedures are followed. Noncompliance occurs whenever the IRB deviates from the duties required of it by federal regulations. The deviations may include (1) inadequate review of research protocols, (2) failure to ensure the consent document and process provide sufficient information to allow prospective subjects to make an informed decision about whether to participate in the research, (3) failure to ensure that the research design includes adequate monitoring of the data and any additional safeguards necessary to protect the welfare of particularly vulnerable subjects, and (4) failure to conduct continuing review of research at intervals appropriate to the degree of risk. IRBs must also uphold their regulatory record keeping responsibilities[1(Chap.IB)] and only make research-related decisions with appropriate quorum and attendance of sufficient nonscientific and non-affiliated members.[7(Sec.107)]

If the three partners—institutional official, investigator, and IRB—embrace and express *The Belmont Report,* they will create a culture that is free of hostility and one in which the importance of IRB review and compliance with the regulations is readily acknowledged. The integration of the three ethical principles of Belmont with the three levels of responsibility for the protection of the rights and welfare of research subjects will result in program accountability as well as commitment to the federal assurance, ultimately benefiting all stake holders and promoting justice. The institution, the investigator, and the IRB complete the Belmont circle by applying the principles in the following manner:

1. *Respect.* Respectful interactions between the institution, the IRB, and the investigator will build a culture of respect for and understanding of the importance of the ethical review and conduct of research.

2. *Beneficence.* It is incumbent on the institution, the IRB, and the investigator to apply the concept of beneficence to their relationships with each other. Ineffective accountability harms the institution and fellow researchers and puts research at risk. Additionally, maximizing benefit through acknowledgment of institutional accountability will help create a culture of understanding and trust. In other words, all parties should agree that minimizing the risk of noncompliance and maximizing the benefits of collegial interactions will lead to a common goal: an environment that ensures continued research through the protection of the rights and welfare of human subjects. To build a program that upholds respect for human dignity, the concept of beneficence must have primacy, even if that means deciding that the potential risk of the institution's participation in a project outweighs the possible benefits in academic promotion, extramural funds, etc. Ultimately, a lack of unity in the acknowledgment of the importance of the letter and spirit of Belmont

and the federal regulations poses great risk to the success of the IRB process and the general research program.

3. *Justice.* The application of justice requires that no single party carries an unfair burden and that there is an equal distribution of responsibility. The IRB cannot ensure compliance alone. The function and support of the IRB and membership on the IRB should not be an "unfunded mandate." The IRB and investigators should be supported through appropriate education regarding their responsibilities and obligations. Without appropriate education, it is impossible to ensure a respectful research environment. Furthermore, all members of the institution's human research community should actively participate in the IRB process through revolving membership that will act as an educational tool and allow for an equitable distribution of the burden of membership.

Conclusion

In spite of past and recent problems in the conduct of human-subject research, society continues to allow investigators to engage in human experimentation because specific parameters are in place to ensure the protection of the participants. An institution that takes responsibility for the review and conduct of human research positions itself to engage the trust and support of the scientific community. In addition, it attracts additional financial support for research because it can assure ethical conduct and safety, and it creates an environment for successful collaboration with the community of potential research subjects. The responsibility of local review obliges all institutional parties to acknowledge a collective responsibility for the creation of a culture of intramural and extramural community participation, mentoring, and accountability. The local system of review is most effective when the institutional official sets the highest ethical standards for the research community and insists on an institutional culture that demonstrates support for the charge of the IRB, namely, respect for human dignity.

Acknowledgment
Sections of this chapter were adapted from Steven Peckman, *Local Institutional Review Boards,* National Bioethics Advisory Commission, 2001, as well as from "Developing a Program of Human Subject Protection Before an FDA Inspection or OPRR Site Visit," *Balancing the Belmont: Human Subjects and Future Research,* Wayne State University/OPRR/FDA Conference, Keynote Address, September 16, 1999.

References
1. Penslar RL, Porter JP. Office for Human Research Protections. *Institutional Review Board Guidebook.* Updated 6 February, 2001. Access date 29 March, 2001. http://ohrp.osophs.dhhs.gov/irb/irb_guidebook.htm
2. Moore FD. Therapeutic innovation: Ethical boundaries in the initial clinical trials of new drugs and surgical procedures. In: Freund PA (ed.). *Experimentation with Human Subjects.* New York: George Braziller; 1970:375.

3. Levine RJ. *Ethics and Regulation of Clinical Research*, 2nd ed. Baltimore, MD: Urban and Schwarzenberg; 1986.

4. National Commission for the Protection of Human Subjects of Biomedical and Behavioral Research. *The Belmont Report: Ethical Principles and Guidelines for the Protection of Human Subjects of Research*. In DHEW Publication No. (OS) 78-0013 and (OS) 78-0014.4, 18 April, 1979. Access date 22 March, 2001. http://ohsr.od.nih.gov/mpa/belmont.php3

5. National Commission for the Protection of Human Subjects of Biomedical and Behavioral Research. *Report and Recommendations: Institutional Review Boards* (DHEW Report No. OS 78-0008). 1978. Washington, DC: Department of Health, Education, and Welfare.

6. Hammerschmidt D. There is no substantive due process right to conduct human subject research: The saga of the Minnesota Gamma Hydroxybutyrate Study. *IRB: A Review of Human Subjects Research* 19(3, 4):13–15, 1997.

7. Code of Federal Regulations. Title 45A—Department of Health and Human Services; Part 46—Protection of Human Subjects. Updated 1 October, 1997. Access date 18 April, 2001. http://www4.law.cornell.edu/cfr/45p46.htm

8. Advisory Committee on Human Radiation Experiments. *The Human Radiation Experiments: Final Report*. New York: Oxford University Press; 1996. http://tis.eh.doe.gov/ohre/roadmap/achre/report.html (DOE 061-000-00-848-9)

A Brief History of Public Responsibility in Medicine and Research and Institutional Review Board Education

Joan Rachlin

INTRODUCTION

As the long-time executive director of the nonprofit organization Public Responsibility in Medicine and Research (PRIM&R), I am one of a small but stalwart group of institutional review board (IRB) "lifers," or at least a member of the Quarter Century Club. Over the past 33 years, there has been tremendous change in the world of research regulation, particularly in the IRB system. I am not a historian, but I am—and have always been—an avid IRB watcher; therefore, my perspective may be of interest to IRB newcomers and may evoke warm memories in IRB veterans.

Beginnings of PRIM&R

PRIM&R and IRBs grew up together, and therefore, the history of one is a window on the history of the other. When I first came to work at PRIM&R, I was an idealistic young law student working part-time for a firm specializing in health care law. I began working in the law firm in late 1974, just as PRIM&R was being incorporated. As I was the low person on the firm's totem pole, the tasks associated with this pro bono effort were left to me. PRIM&R's initial mission was to improve, and proactively influence, the level of both governmental and public understanding on issues relating to research. Another objective was to improve the general image of and climate for research, but in truth, none of us knew how to approach either of those very theoretical goals.

One of the hot research topics in the 1970s was the growth of IRBs and federal involvement in their regulation. Federal funding of clinical research had grown exponentially after World War II, and the National Institutes of Health (NIH) opened their Clinical Center in 1953 to accommodate that growth. The NIH Clinical Center insisted on committee review of all proposed research protocols in its intramural program but, along with a handful of teaching hospitals, was unusual in this practice.

Then, in 1966, the U.S. Surgeon General required prior local review of all clinical research involving human subjects funded by the U.S. Public Health Service. This review was to take into account the rights and welfare of subjects and the potential risks and medical benefits of the research. In 1974, these policies and guidelines were revised and issued as regulations mandating that institutions establish diversely constituted review boards consisting of at least five members. Thus, 1974 was a milestone year in IRB history! The IRB regulations were first issued, and both the National Commission (a federal advisory committee) and PRIM&R were born.

One of the key missions of the National Commission was to consider procedures for evaluating and monitoring the performance of the previously described IRBs after their establishment by the National Research Act of 1974 and to recommend appropriate enforcement mechanisms. The commission issued a report and recommendations on IRBs in 1978, and along with *The Belmont Report* and Jay Katz's seminal work, *Experimentation in Human Beings,* it became one of our three early bibles. It is haunting that the question Jay Katz articulated in the early 1970s—"When may a society expose some of its members to harm in order to seek benefits for others?"—is still the fundamental question that researchers and IRBs struggle with today.

I remember hearing many observers predict back in the mid-1970s that IRBs, after widely adopted and well developed, would solve many, if not most, of the ethical and "public perception" problems in research. Would that it were so easy. I heard a talk by Jeremy Sugarman of Duke University in which he humorously referred to a scene from the movie *Pulp Fiction* when describing the situations in which IRBs often find themselves today. The analogy Sugarman invoked described the plight of the "clean-up crew" called to the scene after a significant amount of blood had already been shed. The leader of the clean-up crew said to his would-be employer, "We don't *do* the cleaning; we show *you* how to do it"— words to that effect. So, too, with IRBs—a small, often underfunded and always overworked committee, no matter how dedicated and competent, cannot "clean up" the problems that plague the research programs and cultures at many institutions. However, that reality did not stop many of us idealists from having high hopes when the IRB system was young. Thus, the journey began.

Administering the IRB

The task of administering IRBs fell to an early collection of mostly unwitting individuals who answered job descriptions that plunged them down the rabbit hole quickly and deeply. The IRB professionals who have endured and established credible programs are an intelligent, patient, well-organized, and committed lot, who are also (1) able to keep many balls in the air without missing a beat, (2) determined to keep many investigators and institutional officials grounded without their feeling attacked and unappreciated, (3) capable of keeping many protocols moving without incurring the wrath of the investigators on the one hand and the sponsors on the other, and (4) willing to, in his or her "spare" time, read, read, read, and then read some more because there is always so much to learn.

In the hope of improving the quality of research by protecting the rights of those who participate as subjects, a core group of people did meet these criteria and have dedicated themselves to building effective IRBs at their institutions. These are people of remarkable character, competence, and personal courage who have made the IRB community what it is today. This is an unusual group of professionals, and it is one of the main reasons that I and so many others have remained connected to the IRB world for as long as we have.

Developments in the Late 1970s

On to more history! In the early days of the IRB system, no one knew how to establish an IRB, whom to recruit, how to structure IRB reviews, and most urgently, how to interpret and apply the regulations. Recognizing the need for education in basic aspects of IRB function, PRIM&R decided to launch an educational campaign with its first IRB conference—for that matter, the first IRB conference anywhere—in April 1977. The meeting was held in the Suffolk Law School auditorium, and lunch cost $3.75 per person. We had no idea how many people would attend

the conference because we had no idea if anyone was interested enough in IRB issues to travel to Boston. We invited Donald Chalkley, the first director of the Office for Protection from Research Risks (OPRR), to be one of the speakers, and he obliged. We sent out our very primitive brochures and waited. Hoping for 75 to 100 attendees, we were delighted to welcome 175, and the PRIM&R IRB conference tradition was launched.

Shortly after this first PRIM&R conference in 1977, what has fondly become known as the "Charlie McCarthy" era arrived. Dr. Charles McCarthy took over from Don Chalkley in 1978 and led OPRR for the next 14 years with a thoroughly enchanting and effective blend of wit, warmth, determination, and wisdom. Dr. McCarthy was an ideal leader of OPRR during its formative years. He was one part ethicist, one part federal emissary, one part negotiator, and one part educator. He filled each role with competence and grace, and both the promulgation and widespread adoption of 45 CFR 46 in 1981 are rightly credited to him. Dr. McCarthy not only mediated the many battles that raged when the proposed regulations were first published in 1979, but he implicitly understood the need for community buy-in and worked tirelessly to achieve that through education and ready access to his office.

The next hallmark on our timeline was 1980, when the President's Commission was impaneled. Although it was the federal successor to the National Commission, it had an expanded mandate to look at issues outside the NIH. The President's Commission portfolio included reporting on the adequacy of human-subjects regulations, gene transfer, compensation for research-related injuries, and whistleblowing. Its recommendations include these requests:

1. All federal agencies should adopt common regulations.
2. The Department of Health and Human Services (DHHS) secretary should establish an office to coordinate and monitor implementation of the human-subject protection regulations.
3. Each federal agency should apply one set of rules consistently to all of its subunits.
4. Principal investigators should be required to submit annual data on the number of subjects in their research and on the number and nature of adverse events.
5. Action should be taken on the National Commission's recommendations for added protections in research with children and mentally disabled persons.
6. Institutions should be free to handle misconduct through mechanisms other than IRBs.
7. A procedure should be adopted for debarring grantees found guilty of serious misconduct and for sharing each agency's results.

Sound familiar? The more things change, the more they stay the same! Perhaps the most directly relevant connection between the work of the President's Commission and this book is that the commission contracted with PRIM&R to develop a guidebook for IRBs, which we did with gusto and pride in 1979. *The Official IRB Guidebook* took many of you far and served many of you well, but its time had long since come, and this book is a welcome and long overdue successor to that ground breaking volume.

The 1980s and Beyond

In 1986, one of the most significant events on the timeline occurred when PRIM&R formed its membership affiliate, Applied Research Ethics National Association (ARENA), which has filled a huge void in the leadership and information vacuum for the IRB community. I know that many of the chapters in this book are the result of ARENA initiatives and have been penned by ARENA leaders and members. The formation of ARENA and the subsequent achievements of this organization are PRIM&R's greatest "reflected" accomplishments.

In 1994, Dr. Gary Ellis assumed the leadership of OPRR after Dr. McCarthy's retirement, and he built on the foundation of outreach and education with his own brand of activism and unswerving principle. Dr. Ellis understood that OPRR's stewardship had entered a new era, in part because of the growing complexity of research itself and the financial ties between researchers and sponsors. He was a courageous and tireless leader of the office as it sought to reform, correct, revise, and improve the dynamic system that keeps those who are enrolled in research out of harm's way. Like Dr. McCarthy, his belief in the value of and need for education was fierce. He preached his own version of the "trickle-down" theory in which conscientious and committed institutional leaders set the tone for the ethical conduct of research at their respective facilities. Under Dr. Ellis's direction, OPRR's compliance site visits increased despite acute staffing shortages and increased workload. The results of

those site visits are widely credited with improving the research community's willingness to staff more adequately and otherwise fund IRBs.

Conclusion

We now find ourselves in the 21st century, with the conversion of an NIH-based OPRR to a DHHS-based Office for Human Research Protections (OHRP). The new office possesses broader authority, a larger budget, and a strong public mandate to improve the protection of research subjects. However, despite the passage of time, the problems that led to the formation of IRBs almost 30 years ago are still among the main issues with which IRBs struggle today.

As we all know, progress never comes easily, but as I look back on the past 30 years I am proud of everything that has been accomplished and excited about the possibilities for the future. Today the opportunity has never been greater for IRBs to impact the conduct of research in a way that we only imagined could be possible in the early days of this field. As I look around the room at the meetings and other discussion forums I attend and/or organize around the country, I see nothing but good things: energy, determination, and commitment to the fundamental ideals of research ethics. The protection of research subjects has never been in better hands owing to the coming of age of a community of committed and principled IRB professionals. Thank you for keeping the flame burning and for caring enough to never stop learning, to never stop teaching, to never stop asking! May it always be so, for your vigilance ensures "their" protection, and no one could ask for anything more.

The Institutional Review Board: Definition and Federal Oversight

Robert J. Amdur and Elizabeth A. Bankert

INTRODUCTION

An institutional review board (IRB) is a committee whose primary responsibility is to protect the rights and welfare of human research participants. Currently, no federal law or national directive requires all research to be reviewed in a uniform way regardless of researcher affiliation or funding source. In situations in which research is subject to federal regulation (e.g., involves the use of federal funds), the definition of an IRB and the procedures for research review are described in detail in the Code of Federal Regulations. When research is not subject to federal regulation, researchers are under no legal obligation to monitor the ethical aspects of research, but many elect to do so with a system modeled after the federal IRB system.

The distinction between a federally regulated and non–federally-regulated IRB is important because the purpose of this book is to explain how an IRB should function. In an effort to focus the discussions presented in this book, a decision has been made to use federal research regulations as the reference standard for IRB practice. All explanations and recommendations about IRB policy are organized for readers who want to understand how to conduct IRB activities in compliance with federal research regulations.

The two segments of the federal government that tell the IRB what to do and how to do it are the Office for Human Research Protections (OHRP) and the Food and Drug Administration (FDA). It is important to understand when and how these agencies interface with the IRB. These are the federal authorities that determine performance standards and enforce compliance with federal research regulations.

OHRP

The mission of the OHRP is to monitor and promote compliance with regulations promulgated by the U.S. Department of Health and Human Services (DHHS) that relate to the ethical standards of research involving human subjects (45 CFR 46).[1] Before 2000, this office was called the Office for Protection from Research Risks and administratively was located in the Office of Extramural Research in the National Institutes of Health (NIH). However, in September 2000, the office was reconstituted as OHRP and moved from the NIH to the Office of Public Health and Science within the Office of the Secretary of DHHS. The administrative location of OHRP was changed to eliminate the situation in which a research regulatory office reported to the director of an

agency whose primary mission is to conduct research (NIH). In addition to changing the administrative location so that the OHRP's viewpoint can now be communicated directly within the highest levels of DHHS, the status of the OHRP director was upgraded to the Senior Executive Service, which is the highest level of nonpolitical civil servant.

The OHRP monitors compliance with DHHS research regulations by establishing a type of contract called an *assurance* with institutions that conduct research that is funded by or otherwise subject to DHHS regulation. The assurance is a type of contract between the institution and OHRP that specifies when and how the institution will comply with DHHS research regulations. IRB leadership should understand any assurances that the institution has with OHRP.

OHRP does not routinely audit institutions for compliance purposes. OHRP usually does not audit IRB activities without provocation. With most institutions, OHRP documents compliance by recording the assurance agreements previously mentioned. If your institution has an OHRP assurance, OHRP needs no justification for investigating your institution's research program for the purpose of evaluating compliance with DHHS regulations. Common examples of events that trigger an OHRP investigation include an adverse event that receives national publicity, a complaint by a research subject or someone connected with the research program, and review of publications that describe research that is of concern to OHRP officials. OHRP has the final word on when an institution is not complying with DHHS regulations and what the institution must do to correct the problem. An OHRP contact may range anywhere from a simple phone call seeking clarification about a specific issue to a comprehensive, formal investigation, including a site visit. Any time that OHRP launches an official investigation, the institution is notified in writing and provided the opportunity to respond.

When OHRP determines that an institution has not complied with the terms of its assurance, OHRP officials present a representative from the institution (usually the OHRP assurance signatory) with a list of corrective actions that must be followed to maintain an approved OHRP assurance of compliance with DHHS regulations. The threat to restrict or suspend approval of an OHRP assurance is a powerful motivation for an institution to change its research review program. A restricted OHRP assurance can dramatically increase the administrative work associated with the review of research (e.g., when an assurance is restricted such that the IRB may not use the expedited process to approve research). Suspension of DHHS approval of an institution's OHRP assurance means that, with the stroke of a pen, DHHS funding for ongoing or previously approved research is suspended.

FDA

Any research involving a drug, a biologic, or a medical device is subject to FDA regulation. In many situations, research that is not funded by a federal agency is subject to FDA regulation. To understand the authority of the FDA over IRBs, it is important to realize that although the FDA is an agency within DHHS, the FDA and DHHS have separate regulations that apply to research involving human subjects and the IRB function. OHRP is the office within DHHS that is responsible for overseeing the implementation of DHHS research regulations.

DHHS and FDA regulations related to IRB responsibility are presented in the Federal Code of Regulations at 45 CFR 46[1] and 21 CFR 50,[2] 56,[3] respectively. Fortunately, the regulations that concern the IRB are similar for DHHS and FDA, but they are not identical. The important differences that the IRB should be aware of between DHHS and FDA regulations are discussed in a chapter in this book. For the purposes of this chapter, the point is that when research is subject to both DHHS and FDA regulation, an institution has two masters to satisfy when considering the need for, and process of, IRB review. In this situation, IRB review must be in compliance with the regulations of both of these federal authorities.

The factors that determine DHHS authority over an IRB have been discussed previously and basically consist of an assurance of compliance with OHRP. FDA regulations are cited in the reference section of this book.

The FDA system of compliance evaluation differs in several ways from that of OHRP. First, the FDA compliance program includes a plan to audit the IRBs at all institutions that conduct FDA-regulated research at regular intervals. Although an FDA investigation may be triggered by a concern about noncompliance, most FDA audits are done for routine evaluation. The standard program is for the FDA to audit each IRB that is subject to FDA regulation approximately once every 4 years. A second difference between the FDA and OHRP is that with the FDA, the processes for determining noncompliance and penalties are specified in some detail by the regulations.[3(Sec.121–124)] As is true with OHRP, FDA compliance officials have a wide range of options when directing a change in an institution's regulatory program. With the FDA, the leverage to change institutional behavior comes from FDA authority under the Food, Drug, and Cosmetic Act to impose civil penalties on an institution that does not comply with FDA regulations.

References
1. Code of Federal Regulations. Title 45A—Department of Health and Human Services; Part 46—Protection of Human Subjects. Updated 1 October, 1997. Access date 18 April, 2001. http://www4.law.cornell.edu/cfr/45p46.htm
2. Code of Federal Regulations. Title 21, Chapter 1—Food and Drug Administration, DHHS; Part 50—Protection of Human Subjects. Updated 1 April, 1999. Access date 18 April, 2001. http://www4.law.cornell.edu/cfr/21p50.htm
3. Code of Federal Regulations. Title 21, Chapter 1—Food and Drug Administration, DHHS; Part 56—Institutional Review Boards. Updated 1 April, 1999. Access date 27 March, 2001. http://www4.law.cornell.edu/cfr/21p56.htm

The Limits of Institutional Review Board Authority

Robert J. Amdur

INTRODUCTION

The mission of an institutional review board (IRB) is to protect the rights and welfare of human research participants. Such a mission makes it difficult to limit the scope of IRB activities. In the world of research ethics, there is no finish line when it comes to quality improvement. There is no limit to the amount of time and energy an IRB could spend on protocol review, research monitoring, continuing education, and the process of informed consent. Federal regulations require an institution to provide for "meeting space and sufficient staff to support the IRB's review and record-keeping duties."[1[Sec.103(b)(2)]] Few IRBs operate in an environment without pressure to improve efficiency and prioritize the allocation of limited resources. Several reports have been critical of the IRB function in important aspects of research review (e.g., monitoring of ongoing studies) and the ability to manage heavy workloads.[2] These realities make it important for institutional and IRB leadership to realize that the IRB cannot afford to spend time on activities not required for protection of human research subjects in compliance with federal research regulations.

At most institutions, anything that distracts the IRB from its fundamental responsibilities will compromise the IRB function. Although this concept may seem straightforward, in practice, it is often difficult to apply. IRBs often find themselves in the position of being the most convenient or qualified group to take responsibility for important administrative responsibilities that from the regulatory standpoint could be handled by another administrative body. Most of this book is devoted to helping the IRB understand what it must do to comply with federal regulations. However, at some institutions, understanding what the IRB does not have to do is a critical factor in improving IRB function.

The IRB Is Not an Editorial Service

The IRB reviews the consent document to see that it clearly and accurately describes the essential elements of informed consent in language appropriate for the study population. When the IRB thinks that it is important to revise the consent document, such changes are made a requirement for approval of the study. Some IRB members are extremely demanding about the wording of the consent document, whereas others have a high threshold for requiring editorial changes. The amount of time and energy that the IRB spends on the consent document is an important issue because it may limit the thoroughness of review of other components of the research process. This topic is discussed in a later chapter.

When the IRB requires a change in the consent document, a decision has to be made about the role of the IRB in drafting the revision. Whenever possible, the IRB should be as explicit as possible about required changes, but the IRB is under no regulatory obligation to direct the revision process. When problems with the consent document are extensive or complex, it is appropriate for the IRB to simply describe the problems in a general sense and then require the investigator to figure out the details of the revision. A researcher who is not motivated to improve the consent document or who does not understand the basic goal of the consent document should not be doing research. The IRB should help the researcher whenever possible, but it is important for everyone to understand that it is not a productive use of institutional resources for the IRB to function as an editorial service for investigators or protocol managers.

Example

Revise the consent document so that it is in "lay language." It is not unusual to see language used throughout a consent document that is too complex for the target population. The meaning of "too complex" and "lay language" will vary with the IRB and study population and need not be formally defined. When complex language is used throughout a consent document, the IRB should instruct the investigator to revise the document. This is to present complex terms and explanations in "lay language," meaning in a manner that is likely to be understood by the general public. The IRB need not be more explicit.

The IRB Is Not the Office of the Medical Director

At most medical centers, the medical director is the administrative authority that is responsible for making the rules of medical practice. When the IRB identifies the need for guidelines regarding activities that involve both research and nonresearch practice, the IRB may be asked or encouraged to administer policy that is more appropriately handled by the office of the medical director. An example of a situation that recently occurred at a major U.S. medical center will aid in understanding this issue.

Example

The IRB reviews a research protocol involving genetic testing. Study procedures do not specify whether genetic test results will or will not be recorded in the hospital medical record. Before approving the protocol, the IRB requires that the investigator establish a clear policy regarding the reporting of test results. In addition, if genetic results are going to be recorded in the medical record, they need to provide for genetic counseling and explanation of risks in the initial consent process.

As part of the process of evaluating this study, the IRB learns that no institutional policy exists regarding the reporting of genetic test results. Several members of the IRB believe strongly that patients who undergo genetic testing outside the setting of a research protocol should have the same protections as research participants. They recommend that the establishment of institutional policy on genetic testing be made a requirement for IRB approval of the research protocol.

If the IRB follows this recommendation, it will be in the position of forcing the institution to make policy for nonresearch activity. The IRB will be committed to spending time and energy directing or critiquing such policy as part of the research approval process. The IRB does not want to take responsibility for something that would distract it from the mission of protecting the rights of human research subjects. Recognizing the limits of IRB authority in this setting, the IRB approves the protocol with the appropriate changes. IRB approval is not made contingent on the development of an institutional policy on genetic testing. In an effort to improve patient care at their medical center, the IRB sends an unsolicited letter to the office of the medical director. The letter explains the issues related to the reporting of genetic test results and recommends that institutional policy on this subject be established.

The IRB Is Not the Medical Records Department or Confidentiality Committee

The problem of determining the need for and process of IRB review of projects that involve analysis of confidential information from the medical record is discussed in detail in later chapters. The bottom line for this discussion is that it is important for the IRB to recognize that (1) many projects that involve a systematic investigation of medical records are appropriately classified as something other than research (e.g., quality assessment, education, outcome evaluation, or utilization review), and (2) recording private information from the medical record with linkage to personal identifiers puts people at risk for the problems associated with a breach in confidentiality, regardless of whether medical information is collected for research or nonresearch purposes.

When data from the medical record are being collected for research purposes, federal regulations unquestionably require that the IRB approve the conditions for access to the medical record and the procedures for protecting confidentiality. However, when medical record review is being done for something other than research, the IRB has no regulatory authority over the activity. To avoid distracting the IRB from its mission of research regulation, a division of the medical records department or a separate "confidentiality committee" should oversee the use of confidential information from the medical record. The IRB and other segments of the medical center will need to work together to make medical record policy uniform throughout the medical center. Procedures for screening and triaging projects that require access to the medical record are discussed in the chapters mentioned earlier.

The IRB Is Not the Risk-Management Department

The term *risk-management department* is used in this section to describe the institutional authority that is responsible for advising institutional leadership on ways to avoid or minimize problems that could lead to charges of criminal activity, civil misconduct, or regulatory noncompliance. Risk-management advisors are usually lawyers who are familiar with the laws and regulations that apply to the activities that go on at their institution. At some institutions, a member of the risk-management team advises or serves on the IRB.

When an institution conducts research regulated by the federal government, some overlap occurs between the risk-management department and the IRB because the penalties may be significant if the IRB process does not comply with applicable federal regulations. The purpose of this section is to clarify the distinction between the IRB and an institution's risk-management department. This distinction is important when situations occur where IRB review of a research protocol identifies a practice pattern that could represent a legal liability for the institution. In many of these cases, the problematic activity is not limited to research; simply modifying or not approving the research study will not eliminate liability exposure for the institution. In this setting, there may be a tendency to use the IRB as a tool to draw attention to the problem or to advance the policy agenda of the risk-management department. The IRB should avoid this position because it does not support the IRB mission of protecting the rights and welfare of human research subjects. An example will help to illustrate the issue of IRB versus the risk-management department.

Example
An IRB reviews a research protocol involving an investigational medical treatment for patients in a coma after brain injury. Because eligible patients are in critical but stable condition, this is not an emergency research situation. However, the subjects of research will not be competent to give informed consent to study participation. State law is not definitive about who may or may not serve as a surrogate decision maker in this setting.

The IRB consults the risk-management department for help in understanding who qualifies as a legally authorized representative for an incompetent patient when it comes to enrolling in a research study. The risk-management advisor explains that the surrogate decision-maker issue is one that raises a concern about legal liability for the institution regardless of whether patients are involved in research. The risk-management department would like to see an internal institutional policy on the hierarchy of people (spouse, adult child, parent, sibling, etc.) who may serve as a surrogate decision maker when a patient is not competent to give informed consent for medical treatment. The risk-management representative advises the IRB to make IRB approval of the research protocol contingent on the establishment of institutional policy on this subject.

The IRB should not make modification of general institutional policy a condition for IRB approval of a research study. As discussed previously, such a decision puts the IRB in the position of directing or critiquing policy that is primarily aimed at nonresearch activity. The IRB does not need an institutional policy to decide on conditions for approval of the research project in question. In the example described previously here, the IRB approves the project with changes suggested by the risk-management consultant. The IRB leaves it to the risk-management department to establish institutional policy regarding surrogate consent as they think appropriate.

The IRB Is Not the Office of Patient Financial Services

The role of the IRB in evaluating the explanation of the costs of medical treatment delivered on a research protocol is currently not well defined. In Chapter 6-10, this issue is discussed in detail. The reason to mention it here is that few IRBs have the resources to administer a system that documents research versus nonresearch costs to

the degree that may soon be required by federal health insurance programs. IRBs are struggling with this issue because federal regulations require the investigator to explain "any additional costs to the subject that may result from participation in the research"[1][Sec.116(b)(3)] as part of the consent process. How the IRB interprets this regulation will determine whether the IRB has time to focus on other aspects of the research process.

The IRB Is Not a Data Safety Monitoring Board

A problem for many IRBs is the management of adverse event reports for multicenter medical research studies. In Chapters 7-3 and 7-4, this issue is discussed in detail. The reason to mention adverse event reporting in this section is to remind readers that the IRB cannot and should not attempt to function as a data safety monitoring board. During initial review of a protocol, Department of Health and Human Services regulations require that the IRB determine that the study design provides for an appropriate system for monitoring the study from the point of view of reacting to unexpected reports of inefficacy or toxicity. The role of the IRB is to document that an appropriate monitoring system is in place, but the IRB is not required to oversee the monitoring process.

Conclusion

At most institutions, anything that distracts the IRB from its fundamental responsibilities will compromise IRB function. IRBs often find themselves in the position of being the most convenient or qualified group to take responsibility for important administrative responsibilities that, from the regulatory standpoint, could be handled by another administrative body. At some institutions, understanding what the IRB does not have to do is a critical factor in improving IRB function. To this end, it may be useful for some IRBs to recognize the following:

1. The IRB is not an editorial service.
2. The IRB is not the office of the medical director.
3. The IRB is not the medical records department or confidentiality committee.
4. The IRB is not the risk-management department.
5. The IRB is not the office of patient financial services.
6. The IRB is not a data safety monitoring board.

References

1. Code of Federal Regulations. Title 45A—Department of Health and Human Services; Part 46—Protection of Human Subjects. Updated 1 October, 1997. Access date 18 April, 2001. http://www4.law.cornell.edu/cfr/45p46.htm
2. Office of Inspector General. Institutional Review Boards: A Time for Reform (OEI-01-97-00193). Department of Health and Human Services, June 1998. Access date 27 March, 2001. http://www.dhhs.gov/progorg/oei/reportindex.html

PART 2

Organizing the Office

Administrative Reporting Structure for the Institutional Review Board

Ernest D. Prentice, Sally L. Mann, and Bruce G. Gordon

INTRODUCTION

The purpose of this chapter is to discuss the reporting structure of the institutional review board (IRB). In this context, reporting structure refers to the administrative home of the IRB, the administrative superiors of the IRB chair and administrative director, and the position(s) in the organization that controls IRB resources. The reporting structure of the IRB is important because it may have significant influence on the quality and efficiency of IRB function. The reporting structure of the IRB is related to the topic of conflict of interest, which is discussed in detail in Part 5 of this book.

Tension Between Conflicting Goals

Some IRBs function well with a reporting structure in which the IRB is a division of an office that is organized for the primary purpose of promoting research at the IRB's institution. The criticism that has been raised about this kind of organization is that it creates the potential for conflict between the mission of the IRB and the mission of the IRB's administrative superiors. For an IRB to function effectively, it is essential for the IRB to have adequate resources and work in an environment where there is support for the IRB to make independent decisions related to the protection of research subjects. IRB leaders who function well in organizations in which the IRB is administratively housed in a grants and contracts or sponsored research office explain that the primary goals of their administrative superiors are not only to increase research volume but, more importantly, to manage the overall research enterprise according to the highest of ethical and regulatory standards.

Federal regulations do not address the reporting structure of the IRB to a degree that answers the question of whether it is acceptable for the IRB to be part of the grants and contracts or sponsored research office. Regardless of the name of the office that administers the IRB, the important thing is that the IRB reporting structure must be organized so that no real or perceived conflict of interest compromises IRB function or credibility. In the absence of definitive federal guidance, it is our recommendation that the IRB be administratively independent from offices that have any direct responsibility for the recruitment of research dollars to the institution.

Institutional Official

Each institution should appoint a high-ranking administrative officer who is authorized to act for the institution and assume overall responsibility for compliance with the federal regulations for the protection of human subjects. This individual is designated as the "Institutional Official" (IO) and is the person who signs the Office for Human Research Protections Federalwide Assurance. In many small- to medium-sized institutions, the chief executive officer serves as the IO. Large institutions usually assign administrators such as a vice-president, vice-chancellor, associate dean, or other senior administrator. Regardless of who is chosen to serve as the IO, it is of paramount importance that he or she has the knowledge, authority, and ability to commit the resources needed by the IRB.

As alluded to earlier, we think that problems are more likely to occur if the sponsored programs or grants and contracts director serves as the IO. Many perceive these departments to have an unacceptable conflict of interest because the primary role of the IRB is to protect research subjects. In contrast, the major role of any office that deals with funding programs is necessarily focused on increasing the amount of research funds awarded to the institution and its investigators. Although a vice-president or vice-chancellor for research may also be involved in obtaining grant funds, such individuals usually have broad-based responsibility for many aspects of the research infrastructure, such as chemical safety, radiation safety, and the animal facilities. Thus, any potential conflict of interest should effectively be reduced to an acceptable level. The rights and welfare of human subjects must always take precedence over the needs of science or fiscal considerations. All IOs should recognize this ethics-based mandate and take all necessary steps to ensure the integrity and functionality of the institution's program for the protection of human subjects.

Lines of Authority

IRB Chair
Although in many organizations the IRB chair currently reports to a subordinate of the IO, in our opinion, this is not the optimal arrangement. The IRB chair acts on behalf of the IRB, and the IO acts on behalf of the institution. It is, therefore, essential that there be direct reporting and regular communication between these two individuals. For this reason, we recommend that the IRB chair report directly to the IO. The IRB chair should not report to a committee such as the "executive committee of the medical staff" or the "dean's council" except to provide information and respond to questions. It is important to preserve the autonomy of the IRB and insulate it from pressure exerted by individuals or groups with special interests that are inconsistent with the mission of the IRB. The IRB must be able to act as an independent and objective body without answering to multiple masters who may have different agendas.

Reporting Line for the Chief IRB Administrator
The chief administrator of the IRB is usually the director of the IRB's support office. He or she should report to the IO or other high-level officer who can act on behalf of the IO on matters related to the administrative operation and support of the IRB. Normally, the director should not report to the IRB chair. This is because the IRB chair is usually a faculty member who serves as the chair on a voluntary and part-time basis. Thus, the chair is usually not in a position to deal with personnel issues, budgets, and other administrative matters. The director and IRB chair must obviously work closely together on policy development, protocol reviews, and other activities of the IRB. The effectiveness of this interaction, however, is not dependent on a direct reporting relationship. Indeed, quite the opposite may be true.

When the IRB chair is not responsible for potentially contentious personnel decisions such as promotions, salary increases, and budgets, the chair and administrators are able to focus their efforts on protecting research subjects without the interpersonal tension that often accompanies a supervisor–subordinate relationship.

Reporting Line(s) for the IRB Staff
The volume and nature of research requiring IRB review should determine the number of IRBs required by a given institution and the size of the IRB staff. A small institution may have only one IRB and one or two IRB staff persons, whereas a large institution may have four or more IRBs and 30 or more IRB staff. The administrative reporting structure and IRB personnel classifications obviously vary among institutions. Regardless of the size of the institution, however, all IRBs should employ a management system that allows the IRB to perform quality reviews that are both efficient and consistent.

The IRB management systems adopted by large institutions with multiple IRBs are usually more complex than the systems used by smaller institutions. One common model employed by large institutions is to provide each IRB with its own designated staff. For example, an institution with four IRBs may have a support office with a director, associate director, and four assistant directors. Each assistant director would report to the associate director and be responsible for one of the four IRBs. Each IRB, in turn, would have three protocol analysts and one secretary. Thus, each of the four IRBs would have five staff. The IRB support office would have a total of 22 personnel. To promote consistency and common standards of review, the director and/or associate director would normally attend all IRB meetings.

Conclusion

The IRB should occupy a highly visible and elevated position within the administrative structure of the institution. A culture of compliance is best established from the top down, and ideally, the chief executive officer or other high-ranking official should serve as the IO and play an active role in fostering the important work of the IRB. When an institution's IRB does not command the respect and support of the highest administrative officials, its effectiveness and credibility are jeopardized. Thus, it is incumbent on the institution to establish an administrative reporting structure for the IRB that will allow it to operate in a highly functional manner that best serves the institution, its investigators, and research participants.

Documentation, Policies, and Procedures

Celia S. Walker and Deborah Barnard

INTRODUCTION

This chapter focuses on institutional review board (IRB) policies and procedures. Procedures are differentiated from policies, and suggestions are offered about how to produce written procedures. Most importantly, however, the chapter emphasizes the importance of creating and using written procedures in IRB administration. This entails a systematic and thorough approach to transparent, concise, and thoughtfully presented standard operating procedures for the IRB staff, researchers, and the parent institution.

Differentiating Procedures from Policies

Policies and procedures are such stock words that we might not stop to discriminate between the two or consider their deeper meanings. In general, they are explanations of why and how matters are handled a specific way. They describe how the IRB operates. Policies tend to be general statements of broad principles, strategies, and philosophic guides. They often deed authority. Procedures, on the other hand, are practical, specific, step-by-step tactics and detailed directives about how to implement a policy. Policies provide overall guidance, but procedures are what an IRB, its administrative staff, and the institution's researchers consult every day (Table 2.2.1).

This chapter concentrates on procedures instead of policy, but many institutions promulgate both, either separated or combined. The University of Minnesota's web-based policy library exemplifies broad policy dissemination at an institutional level (http://www.fpd.finop.umn.edu/).[1] The policies typically refer to more complete sets of procedures that are more likely to be developed at the unit level, rather than at the institutional level. Another format would entail an integrated document, with the policy as opening paragraph, followed by higher level procedures that implement the policy.

Why Have Written Procedures?

There are two responses to this question. First, written procedures are required by federal regulation and anticipated accreditation processes. Second, and more importantly, written procedures are required because of what they accomplish. Written procedures are the references used to instruct or remind.

Federal Requirements

Among the Office for Human Research Protections (OHRP) Common Findings,[3] the list of deficiencies commonly found in audits, appears No. 67:

Written IRB Guidelines and Procedures. OHRP strongly recommends that institutions develop and distribute a handbook of IRB guidelines for research investigators. The handbook should include detailed information concerning (a) federal and institutional requirements for the protection of human research subjects, (b) the

Table 2.2.1 Policies versus Procedures

	Cooking	IRB
Policy	Creating meringue	Decisions are made at properly constituted meeting.
Procedure	Beat 2 egg whites in a bowl with a mixer until stiff. Be sure there is no grease in the bowl. Add 2 tablespoons of sugar slowly when the egg whites have begun to stiffen.	An IRB quorum consists of one half of the regular membership plus one person. If a quorum is present, and a nonscientific member is in attendance as a part of the quorum, a meeting is considered properly constituted.

IRB's role and responsibilities, (c) the requirements and procedures for initial and continuing IRB review and approval of research, (d) the rationale and procedures for proposing that the research may meet the criteria for expedited review, (e) the requirements and procedures for verifying that research is exempt from IRB review, (f) the responsibilities of investigators during the review and conduct of research, (g) requirements and procedures for notifying the IRB of unanticipated problems or events involving risks to the subjects, as well as any other expected or unexpected adverse events, (h) an explanation of the distinction between Food and Drug Administration (FDA) requirements for emergency use of test articles versus HHS regulations for the conduct of human subjects research, (i) relevant examples and user-friendly forms for providing information to the IRB, and (j) a copy of the institution's multiple project assurance (MPA), the HHS human subjects regulations (45 CFR Part 46), and The Belmont Report. Where appropriate, the OHRP also recommends that IRBs develop written operating procedures to supplement its guidelines for investigators.

Accreditation standards likewise insist that an institution have developed written procedures for IRB functioning. For example, AAHRPP's Standard 1.7 requires written procedures: "The organization must follow written policies and procedures governing all research involving human subjects. The policies and procedures specify to whom they apply and how they are disseminated. The policies and procedures must be reviewed periodically and updated as necessary." Subsequent sections refer to a variety of situations for which the institution must have and follow procedures, such as addressing allegations of noncompliance.

The FDA regulations mirror the Common Rule requirements, but with a critical difference in interpretation. Although OHRP in the past has accepted the written procedures appearing in an MPA as being adequate, the MPA mechanism is no longer available, and the FDA format does not include detailed procedures. The FDA has a record of requiring a separate document of written procedures when it audits programs. A survey of FDA audit-finding letters sent to sanctioned IRBs shows almost every one with a finding of "failure to have and follow written procedures for IRB functions and operations in accordance with 21 CFR 56.108 and 812.66."

Likewise, the terms of a federalwide assurance include a requirement to establish within 90 days and provide OHRP on request, written procedures, including specific items.[3] In light of the emphasis in the accreditation standards and changes in the assurance process, the distinction becomes moot, and a set of written procedures is required by both the FDA and OHRP.

The FDA additionally provides a checklist for evaluating procedures. This allows an institution to assess the completeness of its procedures before any kind of audit or accreditation visit. The entire list can be obtained from the FDA's website[4] and is discussed later here.

In summary, institutions should have been using written procedures for a variety of audiences because they are required by federal regulation. That requirement does not appear likely to change.

What Written Procedures Accomplish

Although we all use *unwritten* procedures to some degree, they are not as effective or desirable as written ones. Institutions operating solely with unwritten procedures may be viewed as unorganized, understaffed, unknowledgeable, or inconsistent and certainly would not be viewed by federal oversight agencies as adequate. Unwritten procedures should be formalized into written ones as soon as possible for use.

It might be tempting to maintain that the singular goal of written procedures is to maintain institutional compliance with federal regulations: "Written procedures are required, and we have them." However, just having them is not sufficient to constitute compliance. Having but not following those written procedures will be cited as a deficiency by federal audit agencies just as quickly as not having written procedures in the first place. The procedures are not a mantelpiece just for display; they should become an integral, practical description of the various IRB functions. Finally, they engender many positive outcomes.

1. They will establish consistency in how situations are handled. This is especially valuable for instances that may not occur frequently enough for the handling to become a well-learned pattern. Researchers appreciate greater consistency and view IRB decisions more credibly.

2. They result in an overall reduction in errors. It is harder to overlook critical procedural aspects if they are in writing.

3. They provide clarity about who is responsible for what. For those tasks that are left undone because neither the chair nor the administrator realizes it is his or her responsibility, the written procedures explicitly address responsibilities.

4. They lead to faster and improved training for new faculty, IRB members, and IRB staff. New staff members have a reference manual, and new IRB members have a complete procedural framework on which to structure their review of protocols.

5. They provide a partial defense against complaints, grievances, or lawsuits about inequitable treatment with respect to IRB determinations.

Policies and Procedures for Whom?

The federal regulations tend to be interpreted as requiring written procedures for researchers. In fact, three sets of interlocking procedures need to be developed, including those for the IRB itself.

IRB Administrative Office

This set is an expanded "desk reference" for all staff serving the IRB. In it might appear application intake procedures, schedules, contacts, application routings, procedures for operating and maintaining any database, the protocol for assigning approval numbers, and a catalog of applicable document files. It can even include procedures for producing procedure manuals, with the frequency and method for revising them. The administrative manual is useful for training new staff and is critical for maintaining consistency in handling protocols.

Researchers

Often called an *institutional handbook* or *manual*, it informs researchers about the application process, researcher responsibilities, and specific techniques such as obtaining a child's assent. It would be useful to include the location of core resources such as *The Belmont Report*, the federal regulations, and other institutional procedures (such as for graduate advisors). The web is generally an effective way of distributing such a handbook, in part because the web is so widely available and in part because changes can be made centrally so that any subsequent access shows the new information.

The IRB

The IRB's procedures will begin with the governing federal regulations. However, they will be expanded to include the institutional and committee interpretations and implementations of those regulations.

How to Produce Written Procedures

It is rarely necessary to start from scratch. It is almost always easier to begin with some existing written procedures and modify them for your purposes. Contact IRB administrators at other institutions similar to yours and ask whether you could receive a copy of their written procedures to adapt. Likewise, consult the web for the procedures of other institutions to see what topics they include. IRB administrators are typically quite generous in allowing use or adaptation of their documents; it is a courtesy to acknowledge the source in your finished product.

The FDA self-evaluation checklist, available from their web page, offers a helpful start with respect to topics that might be covered.[4] For institutions not engaged in FDA-regulated research, there are obviously sections that would not need to be covered in your procedures (such as provisions for emergency use at X.C.3), as well as institution-specific processes that differ. In addition, FDA references would need to be converted to Common Rule references. This checklist affords a workable map for comprehensive IRB procedures. The following is a comprehensive outline of policies and procedures related to IRB function. Use this list to create a procedures manual applicable to your organization.[4]

I. The institutional authority under which the IRB is established and empowered.
II. The definition of the purpose of the IRB, that is, the protection of human subjects of research.
III. The principles that govern the IRB in assuring that the rights and welfare of subjects are protected.
IV. The authority of the IRB.
   A. The scope of authority is defined, that is, what types of studies must be reviewed.
   B. Authority to disapprove, modify, or approve studies based on consideration of human subject protection aspects.
   C. Authority to require progress reports from the investigators and oversee the conduct of the study.
   D. Authority to suspend or terminate approval of a study.
   E. Authority to place restrictions on a study.
V. The IRB's relationships to
   A. The top administration of the institution.
   B. The other committees and department chairpersons within the institution.
   C. The research investigators.
   D. Other institutions.
   E. Regulatory agencies.
VI. The membership of the IRB.
   A. Number of members.
   B. Qualification of members.
   C. Diversity of members (e.g., representation from the community, and minority groups), including representation by:
      1. Both men and women
      2. Multiple professions
      3. Scientific and nonscientific member(s)
      4. Not otherwise affiliated member(s)
   D. Alternate members (if used).
VII. Management of the IRB.
   A. The chairperson.
      1. Selection and appointment
      2. Length of term/service
      3. Duties
      4. Removal
   B. The IRB members.
      1. Selection and appointment
      2. Length of term/service and description of staggered rotation or overlapping of terms, if used
      3. Duties
      4. Attendance requirements
      5. Removal
   C. Training of IRB chair and members.
      1. Orientation
      2. Continuing education
      3. Reference materials (IRB library)
   D. Compensation of IRB members.
   E. Liability coverage for IRB members.
   F. Use of consultants.
   G. Secretarial/administrative support staff (duties).
   H. Resources (e.g., meeting area, filing space, reproduction equipment, computers).
VIII. Conflict of interest policy.
   A. No selection of IRB members by investigators.
   B. Prohibition of participation in IRB deliberations and voting by investigators.
IX. Functions of the IRB.
   A. Conducting initial and continuing review.
   B. Reporting, in writing, findings and actions of the IRB to the investigator and the institution.
   C. Determining which studies require review more often than annually.
   D. Determining which studies need verification from sources other than the investigators that no material changes have occurred since previous IRB review.

E. Ensuring prompt reporting to the IRB of changes in research activities.

F. Ensuring that changes in approved research are not initiated without IRB review and approval except where necessary to eliminate apparent immediate hazards.

G. Ensuring prompt reporting to the IRB, appropriate institutional officials, and the FDA of:
   1. Unanticipated problems involving risks to subjects or others
   2. Serious or continuing noncompliance with 21 CFR parts 50 and 56 or the requirements of the IRB
   3. Suspension or termination of IRB approval

H. Determining which device studies pose significant or nonsignificant risk.

X. Operations of the IRB.
   A. Scheduling of meetings.
   B. Premeeting distribution to members of, for example, place and time of meeting, agenda, and study material to be reviewed.
   C. The review process.
      1. Description of the review process ensuring that
         a. All members receive complete study documentation for review (see XI.B);
         b. Or one or more "primary reviewers"/ "secondary reviewers" receives the complete study documentation for review, reports to IRB and leads discussion; if other members review summary information only, these members must have access to complete study documentation
      2. Role of any subcommittees of the IRB
      3. Emergency use notification and reporting procedures
      4. Expedited review procedure
         a. For approval of studies that are both minimal risk and on the FDA-approved list
         b. For approval of modifications to ongoing studies involving no more than minimal risk
   D. Criteria for IRB approval contain all requirements of 21 CFR 56.111.
   E. Voting requirements.
      1. Quorum required to transact business
      2. Diversity requirements of quorum (e.g., requiring at least one physician member when reviewing studies of FDA-regulated articles)
      3. Percentage needed to approve or disapprove a study
      4. Full voting rights of all reviewing members
      5. No proxy votes (written or telephone)
      6. Prohibition against conflict-of-interest voting
   F. Further review/approval of IRB actions by others within the institution (override of disapproval is prohibited).
   G. Communication from the IRB.
      1. To the investigator for additional information

2. To the investigator conveying IRB decision
      3. To institution administration conveying IRB decision
      4. To sponsor of research conveying IRB decision
   H. Appeal of IRB decisions.
      1. Criteria for appeal
      2. To whom appeal is addressed
      3. How appeal is resolved (override of IRB disapprovals by external body/official is prohibited)

XI. IRB record requirements.
   A. IRB membership roster showing qualifications.
   B. Written procedures and guidelines.
   C. Minutes of meetings.
      1. Members present (any consultants/guests/ others shown separately)
      2. Summary of discussion on debated issues
      3. Record of IRB decisions
      4. Record of voting (showing votes for, against, and abstentions)
   D. Retention of protocols reviewed and approved consent documents.
   E. Communications to and from the IRB.
   F. Adverse reactions reports.
   G. Documentation that the IRB reviews adverse reaction reports.
   H. Records of continuing review.
   I. Record retention requirements (at least 3 years after completion for FDA studies).
   J. Budget and accounting records.
   K. Emergency use reports.
   L. Statements of significant new findings provided to subjects.

XII. Information the investigator provides to the IRB.
   A. Professional qualifications to do the research (including a description of necessary support services and facilities).
   B. Study protocol that includes/addresses.
      1. Title of the study
      2. Purpose of the study (including the expected benefits obtained by doing the study)
      3. Sponsor of the study
      4. Results of previous related research
      5. Subject inclusion/exclusion criteria
      6. Justification for use of any special/vulnerable subject populations (e.g., the decisionally impaired, children)
      7. Study design (including as needed, a discussion of the appropriateness of research methods)
      8. Description of procedures to be performed
      9. Provisions for managing adverse reactions
      10. The circumstances surrounding consent procedure, including setting, subject autonomy concerns, language difficulties, vulnerable populations
      11. The procedures for documentation of informed consent, including any procedures for obtaining assent from minors, using witnesses, translators and document storage

12. Compensation to subjects for their participation
13. Any compensation for injured research subjects
14. Provisions for protection of subject's privacy
15. Extra costs to subjects for their participation in the study
16. Extra costs to third party payers because of subject's participation
C. Investigator's brochure (when one exists).
D. The case report form (when one exists).
E. The proposed informed consent document.
    1. Containing all requirements of 21 CFR 50.25(a)
    2. Containing requirements of 21 CFR 50.25(b) that are appropriate to the study
    3. Meeting all requirements of 21 CFR 50.20
    4. Translated consent documents, as necessary, considering likely subject population(s)
F. Requests for changes in study after initiation.
G. Reports of unexpected adverse events.
H. Progress reports.
I. Final report.
J. Institutional forms/reports.
XIII. Exemption from prospective IRB review.
A. Notify IRB within 5 working days.
B. Emergency use.
C. Review protocol and consent when subsequent use is anticipated.
XIV. Emergency research consent exception.
A. The IRB may find that the 50.24 requirements are met.
B. The IRB shall promptly notify in writing the investigator and the sponsor when it determines it cannot approve a 50.24 study.
C. The IRB shall provide in writing to the sponsor a copy of the information that has been publicly disclosed under 50.24(a)(7)(ii) and (a)(7)(iii).
D. In order to approve an emergency research consent waiver study, the IRB must find and document:
    1. Subjects are in a life-threatening situation, available treatments are unproven or unsatisfactory and collection of scientific evidence is necessary
    2. Obtaining informed consent is not feasible because:
        a. Medical condition precludes consent
        b. No time to get consent from legally authorized representative
        c. Prospective identity of likely subjects not reasonable
    3. Prospect of direct benefits to study subjects because:
        a. Life-threatening situation that necessitates treatment
        b. Data support potential for direct benefit to individual subjects

c. Risk/benefit of both standard and proposed treatments reasonable
4. Waiver needed to carry out study
5. Plan defines therapeutic window, during which investigator will seek consent rather than starting without consent. Summary of efforts will be given to IRB at time of continuing review.
6. IRB reviews and approves consent procedures and document. IRB reviews and approves family member objection procedures.
7. Additional protections, including at least
    a. Consultation with community representatives
    b. Public disclosure of plans, risks, and expected benefits
    c. Public disclosure of study results
    d. Assure an independent data monitoring committee established
    e. Objection of family member summarized for continuing review
8. Ensure procedures in place to inform at earliest feasible opportunity of subject's inclusion in the study, participation may be discontinued. Procedures to inform family the subject was in the study if subject dies.
9. Separate investigative new drug (IND) or investigative device exemption (IDE) required, even for marketed products.
10. IRB disapproval must be documented in writing and sent to the clinical investigator and the sponsor of the clinical investigation. Sponsor must promptly disclose to FDA, other investigators and other IRBs.

How to Create Written Procedures

One of the largest hurdles faced by an IRB administrator in writing procedures is simply getting started. The task seems insurmountable, the necessary "handle" missing. After one has broken into the assignment, it will begin to seem much more manageable. Adapting another institution's procedures to make them complete and pertinent to your institution is one expedient way of beginning. There are several resources available to help.[5-7]

It is likely, however, that some sections will need to be written from "scratch." To get started, use the guidelines that follow.

1. Brainstorm a list of all the topics that need to be covered. Pay no attention to order. Do not worry about including too much; extraneous topics can be weeded out later. Attempt to capture every related aspect.

Example
Appointing new members. Should not be appointed by researchers. Authorized institutional official (IO) makes final decision. Existing IRB makes recommendations. Involve deans. New members need to train. Need to represent research areas reviewed by IRB. Pay attention to diversity (gender, ethnicity).

Watch balances on IRB (longevity, scientist/nonscientist, physicians, prisoner representative, community membership). Have an order in which various bodies are consulted. Make the appointment in writing from institutional official. Get current curriculum vitae. IRB administrative office provides instructional materials and basic orientation.

2. Order the topics by grouping them into logical relationships, chronologic sequence, or some other system.

Example
Selecting ⟶ *Appointing* ⟶ *Finalizing the appointment*

3. Create an outline of the topics that is a further refinement of the grouping.

Example
1.0 Procedure for Appointing New IRB Members

   1.1 Selecting candidates

      1.1.1 Timing

      1.1.2 IRB starts process

      1.1.3 Get Deans' input

      1.1.4 Can the IRB propose? Can researchers select?

      1.1.5 Prioritizing and getting list to authorized institutional official (IO)

      1.1.6 The appointment

      1.1.7 Communicating to new member and IRB

4. Then, finalize and "polish" each procedure.

   a. Assess the situation needing a written procedure. Think through the variations and exceptions that can occur.

   b. Gather and review background material: existing procedures, laws and regulations from federal, state, and local sources; previous IRB actions (both those that worked and those that did not).

   c. Draft the procedure. Write rapidly and do not worry about grammatical precision. Get it down in a train of thought. Organize by introductory paragraph containing policy, description of procedure, summary of main points. Depending on the ultimate audience and use of the procedures, you may wish to cite pertinent regulations.

   d. Let the draft procedures rest at least 24 hours. When you return to them, you will see them with new eyes and are likely to see aspects you missed in the first draft.

   e. Test the procedure. "Drop" actual situations through the procedure to see whether it works. You may identify gaps or needed variations or additions, some of which may require IRB action to rectify processes or approve new ones.

   f. Revise procedures as necessary.

Example of Result
1.0 Procedure for Appointing New IRB Members

   Members shall be appointed to the IRB such that requirements of Common Rule § 107 are met.

   1.1 Selecting candidates

      1.1.1 The selection process for routine appointments shall begin approximately 3 months before the appointment date; ad hoc appointments needed to fill unanticipated vacancies shall begin as soon as possible after the announcement is given.

      1.1.2 The IRB shall ascertain what attributes a new member needs to possess (community member, scientist/nonscientist, duration of term, diversity, representation for vulnerable populations, academic standing, research arena).

      1.1.3 The IRB administrator will communicate these attributes to the college deans either by memo or e-mail, asking on behalf of the IRB for suggested candidates. A response date needs to be stipulated.

      1.1.4 The IRB shall likewise suggest candidates.

      1.1.5 At a convened meeting, or using an appointed subcommittee process, the IRB shall prioritize the list of candidates generated by deans and the IRB, listing briefly the reasons for the priority ranking. The IRB administrator will communicate the listing to the authorized IO within 3 working days of receiving the list.

      1.1.6 The IO shall appoint the new member. The IO retains this responsibility exclusively; researchers may not appoint new members; the IRB and college deans may recommend, but may not appoint.

      1.1.7 The IO shall convey in memo or e-mail his/her appointments to the IRB administrator, who shall

         1.1.7.1 Notify the IRB chair of the selection.

         1.1.7.2 Prepare the official appointment letter to the new member, using the model retained electronically at c:/appointments/appointment memo, with alterations as needed to fit the circumstances.

5. Have others review the procedures. You may wish to use several reviewers, including a "typical user" as well as a knowledgeable colleague.

6. Determine a workable layout: numbering system; format (outline, paragraph, play script); fonts; headings; how to handle graphics and appendices; issue and revision numbers and/or dates; pagination scheme; logo/institutional name; how new material will be inserted; front and back matter such as preface, table of contents, index, glossary, appendix; headers and footers; justification style. Be sure the format accommodates revisions, additions, and withdrawn procedures. Be sure there is a procedure for making these changes as well.

7. Produce final version. Consider whether multiple venues are necessary: web, printed, office manual.

8. Promulgate the procedures among the target audience.

9. Follow procedures.

10. Revisit procedures on schedule to ascertain if they continue to be current.

11. Revise procedures as needed.

What Contributes to Good Procedures

Simply *having* procedures—meeting the letter of the law—is not adequate. Unduly complex or unrealistic procedures are difficult to follow. They may actually misinform or introduce ambiguity. Precise language and concision are vital; provide enough detail so that individuals unfamiliar with your institution (be they new researchers or OHRP) can follow your procedures and understand your process. High-quality written procedures will have several characteristics.

1. They will be appropriate to the audience in terms of content, detail, and tone.

2. They will be concise: Users do not get lost in verbiage or unnecessary detail.

3. They will be clear: "10 days" raises the question of working days or calendar days and 10 days from what event?

4. They will use the active voice: "Mail the approval letter" instead of "The approval letter is mailed." The active voice is more dynamic and readable and reduces ambiguity surrounding who does what.

5. They will be coherent. The organization needs to be obvious, complete, and typically sequential.

6. They will be factual. The procedures reflect what is accurate and actually will be implemented.

7. They will avoid vague, superfluous words such as the superlatives *really*, *actually*, and *very*.

8. They will explain acronyms, slang, special terms and shortcuts to the reader before using them. A glossary and index may be in order.

9. They will avoid repetition unless necessary.

10. They will use a positive rather than a negative tone (e.g., "Use the provided form," instead of "Do not use forms other than the provided one").

11. They will use bullets, numbers, flow charts or special formatting to increase readability. For printed formats, wider margins allow for notes. Online venues can effectively use embedded links to provide additional details, cross-references, and immediate definitions.

12. They will judiciously employ cross-referencing to place the procedures in a broader context and reduce repetition.

Overuse of cross-referencing may make the procedures difficult to follow.

Conclusion

Producing, maintaining, and using written procedures for the IRB, its administrative staff, and researchers are obligatory. Although the task may seem daunting, its alternatives are distinctly unappealing and could culminate in federal sanctions against the institution. A methodologic approach is available that, although time consuming, has a high probability of generating workable procedures. After developed, the procedures must be followed, revisited on a regular basis, and revised as necessary.

References

1. University of Minnesota. University of Minnesota Web-based policy library. Access date March 10, 2005. www.fpd.finop.umn.edu

2. Travis AB. *The Handbook Handbook: The Complete How-To Guide to Publishing Policies and Procedures.* New York: R.R. Bowker Company; 1984.

3. Office for Human Research Protections. Compliance Oversight, 12 December, 2000. Access date 20 March, 2001. http://ohrp.osophs.dhhs.gov/compovr.htm

4. Food and Drug Administration. A Self-Evaluation Checklist for IRBs (1998), 16 April, 2001. www.fda.gov/oc/ohrt/irbs/irbchecklist.html

5. Campbell NJ. *Writing Effective Policies and Procedures: A Step-by-Step Resource for Clear Communication.* New York: Amacom; 1998.

6. Lunine LR. *How to Research, Write, and Package Administrative Manuals.* New York: American Management Association; 1985.

7. Page SB. *Business Policies and Procedures Handbook: How to Create Professional Policy and Procedure Publications.* Englewood Cliffs, NJ: Prentice-Hall; 1984.

Tracking Systems Using Information Technology

Patricia M. Scannell and Denise Niles Canales

INTRODUCTION

A systematic, dependable, and user-friendly tracking system is essential to successful institutional review board (IRB) operations. Thus, IRBs are increasingly turning to technology to assist them in tracking their work. This chapter looks at the trend toward using information technology (IT) to support IRBs, types of technology being used in the field, and how technology affects the IRB's human as well as material resources. In addition, we cover topics relevant to the implementation process itself. This chapter is written based on the experiences of several institutions that have gone through the conversion process from paper-based to web-based systems and is a collaborative effort by representatives of academia and industry.

History

Just a few years ago, most IRBs functioned with paper-based processes. In a relatively short period of time, however, many institutions have begun using partial or fully electronic IT systems to make their IRBs more efficient and to ensure better compliance with federal regulations. Today, many IRBs are turning to technology to address the challenges of tracking: protocols, adverse event, progress reports, ongoing reviews, revisions, and amendments, as well as all correspondence associated with each protocol for which they are responsible.

IT solutions to IRB paperwork have become more affordable, and qualitative evidence from institutions that have gone through a conversion suggests that the use of IT in tracking protocol activity is cost effective. Not all development projects are full range, completely web-based, paperless systems—there are hybrid options for institutions that choose to progress gradually toward an electronic tracking system. While larger institutions continue to seek technical enhancement in record numbers, we are also seeing an increasing number of small- to mid-sized IRBs turning to technology to enhance their research enterprise and the function of their IRBs as well.

Why Have an Electronic IRB?

In the present research environment, competitive demands are forcing organizations to reassess their business strategies to be more efficient. Industry sponsors require rapid turnaround, or they will take their research elsewhere. The International Conference on Harmonization requires reliable data that complies with regulations and adheres to ethical principles to insure valid outcomes to costly research activities. Using technology to help ensure an efficient and effective IRB is one way to do that.

Having an electronic IRB allows institutions to use technology to do the following:

- Establish more efficient business processes
- Maximize the use of available data
- Make consistent decisions that comply with all relevant regulations and institutional policies

All institutions have their own unique history of competence and inefficiencies; thus, specific reasons for seeking technical support vary. The most common reasons that IRBs seek IT support include the following:

- A reduction in human error
- A desire to automate established procedures
- Data safety (data are continually backed up)
- More efficient record keeping
- Automation of key events such as renewal notifications
- Availability of data to ancillary committees, for example, biosafety and scientific review via a single research submission
- Elimination of redundant data entry and thus better use of staff and investigator time
- Elimination of printing and mailing documents resulting in conservation of human and material resources
- Better service for research faculty and staff

Table 2.3.1   Technology and Common IRB Uses

Technology	Common IRB Uses
E-mail	Exchange of documents and correspondence between IRB and investigators
	Ability to keep documents in electronic format or to print only as needed
Instant Messaging	Accelerate communication among IRB members or between various user groups such as ancillary committees and the IRB staff members
	Increase communication within the IRB office providing automated documentation of communications
Websites	Provide standard operating procedures (SOPs), links to federal and state sites, and internal guidance documents and facilitate education and document key participants' educational requirements
	Make current versions of IRB forms easily accessible and make modified forms available to the community instantly
Compact Disc	Distribute standardized forms and guidelines to user groups
	Store records such as closed protocols and meeting minutes
Spreadsheet Software	Track dates and demographic data about IRB protocols and processes
Diagramming Software	Prototype forms and get user group buy-in before making changes effective
	Business process modeling and/or workflow diagramming (which can be an effective training tool because it is easier to *see* the process rather than to *describe* the process of IRB work with text)
Databases	Provide greater capabilities than spreadsheets or word processing programs
Web-Enabled Databases	Full system electronic submission programs have databases that store IRB forms and provide processes that track protocols from their inception (including all required reviews) through study closure
	IRBNet, developed by Dartmouth and Children's Hospital of Philadelphia, is a ***communication and cooperation system between IRBs*** reviewing the same protocol to promote efficiency and effectiveness. The cooperative review facilitated by IRBNet can be initiated by any researcher and/or study site (and the responsible IRB) and thus potentially can be extended to any condition, subject population, or phase of research. IRBNet thus seeks to combine the efficiencies of centralization and electronic communication with the effectiveness afforded by the diverse scientific and ethical expertise of individual IRBs. IRBNet can be accessed at www.irbnet.org.
Hybrid of the Above	Most institutions use a combination of the above technologies effectively

Types of Technology

IRBs have options in how they integrate technology into their business practices. Electronic systems can support a full range of IRB work or a specific aspect, such as adverse event reporting. You can develop your system at one point in time or in stages. Table 2.3.1 lists various technologies that IRBs use in support of their operations and some common ways they are used.

Determining the Level and Type of Technology Needed

In today's paper environment, electronic submission is not difficult to sell. Most users are eager to see the process of IRB submission become more efficient and expeditious. However, many institutions seeking technical enhancement may errantly assume that if they cannot afford a full-range, web-based system they should remain in the paper world. Today, a variety of options are available to clients seeking web-based solutions.

As such, it is beneficial for institutions to evaluate areas critically where their existing process works well and areas in which improvement is required. Stepping into technology in stages rather than at one point in time may provide the middle ground that an IRB director or administrator needs to use some technology, show improved process and functioning in identified areas of weakness, and with that gain administrative support for future development projects.

Whether you choose to step into an automated system in phases or jump into a full system all at once, it is essential to obtain the assistance of an experienced IT consultant or solicit input from a peer who has already been through an IT implementation project. Getting a consult from someone with experience will help you define your immediate needs and plan your long-term transition most efficiently. You can learn from the successes and errors of others.

Your Vendor or In-House IT Team

Because of the vast scope of electronic-submission projects, both human and financial resources must be considered. When determining whether to employ a vendor or develop software in-house, decisions regarding the use of in-house IT personnel or outside consultants should be made. Institutional funding or outside resources (grants), above and beyond routine operating budgets, must be obtained. You must plan to allocate funds for the continued operation of your new IT systems over time.

Most systems will increasingly provide savings and efficiencies in many areas, but they themselves will require upkeep and maintenance. Also, after an institution has an electronic system in a production environment, it is very likely that they will choose to enhance the functionality of the system over time because they will see the power and possibility of the electronic system itself.

It is essential that the initial steps in developing an electronic system include the following:

- An in-depth evaluation of the existing paper process and requirements for the e-submission system

- Development and analysis of a business process model and/or workflow diagram of areas that are to be automated and streamlined

- Prioritization of and identification of what development is essential and what development may need to wait until time or funds are available

Prioritizing is imperative and ensures that the fundamental needs of the IRB will be met by the system. After the top-priority items have been accomplished, the foundation is set, and attention can be focused on lower priority amenities that will make the system even more efficient and exciting for everyone involved in the research arena.

If you are planning to use a vendor, you may choose to hire an outside consultant or use an internal source to analyze the top vendors' capabilities and match them to your needs. Be sure to talk with involved, high-level personnel who have worked with the vendors and assure them that you will keep whatever they share confidential.

Ask important questions such as these:

- Did you have to do a request for proposal or a sole source agreement? (If yes, ask to see a copy of the document. Using a request for proposal as a reference can save you a tremendous amount of time!)

- Why did you choose one vendor over another?

- What is your overall impression of the selected vendor?

- What do they do well? Where are they weak?

- How do they react when there is a difficult situation or problem?

- Do and did they understand your business?

- Are they responsive to your communications, questions, and requests?

- What would you do differently if you could do it over again?

- Was the project what you anticipated? If not, please explain.

- If your system is in production, are they providing support? If yes, do they respond in a timely manner? Are they knowledgeable? Are they friendly?

- Do they provide consulting and training in addition to software/IT work? Have you used them in this capacity? If yes, what is your impression of these other services?

- Are there any other advice, tips, and suggestions that you could offer to an institution considering starting an IRB/IT project?

- Was the project completed in accordance with agreed-on timeline and within the proposed budget?

Throughout the project, the IRB and IT teams must work together—continually reassessing and clarifying expectations. If you choose a vendor, you should be confident that you could establish such an interactive relationship. Whether you choose a vendor or an in-house development team, communication is the key to having your expectations met. As the customer, you have much to say in how your project is planned and how it progresses.

Regardless of your choice, you must design and implement your system such that you ensure flexibility because needs and regulations change over time; your forms will need to be modified—ideally, you need a product and a process that can flex with only minimal effort for selected IRB staff.

Beyond the Technology

Regarding implementation projects, it is the integrated development of teams, technologies, and organizational structures that creates high performance. It is not the technology that will transform your operations—it is the interaction of the software, the people, and the process. A successful implementation project involves more than choosing the right application. It takes the right application, the right team, and the right process.

If the system is successful, it will function as planned, reduce the IRB's challenges, and enhance the IRB's assets. The system must be user friendly, and adequate training must be provided before the system is implemented. It is essential that adequate support and continued training are provided after the system is implemented.

Human Resource Considerations

It is ideal if you are able to work with a technical group that is aware of IRB processes; if this is not possible, a good deal of time will be required to educate the IT team. This team must take on the IRB's vision. It must also have initiative and commitment in order to exceed the existing paper standard.

In addition to enlisting the technically savvy and taking all preparatory steps required to bring your project to fruition, you need to determine who from your IRB staff members are best suited to work with the technical team. This is important because IT experts and people who are knowledgeable about the IRB will work together throughout development and implementation.

Some institutions use IRB and IT staff members who continue to do their routine work and add the IT project to their list of responsibilities. This is a more challenging approach but can be accomplished with the right people. Other institutions are able to move resources such that they have devoted staff members working only on the IT project. This arrangement results in a faster implementation project, but the prior arrangement is "doable" with the right resources.

The following skills are essential to your key project team members:

- Self-motivation
- Ability to produce in high volume and work long hours
- Interested in learning new things
- Comfortable with trial-and-error learning and challenges
- Low frustration threshold
- Excellent written and verbal communications skills
- Comfort with technology and multitasking
- Critical and analytical thinking patterns
- Customer service and detail oriented
- Able to sustain high focus work over long periods of time

Developing electronic submission in the IRB is much like changing the wheels on a moving train; the IRB must involve its best employees, in full or in part, and allow them to focus on the project. These people will remain, in one way or another, responsible for the system and the system's users after the project is complete.

Having a project manager who knows how your IRB functions and selected IRB staff who are subject matter experts will reduce the time and expense of your project and make your experience much less stressful. Basically, you begin the project speaking the same language. The inverse logic also holds true; you need to have IRB staff on your team who understand IT and software development. If you cannot use an institutional IT resource to fulfill this need, you may want to consider hiring a project manager from a consulting firm or negotiating a dedicated project manager from your vendor.

Continually verbalizing your satisfaction or concerns about the project with your development source is essential. There must be open, honest communication between the IT development team and the IRB team. It is the project manager's responsibility to keep such communication flowing. The project manager must also see that timelines are met and that responses to requests for modifications are implemented in a timely manner.

Postimplementation: New Operations and Continued Evolution

Assess your users' (investigators, research staff, IRB staff, and IRB members) state of preparedness for this major change in operation. In addition to requiring computer skills, logistical considerations will impact the success of the system (e.g., access to scanners, sponsors' willingness to provide confidential documents electronically, difficulties in electronic transference of data between MACs, PCs, and the high-speed Internet server). Be aware of these potential difficulties, and take steps to address them early in the development process.

Keep communication open between your users and your e-submission team during all phases of the project. User buy-in is critical to success! Communication during all phases can be achieved by requesting comments from users via e-mail, campus mail, and open-forum sessions and by initiating a user group that meets periodically to discuss system enhancements. Additionally, IRB staff should be receptive to comments offered in individual interactions and should log all comments in a common place for consideration by the e-submission team.

For several months before and 3 to 6 months after the system is activated, the need for user education and support is intense. Most education work consists of teaching users how to conduct business in the new electronic environment. Regardless of your best efforts, there will likely be some staff members who find other positions and members who resign from the IRB because change can be challenging. As time passes and the system evolves, education will focus on teaching new processes and system enhancements. System enhancements are inevitable because they provide continued quality improvement.

Another consideration is that IRB staff members may be concerned that the new technology will put their positions in jeopardy. The reality is that ordinarily electronic submission will simply change their position descriptions to include help-desk responsibilities, providing support, teaching, and the ability to offer greater attention to pre-screening submissions for compliance with regulatory and institutional requirements. In addition, most IRBs are understaffed; thus, technology will usually not result in a reduction of staff. In hiring new employees, the IRB will likely look for a different set of qualifications and skills than in the past. Also, staffs with experience in an electronic system will find that they are even more valuable resources because that experience enriches what they can bring to current and future employers.

The Future

Technology is evolving with incredible speed. One key to being an institution that maximizes technology is to ensure (regardless of the level of automation at which you currently find yourself) that you make good choices in products and services. Standardizing your systems and working with technical groups, either in-house or hired consultants that understand your long-term vision, is critical.

The future of electronic IRBs will be in sharing data and facilitating the research process from protocol creation through clinical implementation. With new technology, users can generate data and reports in wonderfully productive ways; moving toward using a system to connect various points in the full continuum of human subject research is the next step.

Summary

Technology can provide the transfer of data and storage of all protocol-related materials and assist the research investigator and IRB staff in sharing pertinent information. Such greatly increases efficiencies in an institution's research enterprise. IT can provide research staffs with a single data-entry point, thus further saving the IRB staff time and material resources. This is good. This is a tremendous step forward for our field, but no electronic system provides the silver-bullet solution, and that point should not be forgotten, even when in the middle of an exciting and challenging IT project.

Thus, the most important thing to remember regarding electronic systems is ironically that decisions and the thoughtful exceptions to the rules are still necessary. The need for dedicated IRB staff and committee members will continue in order to protect human subjects optimally, which is, after all, the purpose for doing what we do. The technology is but one means to that end.

Support Staff

Helen McGough

INTRODUCTION

There are many pieces to the puzzle of how to staff an institutional review board (IRB) office: the size, nature, and culture of the institution; the numbers and kinds of protocols reviewed; and the budget, space, and other resources available. The shape and configuration of these pieces must be matched with the tasks that an IRB office staff can perform to keep the IRB operating efficiently and effectively. Some IRBs operate with no staff at all, some with part-time staff whose other responsibilities are partially or completely separate from the IRB office, and some with one or more staff members dedicated solely to the IRB.

The purpose of this chapter is to help the reader put the puzzle together and come up with answers on how to staff an IRB office. I identify regulatory requirements for support, what tasks the staff must be prepared to handle, and what kinds of qualifications staff should have to carry out these tasks. Finally, I outline a number of different strategies for staffing the IRB office. An appendix to this chapter includes sample job descriptions for a variety of IRB staff positions.

Why Is Staffing Important?

Proper staffing is crucial to the effective operation of an IRB. In most cases, IRB members and chairs are volunteers from within and from outside the institution hosting the IRB. The time that they have to devote to the everyday functions required of the IRB is quite limited. It is unrealistic to expect that members and chairs will have the time and resources to prepare and distribute IRB protocol materials before the meeting, take and distribute IRB meeting minutes, and provide advice and information daily to researchers, sponsors, and research subjects. To manage these and the many other tasks required to assist the IRB in its mission of the protection of human subjects, an institution hosting an IRB must be prepared to devote sufficient resources to hiring qualified staff.

Federal Regulations

All of the regulatory authorities imply that an IRB is supported by an infrastructure. IRB members must be appointed. Policies and procedures must be developed and disseminated. Members and researchers must receive training and education about the protection of human subjects, and records must be prepared and maintained. Beyond these general rules, there is relatively little direct regulatory guidance on how to staff the IRB office.

In 21 CFR 56, which addresses the Food and Drug Administration (FDA) regulations pertaining to IRBs, there are no specific references to the staffing of the IRB office. One section mandates the records that an IRB or its institution must maintain, the records retention period required, and the requirement to allow an FDA audit of the IRB records.[1(Sec.115)]

In 45 CFR 46, which includes the Department of Health and Human Services' regulations pertaining to IRBs, the regulations state that resources and space must be sufficient to support the IRB but do not specify staffing in particular. In 1993, Dr. Gary B. Ellis, then director of the Office for Protection from Research Risks, stated his opinion that the ratio of support staff to number of protocols reviewed should be 1:300. It is also clear in its investigations that the Office for Protection from Research Risks, now known as the Office for Human Research Protections, regards adequate staffing of the IRB office as a necessary condition.

The International Conference on Harmonization (ICH) has developed a set of guidelines for the conduct of research involving human subjects. This is to be used by those agencies that are not regulated by the FDA but that wish to market their products in the United States and other countries. These guidelines have been accepted by the FDA and also underscore the importance of adequate staffing for the IRB office. ICH guidelines are the subject of Chapter 8-3.

Functions of the IRB Office

The staff of an IRB, as opposed to its chair and members, can perform a variety of functions. The assumption in this section is that staff members will not hold membership on the IRB itself. The tasks that follow, therefore, do not include those for which formal IRB action is required. This section describes each function and illustrates how appropriate staffing can facilitate the work of the IRB. These functions may also be used as job descriptions for the various staff positions an IRB might consider incorporating into its structure.

Screening Protocols Before IRB Review

Most IRBs require that researchers complete application forms or follow fairly specific instructions about what information the IRB will need to complete its review. An important staff function that can improve the efficiency of IRB review is screening the applications or submissions for completeness and accuracy before review. This screening process can be as rudimentary as making sure that the forms have been completed and the appropriate attachments are in place. More sophisticated screening responsibilities can include reviewing the consent forms to make sure that the required elements have been addressed and the language level is appropriate for the intended research population. Experienced staff members can review the actual content of the submissions to make sure they provide enough detail to allow adequate review. For example, most applications ask the researcher to identify the background and purpose of the review. If a researcher answers, "The purpose of this study is to test X drug for safety and efficacy," a competent screener can recognize that this is not an adequate answer and can request a more detailed description from the researcher before the protocol goes to the board for review.

Agenda Preparation

IRB members must be provided sufficient time to review the submissions before the meeting actually takes place. This means that the applications must be made available to them, whether electronically through secure e-mail attachments or a secure website or on paper through the mail system or via messenger. An agenda for the meeting must be prepared and the submissions copied and sent to each member. In some cases, the staff may assign primary and secondary reviewers to each submission. If this is the case, the staff must be familiar enough with the expertise of each member to make appropriate assignments.

Taking Minutes

Minutes in sufficient detail to provide information about the number of members present at the review of each submission, the vote, and a description of any controverted issues are required by the regulations. Usually, this responsibility is assigned to an IRB staff person. The staff member must be sufficiently skilled to take notes that reflect the discussion and disposition of each submission reviewed. An alternative is to make an audio recording of the meeting and have it transcribed afterward. Although this method would appear to require less skill on the part of the staff member, it requires transcription time, a transcriptionist who is at least familiar with the functions of an IRB, and staff and IRB member time to review the transcript for accuracy. The transcript

will usually not include the number of members who voted for and against the submission, the number of abstentions, and who was actually present.

Drafting Correspondence

After the meeting, correspondence must be sent to the researchers to inform them of the IRB's disposition. Ideally, the IRB chair prepares this correspondence. In many cases, however, the chair does not have the time to perform this task, which then falls to a staff person. This responsibility requires that the staff person either attends the IRB meetings or has immediate access to detailed meeting minutes. It also requires that the staff person has sufficient experience with biomedical or behavioral research to draft correspondence that describes the IRB's concerns correctly.

Triage of Amendments and Modifications

Unless the IRB is a fairly small operation, the chair and members will not have time to review requests to amend or modify approved protocols. IRB staff can assist in this process by making determinations about which requests require full IRB review and which can be reviewed using the expedited process.

Mail and Reception

These information-flow management functions may be handled at a simple level (office hours, contact information, and meeting dates) by IRB staff or may involve transmission of more complex advice about submission preparation, status of review, and regulatory information.

Database and Information Management

As with any regulatory and compliance function, much of the success of the operation depends on managing information flow. The IRB office requires a staff person who can establish and maintain a database and staff to make sure that documents coming to and from the IRB can be tracked and located. Even if construction of a database is contracted, a staff member must be able to troubleshoot and correct minor problems.

Triage of Adverse Event and Safety Reports

As with amendments and modifications, the IRB staff can simply transmit the information to the IRB chair and members. In addition, it can be assigned the task of triaging these reports for presentation to the IRB chair or full board. At the very least, the staff can assist the IRB by separating reports into "on site" and "off site." Staff can also pull relevant files, flag consent forms, and generally make the IRB's huge task a little more manageable.

Staff Supervision

In an IRB office with more than one person, one or more of the staff will have to assume supervisory responsibilities over the others. This may include recruitment and hiring of new staff, training, ongoing evaluation, maintaining time records, and other personnel issues. A well-staffed IRB office may require that more than one person assume some or all of these responsibilities.

Responding to Subject Concerns

Most commonly, research subjects are directed during the consent process to contact the IRB office if they have questions about their rights. The IRB office may be assigned the responsibility of answering participants' questions about the research, about whom to call in case of an adverse event, and about who will provide treatment for adverse events. The assumption of one or more of these responsibilities requires IRB staff members who are able to respond quickly and appropriately to these inquiries. Staff may be required to negotiate a research subject's concerns with a billing department, with risk management, with the researcher or the researcher's staff, and with legal counsel.

Triage of Protocol Violations

Reports of protocol violations may come directly to the IRB chair or its members. However, if the IRB staff has high visibility within the institution, these problems may be directed first to the IRB office. Staff members must be able to determine what the violation consists of and how it should be directed for consideration. Reports of noncompliance within the institution may come from research and other staff who feel more at ease making their reports to IRB staff rather than to the IRB chair and members. At a minimum, IRB staff must be trained to handle these reports appropriately.

Office Procedures

Many of the procedures that the Office for Human Research Protections, the FDA, and research sponsors are concerned about are directed at how the IRB accomplishes its work. However, some ancillary procedures are also auditable and are more appropriate to the staff than to the IRB chair and members. These may include establishing procedures for putting an agenda together, entering protocol data into a database, establishing a filing system, a file-purging system, protocols for security, information referral, and all of the other tasks listed in this chapter. IRB staff should be able to develop office procedures and train other staff members in their application.

IRB Policy and Procedures

Every IRB operates according to policy consistent with its regulations and must make its procedures available to researchers. When regulations and policies outside the IRB change, the IRB must be able to respond to those changes promptly and appropriately. An institution may want to consider using its IRB office staff to develop and recommend policy and procedures with regard to IRB operations. Often IRB chairs and members rotate frequently enough that there is relatively little "institutional memory" located in the IRB itself. However, long-term staff may understand both the implications of regulatory changes and the culture of the institution in which the IRB functions and, therefore, be in a good position to recommend policies that satisfy both. For example, when a regulatory agency issues new guidance information, someone knowledgeable about the IRB must be able to analyze the guidance and explain how it differs from current policy and procedures. He or she can recommend changes that must be made to bring the IRB into compliance with the new guidance.

Education and Training

At a minimum, each institution conducting research with humans must also make sure that its IRB members and researchers (from principal investigators to research administrators to research staff) are knowledgeable about the ethics and regulations pertaining to this kind of research. Although a few external sources exist for this kind of education and training, the responsibility for training researchers and their staffs often falls to the IRB members and office staff. If the staff exercises this responsibility, it should have the necessary skills and credibility to do the job well. Even if the staff does not actually deliver education and training, it can be responsible for organizing events and providing the infrastructure for training and education within and outside the institution.

Intrainstitutional Relationships

An IRB cannot operate in isolation. The IRB must coordinate its activities with a variety of other compliance and management groups and individuals within the institution. These include the institutional official, risk managers, researchers, grants and contracts management, and other regulatory committees such as biohazards, radiation safety, and recombinant DNA committees. The IRB office staff can take responsibility for maintaining relationships between the IRB and appropriate persons within the institution. This is to make sure that the IRB is aware of and acts in accordance with the actions and policies of these other groups and to make its own policies and procedures known as appropriate.

External Relationships

IRBs must maintain positive and productive relationships with a variety of agencies and individuals outside of as well as within the institution. These may include regulatory agencies, research sponsors, other IRBs with which it has review relationships, local and state legislators, and community and special-interest advocacy groups. Staff can be assigned tasks such as acting as legislative liaison, drafting assurance documents, negotiating reviews between IRBs, and communicating with nonaffiliated research and advocacy groups.

Meeting Logistics

IRBs have basic needs: a meeting place, transportation and parking, food and beverages, and other support. If the meeting will incorporate members by teleconference or video conference, arrangements for these technologies must be made before each meeting. Nonaffiliated members may require transportation to meetings. IRB staff can be assigned to carry out a wide range of support activities.

Number of Staff Members Needed

There is considerable controversy and a serious lack of reliable information on how many staff members should support an IRB. The following are some options for determining the number of staff members that are necessary to serve the needs of the IRB.

Ratios of Staff to Volume

Although some data show that the ratio of IRB administrators to number of new applications is about 1:300, it is dangerous to leap to the conclusion that this ratio is appropriate for all situations. For example, it might be tempting to assume that an IRB reviewing only 150 protocols per year could manage adequately with only a part-time IRB staff person. However, there appears to be an economy of scale that kicks in only after a certain volume of protocols is reached. As with almost any other activity, one achieves excellence only with practice. It will take a part-time IRB staff member longer to learn the regulations and procedures and longer to achieve an appropriate comfort level with the work. At the other end of the spectrum, certain IRB office activities can be streamlined to some extent through automation, and the ratio of staff to protocols may be higher without ill effect. Even at this end, however, the drafting of correspondence and negotiations with researchers cannot be streamlined.

Number and Type of IRBs

It is recommended that if an institution hosts more than one IRB panel, it should have IRB staff dedicated to each board. This is especially true if the IRBs operate in different spheres within the institution. For example, in a college or university setting, one IRB may be dedicated to the review of biomedical research and one to the review of behavioral research. The skills required to support these two kinds of IRBs may be quite different in terms of the protocols reviewed and the culture of the community of researchers. IRB staff with familiarity with the subject matter and the subject populations may ease the path for the IRB in carrying out its responsibilities.

Time Allocation for Chair and Other IRB Members

IRB chairs and members who are paid for their services will need less support than those who are volunteers. Given the relative costs of staff versus faculty, most institutions will make the choice to hire dedicated staff rather than to pay faculty or researchers for the time that they devote to the IRB. A volunteer chair and members will not have the time to draft IRB correspondence, prepare and distribute agendas, take and prepare minutes, maintain a database, maintain intrainstitutional/interinstitutional relationships, and keep up on regulatory changes. A qualified dedicated staff can perform these functions at less cost to the institution than if faculty were paid to do them.

Expertise of Investigators

If an institution's researchers demonstrate a high level of expertise in the area of research ethics and if an effective training system and a good mentoring program for new members of the institution exist, then the IRB will need fewer staff. In addition, if the institution is young, lacks experience, or has a culture of noncompliance, the IRB will

(at least initially) require more staff support. This will help create a culture in which the ethical conduct of research is valued and the training and advising requirements are more limited.

Resources Available

Although it is clearly not reasonable to deprive research subjects of adequate protections because of lack of resources, it is also clear that some institutions are better endowed than others to be able to absorb the costs of running a protection program. Institutions with lower levels of funding available for the IRB will have to resort to other sources of support for the IRB staff: work-study students, hospital volunteers, retired staff members, and community volunteers, for example.

Turnover

A higher rate of staff turnover places increased demands on existing staff to hire and train replacements. An institution having high turnover will have to consider a higher staffing ratio. An institution in which IRB staff turnover is low will be able to use the experience of its staff more effectively and may be able to employ fewer staff members.

Staff Qualifications

Another controversial area is what characteristics IRB staff should have. Requirements for assessing staff fall into several areas.

Educational Requirements

The qualifications of IRB staff depend largely on the level of responsibility they are expected to assume. It is clear that what is important in good IRB staff are personality characteristics as well as areas of expertise. Candidates for IRB staff positions should demonstrate high levels of skill in the following areas:

1. Oral and written communication
2. Interactions with people from a wide variety of educational, occupational, and ethnic backgrounds
3. Management of high volumes of work with limited turn-around time
4. Ability to learn complex concepts (regulatory, ethical, and scientific)

In an IRB office in which staff is expected to operate at a high level of interaction with researchers and board members, a PhD or MD may be required. However, an individual with a bachelor's degree or even a high school diploma plus years of regulatory and management experience can also function effectively.

Certification

Several certification programs are available for IRB office staff. The institution may want to investigate these programs to evaluate their suitability for a particular IRB's needs. Certification is one way to measure the qualifications of new staff and to provide ongoing assurance that existing staff is knowledgeable about current regulations and IRB office management.

Conflict of Interest

IRB staff should understand the principles of conflict of interest so that they can assist the IRB in determining when such a conflict exists for themselves as well as for the IRB members.

Models for Staffing

A variety of models may be used to staff an IRB office.

Team Model

This staffing model may work very well in an institution in which more than one IRB panel functions. In this case, each IRB panel has its own IRB coordinator and one or more clerical support persons. The advantages of this model are that the IRB staff has a smaller number of protocols to work with and can share the tasks associated with supporting the IRB and facilitating the review of proposals more effectively. Members of one team can substitute for equivalent members of another team in an emergency. The teams could be located in one office or could be located where the IRB is housed. This model can be decentralized in a situation in which, for example, a school of medicine has an IRB that operates independently of the IRB for a school of social work. The disadvantage of the team model is that consistency between IRBs may decrease. It is, therefore, appropriate to include an overall administrator in the team model whose responsibilities include maintaining consistency.

Traditional Model

The more traditional model of staffing an IRB office is stratified and hierarchical. In this model, there is usually an administrator whose responsibilities include managing the IRB office, one or more IRB coordinators (depending on how many IRBs there are), and clerical staff who function to support all of the IRBs within an institution. Some economy of scale is achieved with this kind of staffing model, and it is easier to maintain consistency if there is more than one IRB. The disadvantage of this model is that functions become more discrete and cross-training becomes more time consuming, and it is not as easy to ask one staff member to take over the functions of another in an emergency situation.

Conclusion

An appropriately qualified and trained IRB staff can reduce the burden of review for both researchers and the IRB chair and members. The more responsibility staff members assume, the more responsibility the institution assumes for making sure that they are qualified and able. A high-functioning IRB staff increases the ability of the IRB chair and members to focus their attention on the business of protecting human research subjects.

Reference

1. Code of Federal Regulations. Title 21, Chapter 1—Food and Drug Administration, DHHS; Part 56—Institutional Review Boards. Updated 1 April, 1999. Access date 25 April, 2001. http://www4.law.cornell.edu/cfr/21p56.htm

Appendix:
Sample Job Descriptions

Job Description: IRB Administrative Assistant

This position will share responsibility for the administration of the operation of the IRB program with the director. Primary administrative responsibilities include assisting the director and IRB coordinators with implementation of the program to researchers, external researchers, and sponsors.

Job responsibilities include assisting the director and coordinators with the following:

1. Interview, hire, train, and supervise IRB staff
2. Negotiate administrative modifications to existing IRB applications
3. Perform ethical and technical review of IRB applications meeting criteria for exempt review
4. Provide consultation, assistance, and dissemination of information regarding the review process
5. Provide information on technical and ethical requirements for conducting research involving human subjects
6. Provide assistance to researchers to bring proposals into compliance with minimum review standards (screening)
7. Provide assistance with development of written guidelines to improve communication and understanding of human research requirements
8. Provide assistance with development of written office procedures
9. Prepare certification of compliance with review requirements for funding agencies
10. Assist with review of IRB applications eligible for expedited review
11. Receive adverse effect reports and forward to director and coordinators
12. Receive closeout reports and review for signature by director
13. Other duties as requested

This job requires a person who is able to learn the program function, is skilled in interpersonal relationships, oral and written communication, and is able to deal with seasonal high volume and rigid deadlines. Required computer skills include data entry, word processing, and database management. Attention to detail and research experience are valuable assets.

Job Description: IRB Administrator

This position will manage the privileged and confidential institutional review and approval process of all proposed research activities involving human subjects to protect their safety, rights, and welfare.

Under administrative direction, the IRB administrator will serve as a member, with vote, on the Institutional Review Board; perform highly complex duties to facilitate the review and approval process, such as use of independent judgment in interpreting and applying relevant federal and state laws, regulations, and institutional policies and guidelines; conduct literature reviews and prepare reports on scientific topics and on regulatory precedent and changes; instruct IRB chairs, members, and researchers on the regulations and ethical principles essential to the review process; provide training and advice to faculty, staff, and student researchers on the regulations and on preparation of applications and consent forms; and review and approve administrative and procedural modifications of applications.

Typical work includes the following:

1. Serve as ex-officio member, with vote, on IRB(s)
2. Interpret and apply federal and state laws, regulations, institutional policies, and guidelines to protect human subjects and to ensure institutional compliance
3. Conduct literature reviews and prepare reports for the IRBs on scientific, ethical, and existing and proposed regulatory topics
4. Draft correspondence that conveys IRB deliberations and contingencies for approval of research activities involving human subjects
5. Signatory authority for certifications documenting IRB approval for funding agencies (federal and nonfederal)
6. Independently review correspondence to the IRB, review and approve administrative and procedural modifications, reconcile proposals for funding with approved IRB applications, and facilitate approval for emergency or unique research opportunities
7. Provide regulatory, ethical, and method advice to individual faculty, staff, and students in preparation of applications for research proposals involving human subjects and consent documents

8. Direct the work of others

9. Develop and present materials and training programs for faculty, staff, and students on the ethical conduct of research involving human subjects

10. Provide orientation and training to IRB members

11. Assist in program development, implementation, and evaluation

12. Act in the absence of the director

13. Perform related duties as required

This job requires a person who can learn the program function, who is skilled in interpersonal relationships and in oral and written communication, and who is able to deal with high volumes and rigid deadlines. Familiarity with research ethics and methods and the ability to conduct independent literature research (including Internet-based research) are required. Computer literacy is a necessary skill. A master's degree and 2 years of applicable work experience or a bachelor's degree and equivalent education/experience are required. Previous research experience is desirable.

Job Description: IRB Program Coordinator

This position will share responsibility for the coordination of the operation of the IRB program. Primary coordination responsibilities include representation and assistance with implementation of the program to researchers and external researchers and sponsors. Based on experience and knowledge of the program, the incumbent will disseminate information about and assist investigators in the preparation of IRB applications. The incumbent will coordinate the preparation of applications for presentation to the IRBs and will independently determine adequacy of the application and level of review required.

This job requires a flexible person who has experience in IRB review, who is skilled in interpersonal relationships, and who is able to deal with seasonal high volume and rigid deadlines. Computer literacy, word processing, and computer entry skills are required. Attention to detail is a valuable asset. Specific job tasks include the following:

1. Log in and complete new and renewal applications: computer entry and hard-copy entry

2. Screen new and renewal applications: contact and advise investigators in preparation and completion of application process

3. Prepare meeting agendas: assign applications to committees, prepare agenda, and prepare member packets

4. Maintain renewal system: prepare tickler report and prepare and mail reminders and forms

5. Close out applications: prepare final reports for closure

6. Withdraw applications: prepare applications at several stages of withdrawal

7. Prepare finalized applications for filing: prepare applications and certifications

8. Enter information into the computer for modified applications and adverse effect reports

9. Prepare subcommittee (biomedical and behavioral) agendas

10. Prepare final meeting reports for biomedical and behavioral IRBs and subcommittees

11. Maintain record and filing system: paper and computer-based files

12. Assist internal and external sponsors to assure human subjects compliance

13. Provide lead for office assistant, hourly; assign work when necessary

14. Assist other program coordinators when necessary

15. Assist IRB coordinators with modifications when requested

16. Open, date stamp, and sort mail

17. Answer and refer telephone calls

18. Filing and copying as requested

19. Proof and edit IRB correspondence as requested

20. Coordinate supply orders, physical plant, and other on-campus coordination

21. Other duties as requested

Job Description: IRB Director

The director has responsibility for implementing university policy and procedures, federal and state statutes, and regulations on the protection of human subjects for the university and several of its affiliates. In this capacity, the following duties are performed:

1. Functions as chief administrative and programmatic support for the IRB

   - Administers policy on the protection of human subjects

   - Recruits and interviews prospective IRB chairs and members; makes recommendations to the appropriate department chair for appointments; supervises training and orientation of new members to the technical and ethical literature, appropriate policy, statutes and regulations, and duties as IRB members

   - Provides technical consultation to IRBs concerning review of ethically and scientifically complex research involving vulnerable client and patient populations and sensitive research

   - Advises IRB members of review requirements based on policy, regulation, statute, and legal precedent; monitors changes and recommends appropriate revisions in policy and procedures

   - Represents the university in audits and deliberations with federal, state, and local agencies and organizations

   - Advises on handling of subpoenas for the release of study data filed against researchers.

   - Supervises ethical and technical review of proposals meeting criteria for exempt and expedited review

   - Coordinates with grant and contract services regarding compliance on new, continuing, and competing proposals with human subjects' regulations and policies

   - Provides advice on regulatory compliance to deans, directors, chairs, and the office of the president within the university and federal regulatory agencies as requested

   - Maintains liaison with federal regulators

- Serves on university-level committees and task forces as required

2. Provides consultation, assistance, and dissemination of information regarding the review process:

   - Provides information on technical and ethical requirements for conducting research involving human subjects to faculty, staff, and students at all three campuses and affiliate institutions
   - Provides advice and assistance to researchers to bring proposals into compliance with minimum review standards
   - Develops written guidelines to improve communication and understanding of human research requirements
   - Develops and presents formal and informal workshops upon request on the review process in general and on topics of particular interest to university and nonuniversity audiences
   - Provides liaison with the state legislature and other community agencies on human subjects' issues such as privacy and genetic research
   - Participates in professional conferences and training opportunities to improve knowledge of technical and ethical aspects of research with human subjects

3. Directs, coordinates, and supervises the administrative and clerical functions of IRB office

- Supervises maintenance and updating of database
- Prepares annual reports on IRB office activities
- Prepares budget recommendations for IRB office; approves expenditures, requisitions, and vouchers
- Prepares certification of compliance with review requirements for funding agencies
- Responsible for hiring, training, evaluating, disciplining support staff; establishes work priorities and deadlines
- Provides technical and ethical information to staff members responsible for screening and reviewing applications
- Receives and triages adverse effect reports and complaints from subjects and researchers
- Attends IRB meetings as necessary

Minimum requirements are as follows: bachelor's degree in relevant field, but master's degree preferred. At least 2 years of experience are required in program administration and personnel management. Computer literacy and word processing skills are required. Experience in the conduct of basic or applied health, social, or behavioral research is preferred. Demonstrated ability in effective oral and written communication is necessary.

Audit Systems

Ernest D. Prentice, Ada Sue Selwitz, Gwenn S. F. Oki, and Judi Kuhl

INTRODUCTION

One strategy for improving the quality of a human subjects protection program is to implement an internal audit process. An audit process can heighten investigator and institutional review board (IRB) awareness of regulatory requirements and improve the ethical conduct of research. Traditionally, IRBs have not had a structured research audit program in place, largely because IRBs were and still are underresourced and overloaded with work. There is now, however, an enhanced Office for Human Research Protections (OHRP) and Food and Drug Administration (FDA) emphasis on monitoring research processes and maintaining compliance, which has pressured more IRBs to engage in auditing functions. Auditing of research can be a key component of an institution's program for the protection of human subjects.

The purpose of this chapter is to discuss quality improvement in human subject protection through auditing of research and to describe the basic components of a successful audit program. The focus is on the audit of investigator research records and the corresponding IRB files. This chapter does not describe the procedures for assessing an institution's total human subjects protection program, which would include an evaluation of the organization and its reporting structure, the infrastructure, written policies, procedures, training, databases, file records, and overall efficiency. All IRBs, however, can benefit from routine general audits that can be performed using the 1998 FDA Information Sheets as a guide,[1] or the OHRP's "Quality Assurance Self-Assessment Tool,"[2] which is accessible via their website. In addition, IRBs may wish to consult the OHRP[3] and FDA[4] websites to review citation letters, which can be very instructive.

Regulatory-Based Authority for the Research Audit Program

In 1991, 17 federal agencies and departments adopted the Federal Policy for the Protection of Human Subjects (Federal Policy, also known as the Common Rule). The FDA adopted a modified version of the Common Rule, codified at 21 CFR 50 and 56. For the purpose of avoiding multiple but equivalent regulatory citations, only Department of Health and Human Services (DHHS) and FDA regulations for the protection of human subjects will be referred to in this chapter.

DHHS regulations at 45 CFR 46[5[Sec.109(e)]] and FDA regulations at 21 CFR 56[6[Sec.109(f)]] state, "An IRB shall conduct continuing review of research covered by this policy [regulation] at intervals appropriate to the degree of risk, but not less than once per year, and shall have authority to observe or have a third party observe the consent process and the research." The IRB is also required by 45 CFR 46[5[Sec.111(a)(6)]] and 21 CFR 56[6[Sec.111(a)(6)]] to ensure that "when appropriate, the research plan makes adequate provision for monitoring the data collected to ensure the safety of subjects." These provisions are currently interpreted as granting the institution, the IRB, and/or its representative(s) the authority and responsibility to audit research.

Institutions that hold an OHRP Federal Wide assurance are required to have procedures that "include formal mechanisms for monitoring compliance with human subject protection requirements." Research audit programs provide one mechanism for ensuring compliance with this requirement.

Characteristics of a Sound Research Audit Program

A research audit program might include any or all of the following: review of investigator records, monitoring of ongoing research on site, observation of the consent process from initiation to documentation of the subject's consent, and interview of investigators, staff, or subjects.

A research audit program should be proactive, nonpunitive, and focused on educating investigators about their ethical and regulatory responsibilities in the conduct of research. Ideally, the audit program should be accepted, if not embraced, by investigators and their research staff. The program should also be as comprehensive as possible, given any limitations imposed by the available personnel and resources that can be devoted to audit functions.

Research audit responsibilities may be delegated to the IRB staff and/or IRB members, or a separate but linked office can be established solely for assessment of the institution's human subjects protection program, including the audit of research. The decision about the appropriate assignment of the audit function depends on a number of variables such as the size and nature of the research program, organizational structure of the institution, resources available, and the goals/objectives of the audit program. Consideration should be given to assigning the audit function to an independent position that is administratively separate but, nevertheless, linked to the IRB, because the auditing program should include an assessment of IRB records.

The Administrative Structure

The administrative structure of a research audit program is obviously dependent on the needs and the nature of the institution itself. Nevertheless, aside from the administrative entity that is assigned audit responsibilities, there are certain characteristics that successful research audit programs display. Based on the experience of institutions or IRBs that have initiated research audit mechanisms, the following six principles have proved to be critical to the success of the programs:

1. Develop an organized audit research plan based on immediate objectives and long-term goals that fit the institution and its needs. A copy of the University of Kentucky (UK) Quality Improvement Program and other UK Audit Forms can be found at http://www.research.uky.edu/ori/QIP/QIP%20Main.htm.

2. Obtain administrative endorsement and support of the research audit program by senior institutional officials. This should include allocation of adequate resources.

3. Ensure that the program is adequately staffed and that personnel involved in the research audit have the requisite scientific and regulatory experience as well as the necessary interpersonal skills.

4. Ensure that the research audit program is proactive and educational in nature. To facilitate this, the audit program should use a positive title, such as "Quality Improvement Program for Human Subjects Research."

5. Ensure that all investigators and their staff are educated about the goals of the research audit program and that they do not feel disenfranchised or disengaged from the audit process. Input from key investigators should be obtained during the development of the audit program.

6. Perform an ongoing quality control assessment of the research audit program and make changes as necessary.

The Research Audit Program

In developing a research audit program, institutions together with their IRBs should consider the following procedures that can be adapted or modified to suit the specific needs of the institution and their research portfolio.

1. The program should establish the criteria for selecting the studies to be audited. The selection criteria will be impacted by resources available to conduct audits and the nature of the research conducted at the institution or reviewed by the IRB. For example, audit personnel could randomly select categories of research from which a specified number of studies would be audited. Depending on the institution's research activities, categories of studies that should be considered for auditing include investigational new drug studies; investigational device exemption studies; research involving children, decisionally impaired subjects, or prisoners; research conducted under an emergency waiver of informed consent; research approved by expedited review; and exempt research. Examples of study-specific criteria that could be used in selecting studies for audit include the following: the number of subjects enrolled (e.g., select only studies that have enrolled four or more subjects), IRB approval status (e.g., select only studies that are currently active and received approval during the past 3 years), and the funding status (e.g., select federally funded studies and drug company-sponsored studies).

2. The audit personnel should carefully review, in advance, the entire IRB file for each protocol selected for audit.

3. The audit should be scheduled at a time that is convenient for the investigator and his or her research staff. Unannounced audits are generally counterproductive.

4. Investigators should be informed in writing about the research audit, including the date, time, place, and protocol(s) selected for audit. They also should be given a description of the audit process and criteria. A comprehensive research audit would normally include a review of the investigator's study records, observation of the consent process, and interviews with both the investigator and his or her research coordinators. Although less typical, some programs even include an interview or survey of research subjects to determine whether they understood that they were actually participating in research. If the audit program includes either observation of the consent process or an interview with the subject, procedures should be developed to address protection of privacy and confidentiality. In this case, the consent form should disclose the possibility of a requested interview as well as IRB and auditor access to the subject's research record and/or medical record.

5. A reasonable time frame should be established for completing the audit and producing the audit report.

6. The role of the institution and/or the IRB in reviewing, approving, or taking further action on the final audit report should be delineated and included in the IRB written procedures.

Mechanics of the Research Audit

The mechanics of a research audit are critical to a successful quality improvement program. The following questions address the criteria that should be used in evaluating compliance. The criteria are based on the FDA and DHHS regulations that focus the audit on goals of increasing investigator and IRB awareness of regulatory requirements.

Audit of IRB Records

1. Does the IRB protocol file contain all of the records required by 45 CFR 46[5(Sec.115)] and 21 CFR 56[6(Sec.115)] in sufficient detail to demonstrate compliance and performance of a substantive review(s)? These records include the following: IRB application, detailed protocol, investigator's brochure if applicable, DHHS grant application if applicable, informed consent/assent forms, consent addenda (e.g., significant new findings), amendments, reports of adverse events or unanticipated problem(s), reports of protocol deviations, continuing review reports, and all correspondence between the IRB and the investigator.

2. Are the IRB minutes pertaining to the protocol(s) in question sufficiently detailed per 45 CFR 46[5[Sec.115(a)(2)]] and 21 CFR 56?[6[Sec.115(a)(2)]] For example, the IRB meeting attendance is recorded; the vote on the protocol is recorded (number for, against, and abstaining), and recusal of IRB members with a conflict of interest is documented. Where appropriate, additional protections for vulnerable subjects are documented in accordance with 45 CFR 46.[5(Subparts B,C,D)] In addition, there should be documentation of appropriate protections for other vulnerable subjects not specifically covered by the previously mentioned subparts. For example, subjects who are homeless, economically disadvantaged, or from a foreign culture may be vulnerable. The minutes should also include a reasonably detailed summary of the IRB's discussion of any controverted issues and their resolution.

3. Is the consent form approved by the IRB in compliance with 45 CFR 46[5[Sec.116(a),(b)]] and 21 CFR 50[7[Sec.25(a),(b)]]

4. Were the IRB's initial review and subsequent reviews (e.g., amendments and adverse events) and the IRB office's handling of the review timely and efficient?

5. Was continuing review substantive per the requirements of OHRP July 2002 Guidance[8] and the 1998 FDA Information Sheets?[1] Was the continuing review conducted within the annual time limit or earlier, as required by the IRB?

6. Were adverse events or other unanticipated problems involving risk to the subject or others promptly reported to OHRP and/or the FDA per the requirements of 45 CFR 46[5[Sec.103(b)(5)]] and 21 CFR 56?[6[Sec.108(b)(1)]]

7. Was serious or continuing noncompliance promptly reported to OHRP and/or FDA per the requirements of 45 CFR 46[5[Sec.103(b)(5)]] and 21 CFR 56?[6[Sec.108(b)(2)]]

8. Were IRB review activities conducted under expedited review processes permissible under 45 CFR 46?[5(Sec.110)] Is the expedited review category documented?

9. Was research that was exempted permissible under 45 CFR 46?[5[Sec.101(b)]] Is the applicable exempt category documented?

Audit of Study Records

Does the investigator have a comprehensive and secured file containing the following records?

1. The IRB-approved application and detailed protocol

2. The investigator's brochure, if applicable, and the IRB-approved amendments

3. A current IRB-approved stamped copy of the consent form and copies of all investigational new drug safety reports, adverse event reports, and other relevant safety information.

4. Records of continuing reviews and copies of all correspondence between the investigator and the IRB (e.g., IRB review and approval letters)

All of these records should also be present in the IRB protocol file.

Did the investigator implement the protocol as approved by the IRB according to the following criteria?

1. The current IRB-approved version of the consent form was used.

2. The consent form(s) were signed and dated by the subject and by a person authorized to obtain consent.

3. IRB-approved inclusion and exclusion criteria for subject accrual were met.

4. The date of the first intervention(s) is consistent with the date that the consent form was signed.

5. All research-related procedures performed were described in the IRB-approved protocol.

6. Subjects received only the approved dose range(s) of the study drug(s), and all adverse events or unanticipated problems were promptly reported to the IRB.

7. All protocol modifications or deviations/exceptions were implemented only after IRB approval, except when in the immediate medical interest of the subject.

8. The number of valuable subjects accrued was within the IRB approved limit.

9. The procedures for ensuring privacy and monitoring the confidentiality of data were implemented as approved by the IRB.

The number of individual subject records to be audited can vary. If four to six subject records are audited and no major problems are identified, this would normally be sufficient. However, if problems are identified, it would be prudent for the auditors to review additional and perhaps even all of the study records. Review of records may include case report forms used in FDA-regulated research, original data, and/or pertinent portions of the medical records.

Observation of the Consent Process

1. Was the environment in which the consent process took place conducive to rational and thoughtful decision making on the part of the subject?

2. Was the length of time devoted to the consent process sufficient?

3. Was the subject given adequate opportunity to ask questions?

4. Was the subject given an adequate explanation of the research using appropriate simplified language?

5. Did the subject demonstrate an acceptable understanding of the research before signing the consent form?

Interviews with the Investigator and Research Personnel

1. Did the investigator encounter any problems in recruitment, subject retention, or other areas? If so, what was the nature of the problem, and how was it addressed?

2. Did any subject suffer a serious, unanticipated adverse event? If so, what was the nature of the event, and how was the subject treated?

3. Do the investigator and/or research staff have any problems with the IRB, IRB staff, or IRB reviews? If so, what are the problems and proposed solutions?

The interview is a time when problems identified during the records review can be discussed and any necessary clarifications obtained. It is also an ideal time to educate the investigator and his or her staff.

Preparation of the Audit Report and Follow-up

The audit personnel should use standardized specific forms to record audit findings. After the audit is complete and all findings are analyzed and determined to be valid, a written report should be developed. It should be structured to be proactive and educational in nature by providing comments concerning strengths and recommendations on how deficiencies can best be corrected, with appropriate citations of the federal regulations and institutional policies. The report should be completed in a timely manner, and a copy of the report should be provided to the IRB and/or the institution for review, approval, or initiation of additional action. If evidence of serious or continuing noncompliance is found, this must be promptly reported to the appropriate institutional official and the OHRP per the requirements of 45 CFR 46.[5][Sec.103(b)(5)] Noncompliance must also be reported to the FDA when the study involves use of an FDA-regulated product per the requirements of 21 CFR 56.[6][Sec.108(b)(2)] Obviously, such a report may be viewed by the investigator with a certain degree of concern and alarm that may interfere with the intended collegiality of the audit. Nevertheless, if such deficiencies are identified, they must be corrected immediately and reported to the appropriate federal agency as specified by the regulations.

The audit program should include appropriate follow-up to ensure that deficiencies are corrected in a timely manner. This follow-up may include only a written report of corrective action(s) implemented by the investigator, or it may require additional auditing or monitoring by the IRB. In some cases, it may be appropriate to require the investigator to undergo specific training in order to help him or her achieve the desired level of compliance.

Conclusion

Quality improvement in an institution's program for the protection of human subjects can be achieved through a variety of mechanisms, including audit of research. A research audit program can be an integral component of an institution's efforts to enhance the ethical quality of its research. It can also ensure that compliance with applicable federal and state regulations is maintained. Considering the evolving nature of the ethics and regulation of research, however, the audit program must be progressive, up-to-date, and educational in nature. Indeed, education of the investigator and the IRB that results in the enhancement of the quality of human subjects protection is the most important product of a research audit program.

Acknowledgment
The authors thank Steven Hansen, PhD, for his help in editing this chapter.

References

1. Food and Drug Administration. Information Sheets: Guidance for Institutional Review Boards and Clinical Investigators, September 1998. Access date 9 April, 2001. http://www.fda.gov/oc/oha/IRB/toc.html

2. Office for Human Research Protections. *Quality Assurance Self-Assessment Tool.* http://www.hhs.gov/ohrp/human subjects/qip/qifedreg.pdf Federal Register: 8 May, 2002 (Volume 67, Number 89).

3. Office for Human Research Protections. Dear Colleague Letters, 20 March, 2001. Access date 12 January, 2005. http://www.hhs.gov/ohrp/dearcoll.htm

4. Food and Drug Administration. *A Self-Evaluation Checklist for IRBs,* 16 April, 2001. Access date 2 August, 2001. http://www.fda.gov/oc/ohrt/irbs/irbchecklist.html

5. Code of Federal Regulations. Title 45A—Department of Health and Human Services; Part 46—Protection of Human Subjects. Updated 1 October, 1997. Access date 18 April, 2001. http://www4.law.cornell.edu/cfr/45p46.htm

6. Code of Federal Regulations. Title 21, Chapter 1—Food and Drug Administration, DHHS; Part 56—Institutional Review Boards. Updated 1 April, 1999. Access date 27 March, 2001. http://www4.law.cornell.edu/cfr/21p56.htm

7. Code of Federal Regulations. Title 21, Chapter 1—Food and Drug Administration, DHHS; Part 50—Protection of Human Subjects. Updated 1 April, 1999. Access date 18 April, 2001. http://www4.law.cornell.edu/cfr/21p50.htm

8. Office for Human Research Protections. Guidance on Continuing Review. Updated 11 July, 2002. Access date 10 January, 2005. http://www.hhs.gov/ohrp/humansubjects/guidance/

Charging for Institutional Review Board Review

Ernest D. Prentice, Sally L. Mann, and Bruce G. Gordon

INTRODUCTION

This chapter explores the issue of charging a fee for local institutional review board (IRB) review. Concern has often been expressed that if IRBs are not adequately funded, these institution-based oversight boards will be unable to carry out successfully their federally mandated responsibility to protect the rights and welfare of research participants. In 1978, the National Commission for the Protection of Human Subjects of Biomedical and Behavioral Research recommended that IRBs receive direct funding as opposed to relying on support from indirect cost mechanisms.[1] Unfortunately, the commission's recommendation was not implemented.

In the 1980s, many academic medical center (AMC) IRBs began to experience problems related to inadequate staffing and operational budgets. Institutions, however, were generally not very sympathetic to the needs of the IRB, which largely remained unmet. Consequently, the possibility of charging an IRB review fee for commercially sponsored research was explored by an increasing number of IRBs. After consideration of a review fee for commercially sponsored research as a form of supplemental funding for their IRBs, some AMCs then decided to implement such a fee. The common prevailing concern at the time, however, was one of fear that institutions that charged for IRB review would be less competitive for award of commercial contracts than those that did not charge. In addition, some IRB members expressed concern that charging an IRB review fee would create a conflict of interest that, in turn, could bias IRB reviews at worst and raise questions about the board's objectivity and independence at best. Thus, during the decade of the 1980s, there was little movement in the direction of charging for IRB review.

As the clinical research enterprise moved into the 1990s, most AMCs experienced a significant increase in their research volume. This, in turn, exerted even more pressure on IRBs, which found themselves without the necessary staffing and resources to handle the workload effectively. IRB review turnaround times were often inordinately slow, and protocol reviews were all too often characterized as overly cumbersome. It was, therefore, not surprising when commercial sponsors began relying, more than ever before, on physicians in the private sector to conduct many of their clinical trials. This, in turn, created an increased demand for the services of independent IRBs, which operated in an efficient business mode and, obviously, charged for their reviews. Questions about conflict of interest were invariably raised, but no data were ever presented to substantiate such concerns.

By the mid-1990s, many AMCs were suffering from the budgetary throes of managed care. The Balanced Budget Act of 1997 generally resulted in reductions in net clinical income.[2] AMCs struggled to remain fiscally sound, and downsizing or mergers were common. At the same time, the workload of their IRBs grew because of increased research and escalating compliance requirements from the Office for Protection from Research Risks (now the Office for Human Research Protections) and the Food and Drug Administration. In the face of restricted budgets and inadequate resources, AMC IRBs across the country began to examine or re-examine the issue of charging for IRB review. Support for initiating such a fee was indirectly provided by the Office of the Inspector General, which called attention to the critical shortage of IRB resources.[3] Although the same concerns expressed previously about charging for IRB review were still present, opposition was clearly not as strong. Many IRB members, research administrators, and investigators began to realize that when an IRB charges a review fee, the quality and integrity of its review are not compromised; commercial sponsors do not object to paying a reasonable review fee, and institutions that charge for review are no less competitive. Indeed, charging commercial sponsors for IRB review has become the norm and is no longer the exception. Although there are no data to indicate the percentage of IRBs that charge a review fee, it is reasonable to suggest that most AMC IRBs either currently charge a review fee or will do so in the near future.

The IRB Review Fee

A number of limited and unpublished surveys of IRB review fees have been conducted. Data obtained in a 2000 survey indicate that AMC IRBs typically charge between $500 and $2,000 for initial review, with an average fee of $1,130.[4] The University of Nebraska Medical Center (UNMC) IRB administrative office indicated that fees ranged between $700 and $2,000 for initial review in 2000. Some IRBs charge for only initial review, although others also charge a fee for continuing review and amendments. A few institutions also charge for review of studies qualifying for exempt and expedited review. The data also indicate that IRB review fees are routinely increased over time. For example, the UNMC IRB began charging a review fee of $650 in 1995, which was increased to $700 in 1998 and to $1,250 in 2001. It should be mentioned that some institutions have discussed extending the fees to federally sponsored projects. Importantly, however, in 2003, the National Institutes of Health issued NOT-OD-03-042 that reminded institutions "that no costs associated with the review of human research protocols by an Institutional Review Board (IRB) may be charged as direct costs for NIH-funded research involving human participants, unless such costs are not included in the institution's facilities and administrative rate (F&A)."[5]

Finally, it is not uncommon for institutions with a clinical trials office (CTO) to charge a fee to offset the costs of reviewing and processing the contract. An unpublished survey of 32 institutions conducted by the UNMC CTO in 2000 indicated that 50% of institutions surveyed have a CTO fee, and the average fee is $1,500.

Collection of Fees

It is not surprising that institutions employ various methods of collecting IRB review fees. For example, some institutions collect fees from investigators up front, before IRB review, whereas other institutions bill the investigator on completion of the initial review but before final approval is granted. In the latter case, final approval may be contingent on actual receipt of the fee or receipt of a promissory note from the investigator payable on establishment of the research account. Some institutions, however, bypass the investigator and directly bill the commercial sponsor, either up front or on completion of the IRB review. Other institutions rely on the investigator to bill the sponsor directly. Regardless of which collection method an institution chooses to use, it is imperative that if a review fee is assessed, it should be collected routinely, even when an IRB chooses to disapprove a protocol. It is obviously inappropriate to collect a fee only if the protocol is ultimately approved. However, it is also desirable for institutions to allow a waiver of the IRB review fee for studies funded by small contracts or when there are extenuating circumstances. The point is that the IRB fee should never be an obstacle to the conduct of important research. IRB policy regarding the IRB review fee should clearly provide for waiving of the fee when it would create a meaningful obstacle to research conduct.

Preservation of the IRB Budget

Budget cutting is a way of life at many institutions. The IRBs that generate revenue by charging for reviews should be wary of the possibility that the administration of the institution may find it easier to cut its support of the IRB during financially hard times. This, in turn, may ultimately force an IRB to rely too much on the money generated from review fees to carry out little more than the basics of its daily operation. Therefore, it is extremely important for the IRB to have an adequate and ongoing budgetary commitment from the institution without excessive reliance on review fees. In this age of enhanced emphasis on maintaining compliance, no institution can afford to underfund its IRB.

Conclusion

Charging an IRB review fee for commercially sponsored research is a common way for an IRB to supplement the operating budget provided by the institution. Sponsors do not object to paying reasonable IRB review fees, and the additional revenue can be used by the IRB to improve the quality and efficiency of its service. Clearly, an adequately resourced IRB is a benefit to the sponsor as well as to the institution, its investigators, and, most importantly, the subjects who participate in research.

References

1. National Commission for the Protection of Human Subjects of Biomedical and Behavioral Research. Report and Recommendations: Institutional Review Boards, (OS)78-0008. Washington, DC: Department of Health, Education, and Welfare; 1978.

2. 105th Congress. Balanced Budget Act of 1997. Public Law 105-33. 5 Aug, 1997. Access date 2 August, 2001. http://www.access.gpo.gov/nara/publaw/105publ.html

3. Office of Inspector General. Institutional Review Boards: A Time for Reform (OEI-01-97-00193), June 1998. Access date 27 March, 2001. http://www.dhhs.gov/progorg/oei/reportindex.html

4. Office of Research. Fees for IRB Review—Baylor College of Medicine. Access date 2 August, 2001. http://research.bcm.tmc.edu/Whats_New/whats_new.html

5. NIH Grants and Contracts. NIH Policy on Director Cost Charges for IRB Review. Access date 5 January, 2005. http://grants2.nih.gov/grants/guide/notice-files/NOT-OD-03-042.html

PART 3

Organizing the Institutional Review Board Committee

Reflections on Chairing an Institutional Review Board

Robert J. Levine

INTRODUCTION

In 1961, I accepted the invitation of Dr. Paul Beeson, Chair of the Department of Medicine at Yale University School of Medicine, to leave the National Institutes of Health to be chief resident at the Yale-affiliated Veterans Administration Hospital in West Haven, CT. About 8 months later, when I was preparing to move to West Haven, I was stricken with anxiety. I did not have the slightest idea of how to be a good chief resident. My principal role model was Dr. Buris Boshell, who had been chief resident in medicine at the Peter Bent Brigham Hospital when I served on that service as an intern. (Actually, in those days, we were called "house officers.") He gave me much good advice. I will now adapt the advice he gave me on being a good chief resident to make it fit the job of institutional review board chair. In principle, it is almost the same. Most importantly, he said that I should always strive to "make molehills out of mountains."

Solve Problems When They Are Small

Always be alert to detect problems when they are so small that almost nobody else has noticed them. Small problems that are not satisfactorily dealt with have a tendency to become larger problems. When they get large enough that many others can recognize them, the range of options available to the chair for their resolution is often diminished.

Handle each problem at the lowest permissible level in the administration of your institution. The regulations require that you report serious or continuing noncompliance by investigators to appropriate institutional officials and to the federal government. After you have detected a problem early—one hopes before it becomes serious—you should try to resolve it before it becomes necessary to report it. If it is necessary to report it, you should send a letter to the deviant investigator with a copy to his or her immediate supervisor. With physician–investigators, this usually means the section or division chief. Your letter should state why the copy is being sent to the section chief and that, if it is necessary to send another to the same investigator, a copy of that one will go to the next level, usually the department chair. Now you have two individuals working with you to prevent future noncompliance. Also, by limiting the scope of the embarrassing exposure, you preserve the possibility that these two people—the investigator and the section chief—will be motivated in the future to work with you as colleagues.

Assemble the Right Team

Surround yourself with people who are highly intelligent and devoted to doing the work of the institutional review board (IRB). This, of course, includes a high-quality staff and IRB members. It also should include many other members of the institution's faculty, staff, and students. When an IRB has a high degree of credibility within its community, one sees the development of rather extensive *informal monitoring systems* in the form of unsolicited reports by students, physicians, nurses, and others. An IRB without credibility is not likely to have this large network of volunteers assisting it. Payment of equally efficient and effective replacements, if such could be found, would be very expensive.

The IRB chair should see to it that the IRB staff and its members have an adequate degree of familiarity with the applicable federal, state, and local laws and regulations. Although they should be conversant with the major themes in the regulations, they should be allowed to rely on one or two of their fellow members to provide the detailed knowledge needed to resolve some difficult issues. There is no need to make the cardiologist–member an expert on the law. By the same token, the lawyer does not need to have an intimate knowledge of cardiac electrophysiology. The layperson–members should be assured that each and every IRB member is a part of the laity with regard to the specialties of some or all others. They should work together in a climate of trust that each will contribute according to his or her abilities to the overall function of the IRB.

The IRB Is an Agent of Its Own Institution

Even though it is necessary to be sufficiently familiar with relevant law to avoid inadvertent violations, an effort should be made to promote within the institution the attitude that the IRB is an agent of its own institution; its purpose is to uphold the value system of the institution. Respect for persons, beneficence, and justice are (or should be) principles that your institution values greatly and not just because they were once published in *The Federal Register*. IRBs began to function in most institutions before *The Belmont Report* was published in 1978 by the National Commission for the Protection of Human Subjects of Biomedical and Behavioral Research.[1] Historical evidence suggests that in the 1960s (even earlier in many institutions), the forerunners of IRBs were conducting their business as if they were being responsive to basic ethical principles. In passing, it is worth recalling that Congress instructed the National Commission to identify the ethical principles that should underlie the conduct of research involving human subjects—identify, not invent.

Do Not Blame the Feds for IRB Policy and Practices

IRB personnel should scrupulously avoid saying, in effect, "Don't blame us for enforcing these rules; it's all the feds' fault." Such statements diminish the credibility of the entire system. The IRB that relies on this "justification" for its decisions loses its ability to make decisions that are not explicitly required by federal regulations. IRBs have the authority and responsibility to be able to exercise judgment in making their decisions; they should exercise this authority wisely and be willing to be held accountable for their decisions.

Treat Researchers as Trusted Colleagues

The authority of the IRB to monitor the activities of investigators should be exercised with great caution. There is generally not much of a problem with conducting "for-cause" audits. An effort should be made to bring "whistle-blowers" into the process of investigating the complaint; in this way, they can be satisfied that you are taking their complaints seriously. For-cause audits should begin with an assumption that there is a misunderstanding, perhaps a miscommunication, and not that someone has violated institutional policy. Every aspect of the IRB's interaction with its community should be grounded in the belief that all participants in the research process can be trusted—at least until the accuracy of any contrary evidence is confirmed.

Routine audits are more problematic. It is very difficult to avoid projecting an attitude of distrust in the investigator. To the extent that such audits are perceived in the community as similar to the audits of the Internal Revenue Service, there is an increasing probability that the IRB will be treated like the IRS in its dealings with the investigators. This would essentially close down the informal monitoring system.

Continuing Education

IRB chairs and members should be conversant with the major themes in the current commentary on research ethics, particularly those that have a bearing on the interpretation and revision of the policies and practices of IRBs. There are some concepts in the field that do not have precise definitions. For example, what is a "minor increase over minimal risk?" Even though no clear definition of this standard exists, we can learn by reading reports of actual decisions reached by IRBs in their consideration of actual cases. By reading such cases, we learn that IRBs consider as a minor increase the risk attached to such procedures as lumbar punctures and bone marrow biopsies; it is less than the risk presented by liver biopsies.

I suppose you are thinking, "How can I possibly keep up with the current deluge of information?" You cannot. It is necessary to be selective. The most reliable sources of information on the policies and practices of IRBs and the underlying rationale for them are peer-reviewed periodicals. Authoritative sources of current policies and practices of federal regulators are the information sheets and other documents prepared by the federal regulators for the guidance of IRB members. Some books are very helpful and some are not. Those that are well documented by references to peer-reviewed literature tend to be more reliable than the others.

The spontaneous contributions of individuals in such places as Internet chat groups tend, in general, to be less reliable. Although some good information is made available in such forums, many Internet offerings are incorrect facts or idiosyncratic opinions. One needs a high level of expertise to distinguish the wheat from the chaff.

What about going to conferences designed for the continuing education of IRB members? Again, there are good ones and bad ones. I think those presented by Public Responsibility in Medicine and Research (PRIM&R) are clearly the best. However, as I am a member of its board of directors, what else would you expect me to say?

Conclusion

Chairing an IRB is a demanding job. To function optimally, an IRB chair should focus on achieving seven fundamental goals:

1. Solve problems promptly before they become so large and visible that they attract widespread attention.

2. Try to resolve problems at the lowest level permissible within the academic and administrative hierarchy.

3. Assemble the right team; this includes IRB members and staff.

4. Support the concept that the IRB is an agent of its own institution.

5. Take responsibility for the IRB's decisions; do not blame them on the federal government.

6. Treat researchers as trusted colleagues unless and until there is reliable evidence to the contrary.

7. Make continuing education a priority.

Reference

1. National Commission for the Protection of Human Subjects of Biomedical and Behavioral Research. *The Belmont Report: Ethical Principles and Guidelines for the Protection of Human Subjects of Research* (DHEW [OS] 78-0012). Washington, DC: U.S. Government Printing Office; 1978. Access date 22 March, 2001. http://ohsr.od.nih.gov/mpa/belmont.php3

The Institutional Review Board Chair

Robert J. Amdur and Robert M. Nelson

INTRODUCTION

The person who directs the proceedings of an organized meeting is referred to as the chair, chairman, or chairperson. The word chair may be used as a noun or a verb. When used as a noun, the words chair, chairman, and chairperson are synonyms. Therefore, it is correct to say either, "The chair called the meeting to order," or "The chairperson called the meeting to order." Chair may also be used as a verb to describe the act of directing the meeting process: "Dr. Jones chaired the institutional review board (IRB) meeting." The purpose of this chapter is to discuss the role and responsibilities of the IRB chair in the overall IRB organization.

Different Models for the IRB Chair

The roles and responsibilities of the IRB chair vary widely across the IRB community. Some IRB chairs direct every important aspect of the IRB process; many share the decision-making responsibility with other members of the leadership team, and some view their job to be limited to directing the full IRB committee meeting. Recognizing that many different options are possible, it is conceptually useful to discuss the role of the IRB chair in terms of two basic models.

Director of the Full-Committee Meeting

An important responsibility of an IRB chair is to direct the full-committee meeting. Specific tasks are discussed later here. The job of directing meeting discussions, keeping the membership focused on the established agenda, and reminding IRB members of the basic guidelines for the IRB meeting procedure is critical to the process of full-committee protocol review. Although all IRB chairs take primary responsibility for directing discussion at the full-committee meeting, some view this as the only absolute requirement of the chair position. In our view, it will be difficult for an IRB to function optimally without additional leadership from its chair.

An IRB may function well with a chair whose role is limited to that of a meeting director if other members of the organization provide expertise in, and take responsibility for, the other activities that are required for the IRB to function properly. IRB members may understand the ethical issues associated with the studies they review well enough to make excellent decisions without insight from the IRB chair. In some organizations, the IRB administrative director is the best person to direct the overall IRB process,

establish IRB policy, evaluate compliance with federal research regulations, and interact with other segments of the research and administrative community. Some organizations employ an attorney (separate from the IRB administrative director) specifically to instruct the IRB about federal research regulations and to represent the IRB in policy decisions that involve other segments of the organization. In addition, an individual with expertise in research ethics may serve as a full-committee member or IRB consultant, either on a voluntary or compensated basis. At some institutions, administrators—such as the director of sponsored research, vice-president for research administration, or dean of research—make decisions about the process of research regulation with or without input from the IRB and IRB chair. Within this model, an IRB chair does little more than direct the full-committee meeting.

Comprehensive IRB Professional

All IRB chairs are expected to direct the full-committee IRB meeting. In many organizations, the IRB chair also is expected to play a major role in other areas of the IRB system. For the sake of this discussion, the term comprehensive IRB professional is used to describe the model in which the IRB chair is expected to provide expertise and leadership in a wide range of areas related to IRB function. Discussion with IRB chairs and administrative directors at several busy research organizations suggests a similar group of expectations for the IRB chair.

Responsibilities of the IRB Chair

1. The chair should play a leadership role in establishing and implementing IRB policy. As a primary representative of IRB decisions, the IRB chair should have shared authority

over all IRB policy and procedures in collaboration with the institutional official and/or IRB administrative director.

2. The chair should represent the IRB in discussions with other segments of the organization.

3. The chair should represent the organization in discussions with federal authorities.

4. The chair should review all protocols presented to the full committee. The IRB chair is expected to have read each full-committee protocol and to communicate with other reviewers so that important IRB issues are identified or resolved before the full-committee meeting. For example, at the University of Washington, the IRB chair is formally listed as the primary or secondary reviewer for all full-committee protocols.

5. The chair should direct the proceedings and discussion of the full-committee meeting. This includes keeping the discussion focused on important IRB issues and seeing that the full-committee meeting process is both efficient and effective.

6. The chair should vote at the full-committee meeting. Most IRB chairs routinely vote on protocols at the full-committee meeting. However, there are experienced IRBs that use a process in which the IRB chair serves as a full-committee IRB member but does not vote at the full-committee meeting (personal communication with Ernest Prentice, University of Nebraska, November 2000). This is discussed in more detail in Chapter 5-14.

7. The chair should have an in-depth understanding of the ethical issues, state law, institutional policy, and federal research regulations that are applicable to studies that are reviewed by the IRB. The IRB chair is not expected to be the only, or ultimate, authority on compliance issues. The IRB administrative director or other members of the IRB organization also take responsibility for compliance verification, but the IRB chair is expected to be an active and knowledgeable partner in this aspect of the IRB system.

8. The chair should assist IRB administration in the drafting of letters from the IRB to researchers regarding IRB decisions.

9. The chair should review and sign IRB response letters in a timely fashion.

10. The chair should review and make decisions about responses to conditions for IRB approval of research in a timely fashion. In some situations, this task is shared with the IRB administrative director.

11. The chair should serve as the reviewer for research that is reviewed by an expedited process. This task is often shared with other members of the IRB, depending on expertise.

12. The chair should represent the IRB in defending or discussing IRB decisions with researchers.

Skills, Qualifications, and Time Commitment

Meeting Skills

At a minimum, the IRB chair should have the leadership and management skills to direct discussion at the full-committee meeting. Ideally, the IRB chair would have experience chairing similar kinds of meetings, but this should not be an absolute requirement. The ability to foster open and collaborative discussion among IRB members while maintaining a directed focus on the issues at hand is an important skill for the IRB chair.

Interpersonal Skills

To be effective, an IRB chair should be able to interact under difficult circumstances with people from many different backgrounds and levels of experience. In most settings, the IRB functions with the culture of a volunteer committee such that it will not be productive for the IRB chair to force the membership into functioning a certain way. Making good IRB decisions in an efficient time frame requires that IRB members discuss issues in an atmosphere that encourages new insights and trust. It is not easy to maintain an atmosphere that promotes consensus on the issues that are critical for the IRB to evaluate. An IRB chair whose interpersonal style leads to tension or disorganization will inhibit the IRB review process.

An IRB chair must work closely with the IRB administrative director and other administrative staff under conditions that involve time pressure and other stressful influences. Each group will have its own dynamics, but optimal IRB function requires that all members of the IRB leadership work as a team to improve the protection of human research subjects and operate the IRB in compliance with all applicable laws and regulations. It will be difficult for the IRB to function well if the IRB chair and administrative director do not work well together.

Another challenge to the IRB chair's interpersonal skills lies in his or her interactions with researchers. In many organizations, the IRB chair is expected to discuss IRB concerns with investigators and/or protocol directors in moderately contentious situations that may develop between the IRB and the research community. This is often a difficult job under the best of circumstances, and an IRB chair with the wrong background or weak interpersonal skills will not be able to manage things in a way that leads to an environment that promotes the conduct of ethical research.

Leadership and Respect

It is important for the IRB chair to have a background and reputation that encourage respect from both the IRB membership, the administration, and local researchers. The respect of the IRB membership is a precondition of the role of the IRB chair in directing the full-committee meeting, but the respect of administration and researchers is also extremely important. To have a meaningful impact on the protection of human subjects, the IRB must promote a culture of respect for the IRB process and for issues related to research ethics. It is difficult to do this if researchers do not respect the IRB leadership, especially the IRB chair. For this reason, it is important for the IRB chair to be a person who is able to command the respect of most of the research community. The IRB chair should be recognized as an authority on the protection of human research subjects. To this end, it is highly desirable for the IRB chair to have a strong background, knowledge, and expertise in research involving human subjects.

An IRB chair who is familiar with the practical aspects of the type of research that the IRB will be reviewing will be able to focus the IRB on the important ethical issues and support the view of the IRB as a respected member of the peer-review process. Although there are other attributes that engender respect, it may be helpful if the IRB chair is or has been actively involved in clinical research in the community where the IRB reviews research. Although this is not the case with many respected IRBs, it is a factor that will tend to improve the effectiveness of an IRB. Although having a researcher in a leadership position on the IRB may appear to create a conflict of interest, the rote application of this line of thinking fails to appreciate the importance of an IRB chair's reputation to the effectiveness of an IRB. An IRB chair who is a respected colleague of local researchers is likely to facilitate the ability of the IRB to make difficult decisions and will enhance respect for the IRB within the research community.

Profession

For the IRB chair to possess the requisite knowledge and expertise, it may be desirable to have the IRB chair be from the same profession as the majority of researchers who will interact with the IRB. If the IRB reviews only social science research, the IRB chair should be an accomplished social scientist. Similarly, if the great majority of full-committee reviews involve psychology research, then it will be useful for the IRB chair to be a psychologist. If the IRB mainly reviews nursing research, then it would be ideal to recruit an accomplished nurse–researcher to be the IRB chair. For IRBs that review a large volume of biomedical research conducted by physicians, it is important to appoint a physician as the IRB chair. As discussed in other chapters, the situation in which a single IRB reviews both social and biomedical research may present some challenges related to respect for the IRB process. In this situation, it may be desirable to have an individual IRB member, or subcommittee of IRB members, from the appropriate field of expertise as the primary reviewers for research protocols that are directed by investigators who are from a field of research that is different from that of the IRB chair. Whether the focus is the IRB chair or the overall IRB committee, everyone must possess sufficient knowledge and expertise either individually or as a group to be able to conduct an effective protocol review and to communicate that review to researchers in a manner that engenders respect for the IRB process and decisions.

Time Commitment

The time commitment required to serve as an IRB chair will depend on the volume of IRB activity that the chair is responsible for and the model of responsibility of the chair position. Reliable data on IRB staff-volume relationships are not available for the IRB chair (or support staff). Based on the experience of the authors and conversations with chairs and administrators of IRBs that operate in a variety of research environments, it is possible to make some general statements about the time commitment that is required for an IRB chair to function as a comprehensive IRB professional.

A minimum of 5 hours per week is required for an IRB chair to direct an IRB that conducts a full-committee review of approximately 200 new protocols per year. This volume of full-committee reviews usually means that there are approximately 25 full-committee meetings per year and approximately 1,000 active full-committee protocols in the IRB office at any time. Depending on the process for expedited reviews and IRB correspondence, an IRB chair of such a committee would likely spend 1 full day per week on IRB business. The administrative burden and resulting time commitment of the IRB chair may be reduced by adopting a staff-driven model for the IRB system. For example, depending on their level of training and expertise, the IRB staff may be able to work with investigators and other research personnel to address deficiencies before the protocol is reviewed by the IRB chair and/or full committee. In addition, the IRB chair may serve on other committees in the organization that serve to coordinate the various activities that fall under the more general human subjects protection program, such as clinical trials support, compliance oversight, and other research administration.

It is common for university faculty to discuss professional commitments in terms of a unit called an FTE, which stands for "full-time equivalent." IRB chairs in charge of IRBs that review approximately 200 new protocols per year likely spend 0.15 to 0.25 FTE on work directly related to their role as IRB chair. At institutions where the IRB chair receives salary support for IRB service, salary support at the 0.15 to 0.3 FTE level is not unusual. However, the level of salary support should be appropriate for the required effort.

Continuing Education

For IRB chairs who are expected to function as comprehensive IRB professionals, continuing education will be a requirement of the job. Federal research regulations are constantly being revised, and the interpretation of existing regulations is an evolving process. Most IRBs review research that presents a wide range of complex ethical issues. IRBs are under increasing demand to function more efficiently in an environment of limited resources. All of these factors require that the chair of the IRB attends to the disciplines of research ethics and research regulation as to his or her other fields of work. To stay informed, most IRB chairs need to read journals and reference books that specifically deal with IRB issues. Another important source of information is discussion with other members of the IRB community, especially other IRB chairs. IRB chairs should plan to attend a national IRB-related meeting at least once every 2 years. The IRB forum (http://www.irbforum.org) is useful for exchanging ideas and understanding norms of IRB practice.

Academic Rank

An institution must assure that the IRB is able to function in an independent and credible manner. As such, at some academic institutions, professorial rank may be an important factor to consider when choosing or accepting the position of an IRB chair. (The standard categories in ascending order of accomplishment are assistant professor, associate professor, and professor.) Another factor to consider is whether a faculty member's appointment is tenured. In the standard academic model, tenure is given with the appointment to associate professor.

Academic rank may be important for the IRB chair for two reasons. First is the issue of respect, as previously discussed. Academic rank usually parallels seniority and academic accomplishment. In general, therefore, a full professor will have an easier time than an assistant professor in gaining the respect of local researchers and IRB colleagues.

A related, but different, issue is job security. When an IRB is functioning properly, it is not unusual for the IRB to make decisions that are unpopular with powerful researchers or upper-level administrators. An IRB chair with a junior or intermediate academic rank may be concerned that unpopular IRB decisions will compromise chances for promotion in the future. If this is an important factor, an institution should consider whether high academic rank—preferably full professorship with tenure—should be a requirement for the IRB chair.

There are no data on the influence of academic rank on the behavior of IRB chairs. In the authors' experience, most junior IRB chairs are not concerned that unpopular IRB decisions will negatively impact the chance that they will be promoted in the future. IRB chairs from every academic rank explain that the most important factor is to have support for the IRB process from upper-level administrators and a culture of respect for the IRB process. There are IRB chairs at the assistant or associate professor level who routinely support unpopular IRB decisions and policy that may improve the protection of human research subjects.

Another aspect of the academic rank is the negative effect that serving as IRB chair may have on academic productivity. As discussed previously here, serving as an IRB chair is likely to require a major time commitment, on the order of 0.2 to 0.3 FTE. For many faculty members, a commitment of this magnitude will come at the expense of teaching, research, or other activities that have traditionally been required for academic promotion. In our opinion, performing well as the IRB chair should be viewed as an important academic accomplishment on par with getting a major research grant, publishing important papers, or directing an innovative education program. However, it is important to recognize that many promotion committees currently do not give much weight to committee service, including chairing the IRB. Therefore, when a junior or mid-level faculty member is a candidate for chair of the IRB, it is important to consider the effect that the time commitment associated with this service will have on the chance of academic promotion in the future.

Conclusion

The IRB chair is responsible for ensuring protection of human research subjects through the appropriate development and implementation of IRB policy and procedure. In addition, the IRB chair must engender respect for the IRB process by possessing the necessary knowledge and expertise about research practices, ethics, and regulations. The leadership role of the IRB chair within an institution thus requires that the IRB chair has at least shared authority over IRB policy and procedure in collaboration with other institutional officials. Some institutions limit the IRB chair to the role of directing the full IRB committee meeting, with other functions divided among different administrative positions. Although such a system can function effectively in protecting human research subjects, the lack of a strong institutional leadership role for the IRB chair is likely to reduce the overall effectiveness of the IRB in promoting a culture of respect for and compliance with human subject protections. The IRB chair, like the position of the IRB administrative director, should be considered a professional position that requires a comprehensive set of knowledge, skills, and expertise as outlined in this chapter.

The Institutional Review Board Administrative Director

Elizabeth A. Bankert and Robert J. Amdur

INTRODUCTION

From discussions at national institutional review board (IRB) meetings and Internet forums, it is clear that the responsibilities of the IRB administrative director are currently not uniform throughout the country. At one end of the spectrum, the IRB administrative director is expected to function as a comprehensive IRB professional with an in-depth understanding of federal research regulations and the ability to direct or manage all aspects of the IRB process. At the other end of the spectrum, the IRB administrator acts more as an executive secretary with a limited scope of responsibilities that focus on procedural aspects of IRB work. Specific recommendations are made throughout this chapter. The role of the IRB administrator should be that of a knowledgeable and respected partner in the leadership of an organization's overall system for regulating research. In the past few years, the Applied Research Ethics National Association (ARENA) has established a national certification program for IRB administrators. This certification effort requires that an IRB professional master a core knowledge base that includes a detailed understanding of federal research regulations and accepted ethical standards (see Chapter 8-13). In this chapter, we discuss specific responsibilities that IRB administrators have in organizations in which the IRB administrator is expected to function as a comprehensive IRB professional.

Partnership with the IRB Chair

The role of the IRB chair was discussed in Chapter 3-2. In most organizations, the responsibilities of the IRB chair and administrator will overlap in important areas. For an IRB to function optimally, the IRB chair and administrative director(s) must be able to work well together on issues ranging from policy creation to the management of routine committee functions. Open communication between the chair and administrator must exist in an atmosphere of mutual respect and support that facilitates productive leadership. In some situations, the IRB administrative director will have a better understanding of the issue, whereas in others, the IRB chair will be more experienced. The ability of IRB leadership to work together as an administrative team will determine the efficiency and effectiveness of the IRB process. Each relationship will have its own chemistry. The important thing is that both IRB administrators and the IRB chair understand the importance of a partnership in advancing the mission of the IRB.

Establish Compliance with Federal Research Regulations

In organizations that are committed to operating in compliance with federal regulations, the IRB administrative director should be an expert in all regulations that apply to the IRB review of research conducted by the organizations with which the IRB works. Federal regulations that apply to most of the settings in which IRBs function are promulgated by the Department of Health and Human Services (DHHS) and the Food and Drug Administration. Other agency regulations also apply in some instances. DHHS regulations related to the IRB are described in 45 CFR 46[1] and a National Institutes of Health guidance document.[2] FDA regulations related to the IRB are found in four areas: 21 CFR 50,[3] 56,[4] 312,[5] and 812.[6] These regulations are discussed in more detail throughout this book.

Understanding, interpreting, and documenting compliance with research regulations are extremely complex and important responsibilities of the IRB leadership. Many

IRB administrative directors are expected to be the organization's main authority on the regulations pertinent to the IRB and to be sure that the IRB is operating in full compliance with them. This is certainly the case at most of the institutions that direct IRB educational programs and play a leadership role in establishing IRB policy at the national level.

Regulatory Issues

At the other end of the spectrum is the situation in which regulatory issues are primarily the responsibility of someone other than the IRB administrative director. Organizations that do not expect the IRB administrative director to be an authority on the regulations may turn to the IRB chair for this function. However, they more commonly hire an attorney with specialized expertise in this area (see Chapter 3-4). In some organizations, an attorney who is not a member of the IRB committee or administrative office directs IRB policy, procedure, and important aspects of the full-committee meeting. There are organizations that require a consultant attorney to attend each IRB meeting to help the chair identify important ethical issues for discussion. In addition, the attorney instructs the IRB on the criteria for approving research in specific situations and directs the administrative staff (including the IRB administrative director) on how to document things appropriately. With this kind of authority structure, the role of the IRB administrative director is similar to that of an executive secretary. It is certainly possible for multiple people connected with the IRB to understand pertinent research regulations. However, we do not know of IRB administrators with an in-depth understanding of research standards who operate in an organization where they are not responsible for regulatory issues every day.

We strongly endorse an organization in which the IRB administrative director is an expert on policy and regulations that relate to the details of IRB function. In our experience, it often is not possible to apply research standards correctly without an in-depth understanding of the practical aspects of the process of research review for a specific IRB. The IRB administrative director is likely to understand the operational issues the IRB faces better than someone who is peripherally associated with the IRB. In addition, it is the IRB administrator who must manage operational issues every day. An organization in which the IRB administrative director is not an expert in the federal regulations that direct the IRB process is likely to be without the kind of leadership that all IRBs need to function optimally. Educational resources for IRB administrative directors are discussed later in this chapter.

Promote the Image of the IRB as a Partner in the Research Process

As discussed in Part 1 of this book, the best systems for protecting the rights and welfare of research subjects include a culture of respect for the IRB process. Our current IRB system is a direct extension of the review committees that were organized throughout the country by local investigators in an effort to evaluate ethical aspects of their research. The relationship between the IRB and local researchers was never meant to be adversarial, and it is important to recognize that the ability of the IRB to influence the conduct of research will be limited if this is the case.

It is desirable to have members of the local research community on the IRB so that the IRB understands local research standards and has the necessary expertise to evaluate research in specific areas. For a regulatory system to be productive, the IRB must understand the practical aspects of research conduct, and local researchers must understand the operational process of the IRB. Having local researchers on the IRB facilitates this kind of information transfer and helps to solidify the connection between the IRB and the research community. An organization in which the IRB is viewed as a bureaucratic obstacle to the advancement of science has a problem with its system for protecting research subjects. Both researchers and the IRB must approach their work from the point of view that the role of the IRB is to facilitate the conduct of important research according to the highest of ethical standards.

The Importance of Functioning as a Partner

An IRB that understands the importance of functioning as a partner in the research process will interact very differently with researchers, unlike the IRB that views itself as an obstacle that researchers should overcome if they want to conduct research. An IRB that is trying to facilitate research will be as "user friendly" as possible from the administrative standpoint. To emphasize the attitude that should drive the way the IRB interacts with researchers, prominent IRB administrators have urged the IRB office to view itself as a "research service center," which actively assists the researcher in going through the IRB review process. Some IRB offices routinely help the research team write the consent document and prepare the IRB application package. Some IRB administrators spend an enormous amount of time and energy in the days before each full-committee meeting, relaying concerns of IRB members to researchers in an effort to resolve issues that could lead to a delay in protocol approval. Recommendations along these lines were published in the spring 2000 issue of the ARENA newsletter. The section is titled *Twelve Practical Hints for IRB Administrators*.[7] Nine of these points address the way the IRB administrative office should interface with the research community.

1. It should promote an environment that fosters honest feedback from investigators and research staff about the IRB at the institution. Can the office provide better service in accordance with federal regulations?

2. It should ask the investigators to consider the IRB as a collaborator in the research.

3. It should remain flexible. Each protocol may be slightly different. Policies and procedures need to be adaptable.

4. It should let investigators know when an IRB policy changes. It should not wait until it reviews a specific protocol

to advise the investigator that a policy has changed or been implemented.

5. It should consider involving investigators in discussions about establishing new policies and procedures.

6. It should be available and encourage an open-door policy. It should work with investigators, not against them.

7. It should offer to attend departmental meetings for question-and-answer sessions.

8. It should discuss IRB issues with other areas of the institution (like pathology or medical records) in a joint effort.

9. When referencing a policy or practice to investigators, it should help them understand the rationale behind the policy. This helps eliminate the stereotype of a "bureaucratic, paper-pushing office."

Later in this chapter, we discuss the factors to consider when deciding whether the IRB administrative director, or other members of the IRB administrative staff, should serve as a voting member of the IRB. The reason to mention this issue here is that a main argument against an IRB administrator's serving on the IRB is that it may compromise his or her ability to assist researchers in preparing IRB applications.

Develop and Implement IRB Policy

The IRB administrative director should play a major role in establishing or modifying IRB policies and procedures. In most situations, the IRB administrator will work with the IRB chair and/or other members of the organization on policy issues. A good IRB administrator will constantly be looking for ways to improve IRB function and therefore will frequently be the one to suggest policy changes. Examples of situations in which the IRB administrative director should play an important role in establishing policy include staffing requirements of the IRB office, criteria for classifying a project as research, the format of the IRB minutes, the forms required for documentation of IRB activities, management of adverse event reports, and standard wording in the consent document.

Provide Expertise to Other Segments of the Organization

The IRB is not the only segment of an organization that affects research conduct. In most situations, it will be desirable to have close communication between the IRB leadership and other segments of the organization that make policy that may influence research conduct or regulation. In many situations, it will be important for the IRB administrative director to be part of interdepartmental policy discussions. In some cases, the IRB administrative director should provide expertise in the capacity of a consultant, whereas in others, it will be appropriate for the IRB administrator to serve on committees that evaluate issues that may affect the IRB. Interdepartmental responsibilities that IRB administrators have at many university-based organizations include the following:

1. Advise the medical director's office regarding policy related to professional credentials and research activity

2. Advise risk-management and compliance officials regarding institutional policies related to research

3. Advise the medical records department or information services on issues related to privacy and confidentiality of health information

4. Serve as a member of the privacy committee

5. Serve as a member of the hospital or university ethics committee

6. Advise the clinical trials office on a wide range of policy issues

7. Advise undergraduate and graduate course directors on standards for research conducted by students

8. Advise the hospital tumor registry on issues related to access to information for research

9. Advise the cancer center data monitoring committee on the IRB requirements for approval of research

10. Advise the grants and contracts office regarding issues related to payment for research services and conflicts of interest

11. Advise the department of pathology on standards and procedures for access to tissue specimens for research

Represent the Organization in Discussions with Federal Authorities

Federal authorities may evaluate an organization's research program in response to concern about a specific issue or as part of a routine compliance audit. When a federal regulatory agency has questions about research, it is common for the IRB to be a focus of the discussion. In responding to questions related to the IRB, the IRB administrative director commonly plays a major role in drafting the response and assists another member of the organization (the IRB chair, an institutional official, etc.) with this process. In some interactions, the IRB administrative director will be required to speak to federal officials to explain aspects of the IRB system. For all of these reasons, it is important for the IRB administrative director to understand how to document compliance with the regulations related to the IRB. In addition, documentation must be to a degree that allows the organization to demonstrate a high level of competence in interactions with federal authorities.

Administration of the IRB Office and IRB Meetings

The IRB administrative director is the primary person responsible for managing the IRB office and many of the administrative aspects of IRB meetings. These responsibilities are discussed in detail in separate chapters.

Triaging Research Between IRB Review Categories

In many organizations, the IRB administrative director and the IRB chair share the responsibility for determining when a project should be classified as research, when new research projects should be considered exempt from further IRB review, or when research may be reviewed by the expedited versus full-committee process. Similarly, the IRB administrative director frequently shares the responsibility for determining when it is appropriate to use an expedited procedure to review a revision to an approved protocol. When triaging projects, the IRB administrator should always act within the limits of his or her expertise. In view of the complexity of many medical and social science protocols, it will frequently be necessary for the IRB administrator to refer triage decisions to the chair or other designated IRB member.

Approving Research with Expedited Review

In addition to the responsibility for determining the appropriate mechanism for IRB review of research, IRB administrators may have the authority to approve certain kinds of revisions. These are for approved protocols that meet the regulatory criteria for expedited review.[2] To approve research by the expedited procedure, the IRB administrator must be designated to function in this capacity by the IRB chair. In addition, the administrator must be an experienced IRB reviewer and a current member of the IRB committee.[1][Sec.110(b)(2)] For IRBs that use a subcommittee for the expedited review procedure, it is not usual for the IRB administrator to be a member of this group.

Serving as a Voting Member of the Full Committee

Experienced IRB administrators disagree on whether the IRB administrators should serve as voting members of the full committee. When experienced IRB administrators, including several who have directed IRBs at multiple different institutions, were asked for their recommendation on this subject, half of the administrators believed strongly that IRB administrators should serve as voting members for two main reasons. First, an IRB administrator is extremely knowledgeable about research regulation. This expertise is of value to the IRB in making decisions about specific research projects. Second, not serving on the IRB decreases the respect that IRB members have for the IRB staff, especially when it comes to suggesting ways to improve IRB function: "If you don't play the game, you can't make the rules."

Other experienced administrators strongly believed that IRB administrators should not serve on the full committee, also for two main reasons. First, a major role of the IRB administrative staff should be to help the research team prepare its application for IRB review. The IRB administrator should be viewed as an important member of the research team and to some degree must be an advocate for its proposal. By clearly separating the role of the IRB office from the role of the IRB committee, the IRB can be user friendly from the administrative standpoint without compromising the ethical standards for approving research conduct. Second, administering the IRB and working with researchers are full-time jobs. Serving on the IRB demands a considerable amount of time and energy. The mission of the IRB is compromised by anything that distracts IRB administrators from their core responsibilities.

Oversee IRB and Researcher Education Programs

Federal regulations require a structured educational program for IRB members regarding ethical standards and fundamental guidelines for IRB approval of research. In many settings, federal regulations and/or local policy require similar instruction for researchers and upper-level administrators who are responsible for research conduct.

In many organizations, the IRB administrative director is responsible for organizing educational programs related to research regulation. In some cases, IRB administrators teach the sessions, whereas in others, the administrator arranges for someone else (the IRB chair, an outside consultant, etc.) to lead the program. In most organizations, the IRB office is responsible for documenting compliance with educational requirements for IRB members. To accomplish this task, it is important that the IRB administrative director understands the expectations of the federal agencies—mainly the DHHS Office for Human Research Protections—that establish the standards for IRB compliance in this setting.

Continuing Education for the Administrative Director

The scope and complexity of the job of an IRB administrative director require that the person in this position devote a considerable amount of time to continuing education. The standards for efficient and effective IRB function are rapidly evolving. New regulations are being promulgated, and existing regulations are constantly being interpreted in new ways by oversight agencies. A comprehensive list of reference material and contact information related to IRB issues is provided in the appendices to this book. The form and frequency of education should vary with the individual IRB administrator and the research environment in which the administrator works. Many accomplished IRB administrators consider the following four measures foundational to their continuing education program:

1. Membership in an organization specifically geared to the operational aspects of the IRB process. We recommend the organization called ARENA. The ARENA newsletter is particularly useful for learning about practical aspects of IRB administration.[8]

2. A subscription to the journal *IRB: A Review of Human Subjects Research.*[9]

3. Attendance, at least once every 2 years, at the annual meeting organized by the organizations Public Responsibility in Medicine and Research and ARENA. This joint meeting is specifically geared to IRB administrative directors and IRB chairs.[10]

4. Some administrators find that the Internet service IRBFORUM is a useful way to discuss ideas with experienced colleagues.[11] Users of the IRBFORUM should understand that there is no organized quality control regarding the accuracy of the advice given in this setting. IRB administrators should discuss their situation with experienced IRB authorities before making important changes in their work habits based on IRBFORUM advice.

Conclusion

The responsibilities of the IRB administrative director are currently not uniform throughout the country. At one end of the spectrum, the IRB administrative director is expected to function as a comprehensive IRB professional with an in-depth understanding of the federal research regulations and the ability to direct or manage all aspects of the IRB process. At the other end of the spectrum, the IRB administrator acts more as an executive secretary with a limited scope of responsibilities that focus on procedural aspects of IRB work. This chapter has explained the responsibilities that are appropriate for the IRB administrative director to assume. In the authors' opinion, the role of the IRB administrator should be that of a knowledgeable and respected partner in the leadership of an organization's overall system for regulating research.

References

1. Code of Federal Regulations. Title 45A—Department of Health and Human Services; Part 46—Protection of Human Subjects. Updated 1 October, 1997. Access date 18 April, 2001. http://www4.law.cornell.edu/cfr/45p46.htm

2. Office for Protection from Research Risks, NIH, DHHS. Protection of human subjects: Categories of research that may be reviewed by the Institutional Review Board (IRB) through an expedited review procedure. Federal Register 63(216):60353, 9 November, 1998. Access date 3 August, 2001. http://frwebgate.access.gpo.gov/cgi-bin/getdoc.cgi?dbname51998-register5&docid5 fr09no98-109

3. Code of Federal Regulations. Title 21, Chapter 1—Food and Drug Administration, DHHS; Part 50—Protection of Human Subjects. Updated 1 April, 1999. Access date 18 April, 2001. http://www4.law.cornell.edu/cfr/21p50.htm

4. Code of Federal Regulations. Title 21, Chapter 1—Food and Drug Administration, DHHS; Part 56—Institutional Review Boards. Updated 1 April, 1999. Access date 27 March, 2001. http://www4.law.cornell.edu/cfr/21p56.htm

5. Code of Federal Regulations. Title 21, Chapter 1—Food and Drug Administration, DHHS; Part 312—Investigational New Drug Application. Updated 1 April, 1999. Access date 18 April, 2001. http://www4.law.cornell.edu/cfr/21p312.htm

6. Code of Federal Regulations. Title 21, Chapter 1—Food and Drug Administration, DHHS; Subchapter H—Medical Devices; Parts 800 through 898. Updated 1 April, 1999. Access date 18 April, 2001. http://www4.law.cornell.edu/cfr/21p800.htm

7. Twelve practical hints for IRB administrators. *ARENA Newsletter.* Boston, MA: ARENA. Spring 2000.

8. Applied Research Ethics National Association (ARENA). Updated 25 July, 2001. Access date 3 August, 2001. http://www.primr.org/arena.html

9. The Hastings Center. *IRB: A Review of Human Subjects Research.* Updated May 2000. Access date 3 August, 2001. http://www.thehastingscenter.org/irbindex.htm

10. Public Responsibility in Medicine and Research. Updated 18 July, 2001. Access date 3 August, 2001. http://www.primr.org

11. The IRB Discussion Forum (MCWIRB). Updated 21 February, 2001. Access date 3 August, 2001. http://www.mcwirb.org/

The Role of an Attorney

Susan Nicholson

INTRODUCTION

When organizing a new institutional review board (IRB) or evaluating the operation of an existing one, the following question may arise: Does this committee need an attorney? Assuming that question is answered in the affirmative, further questions may follow: Should the attorney attend the meetings of the committee or simply serve as a resource to the committee? If the attorney attends the meetings, should he or she be a voting member of the committee? Does it matter whether the attorney is employed by the organization that operates the IRB or by another organization, such as an independent law firm?

There is no regulatory requirement that IRB membership should include an attorney. Thus, an IRB that lacks an attorney is not out of compliance with the federal regulations for the protection of human subjects as it would be, for example, if the committee lacked a scientist or a nonaffiliated member. Nonetheless, an attorney can play a key role in helping an IRB stay in compliance with all applicable laws and regulations.

The section that follows sets out three different models of how an attorney might function in this regard. Because the choice of model may affect whether an attorney should be a committee member or employed by the institution that operates the IRB, these issues also are discussed briefly.

Three Models of the Role of an Attorney

The three models described later here differ with respect to the manner in which the specialized skills and knowledge of an attorney are used and relied on by an IRB.

Model 1: The Analytical Attorney

Legal education and training are designed to equip attorneys with certain analytical skills and habits of mind. Ideally, an attorney is able to construct logical arguments, identify hidden assumptions, apply principles to complex fact patterns, evaluate opposing arguments in an objective manner, summarize and weigh evidence, and express findings and conclusions in a cogent manner. These skills are content neutral. Consequently, they can be applied in a variety of contexts, even when the attorney has limited knowledge of the underlying science or applicable regulatory framework.

A few examples may serve to illustrate how these skills can be helpful in an IRB context. In a committee discussion of whether a particular protocol presents more than minimal risk, an attorney might be helpful in reminding the committee to refer back to the language of the regulatory definition of minimal risk. The attorney can also summarize the evidence for the conclusion that the study does or does not exceed minimal risk. An attorney who participates over time in a committee's risk/benefit analysis might help to ensure that the analysis takes place within a consistent framework. For example, if the committee excludes indirect benefits from the risk/benefit analysis on some occasions but includes them on others, an attorney may press for a more consistent treatment or may suggest a principled distinction between different types of indirect benefits. In a discussion of possible investigator noncompliance, an attorney might be helpful to the committee in avoiding a precipitous judgment and in suggesting a reasonable process for gathering the relevant evidence for subsequent consideration by the committee.

Because the analytical skills involved are content neutral, the functions previously described can be performed by an attorney even if the attorney practices in a specialized area of the law—such as tax or trusts and estates—that has little substantive relevance to IRB operations. To apply these skills effectively, the attorney should possess a genuine interest in research and human subject protections. He or she must be willing to spend the time required of every committee member to acquire a basic familiarity with relevant ethical principles and federal regulations. Obviously, not every attorney possesses the analytical skills in question, together with an interest in human subject protections. Conversely, many individuals—including scientist–members of the committee—who possess such skills and interest are not attorneys. Consequently, a committee does not have to have an attorney in order to bring analytical rigor to its deliberations. Nonetheless, this is one area in which attorneys frequently make a valuable contribution.

Model 2: The Attorney as Advisor on Ancillary Legal Matters

In Model 1, an attorney contributes content-neutral skills to assist the committee in making reasoned judgments. In Models 2 and 3, an attorney contributes substantive knowledge in areas relevant to the operation of the IRB.

It can reasonably be expected that the administrator and chair of the IRB and, to a lesser extent, IRB members will be familiar with the core federal regulations. The regulations specify the responsibilities of an IRB for protecting human subjects of research. These core regulations consist of the federal Common Rule (45 CFR 46)[1] and the related regulations issued by the federal Food and Drug Administration (FDA) at 21 CFR 50 and 56.[2,3] To implement these core regulations, however, it is necessary to understand certain other laws and regulations with which IRB leadership and members may not be familiar. IRBs frequently rely on an attorney for guidance on these ancillary legal matters. Several examples follow.

To apply the federal regulations protecting children involved as subjects in research, the IRB must know who is considered a child. This is a matter of state law and varies from state to state. Moreover, a person who is below the general age of majority in a particular state may nonetheless be considered by that state to be an adult for certain purposes. In some states, for example, a person below the age of majority can admit himself or herself to a mental health facility for treatment. In the state of Massachusetts, although 18 years is the age of majority, a drug-dependent minor, 12 years of age or older, may consent to treatment for drug dependency (except for methadone maintenance therapy). In addition, a person of any age is considered to be an adult in respect to consenting to a treatment, should he or she be the parent of a child (in which case he or she may also consent to medical care of the child). An IRB may rely on an attorney to know these laws and provide guidance on the extent to which they apply in a research context.

The federal regulations provide that research may not begin until consent has been obtained from the research subject or the subject's "legally authorized representative." The question of who is legally authorized to consent to treatment of persons unable to consent for themselves— for example, a legal guardian, health care attorney, conservator, or next of kin—is again a matter of state law. In some states, moreover, there is no single answer to the question, as the appropriate legal representative may depend on the type of treatment proposed. In the state of Massachusetts, for instance, a legal guardian cannot consent to administration of antipsychotic drugs to an incompetent patient unless there has first been a judicial hearing to evaluate the risks and benefits of the proposed treatment. After the legally authorized representative has been determined for purposes of consent to treatment, the question remains as to whether this representative is also authorized under state law to consent to investigational treatment or to nontherapeutic interventions for research purposes.

The two previous examples illustrate situations in which the IRB needs an understanding of state law in order to make an appropriate application of the core federal regulations for the protection of human subjects. State laws and regulations may themselves contain human subject protections that go beyond those found in the core federal regulations.

For example, the laws of several states, including Massachusetts, prohibit or limit research on fetuses. Because of the way in which the Massachusetts legislature defines the term *fetus*, the prohibition also limits neonatal research. State laws or regulations may also place special limits on or prescribe special procedures that must be followed before conducting research on certain classes of subjects, such as persons who are mentally ill, mentally disabled, or incarcerated. To discharge its responsibility to protect human subjects of research, an IRB must be aware of these state laws and regulations as well.

Still other state laws that do not address research directly may have an indirect impact on it. State laws may, for example, limit the circumstances in which a hospital is permitted to disclose medical record information outside of the institution or prescribe the content of a consent form for the performance of genetic testing. IRBs considering research projects that involve the collection of medical record information or the collection of human tissues for genetic testing may need legal guidance as to the content of these laws and their application to research. Massachusetts has a statute that strictly protects the confidentiality of HIV test information. This law has been interpreted by the relevant state agency as prohibiting access by researchers to HIV records without explicit patient consent, even if the researcher is on the medical staff of the hospital that maintains the records.

Finally, certain federal laws and regulations contain human subject protections that go beyond those found in the core federal regulations. The new federal privacy regulations issued under the Health Insurance Portability and Accountability Act of 1996 are a case in point. The privacy rule specifies the information that must be included in any informed consent for the use or disclosure of protected health information for research purposes and the criteria that must be satisfied in order for an IRB to waive the requirement to obtain an informed consent. These topics are, of course, also addressed by the Common Rule. In both respects, the privacy regulations go beyond the Common Rule, requiring the disclosure of additional information and the satisfaction of additional criteria. Consequently, when reviewing medical records research, the IRB must have knowledge of and meet two separate sets of regulatory requirements.

All of the examples given previously here involve state and federal laws and regulations that are ancillary to the core federal regulations. To reach appropriate judgments about particular protocols, IRBs need reliable advice about these ancillary laws and regulations. To the extent that an IRB relies on an attorney to provide this advice, the attorney is functioning under Model 2.

The attorney's role in Model 1 can be performed by an attorney from any practice area. Model 2 requires substantive legal knowledge and is best performed by an attorney who practices in a specialized area, such as health law.

Model 3: The Attorney as Advisor on the Core Federal Regulations

In Model 1, an attorney contributes content-neutral skills to the committee's deliberations. In Models 2 and 3, the attorney contributes substantive knowledge in particular areas of the law relevant to those deliberations. The distinction between the latter two models is that in Model 2 the committee relies on the attorney's knowledge of federal and state laws and regulations that are ancillary to the core federal regulations. In Model 3, the committee relies on the attorney's specialized expertise with regard to the core regulations themselves.

Because the core federal regulations are not lengthy or complex, one may ask why any specialized expertise is necessary. The answer is that the federal regulations are not self-interpreting. Accordingly, the federal government has issued interpretations of the regulations in the form of guidances or guidelines covering a wide range of topics with which IRBs are expected to be familiar.

To take a simple and straightforward example, anyone reading the Common Rule knows that IRBs are required to conduct continuing review of research not less than once a year. Unless one has also read the guidances on continuing review, issued by the FDA and by the federal Office for Protection from Research Risks (the predecessor agency to the Office for Human Research Protections [OHRP]), one would not be aware of the information that the government expects IRBs to review in order for continuing review to be considered substantive and meaningful, nor would one know that OHRP interprets the 1-year approval period as beginning on the date the research is reviewed by the convened IRB, not the subsequent date on which the IRB chair determines that the research, having met IRB-specified conditions of approval, can begin.

Because the government's interpretations are issued in the form of guidelines, IRBs are not legally bound by them. Nonetheless, an IRB that is unaware of the guidelines and thus unable to provide a reasoned explanation for deviating from them risks being found to be out of compliance with the core federal regulations for the protection of human subjects (see "OHRP Compliance Activities: Common Findings and Guidance."[4(findings 5,7)]

Another example comes from innovative research involving xenotransplantation, the transplantation or implantation into a human subject of live cells, tissues, or organs from a nonhuman animal source. Because the core federal regulations were issued before the development of xenotransplantation, they make no mention of it. Consequently, one must be familiar with the detailed guideline on infectious disease issues in xenotransplantation issued on March 12, 2001, by the federal Public Health Service (PHS).[5] One would otherwise be unaware

of the additional elements of informed consent that are, in the opinion of the PHS, required to obtain an adequate informed consent from research subjects undergoing xenotransplantation. (The PHS is, like the FDA, part of the federal Department of Health and Human Services.) More importantly, one would be unaware that in the view of the PHS, an institution conducting xenotransplantation research cannot adequately protect human subjects unless the institution's biosafety committee and animal care and use committee, as well as the IRB, review and approve the research. In light of the PHS guidelines, an IRB reviewing xenotransplantation research would be well advised to condition final approval on receipt of the necessary additional committee approvals.

Similar guidelines, imposing additional IRB and institutional responsibilities, have been issued with respect to certain categories of human gene-therapy research.[6] As new areas of research are developed, one can expect the federal government to address the human subject protection issues they raise not by amending the Common Rule but by issuing specialized guidances.

An IRB reviewing a moderate to high volume of research will regularly encounter protocols involving the federal guidances listed previously here. For such an IRB, consequently, a thorough understanding of the broad range of government guidances is a necessity. An attorney who provides specialized expertise to an IRB in this regard is functioning under Model 3.

To be effective in this role, an attorney should have experience in advising IRBs as well as comprehensive knowledge of the relevant literature. One need not be an attorney to have this specialized expertise. Rather than relying on an attorney, an IRB might look to its chair or administrator for the necessary expertise. What is important is not who fills this role, but that someone does.

This previous discussion addresses an IRB's need for specialized expertise with respect to the government's interpretations of the Common Rule as reflected in published guidances. Not all provisions of the Common Rule requiring interpretation are the subject of federal guidances. The Common Rule gives rise to a number of interpretative questions that remain the topic of considerable controversy and discussion and about which the government has not yet formulated any guidance.

An example is the question discussed in the most recent report of the National Bioethics Advisory Commission (NBAC) entitled *Ethical and Policy Issues in Research Involving Human Participants.*[7] The NBAC asks whether an IRB should analyze study risks in relationship to the study benefits of a study as a whole or whether they should analyze separately the therapeutic and nontherapeutic components of the study. Another example is the question of how an IRB should conceptualize the possibility of benefit in Phase 1 studies. A related question is whether under the Common Rule an IRB can approve Phase 1 research on children where the research involves more than a minor increase over minimal risk.

An attorney who is functioning under Model 3 may be helpful in developing best practices for the IRB in such controversial areas. An attorney who serves in this capacity should be familiar with the recommendations contained in the various reports on IRBs and human subject protections that have been issued by the Department of Health and Human Services Office of Inspector General and the NBAC.

Finally, an attorney who functions under Model 3 should also be familiar with the recent government suspensions of IRB activity at certain major academic institutions. The attorney will be able to assist the IRB in assessing its own performance against the shortcomings identified at those institutions.

Structuring the Attorney's Role

The three models just described are not meant to be mutually exclusive. An attorney whose knowledge of ancillary legal issues enables him or her to function under Model 2 can also be helpful to the committee by applying analytical skills to the committee's deliberations (the role of an attorney under Model 1). A health law attorney who has developed the specialized expertise in the core federal regulations necessary to function under Model 3 is likely also to be knowledgeable about state and federal law matters that are ancillary to those regulations (Model 2). Consequently, an IRB that wants an attorney in all three roles does not need three attorneys.

Assuming an IRB has decided that it wants one or more of the three roles described previously here to be filled by an attorney, further questions arise.

Should the Attorney Attend the Committee Meetings?
An attorney cannot contribute analytical skills to a committee's discussions unless the attorney is present to hear them. Under Model 1, then, the attorney should attend committee meetings.

If the attorney's primary contribution is knowledge of ancillary legal matters as described in Model 2, it is preferable, but not essential, that the attorney attends committee meetings. If the attorney does not attend, some issues will possibly be missed. If, for example, no one on the committee is aware that a state law limits fetal experimentation, no one will know to ask whether a particular protocol falls under an exemption to that law. An experienced committee, on the other hand, may be able to recognize the protocols that raise ancillary legal issues. In these circumstances, it may be sufficient to have an attorney available outside of the meeting for consultation when necessary.

For IRBs reviewing a moderate to high volume of research, every committee meeting will involve some protocols to which specialized expertise on the core federal regulations is directly relevant. Generally speaking, an IRB that relies on an attorney to provide the specialized expertise described in Model 3 will need that attorney to be present at meetings.

Should the Attorney Be a Voting Member of the IRB?
The lawyer's role in Model 1 is consistent with the ordinary functions of a committee member. Lawyers who function in this capacity frequently serve as nonscientific or nonaffiliated voting members of the IRB. In Models 2 and 3, the IRB relies on the professional advice of a lawyer with regard to the interpretation of laws and regulations. Consequently, the relationship is usually structured as an attorney/client relationship, in which case the lawyer represents, but is not a member of, the IRB.

Should the Attorney Be an In-House or Outside Attorney?
If the attorney's role is limited to the functions described in Model l, it would probably not be an efficient use of the time of an in-house counsel. Such roles are usually filled by volunteer lawyers from the community who, although practicing in other areas of the law, have a special interest in research and human subject protections.

The lawyer's role in Models 2 or 3 could be filled equally well by an attorney employed by the institution that operates the IRB (an in-house attorney) or by a paid lawyer from outside the institution. Some commentators have suggested that the use of outside counsel is preferable, as in-house attorneys might identify too closely with the institution's financial interest in having research go forward or, conversely, may be unduly concerned with protecting the institution from potential liability. Outside counsel, however, is retained by the institution and thus is not ultimately immune from these same pressures. To the extent that the institution's priorities are properly aligned to promote research that protects the rights of research subjects, it should not matter whether the IRB is represented by in-house or outside counsel.

Conclusion

The expertise of an attorney is an important resource for the IRB. There are three basic models of the role of an attorney with the IRB. In Model 1, the attorney provides an analytical perspective on IRB issues that other committee members may lack. In Model 2, the attorney acts as an advisor on ancillary legal matters such as the legal definition of a child or the definition of a legally authorized representative from the standpoint of surrogate decision making. In Model 3, the attorney acts as an advisor on the core federal regulations. For an IRB to function optimally, it is important that the committee understands the potential value of input from an attorney and that an attorney assigned to the IRB understands the role that it is expected to play in the review of research involving human subjects.

References

1. Code of Federal Regulations. Title 45A—Department of Health and Human Services; Part 46—Protection of Human Subjects. Updated 1 October, 1997. Access date 18 April, 2001. http://www4.law.cornell.edu/cfr/45p46.htm
2. Code of Federal Regulations. Title 21, Chapter 1—Food and Drug Administration, DHHS; Part 50—Protection of Human Subjects. Updated 1 April, 1999. Access date 18 April, 2001. http://www4.law.cornell.edu/cfr/21p50.htm
3. Code of Federal Regulations. Title 21, Chapter 1—Food and Drug Administration, DHHS; Part 56—Institutional

Review Boards. Updated 1 April, 1999. Access date 27 March, 2001. http://www4.law.cornell.edu/cfr/21p56.htm

4. Office of Human Research Protections. OHRP compliance activities: Common findings and guidance. Updated 1 September, 2000. Access date 20 April, 2001. http://ohrp.osophs.dhhs.gov/nhrpac/mtg12-00/finguid.htm

5. Public Health Service. PHS guideline on infectious disease issues in xenotransplantation. Updated 12 March, 2001. Access date 8 August, 2001. http://www.fda.gov/cber/gdlns/xenophs0101.htm

6. National Institutes of Health. NIH guidelines for research involving recombinant DNA molecules. *Federal Register* 65(196):60327–60332, 2000. Access date 14 September, 2001. http://www4.od.nih.gov/oba/rac/guidelines.html

7. National Bioethics Advisory Commission. Ethical and policy issues in research involving human participants: Report and recommendations. Bethesda, MD, U.S. Government Printing Office. Updated 20 August, 2001. Access date 31 August, 2001. http://bioethics.gov/human/overvol1.html

Committee Size, Alternates, and Consultants

Robert J. Amdur and Elizabeth A. Bankert

INTRODUCTION

It is often necessary for institutional review board (IRB) leadership to make decisions that affect the size of the IRB. When establishing a new IRB, the size of the committee is an initial step in the organization process. For established IRBs, the question of adding or removing positions from the membership roster is an ongoing issue. Members rotate off the IRB at regular intervals. People with an interest in research regulation ask to join the IRB, and the nature or scope of research changes over time. The need for expertise in the wide range of studies that most IRBs review creates pressure to add additional members to the IRB and to ask for help from people not affiliated with the committee. Often a complicating factor is the desire to improve the efficiency of the IRB meeting. The purpose of this chapter is to discuss factors that are important to consider when making decisions that affect the size of the IRB.

Size of the IRB

The only direct reference to the size of the IRB in the Department of Health and Human Services regulations is the requirement that the IRB consist of at least five members: "Each IRB shall have at least five members."[1][Sec.107(a)] In addition to this regulatory minimum, four main factors are important to consider when making decisions about the size of the IRB.

An Odd Number of IRB Members Makes It Easier to Obtain a Quorum

Federal regulation[1][Sec.108(b)] requires attendance by a majority of IRB members to conduct a full-committee meeting: "In order to fulfill the requirements of this policy each IRB shall . . . (except when an expedited review procedure is used) . . . review proposed research at convened meetings at which a majority of the members of the IRB are present."

The more positions on the IRB full-committee roster, the more people will be available to attend the IRB meeting. However, the larger the committee, the more people there are who have to attend the meeting to make a quorum. Majority means "more than half." An odd number of positions on the membership roster maximizes the number of IRB members for a given quorum requirement. For example, if the IRB has 10 full-committee positions, it takes 6 people to make a quorum. By increasing the IRB membership to 11 positions, the IRB increases the membership workforce without increasing the quorum because 6 is more than half of both 10 and 11. When the schedule of IRB members is such that it may be difficult to make a quorum, the IRB will find it useful to have an odd number of voting positions on the IRB roster.

Adequate Expertise and Diversity

The regulatory requirements for IRB membership are discussed in detail in the next chapter. Basically, the federal regulations[1][Sec.107] require that an IRB include at least one scientist, one nonscientist, and one person not affiliated with the institution and that the IRB have sufficient expertise and diversity to evaluate ethical issues involved in protocols that are sent for IRB review.

Because the regulations go into considerable detail about required areas of expertise and diversity of the IRB membership, these factors often create pressure to add more positions to the IRB roster. Most IRBs review research that may recruit subjects from heterogeneous backgrounds in terms of racial, ethnic, gender, educational, and socioeconomic factors. It becomes difficult for the IRB to know when to stop adding members to comply with this section of the regulations. Similarly, for IRBs that review technically complex protocols from a wide range of medical or behavioral research specialties, the IRB sometimes needs more expertise to evaluate a specific research study. Clearly, the composition of the IRB is an area that requires a high degree of judgment on the part of IRB leadership. An alternative to adding new members to the IRB is to use consultants to advise the IRB on specific issues.

Workload Issues Affect the Size of the IRB

The volume and complexity of the studies that an IRB monitors will be a major factor in determining the size of the IRB. There is no regulatory guideline on appropriate workload. This is the subject of a separate chapter. Ideally, we would have benchmark data from "best practice" IRBs to define national guidelines on the volume of studies per meeting time per IRB member for different research environments (biomedical, social science, etc.). Currently, no formal data of this kind are available.

Logistics of the Full-Committee Meeting

The larger the IRB, the more difficult it will be to support full-committee meetings from the administrative standpoint. Large meeting rooms may be difficult to reserve at a time and location that are convenient for IRB members. When the IRB committee is spread around a large meeting area, it may be difficult for IRB members and support staff to hear what is going on without a sound amplification system. Ideally, the full-committee meeting is a discussion in which people feel comfortable disagreeing with their colleagues or expressing their confusion about an important issue. When a meeting is so large that the members have trouble seeing or hearing their colleagues, it will be difficult for the IRB to function optimally.

The administrative work that must be done to prepare for the full-committee meeting is directly related to the size of the IRB. For most agenda items, each committee member will be given a copy of the IRB forms and supporting documents sometime (usually days) before the meeting. The time that it takes to photocopy, collate, and organize study material will be extensive for large IRBs.

A related issue is the transportation of IRB material to the home or office of committee members in time for them to review it before the meeting. Large IRBs usually have heavy meeting agendas, and getting the necessary documents to members in a timely fashion may require special transportation equipment and full-time employees specifically for this task.

Consultants to the IRB

From the administrative standpoint, consultants have the advantage of providing the IRB with additional expertise or cultural diversity without increasing the requirement for quorum or other factors that are associated with adding additional members to the IRB. There is no standard procedure or published guideline regarding the use of consultants to assist the IRB with the review of specific protocols. An informal survey of IRB directors around the country suggests that this is not a common practice. In our opinion, the use of consultants to help the IRB review a project that the IRB is not comfortable with is an underutilized procedure that has the potential to increase both the efficiency and efficacy of IRB review.

At Dartmouth, we have used consultants many times to help the IRB evaluate issues such as the value of alternative therapy, the choice of the control group, and the potential for coercion in the proposed study population.

The procedure is simple. The IRB chair simply calls a person who is likely to be both unbiased and knowledgeable about the issue in question and asks him or her to provide an opinion to the IRB. The consultant may be a local colleague or may work at another institution. The consultant is given the relevant protocol materials and asked to submit a brief (one-half to one page) opinion in writing (e-mail is acceptable). The consultant's opinion is shown to all IRB members who will be voting on the protocol, and the issue is discussed at the full-committee meeting.

It is best to remove the consultant's name and other identifying information if there is any question that there could be problems if the investigator knows the identity of the consultant. The identity of the consultant may be kept separately in the IRB files. In some cases, it will be appropriate to ask the consultant to attend the IRB meeting, but in our experience, this is rarely necessary.

Administrative Cost

Most IRBs operate in an environment where there is pressure to limit administrative cost. As discussed previously here, the cost of copying and transporting documents related to the full-committee meeting is directly related to IRB size. Similarly, for IRBs that provide meals during regularly scheduled meetings, the cost of food and beverages will be a considerable expense for large IRBs.

When the IRB pays members for the time they spend participating in IRB-related activities, each addition to the IRB roster may have a large impact on the IRB budget. This will be especially true when reimbursement is based on a percentage of the member's salary and high-paid members of society (such as physicians) are recruited for IRB service.

Alternate IRB Members

Federal regulations contain specific instructions on the size and composition of the IRB full committee. The purpose of this section is to explain the use of alternate IRB members. To follow the alternate member discussion, it is important to understand the difference between the IRB membership roster and the IRB membership list. The term *IRB membership roster* refers to the number of voting member positions on the IRB. In federal regulations, instructions about the number and characteristics of the IRB membership refer to voting member positions. For example, when the regulations require that "each IRB shall have at least five members," it means five voting member positions. When the regulations require a majority of IRB members for a meeting quorum, it means that more than half of the number of voting member positions must be represented at an IRB meeting.

The difference between the IRB membership roster and the IRB membership list is the use of alternate IRB members where *alternate* refers to the situation where there is more than one member for an IRB roster position. If your institution holds a Federalwide Assurance (FWA), notification of IRB membership must be submitted to the

Office for Human Research Protections (OHRP) on a regular basis. Contact OHRP for detailed information.

Most IRBs will find it useful to have alternate members for at least some IRB roster positions because the use of alternate members increases the functional capacity and administrative flexibility of the committee. As discussed in other chapters, federal regulations require an approval vote by a majority of the IRB and that the IRB be composed of people with specific characteristics in terms of cultural and professional experience.[1][Sec.108(b)] These constraints often create a situation of competing objectives when selecting the IRB membership. The goal of diverse representation creates pressure to increase the size of the IRB, whereas the majority quorum requirement creates an incentive to keep the IRB as small as possible. The use of alternate IRB members makes it easier for the IRB to satisfy diversity requirements without increasing the number of voting members that must be present to have a full-committee meeting quorum.

Federal regulations and OHRP policy do not limit the overall number of alternate members on an IRB or the number of alternates for any given IRB position. Although most IRBs have only two members for a given roster position (a single alternate member), in some cases, it may be desirable to have more than two people who alternate in providing the IRB with a specific type of representation.

The Nonscientific Member

To approve research at a full-committee IRB meeting, federal regulations require at least one voting member whose primary concerns are in nonscientific areas.[1][Sec.107(c)] If the IRB membership list has only one nonscientific member, the full committee cannot meet if this person is not available for the duration of the meeting. However, if the IRB recruits several people to serve as alternates for the nonscientific voting member position, the IRB has the flexibility to conduct a full-committee meeting anytime that any one of the nonscientific members is available.

Diversity and Issue-Specific Representation

Members who have issue-specific knowledge are required to provide cultural diversity when the IRB routinely reviews research involving diverse populations or populations that are especially vulnerable (e.g., children, prisoners, or persons with mental disabilities).[1][Sec.107(a)] As with the requirement for a nonscience member, the IRB will find it useful to have multiple members for each voting-member roster position that represents important dimensions of the IRB committee.

Alternate Member-at-Large

It is not unusual for IRBs to receive approval from the OHRP to add an "alternate member-at-large" to the membership list. An alternate-at-large position does not change the requirement for quorum because it is not viewed as a regular voting member position. The alternate-at-large only votes at the full-committee meeting when he or she is filling in for another member position. For example, if the IRB roster lists two people in a certain membership position (a regular and one alternate) and neither of these people attends the meeting, then the alternate-at-large may be able to vote in place of these members (and count toward quorum).

The only limitation in terms of the use of an alternate-at-large is that the member-at-large and the voting member for whom he or she is substituting must have the same issue-specific knowledge when such knowledge is required for research review. For example, when reviewing a protocol involving research with autistic children, an alternate-at-large who is not familiar with autistic children is not permitted to substitute for an IRB member who was appointed to provide the IRB with expertise in this area.

Most IRBs that include a member-at-large appoint a person whose primary concerns are in nonscience areas to this position so that there is additional backup for this critical position at the full-committee meeting. Some IRBs appoint an experienced member of the IRB administrative staff as the alternate-at-large so that they know that there will always be a nonscientific member available if there are last-minute or unexpected problems with the members who usually bring this required perspective to the IRB meeting.

Conclusion

The optimal size of an IRB is determined by the following factors:

1. An odd number of members, making it easier to get a quorum
2. The need for adequate expertise and diversity
3. The use of alternate IRB members and IRB consultants
4. IRB workload
5. Logistics of the full-committee meeting
6. Administrative cost

Reference

1. Code of Federal Regulations. Title 45A—Department of Health and Human Services; Part 46—Protection of Human Subjects. Updated 1 October, 1997. Access date 18 April, 2001. http://www4.law.cornell.edu/cfr/45p46.htm

Length, Frequency, and Time of Institutional Review Board Meetings

Robert J. Amdur and Elizabeth A. Bankert

INTRODUCTION

Should the full-committee meeting be scheduled for 8 hours once a month or 4 hours every other week? Should a 4-hour meeting be scheduled from 10 a.m. to 2 p.m. or from 8 a.m. to noon? The schedule of institutional review board (IRB) meetings may seem like a minor detail, but it may have an important influence on the efficiency and effectiveness of IRB function. An informal survey of university-based IRBs suggests that there is no standard template regarding the schedule of IRB meetings. For some IRBs, the meeting schedule has been developed in response to objective constraints, whereas in others, it is "just the way we have always done it." Recognizing that the schedule of IRB meetings is something that should be customized to meet the specific needs of each institution, there are some basic principles to consider when evaluating this aspect of the IRB organization.

Federal Regulations

There is no information in Department of Health and Human Services or Food and Drug Administration regulations about the length, frequency, or time of IRB meetings with the exception of the requirement that continuing review of an approved protocol take place at least once a year.

Length of the IRB Meeting

The IRB meeting should last only as long as necessary to carry out important IRB business and education that require the presence of the full committee. An inefficient IRB meeting wastes committee members' time and creates a situation in which it is difficult to recruit and retain high-quality people for IRB service.

Assuming that IRB meeting time is used productively, the main argument in favor of long IRB meetings (as opposed to shorter meetings at more frequent intervals) is an increase in administrative efficiency. This advantage must be weighed against the tendency for people to lose their ability to concentrate on meeting discussion after an extended time. IRB decisions often require an understanding of complex and controversial ethical or regulatory issues such that even for experienced IRB members the full-committee meeting is usually an intellectually demanding experience. As the integrity of the IRB system depends on an educated opinion from all committee members, it is important that members pay attention throughout the meeting. When the IRB meeting lasts too long, the efficiency and effectiveness of IRB review is likely to be compromised. Although some members may be able to concentrate for lengthy IRB meetings on a regular basis, in our experience, IRB function clearly deteriorates when the meeting lasts more than 4 or 5 hours. For this reason, we recommend scheduling regular full-committee meetings for no more than 4 hours per session.

Frequency of IRB Meetings

After an IRB determines the maximum meeting duration that is appropriate for its membership and agenda, the minimum frequency of full-committee meetings will be determined by IRB workload and the efficiency of the review process. All segments of the research community benefit when research review is completed in a timely fashion. An IRB that is consistently unable to complete a review of all agenda items assigned to a given meeting session will need to improve the efficiency of IRB review or meet more frequently.

For many IRBs, the question is whether the IRB should meet for the maximum time as infrequently as possible or for a shorter period of time at more frequent intervals. For example, many IRBs can effectively manage research review at their institution with a single half-day meeting every 4 weeks (one meeting per month). IRBs in this situation may want to consider changing the meeting schedule so that the IRB meets for a few hours every other week. Similarly, an IRB that is reviewing all submitted review items with a half-day meeting every 2 weeks may consider a shorter meeting every week. Several factors must be considered when determining meeting frequency in this setting.

Research Review Interval

The review interval is the time between the date that a protocol is submitted for IRB review and the date that the investigator is informed of the IRB's final decision (approval or disapproval). This may have important implications for an institution's research program. Excessive IRB turnaround time will compromise an investigator's ability to secure research contracts that benefit both the institution and research subjects, decrease investigator enthusiasm for doing research, and compromise respect for the local IRB system. Although multiple factors may influence the research review interval, it is important for an IRB to recognize when the frequency of IRB meetings is a problem for the research enterprise. When more frequent IRB meetings will meaningfully decrease the time between submission and approval of IRB applications, the IRB should consider changing the IRB meeting schedule accordingly.

Member Availability

The availability of IRB members may determine the frequency of the full-committee meeting. For some IRBs, it will be easier to retain a quorum with high-quality members if the IRB meets frequently for short periods of time, whereas for others, a less frequent but longer meeting will be preferable. An IRB that is having trouble with meeting attendance should consider the possibility that meeting frequency is a source of the problem.

Administrative Efficiency

The main argument in favor of less frequent full-committee meetings is administrative efficiency. The amount of work involved with reserving meeting space, confirming attendance, preparing and delivering information to each member, interacting with IRB members and investigators immediately before the meeting, providing administrative support during the meeting, and generating the postmeeting letters and documentation is such that there is a net loss in administrative productivity with more frequent full-committee meetings.

Alternate Reviewer System

The alternate reviewer system is discussed in Chapter 3-5. The use of alternate IRB members may make it possible to have IRB meetings more frequently than would otherwise be possible. For example, an IRB that would like to meet every week may find it difficult to recruit qualified members who can meet that frequently. If the IRB has two members for each IRB roster position, each member can attend every other IRB meeting, and the IRB will have full-committee attendance at each meeting without increasing the requirement for quorum.

The Time of Day for the IRB Meeting

Factors to consider when deciding on the time of day for the IRB full-committee meetings include several mentioned in the discussions of meeting duration and frequency.

Member Availability

When IRB members are unable to attend the meetings because they are scheduled at a time when the member has an important conflict, it may be advantageous for IRB leadership to move the IRB meeting to a more convenient time. IRBs that are having trouble with meeting attendance should determine whether the time of day of the meeting is part of the problem.

Ability of IRB Members to Concentrate

As discussed earlier, it is essential that all committee members stay alert during the entire full-committee meeting. Some IRBs, especially those with light agendas, seem to function well with late afternoon or evening meetings. However, in our experience, IRB review is more thorough and conducted more efficiently when the IRB meeting takes place at the beginning of the workday. Similarly, meeting times that straddle a major mealtime are likely to be problematic. For example, it is likely to be difficult to keep the committee focused on IRB business in a meeting that goes from 10 a.m. to 2 p.m., especially if a formal lunch is provided at noon. Most people have trouble concentrating on a technical discussion when they are hungry, waiting for food, or recovering from a large meal. When productivity changes during the IRB meeting seem to be related to issues related to the focus and concentration of IRB members, IRB leadership should consider changing the time of day of the IRB meeting.

Conclusion

There is no information in Department of Health and Human Services or Food and Drug Administration regulations about the length, frequency, or time of IRB meetings with the exception of the requirement that continuing review of an approved protocol take place at least once a year. In our experience, IRB function deteriorates when meetings last more than 4 hours. The frequency of IRB meetings should be determined by the research review interval, member availability, and the need to improve administrative efficiency.

Institutional Review Board Subcommittees

Robert J. Amdur

INTRODUCTION

The term *subcommittee* is used in this chapter to refer to a group of institutional review board (IRB) members organized for the purpose of managing a specific task or making a specific type of decision related to IRB function.

The use of subcommittees is extremely variable across the IRB community. Some IRB offices rely on the full committee for essentially all decisions and reviews. Some advocate subcommittees for a fraction of these decisions, and other IRB offices make decisions based solely on the expertise of the IRB chair, IRB administrative director, and/or one other IRB member. In this chapter, we discuss the use of these three options for making IRB decisions and establishing IRB policy and procedure in a variety of areas.

Federal Research Regulations

The Department of Health and Human Services and the Food and Drug Administration regulations related to human research do not contain the term *subcommittee*. The Department of Health and Human Services regulations indirectly address the subcommittee issue in the section on review of research using an expedited review procedure.[1(Sec.110)] Under an *expedited review* procedure, "The review may be carried out by the IRB chairperson or by one or *more* experienced reviewers designated by the chairperson from among members of the IRB."[1(Sec.110(b)(2))] The regulations therefore allow for an IRB to form a subcommittee consisting of one or more experienced reviewers, but the regulations do not imply that multiple reviewers are an important aspect of the expedited review procedure. The regulations stress the importance of *experience,* which implies knowledge of IRB issues and the ability to make decisive judgments in this setting.

Models for Making IRB Decisions

No organizational structure will guarantee efficient, high-quality decision making. Some IRBs function best by assigning decision-making authority to groups of people (subcommittees), whereas others find the group model counterproductive. The alternative to an IRB subcommittee is to have IRB decisions that do not require review by the full committee, made by the IRB chair, by the IRB administrative director (assuming she or he is an IRB member), or by another appropriately qualified IRB member who is not the chair or administrative director. Recognizing that optimal IRB function requires that each IRB customize its organization, there are several points to consider when deciding about the use of a subcommittee.

Efficiency

Scheduling and conducting a meeting that involves several people are usually processes that require considerable time and energy on the part of the committee members and IRB administration. For this reason, a subcommittee is likely to be less efficient than a decision-making process based on an individual such as the IRB chair, an IRB administrative director, or an experienced IRB member.

Workload Distribution

Some IRBs may create subcommittees to improve workload distribution. Although an organization that involves subcommittees may achieve this goal, it is important to understand that workload distribution and subcommittee meetings are two different issues. From the administrative standpoint, it may be easier to distribute IRB work by dividing a specific IRB task among different IRB members, each working independently from the others.

Better Decisions

The main advantage of group decisions is the ability to draw on the experience and expertise of a number of people. A subcommittee creates a forum for ideas to be exchanged, opinions to be challenged, and alternate points of view to be considered. Under ideal conditions, a subcommittee increases the chance that decisions will be free from personal bias and based on sound logic after consideration of all of the important issues. However, in many settings, more people does not translate into a more thorough analysis, better judgment, or other factors that contribute to sound decision making. When one person has the necessary experience and decision-making skills, a subcommittee process is not likely to improve the quality of IRB decisions.

Possible Subcommittees for an IRB

Expedited Review

When specific criteria are met, IRB review may be accomplished with an expedited procedure.[2(pp.60364-60367)] However, for the purposes of this discussion, it is important to remember that the regulations do not permit research to be *disapproved* by an expedited procedure.[1[Sec.110(b)(2)]] Expedited review of research should be done with the understanding that the reviewers should only approve research when there is no concern that an approval decision will meaningfully compromise the protection of research subjects. When a reviewer is uncomfortable with approving research by the expedited procedure, he or she should ask for advice from other IRB members or outside consultants or refer the decision to the full IRB committee.

An IRB may elect to establish one or more subcommittees specifically for the expedited review of research. In our experience, an individual IRB member with expertise in the area of research in question is sufficient for the expedited review procedure, but some IRBs may prefer a group decision in this setting. A situation in which review by a subcommittee or individual specialist may be especially useful is the expedited review of a particular type of research that routinely raises issues that are beyond the expertise of the IRB chair or administrative director. For example, at institutions that manage both social science and biomedical research with a single IRB committee, it may be useful to designate an individual or subcommittee for expedited review of each of these general classes of research.

A format that has worked well at Dartmouth College is that a single IRB reviews both social science and biomedical research, but the IRB designates a member with social science expertise to be the initial review mechanism for all issues involving social science research. This social science research specialist either approves qualified research by the expedited procedure or refers it to the full IRB committee. The IRB chair (a physician) or a member of the IRB with biomedical research expertise (who has been specifically educated about the regulatory guidelines for expedited review) handles the expedited review of biomedical research. To minimize the full-committee workload, we recommend using the expedited review process in all situations permitted by federal regulations.

Determination of Research Versus Nonresearch

In some situations, it is difficult to decide whether a project that uses scientific methods to collect private, identifiable health information should be classified as research or as some form of nonresearch activity. Student survey assignments and medical record reviews are common examples of such activity. The classification of a project as research is obviously important because the IRB system is designed and authorized from the standpoint of federal research regulations to oversee only research. Our recommendation is for the IRB administrator and chair to interact with appropriate departments at the institution, for example, research administration, medical records, and risk management, to generate an institutional policy for classifying projects as research. After guidelines are developed, the IRB chair or administrative director can make the decision for each specific project.

Determination of Review Category

The three main categories of initial protocol review are full committee, expedited, or exempt (from further IRB review). The regulatory criteria for each of these procedures are discussed in separate chapters. The regulations do not explain where the decision regarding the procedure for review should be made in the IRB organization. It is our impression that in most organizations the IRB administrative director and/or the IRB chair decide on the procedure for initial protocol review. However, some IRBs prefer to have this important triage decision made by a subcommittee of IRB members. For this decision, we believe the use of a subcommittee is not an efficient or effective use of time. To streamline this process, our recommendation is to give the responsibility of determination of review category to the IRB administrative director or IRB chair.

Primary Reviewer Subcommittees

Although not described in the federal regulations, the Office for Human Research Protections (OHRP) has approved a process known as the *primary reviewer system*. The primary reviewer system involves one, two, or three full-committee members taking responsibility for a detailed review of a research study. At the time of the full-committee meeting, the primary reviewer(s) provides comments and recommendations to the full committee.

Some institutions have taken the primary reviewer model one step further by designating subcommittees to review each protocol before the full-committee meeting. As in the primary reviewer system, the primary review subcommittee is responsible for analyzing the protocol and IRB application in detail and discussing any unanswered questions with consultants or the researchers before the full-committee meeting. At the full-committee meeting, a representative from the subcommittee presents the final recommendation regarding IRB approval, often with a brief explanation of the important issues that were evaluated. Like the primary reviewer system, the potential advantage of a primary review subcommittee is that it may help the IRB conduct a high-quality review without a lengthy discussion at the full-committee meeting. However, it is important to remember that all members of the full committee must receive the consent form and enough information about the protocol to conduct a substantive review.

Serious Adverse Event Reports

The role of the IRB in reviewing serious adverse event reports (SAERs), especially from multicenter trials, is one of the most controversial issues in the field of research regulation. The Food and Drug Administration held a public hearing related to the *Reporting of Adverse Events to Institutional Review Boards,* Docket No. 2005N-0038 as recorded in the Federal Register, February 8, 2005, Volume 70, Number 25. The results of this hearing are not yet known, however we encourage readers to stay up to date and respond to additional inquires related to this topic. Chapters 7-3 and 7-4 are devoted to this topic. For this discussion, it is sufficient to understand that federal regulations are not specific about the procedure for IRB review of SAERs from ongoing research. Specifically, the IRB does not have clear guidance on the procedure for review or criteria for approval of an SAER. In view of this uncertainty, it is not surprising that the procedure for reviewing SAERs is extremely variable within the IRB community.

In some organizations, all SAERs are reviewed as separate agenda items at full-committee meetings. Some IRBs designate a subcommittee to review SAERs with the understanding that only those SAERs that raise concern are forwarded to the full committee. Our recommendation is for each SAER to be reviewed first by the principal investigator, who must complete a questionnaire indicating his or her assessment of the SAER, and then by the IRB chair. If the IRB chair decides that the SAER may indicate a meaningful change in the risk to research subjects, the chair forwards the SAER for review at the next full-committee meeting. This may suspend IRB approval of the research protocol in the interim. However, when the IRB chair does not have further inquiries about the SAER, then no further IRB review is done until the regularly scheduled time of continuing protocol review, when all SAERs are included in the renewal materials.

Revision Requests

Federal research regulations provide for the use of an expedited procedure to review minor changes to research that has been previously approved.[1(Sec.110)] The use of a subcommittee in this type of review is likely to be less efficient than a review by the IRB chair or designee, without a difference in quality. We also note here that the definition of *minor change* is an opportunity for the institution to carefully review the federal regulations (OHRP and Food and Drug Administration) and document their interpretation in an internal policy document. For example, at Dartmouth College, after reviewing federal regulations, a definition of *minor change* was established that focuses on whether risks to subjects are increased as a result of the revision. Specifically, if the change is not significant and the risks to subjects are not increased, then only the IRB chair or designee reviews the revision, using an expedited process. However, if risks to subjects are increased, then full-committee review is required.

Continuing Review

In 1988, the categories of research that could be reviewed with an expedited process were revised to include continuing review of some studies that were initially reviewed by a full IRB committee.[2(pp.60364–60367)] Expedited review in this setting by an IRB subcommittee, the IRB chair, administrative director, or designated IRB member will increase IRB efficiency and decrease waiting time for ongoing IRB approval.

Compliance Audits

An issue that is receiving increased attention is the need to establish a formal mechanism to audit research records or research practice for compliance with federal regulations and internal IRB policy. Federal research regulations do not require that the IRB conduct an audit outside the scope of the procedures that make up the standard IRB review. However, there are two settings in which an audit system may improve IRB function: the audit of IRB records and the audit of the conduct of research (evaluating the quality of informed consent, verifying that current participants meet the approved inclusion criteria, etc.). Both of these topics are the subject of Chapter 2-5.

For the purpose of this discussion, the point is that auditing IRB records or the conduct of research is a specialized function that goes on outside the framework of other IRB activities. An IRB that wants to make an audit an effective part of its routine procedures must establish audit guidelines and designate people who will manage audit tasks. In many institutions, the IRB administrative director and administrative staff conduct the audits that are limited to the review of IRB records, but some IRBs assign this task to a subcommittee of IRB members or even the full IRB committee.

Because few institutions routinely audit research conduct, it is difficult to make generalizations about the process for this practice. As with other specialized activities, some IRBs will find it useful to audit the conduct of research with a subcommittee, whereas others will assign this job to individual IRB members. In this instance, a subcommittee could serve a useful role in establishing an audit process at your institution. For example, an audit subcommittee could assist in establishing the policy, parameters, and schedule of routine audits as well as to perform the actual audit reviews. As in other settings where subcommittees are used, an audit subcommittee should forward reports and problematic cases to the full committee for evaluation.

IRB Policy and Procedures

IRB work is a dynamic and evolving process. Although some aspects of the IRB function are required to be the same for all IRBs that operate in compliance with federal regulations, in many situations, each individual IRB will need or want to establish its own policy. For example, should the IRB establish subcommittees to perform a preliminary review of research that will be reviewed by the full IRB committee? Should an IRB voting option include tabling a motion? How should the IRB manage SAERs? Should there be standard wording in the consent document when the research involves storage of tissue for future research?

Some IRBs will choose to make decisions about IRB policy and procedure with a subcommittee composed of the IRB chair, IRB administrative director, and other experienced IRB members. IRBs that use this organizational structure often give this type of committee a title like *executive committee*. Certainly the subcommittee approach makes sense in this setting, but many IRBs appear to function extremely well where all decisions related to IRB policy and procedure are made by the IRB chair and administrative director.

Conclusion

Throughout this book, authors are encouraged to analyze a topic and then make recommendations based on their experience managing human research protection programs. In preparing this chapter, we discussed the use of subcommittees with IRB directors at several large not-for-profit and university-based IRBs. As stated in the initial section of this chapter, there is no right or wrong way to use subcommittees in the overall IRB organization. Some institutions function well with subcommittees and others function well without them. With this in mind, it is the recommendation of the authors of this chapter to use subcommittees as little as possible to distribute workload, establish IRB policy, or make important IRB decisions.

References

1. Code of Federal Regulations. Title 45A—Department of Health and Human Services; Part 46—Protection of Human Subjects. Updated 1 October, 1997. Access date 18 April, 2001. http://www4.law.cornell.edu/cfr/45p46.htm

2. National Institutes of Health. Protection of human subjects: Categories of research that may be reviewed by the Institutional Review Board (IRB) through an expedited review procedure. *Federal Register* 63(216):60364–60367, 1998. http://ohrp.osophs.dhhs.gov/humansubjects/guidance/63fr60364.htm

Social Science Versus Biomedical Institutional Review Boards

Robert J. Amdur and Elizabeth A. Bankert

INTRODUCTION

A frequent request at national institutional review board (IRB) meetings is to spend more time on topics related to social science research. At many institutions that conduct both social science and biomedical research, IRB review of these two general categories of research is assigned to separate IRB committees. This organizational structure may suggest that there is a fundamental difference between social science and biomedical research in terms of ethical issues and the process of IRB review. The purpose of this chapter is to challenge this concept. There is no question that many biomedical research issues are not applicable to social science. However, the quality of research review will be enhanced by requiring that members of both disciplines contribute their expertise and unique perspective on research involving human subjects, rather than segregating the discussion of social science and biomedical issues.

Definitions

Social science is "the study of human society and of individual relationships in, and to, society." Academic disciplines that usually conduct social science research include sociology, psychology, anthropology, economics, political science, and history. The terms *behavioral science* and *social science* are used interchangeably.

In contrast to the social science focus on interpersonal relationships, biomedical scientists study human physiology and the treatment or understanding of disease. A dictionary definition of *biomedical science* is "the application of the principles of the natural sciences to medicine."

Why Distinguish Between Social Science and Biomedical Research?

The use of topic-specific IRB committees may be a convenient way to divide the workload at institutions that handle a large volume of research protocols. This section reviews the limitations to a conceptual framework that focuses on the distinction between social science and biomedical research.

Research Regulations Hold Research from All Disciplines to the Same Standards

There is no legal or regulatory basis for making a distinction between social science and biomedical research from the IRB standpoint. Specifically, the U.S. Department of Health and Human Services regulations that focus on the IRB do not mention the terms *social science*, *behavioral science*, or *biomedical research*.[1] The regulations describe ethical standards for research based on the specific characteristic of the risk to research participants, not on the academic field in which research may be classified. The section of these regulations that describes IRB membership requirements[1[Sec.107(a)]] requires that the IRB "have at least five members with varying backgrounds to promote complete and adequate review of research activities commonly conducted by the institution. In addition to . . . professional competence . . . , the IRB shall be able to ascertain the acceptability of proposed research in terms of institutional commitments . . . and standards of professional conduct and practice." Clearly, this means that if an institution conducts social science and/or biomedical research, then it must have individuals with social science and/or biomedical research expertise on the IRB.

Other sections of the regulations go into detail to clarify IRB procedures and approval criteria when research is conducted in a setting with distinguishing ethical characteristics—for example, research involving certain kinds of educational testing, research involving children, and research involving prisoners—but nothing implies a general distinction between social science and biomedical research. The fact that the regulations do not distinguish between social science and biomedical research emphasizes the similarities between these two general types of research in terms of ethical standards and research regulation.

Understanding the Importance of Social Harm

Historically, research regulations and ethical codes were developed in response to situations that resulted in physical harm to research subjects. As social science research usually does not involve a risk of physical harm, some members of the research community may misunderstand the applicability of research standards to both biomedical and social science research. It is still not unusual to read research proposals in which the investigator limits the discussion of risk to the physical harm that may result from research participation. The problem with situations like this, as well as many of the discussions that imply that there are important differences between the ethical standards of social science and biomedical research, is that they ignore the potential impact of social harm on the lives of research participants.

Social harm refers to decreases in quality of life that result from information being created or used in a way that is damaging to the individual in question. Social harm may result in well-defined events such as loss of employability, loss of insurability, and criminal or civil litigation, but more commonly, it disrupts interpersonal relationships by causing embarrassment, humiliation, discrimination, or stigmatization. Social harms are real harms that are just as much a threat to the rights and welfare of research participants as physical harms. To identify the risks of research participation, as well as to structure research to minimize such risk, it may be important to understand the difference between social and physical harm. However, from the standpoint of a conceptual model for thinking about the ethics of research and research regulation, there is no reason to make a distinction between social and physical risks of research participation.

Privacy and Confidentiality

Social science research rarely involves a risk of serious physical harm, but biomedical research often involves an important risk of social harm, either as the primary risk of research participation or in addition to the risk of physical harm. This latter point deserves some emphasis. For those who find it useful to use a social science versus biomedical approach to thinking about research regulation, it is important to understand that modern biomedical research often involves a risk of both social and physical harm. This is especially true with studies that evaluate a condition that is socially stigmatizing, for example, sexually transmitted disease, sexual dysfunction, and psychiatric disorders. A wide range of other aspects of biomedical research imposes a risk of social harm for research participants. Advances in the understanding of the genetic basis of human physiology and disease have been a major factor in focusing attention on the social risk associated with participation in

biomedical research. The importance of this aspect of biomedical research will certainly increase in the future.

Social harm is a result of the creation or transfer of information in a way that may negatively affect the research subject. Whenever the risk of research is related to access to information, IRB review will focus on the protection of privacy and confidentiality. It is for this reason that a major focus of the IRB review of social science research usually involves evaluation of things such as the nature of the information being collected, the mechanism of identifying potential subjects, and the implications of a breach in confidentiality. Other areas of emphasis are the plans for protecting privacy and confidentiality and the likelihood that potential subjects will understand the nature of the social risks associated with research participation. Privacy and confidentiality are also important in biomedical research projects, and IRB review of both social science and biomedical research should consider these important issues.

Considering Separate Social Science and Biomedical IRBs

What specific issues should the IRB leadership consider when deciding whether social science and biomedical research should be reviewed by separate IRB committees? Although we hope that our treatment of this issue is balanced, it is important to recognize that all authors write from a perspective that has been shaped by their experience and training. With this in mind, it may be useful for the reader to understand that the authors of this chapter directed the IRB at Dartmouth College. Dartmouth used a single IRB to monitor a wide range and moderately large volume of both social science and biomedical research. In our experience, the single-committee approach worked well. Indeed, most members of the Dartmouth research community, IRB, and research administration see important advantages to organizing the IRB review in a way that focuses on the similarities between social science and biomedical research.

Specialization

The main argument one hears for separate IRB review of social science and biomedical research is that this type of specialization increases the quality and efficiency of issue specialization by the IRB. Social scientists are intimately familiar with the techniques, theory, and standards of social science research. Similarly, an IRB composed of physicians is more likely to understand the issues pertinent to biomedical research. In theory, organizing an IRB in a way that concentrates issue-specific expertise could increase the efficiency and effectiveness of IRB review. However, given the increasing complexity of both social science and biomedical research and the increased awareness of the importance of the risk of social harm in biomedical studies, the segregation of IRB expertise may be counterproductive. There is now a large degree of overlap in the issues that the IRB must consider when reviewing social science or biomedical research projects. Our current IRB system is based on the concept that input from people with a wide range of expertise and perspective will improve the ethical standards of research. In our experience, an IRB with the expertise to review both social science and biomedical research functions more effectively than either group alone.

Workload

A factor that may influence the decision to use separate IRBs is workload distribution. At institutions where the workload is too high for a single IRB, it will be desirable to divide the work of research regulation between multiple separate IRB committees. When workload requires multiple IRBs and segregating IRB work based on a social science versus biomedical model would result in an acceptable work distribution, then the simplest way to triage protocols may be with a social science versus biomedical approach. However, segregating IRB review based on research type may limit flexibility from the administrative standpoint. The trade-off between these factors at any given institution will depend on the characteristics of IRB members and the scope of the research that is presented for IRB review. In our opinion, the optimal model is to structure all IRBs so that they have the expertise to review both social science and biomedical research.

Conclusion

At many institutions that conduct both social science and biomedical research, IRB review of these two general categories of research is assigned to separate IRB committees. This organizational structure may suggest that there is a fundamental difference between social science and biomedical research in terms of ethical issues and the process of IRB review. There is no question that many biomedical research issues are not applicable to social science. However, the quality of research review will be enhanced by requiring that members of both disciplines contribute their expertise and unique perspective on research involving human subjects, rather than segregating the discussion of social science and biomedical issues. In most situations, the quality of IRB review of research will be enhanced by constructing IRBs so that both social science and biomedical research may be reviewed by the same committee.

Reference

1. Code of Federal Regulations. Title 45A—Department of Health and Human Services; Part 46—Protection of Human Subjects. Updated 1 October, 1997. Access date 18 April, 2001. http://www4.law.cornell.edu/cfr/45p46.htm

PART 4

Review Categories

Exempt from Institutional Review Board Review

Ernest D. Prentice and Gwenn S. F. Oki

INTRODUCTION

Many educational, behavioral, and social science studies present little or no risk to the participants. Likewise, research involving existing data, medical records, and pathologic specimens usually has little, if any, associated risk, particularly if subject identifiers are removed from the data or specimens. Thus, although the rights and welfare of subjects in those studies still require protection, there is usually no need for a detailed institutional review board (IRB) review, the equivalent of the kind performed at a convened meeting of the IRB. Accordingly, certain research activities are exempt from compliance with Department of Health and Human Services (DHHS) regulations for the protection of human subjects.[1] The purpose of this chapter is to assist IRBs in understanding what exempt research means and how to determine what types of research qualify for exempt status.

What Is Exempt Research?

DHHS regulations[1][Sec.101(b)] describe six categories of research that may qualify for exempt status. Although the regulations do not address a maximum risk level, it is implicit within the concept of exempt research that there must be very little, if any, associated risk. Therefore, research that qualifies for exemption from the requirements of 45 CFR 46 must meet the aforementioned risk threshold and fall within one or more of the six exempt categories. Research involving prisoners is, however, not exempt from the federal regulations because this class of subjects is considered vulnerable.[1][Sec.101(i)] Survey research involving children is also not exempt, nor is observation of a minor's public behavior unless the investigator does not participate in the activities being observed.[1][Sec.401(b)] In addition, some IRBs exclude research involving the decisionally impaired from exempt status as well as other subjects who they consider vulnerable, such as the homeless or nursing home residents. However, all of the exemptions are applicable to research involving pregnant women, human fetuses, and neonates, which is a change in 45 CFR 46 Subpart B that occurred in 2001.

Who Determines That a Protocol Is Exempt?

The regulations do not specify who has or does not have the authority to decide whether a research project is exempt. At most institutions, the IRB administrative staff and/or IRB chair/chair designate make this determination. However, the regulations contain no prohibition that would restrict the researcher, department director, or others from determining that a project meets an exempt category. Recognizing that this is an area where federal regulations are silent, the Office of Human Research Protection recommends that the decision to exempt a study from IRB review be made by someone other than a research investigator associated with the project. Many investigators do not have sufficient knowledge of the federal regulations to determine properly, in all cases, whether research is exempt. In addition, investigators have an obvious conflict of interest. To avoid the confusion that may be associated with determining which studies are exempt from IRB review, some organizations choose not to exempt any projects and use either expedited review or review by the full IRB for all human subjects research. An IRB can, however, still classify a study as exempt even though it was reviewed by the full IRB or through the expedited method. This is an important determination that should be documented because research classified as exempt is not subject to continuing review and the other requirements of 45 CFR 46.

Written Policy Regarding Exempt Status

If an institution allows research to be exempt under the provisions of 45 CFR 46,[1][Sec.101(b)] it is important for the IRB to have a clear policy that allows for research that is technically exempt to be referred for further review or even be disqualified from exempt status altogether. Accordingly, any research project submitted by an investigator who requests an exemption should be carefully reviewed to determine whether the project qualifies for exempt status. This review should be designed to identify any potential problems or ethical considerations that may impact the subjects. Any needed clarifications or modifications of the protocol should be obtained from the investigator. A determination should also be made concerning whether informed consent is necessary. The regulations do not require consent for exempt research, but there may be an ethical imperative for full disclosure of the project, even including use of a written consent form that should be submitted to the appropriate IRB representative(s) for approval. Depending on the nature of the research, the consent form may include most of the elements of consent prescribed by 45 CFR 46.[1[Sec.116]]

Food and Drug Administration Regulations Do Not Exempt Research from IRB Review

It is important to understand that Food and Drug Administration (FDA) regulations for the protection of human subjects[2] do not have categories of research that qualify for exempt status like those listed by DHHS.[1[Sec.101(b)]] The FDA does not exempt any research under its jurisdiction from IRB review except in emergency circumstances[2[Sec.104(c)]] and taste and food quality studies[2[Sec.104(d)]] (the same as exemption category 6 under the DHHS regulations). Because the FDA primarily regulates clinical trials involving investigational drugs, biologics, and medical devices, there is no need for expanded exemptions.

Categories of Exempt Research

The following are the six categories of exempt research specified by DHHS.[1[Sec.101(b)]] Because the exempt categories can be problematic in terms of interpretation and application, the authors have included notes that will hopefully assist in making decisions concerning research activities that qualify for exempt status.

Exemption 1: Normal Educational Practices and Settings

Research conducted in established or commonly accepted educational settings, involving normal educational practices, such as (i) research on regular and special education instructional strategies, or (ii) research on the effectiveness of or the comparison among instructional techniques, curricula, or classroom management methods.

Exemption 1 should be limited to the study of normal educational practices that will be conducted in commonly accepted settings such as elementary, secondary, or postsecondary schools. Thus, a study that involves evaluation of a radically new instructional strategy or use of random assignment of subjects to different instructional methods is usually not exempt because the methods employed in the studies deviate from normal educational practices. Certainly, educational research that involves deception or withholding of information from subjects should not be exempt. Exemptions should also not be routinely granted for research on physical education that involves exercise if the activity is altered in a significant way for the purposes of the research. Even though the exercise may still be considered normal educational practice, an element of risk may be introduced with physical activity, particularly if it is intense exercise.

Exemption 2: Anonymous Educational Tests, Surveys, Interviews, or Observations

Research involving the use of educational tests (cognitive, diagnostic, aptitude, achievement), survey procedures, interview procedures, or observations of public behavior, unless: (i) information obtained is recorded in such a manner that human subjects can be identified, directly or through identifiers linked to the subjects; and (ii) any disclosure of the human subjects' responses outside the research could reasonably place the subjects at risk of criminal or civil liability or be damaging to the subjects' financial standing, employability, or reputation.

Exemption 2 clearly reflects concern about protecting the subject's privacy and avoiding any risks associated with breach of confidentiality. Thus, if the research data contain any subject identifiers and if disclosure of data to unauthorized persons could harm the subject in any way, then the research is not exempt. For example, survey research that deals with sensitive and private aspects of the subject's behavior, such as sexual preferences, substance abuse, or illegal conduct, is not exempt if the data are linked to individual subjects. If there are no subject identifiers, then the research is technically exempt. The IRB, however, should consider all potential risks associated with this kind of research in determining exempt status. In the example previously given, there may be more than minimal risk involved even in the absence of subject identifiers. Such surveys often contain invasive questions that may cause the subject to experience emotional distress or discomfort while answering them. Thus, although the research technically qualifies for exemption because there are no subject identifiers, the potential risks of the research should negate exemption. Indeed, such research should use an unsigned consent form that clearly describes the nature and possible risks of the research. Research involving cognitive or diagnostic testing should not normally be exempt if the testing is psychologically invasive in nature (e.g., detailed personality inventory) and could potentially cause the subject some discomfort or distress. Again, although the research is technically exempt if there are no subject identifiers, it should be considered as nonexempt research because of the risk level. Also, IRBs should guard against the possibility that an investigator may inappropriately characterize testing as normal educational practice and apply for exempt status under Exemption 1, which is less stringent in its requirements than Exemption 2.

Exemption 3: Identifiable Subjects in Special Circumstances

Research involving the use of educational tests (cognitive, diagnostic, aptitude, achievement), survey procedures, interview procedures, or observation of public behavior that is not exempt under paragraph (b)(2) of this section, if: (i) the human subjects are elected or appointed public officials or candidates for public office; or (ii) the federal statute(s) require(s) without exception that the confidentiality of the personally identifiable information will be maintained throughout the research and thereafter.

Exemption 3 represents an extension of Exemption 2, but without the same level of oversight of the subject's right to privacy. Personal identifiers can be maintained if there is a federal statute that protects confidentiality or if the subject is either a public official or a candidate for public office. Exemption 3 effectively holds public officials who become research subjects to a different standard by providing less protection of their rights than for other members of society. Nevertheless, despite the loophole created by this exemption, the rights of individuals who hold public office should obviously be protected by conducting a thorough review of the proposed research as previously addressed.

Exemption 4: Collection or Study of Existing Data

Research involving the collection or study of existing data, documents, records, pathological specimens, or diagnostic specimens, if these sources are publicly available or if the information is recorded by the investigator in such a manner that subjects cannot be identified, directly or through identifiers linked to the subjects.

Exemption 4 is the most used and often the most problematic category of exempt research conducted at academic medical centers, particularly because the Health Insurance Portability and Accountability Act or HIPAA Privacy Rule (45 CFR 160 and 164) applies to research involving protected health information but does not recognize exemptions. For research to qualify for exempt status under Exemption 4, the information derived from use of the data, records, or biological specimens must be recorded so that subjects cannot be identified. This means there must be no direct or indirect subject identifiers (e.g., demographic information) that can be linked to the subjects. Some investigators erroneously assume that if they do not have access to the subject's name, which is, however, linked to the data or specimen, the research is exempt. However, the existence of even a one-way identifier, such as a code that can then be used to identify a subject, disqualifies the research from exemption under Category 4. It should also be noted that the research material must be existent ("on-the-shelf") at the time the research begins. Any use of additional research material collected after the research is initiated constitutes a prospective study and obviously disqualifies the study from exempt status. In other words, exempt research under Exemption 4 must be totally retrospective in nature. In addition, IRBs that also serve as privacy boards must consider the HIPAA Privacy Rule (45 CFR 160 and 164)[3] as they relate to use and disclosure of protected health information.

Exemption 5: Public Benefit or Service Programs

Research and demonstration projects that are conducted by or subject to the approval of department or agency heads, and which

are designed to study, evaluate, or otherwise examine: (i) public benefit or service programs; (ii) procedures for obtaining benefits or services under those programs; (iii) possible changes in or alternatives to those programs or procedures; and (iv) possible changes in methods or levels of payment for benefits or services under those programs.

Exemption 5 allows research on public benefit or service programs, such as welfare, Medicaid, unemployment, and Social Security. This research may, however, involve vulnerable subjects such as economically disadvantaged persons or elderly individuals who are decisionally impaired. Research under Exemption 5 may also involve analysis of data that are routinely compiled by the public office that administers the program but would be considered private by the subject. Again, a thorough review of the research project can help protect the rights and welfare of the participants, particularly those who may be vulnerable.

Exemption 6: Taste and Food Evaluation and Acceptance Studies

Taste and food quality evaluation and consumer acceptance studies, (i) if wholesome foods without additives are consumed or (ii) if a food is consumed that contains a food ingredient at or below the level for a use found to be safe, or agricultural chemical or environmental contaminant at or below the level found to be safe, by the Food and Drug Administration or approved by the Environmental Protection Agency or the Food Safety and Inspection Service of the U.S. Department of Agriculture.

Exemption 6 should be limited to taste and food quality evaluation studies that do not involve consumption by the subject of any type or volume of food that has any potential risks such as indigestion or vitamin deficiencies. Clearly, the food consumed by the subject and the time frame in which this is accomplished should constitute reasonable eating behaviors. Studies that involve consumption of alcohol, vitamins, or supplements such as protein power, creatine, and glucosamine chondroitin sulfate should not qualify for exempt status.

Conclusion

Correct application of the exempt categories at 45 CFR 46.101(b) can be one of the most difficult tasks facing the IRB staff and/or IRB chair/chair designee. On the one hand, some investigators regard exempt research as being more or less exempt from any kind of review because DHHS regulations in 45 CFR 46 do not apply. On the other hand, the participants in exempt research are, in fact, human subjects who have rights that must be fully protected. In some cases, research that is technically exempt has associated risk that is greater than minimal. Clearly, such research presents a compelling ethical argument for performing a thorough review and possibly disqualifying the research project from exempt status altogether. IRBs, therefore, should have a well thought out policy concerning exempt research and should remember that 45 CFR 46 sets the minimum standard. Institutions are expected to adopt more stringent requirements for the protection of human subjects as the need arises. Certainly, the area of exempt research is a case in point where IRBs should, at times, look beyond the regulations. Finally, with the promulgation of the HIPAA Privacy Rule, IRBs that also serve as privacy boards must be cognizant of the requirements governing the use and disclosure of protected health information.

References

1. Code of Federal Regulations. Title 45A—Department of Health and Human Services; Part 46—Protection of Human Subjects. Updated 1 October, 1997. Access date 18 April, 2001. http://www4.law.cornell.edu/cfr/45p46.htm

2. Code of Federal Regulations. Title 21, Chapter 1—Food and Drug Administration, DHHS; Part 56—Institutional Review Boards. Updated 1 April, 1999. Access date 27 March, 2001. http://www4.law.cornell.edu/cfr/21p56.htm

3. Code of Federal Regulations. Title 45, DHHS; Parts 160 and 164—Standards for Privacy of Individually Identifiable Health Information.

Expedited Institutional Review Board Review

Gwenn S. F. Oki and John A. Zaia

INTRODUCTION

The Department of Health and Human Services (DHHS) and the Food and Drug Administration (FDA) regulations for the protection of human subjects[1,2] recognize that not all research warrants review by the full institutional review board (IRB) at a convened meeting. Accordingly, DHHS regulations at 45 CFR 46[1] and FDA regulations at 21 CFR 56[2(Sec.110)] permit certain types of research to be reviewed and approved by expedited review. The purpose of this chapter is to assist IRBs in understanding what expedited review means and, in addition, how this type of review should be affected.

Definition of Expedited Review

Expedited review is a type of review that can be conducted by the IRB chair, other IRB members designated by the chair, or a subcommittee of the IRB.[1(Sec.110(b)),2] The IRB members designated to conduct expedited review must be experienced reviewers who are also voting members. Reviewers are empowered by the regulations to approve research qualifying for expedited review or to require modifications of a study to gain approval. The regulations, however, prohibit disapproval of any research reviewed using the expedited method and require that such "proposed disapprovals" be referred to the full board for review and disposition. Therefore, the IRB chair or chair designee(s) may exercise all of the authority of the IRB to review research qualifying for expedited review but does not have the authority to disapprove such research. The full IRB must be notified of all research projects ultimately approved using the expedited review process. Although the regulations are silent on the rationale for this notification, it is clear that the full IRB has the authority to question any approval granted through expedited review.

General Eligibility Criteria for Expedited Review

DHHS[1(Sec.110(b))] and FDA regulations[2(Sec.110(b))] refer to two general categories that can qualify for expedited review: (1) research activities that present no more than minimal risk and are listed in a National Institutes of Health guidance document[3] as an "adjunct" to the DHHS and FDA regulations and (2) "minor changes in previously approved research during the period (of one year or less) for

which approval is granted." In contrast to research activities that can be initially reviewed and approved by the expedited method, a risk threshold for expedited review of minor changes is not specified. The concept of minor, however, implies that the allowable risk associated with the change is either no more than minimum or the risk–benefit relationship of the research is not altered in a way that makes it less favorable.

A major criterion for research that can be initially reviewed through the expedited process is that it must involve no more than minimal risk. Therefore, a review of the definition of minimal risk is warranted. The DHHS regulations[1(Sec.102(i))] and FDA regulations[2(Sec.102(i))] define minimal risk to mean that "the probability and magnitude of harm or discomfort anticipated in the research are not greater in and of themselves than those ordinarily encountered in the daily life or during performance of routine physical or psychological examinations or tests." Based on the interpretation by the Office for Human Research Protections, minimal risk is determined to be relative to the daily life of a normal, healthy person. Therefore, the risk threshold of what constitutes minimal risk cannot increase just because the subject is sick and faces greater risks because of the illness or because of the medical or psychological interventions that would be expected. In fact, just the opposite may be true, and even the normal, healthy person standard of minimal risk may be too high in certain circumstances. For example, a study involving a relatively minor procedure such as a venipuncture, considered to be minimal risk in the life of a normal, healthy individual, would constitute more than minimal risk in the hemophilia population. Therefore, IRBs need to be cognizant of the restrictions and considerations related to determining whether a research project actually is associated with no more than minimal risk.

As mentioned previously, a minor modification of a currently approved protocol can be reviewed by the expedited process. Although the regulations do not specify what types of modifications would qualify as minor changes, common sense dictates that expedited review could be used to approve administrative changes such as routine closure of a study to new subject accrual. In addition, minor clarification of eligibility criteria, consent form clarifications, changes in advertisements, addition of monitoring procedures that are on the adjunct list, and other no more than minimal-risk changes would qualify. Any change that includes an intervention that is greater than minimal risk or that may negatively impact the risk–benefit relationship of the research should normally be referred to the full board for review.

Criteria for Approval of Research Using Expedited Review

In addition to meeting the general eligibility criteria previously indicated, research qualifying for expedited review must also meet the approval criteria defined by the DHHS[1(Sec.111)] and the FDA.[2(Sec.111)] These are briefly summarized as follows:

1. The proposed procedures must be consistent with sound research design, and when possible, procedures already being performed on subjects should be used. For example, obtaining additional blood at the time of routine venipuncture is preferred rather than doing an extra needle stick to obtain the research sample.

2. The risks of the research must be reasonable in relationship to the anticipated benefits, if any, to the subjects and the importance of the knowledge that may be gained.

3. Subject selection must be equitable.

4. Informed consent should be sought and documented unless a waiver of consent and/or documentation of consent has met the waiver criteria at 45 CFR 46.[1(Sec.116(d),117(c))] The requirements for informed consent found at 45 CFR 46[1(Sec.116)] and 21 CFR 50[4(Sec.20,25,27)] have been reviewed extensively in Part 6 of this book. If a waiver of informed consent is granted, IRBs that also serve as privacy boards must consider the Health Insurance Portability and Accountability Act or HIPAA privacy rules (45 CFR 160 and 164)[5] as they relate to human subjects research at 45 CFR 164.512. The criteria for waiver of HIPAA authorization are reviewed later in this book.

5. Where appropriate, there is a plan to collect and monitor data to ensure subject safety.

6. The privacy of subjects and maintenance of confidentiality of data are protected. IRBs also fulfilling the role of privacy board should be cognizant of the HIPAA regulations as they relate to these issues.

7. Where necessary, additional safeguards have been included to protect vulnerable subjects.

Finally, as mentioned previously, research approved by the expedited method must be communicated to the full board. This can be accomplished by providing a list of all such approved studies accompanied by a brief synopsis of the nature of the research and the expedited category under which the research qualifies for review. All IRB members will then have the opportunity to review the list and ask questions and, thus, are kept informed of the activities of the IRB outside of full board deliberations.

Adjunct List of Categories Qualifying for Expedited Review

The "applicability" standards that preface the nine categories of research indicate a strong warning regarding potential risks to research subjects who can be identified. In addition, subjects whose responses could reasonably place them at risk for criminal or civil liability, be damaging to their financial standing, insurability, reputation, or be stigmatizing may be at risk unless appropriate mechanisms to prevent breaches of confidentiality or privacy are in place. Studies that have this potential should be referred for review by the full board, rather than by a designated reviewer.

In consideration of the applicability standards for expedited review and because some of the activities listed could raise issues and problems related to interpretation, the authors have provided relevant examples and guidance under each of the nine categories on the adjunct list that qualify for expedited review.[3] The examples and guidance are not meant to be comprehensive.

Category 1

Clinical studies of drugs and medical devices only when condition (a) or (b) is met. (a) Research on drugs for which an investigational new drug application (21 CFR Part 312) is not required. (b) Research on medical devices for which (i) an investigational device exemption application (21 CFR Part 812) is not required, or (ii) the medical device is cleared/approved for marketing and the medical device is being used in accordance with its cleared/approved labeling.

Although this is an allowable category of expedited review, the authors are hard pressed to find an applicable example. It appears that the minimal risk threshold would be exceeded by the very nature of studies involving drugs and/or devices. Indeed, of the IRB administrators canvassed, none has used this category as justification for conducting expedited review.

Category 2

Collection of blood samples by finger stick, heel stick, ear stick, or venipuncture as follows: (a) from healthy, nonpregnant adults who weigh at least 110 pounds. For these subjects, the amounts drawn may not exceed 550 ml in an 8-week period and collection may not occur more frequently than 2 times per week; or (b) from other adults and children, considering the age, weight, and health of the subjects, the collection procedure, the amount of blood to be collected, and the frequency with which it will be collected. For these subjects, the amount drawn may not exceed the lesser of 50 ml or 3 ml per kg in an 8-week period and collection may not occur more frequently than 2 times per week.

This category description is very detailed and does not appear to require any examples to facilitate understanding.

However, expedited review of research that fits this category that involves very small children and infants warrants a cautionary approach based on health status, frequency of venipuncture, and blood volumes. Although the physical risks in the pediatric population may be very low when the blood volumes to be drawn are safe and appropriate for age and weight, consideration should be given to needle phobia associated with children's real and perceived fear of a venipuncture. Indeed, where minors are concerned, all efforts should be made to obtain the additional research sample at the time of routine venipuncture, rather than necessitate a separate, additional needle stick. Some IRBs have gone so far as to prohibit research venipuncture in minors unless it is done at the time of routine blood draw, thereby completely avoiding an extra needle stick.

Category 3

Prospective collection of biological specimens for research purposes by noninvasive means. Examples: (a) hair and nail clippings in a nondisfiguring manner; (b) deciduous teeth at time of exfoliation or if routine patient care indicates a need for extraction; (c) permanent teeth if routine patient care indicates a need for extraction; (d) excreta and external secretions (including sweat); (e) uncannulated saliva collected either in an unstimulated fashion or stimulated by chewing gumbase or wax or by applying a dilute citric solution to the tongue; (f) placenta removal at delivery; (g) amniotic fluid obtained at the time of rupture of the membrane before or during labor; (h) supragingival and subgingival dental plaque and calculus, provided the collection procedure is not more invasive than routine prophylactic scaling of the teeth and the process is accomplished in accordance with accepted prophylactic techniques; (i) mucosal and skin cells collected by buccal scraping or swab, skin swab, or mouth washings; and (j) sputum collected after saline mist nebulization.

This category description is also very detailed and does not appear to require examples to facilitate understanding. However, any specimens collected for use in research involving DNA testing or in search of a new way to test for pathogenic organisms that could be deemed potentially sensitive should be carefully reviewed. Such studies may ultimately require referral to the full IRB. Clearly, such research may present more than minimal risk to subjects.

Category 4

Collection of data through noninvasive procedures (not involving general anesthesia or sedation) routinely employed in clinical practice, excluding procedures involving x-rays or microwaves. Where medical devices are employed, they must be cleared/approved for marketing. (Studies intended to evaluate the safety and effectiveness of the medical device are not generally eligible for expedited review, including studies of cleared medical devices for new indications.) Examples: (a) physical sensors that are applied either to the surface of the body or at a distance and do not involve input of significant amounts of energy into the subject or an invasion of the subject's privacy; (b) weighing or testing sensory acuity; (c) magnetic resonance imaging; (d) electrocardiography, electroencephalography, thermography, detection of naturally occurring radioactivity, electroretinoraphy, ultrasound, diagnostic infrared imaging, Doppler blood flow, and echocardiography; (e) moderate exercise, muscular strength testing, body composition assessment,

and flexibility testing where appropriate given the age, weight, and health of the individual.

This category contains a number of routine clinical tests that present no more than minimal risk and would routinely qualify for expedited review. Possible exceptions are exercise, strength testing, and flexibility testing. For example, a study on the health effects of moderate exercise over a 6-month period on the overall well-being of senior citizens with mild arthritis, which involves strength testing, noninvasive cardiac monitoring, and use of quality-of-life questionnaires, is research that would qualify for expedited review in Category 4. On the other hand, the same study using a more debilitated subject population would likely not qualify for expedited review because the risks associated with the exercise and strength testing could pose more than minimal risk.

Category 5

Research involving materials (data, documents, records, or specimens) that have been collected, or will be collected solely for nonresearch purposes (such as medical treatment or diagnosis).

Research using retrospectively or prospectively collected, routine medical record information or leftover specimens collected at the time of clinical care would qualify in this category of expedited review, if the information is not considered sensitive and any potential breach of confidentiality would not be damaging to the subject. Research using the medical records of HIV-positive patients is an example of a study that should not be reviewed by the expedited method.

Category 6

Collection of data from voice, video, digital, or image recordings made for research purposes.

Depending on the nature of the study, the IRB must carefully review the types of information that will be recorded. The IRB must determine whether the study would involve information considered sensitive or potentially damaging to the subject's financial standing, employability, insurability, reputation, etc., if his or her voice or (still or moving) image could be identified. The IRB must ensure that appropriate safeguards are in place to prevent any potential harm that may be associated with a breach of confidentiality. For example, if the subject is asked to describe verbally his or her working conditions in a sweatshop and his or her voice could be recognized, appropriate mechanisms should be used to disguise the subject's voice to prevent any potential harm such as loss of employment. Such a study should not be reviewed by the expedited method.

Category 7

Research on group characteristics or behavior (including, but not limited to, research on perception, cognition, motivation, identity, language, communication, cultural beliefs or practices, and social behavior) or research employing survey, interview, oral history, focus group, program evaluation, human factors evaluation, or quality assurance methodologies.

Survey research studies on intelligence or other traits involving specific populations, for example, ethnic groups or patient groups, require careful analysis because this type of research, depending on the nature of the survey questions, could result in stigmatization of a segment of society. For example, the results of research involving standardized IQ scores of a particular ethnic group correlated with their socioeconomic status and the educational levels of their parents may potentially be stigmatizing. This is particularly true if the general cultural background of the subjects becomes known or the patient group can be identified (e.g., women at high risk for breast cancer from a specific geographic area). Although research of this nature clearly fits this expeditable category, many issues, particularly the potential for stigmatization of a class of individuals and issues related to privacy and confidentiality, must be considered so that the subjects are protected. Thus, such research should be reviewed by the full IRB.

Category 8

Continuing review of research previously approved by a convened IRB as follows: (a) where (i) the research is permanently closed to the enrollment of new subjects; (ii) all subjects have completed all research-related interventions; and (iii) the research remains active only for the long term follow-up of subjects; or (b) where no subjects have been enrolled and no additional risks have been identified; or (c) where the remaining research activities are limited to data analysis.

Examples of 8(a) would be a cooperative group clinical trial when the study is closed to new accrual or a study where all subjects have completed active treatment and are in routine clinical follow-up with only the data being used for research. Item 8(b) is somewhat more complex. Although subjects may not have been enrolled during the time period that the study has been open to accrual, the IRB is charged with ensuring that there is no new information about risk. If new risks have been identified, the full IRB must perform continuing review.

Category 9

Continuing review of research not conducted under an investigational new drug application or investigational drug exemption where categories two (2) through eight (8) do not apply but the IRB has determined and documented at a convened meeting that the research involves no greater than minimal risk and no additional risks have been identified.

As indicated previously, initial review of research by the expedited method is limited to only those activities that meet one or more of the categories specified on the adjunct list. However, at the time of full-board review, the IRB may decide that although the research did not appear to qualify for expedited review initially, it is, nevertheless, no more than minimal risk. Therefore, at the time of continuing review, the expedited review process can be used. This determination must be documented at a convened meeting of the IRB and can be implemented if no additional risks are identified when this decision is made.

Conclusion

Some research projects simply do not warrant review by the full IRB in order to protect the rights and welfare of the subjects. Thus, appropriate use of expedited review helps reduce the workload of the full IRB and, ideally, decreases IRB turnaround time. However, whether expedited review actually results in a faster review and turnaround time is, in reality, dependent on the IRB administrative workload and/or the availability of the IRB chair or his or her designee. Nonetheless, it must be stressed that regardless of whether a research proposal is reviewed by the expedited method or by the full IRB, the same regulatory and ethically based standards apply.

References

1. Code of Federal Regulations. Title 45A—Department of Health and Human Services; Part 46—Protection of Human Subjects. Updated 1 October, 1997. Access date 18 April, 2001. http://www4.law.cornell.edu/cfr/45p46.htm

2. Code of Federal Regulations. Title 21, Chapter 1—Food and Drug Administration, DHHS; Part 56—Institutional Review Boards. Updated 1 April, 1999. Access date 27 March, 2001. http://www4.law.cornell.edu/cfr/21p56.htm

3. National Institutes of Health. Protection of human subjects: Categories of research that may be reviewed by the Institutional Review Board (IRB) through an expedited review procedure. *Fed Regist* 63(216):60364–60367, 1998. http://ohrp.osophs.dhhs.gov/humansubjects/guidance/63fr60364.htm

4. Code of Federal Regulations. Title 21, Chapter 1—Food and Drug Administration, DHHS; Part 50—Protection of Human Subjects. Updated 1 April, 1999. Access date 18 April, 2001. http://www4.law.cornell.edu/cfr/21p50.htm

5. Code of Federal Regulations. Title 45, DHHS; Parts 160 and 164—Standards for Privacy of Individually Identifiable Health Information.

Identifying Intent: Is This Project Research?

Robert J. Amdur, Marjorie Speers, and Elizabeth Bankert

INTRODUCTION

Federal regulations give the institutional review board (IRB) the authority to oversee research involving human subjects. The IRB has no regulatory authority to oversee activities that are legitimately classified as something other than research. Many institutions and IRBs prefer to have nonresearch activities handled by an entity other than the IRB so that the IRB can focus all of its time and resources on managing its fundamental mission. To triage projects away from the IRB, it is essential to develop standard operating procedures that describe how an institution decides when it is acceptable to classify a project as a nonresearch activity. After development, it is important for the institution to disseminate the information clearly. The reviewing entity(s), whether it is the department chairman, a quality improvement committee, or the IRB, needs to be aware of the nuances of the levels of review and be able to work together to ensure that each project is handled in a consistent, efficient manner. The purpose of this chapter is to explain the concepts needed to define research intent and to provide discussion related to nonresearch activities.

The Regulatory Definition of Research and Human Subject

Federal research regulations and the Health Insurance Portability and Accountability Act of 1996 (HIPAA) define research as "a systematic investigation, including research development, testing, and evaluation, designed to develop or contribute to generalizable knowledge."[1]

When evaluating a specific project, it is useful to think of this definition as a requirement for two key elements: (1) the project involves a systematic investigation, and (2) the design—meaning goal, purpose, or intent—of the investigation is to develop or contribute to generalizable knowledge.

The first of these two elements—the use of a systematic investigation—may be a characteristic of both research and nonresearch projects. Public health practice, quality assessment (QA) and quality improvement (QI) programs, resource utilization reviews, and outcome analyses are examples of nonresearch activities that frequently use statistical analyses and other scientific methods to collect and analyze data in a manner that is identical to that of research studies. All medical research involves a systematic approach to data collection and analysis, but the use of a systematic investigation does not mean that an activity should be classified as research.

The second element of research is that the primary reason for conducting the activity is to develop or contribute to generalizable knowledge. Just as with the first element of the definition of research (a systematic investigation), this second element is not unique to research activities. For example, the main purpose of most education programs is to bring new knowledge to as many people as possible. Similarly, an integral part of many quality assessment and improvement projects is the dissemination of results to people who may be in a position to benefit from this kind of information.

The regulations require an activity to have two main features to be classified as research. First, the activity must be characterized by a *systematic investigation*, and second, *the primary goal of the activity must be to develop or contribute to generalizable knowledge.* Having only one of these properties means that the activity is *not* research and should not be handled as such from the IRB standpoint.

After a project has been designated "research" as defined by the federal regulations, the next step is to determine whether the project involves "human subjects." DHHS 45 CFR 46[1[Sec.102(f)]] states:

Human subject means a living individual about whom an investigator (whether professional or student) conducting research obtains

(1) data through intervention or interaction with the individual, or

(2) identifiable private information.

Intervention includes both physical procedures by which data are gathered (for example, venipuncture) and manipulations of the subject or the subject's environment that are performed for research purposes. *Interaction* includes communication or interpersonal contact between investigator and subject. *Private information* includes information about behavior that occurs in a context in which an individual can reasonably expect that no observation or recording is taking place, and information which has been provided for specific purposes by an individual and which the individual can reasonably expect will not be made public (for example, a medical record). Private information must be individually identifiable (i.e., the identity of the subject is or may readily be ascertained by the investigator or associated with the information) in order for obtaining the information to constitute research involving human subjects.

In order for a project to require IRB review, it must both be research and involve "human subjects." For more information, please review Office for Human Research Protections (OHRP) guidance at http://www.hhs.gov/ohrp/humansubjects/guidance/decisioncharts.htm#c1

The Defining Characteristic of Research Involving Human Subjects

The requirement that a research activity involves a systematic investigation is usually not difficult to apply. To develop a test to evaluate better the goal of developing or contributing to generalizable knowledge, it is useful to recognize that in the context of research that involves human subjects, the defining characteristic of research is that *a major goal of the activity is to learn something for the purpose of benefiting people other than the research subjects.* In some classes of research, the research subjects may directly benefit from research participation, but benefiting research subjects is never the only, and rarely the primary, goal of a research effort. The terms *innovative therapy* and *nonvalidated practice* describe activities that are designed solely to benefit an individual patient(s), but in which the ability of the activity to result in the desired outcome is to some degree unproven.

Publication of Results Does Not Define a Project as Research

To determine whether a project should be classified as research, some IRBs base institutional policy on the assumption that publication of results in a scientific journal defines a project as research. Project investigators are told that if they "hope to" or "might want to" publish results of their project in a medical journal or present some aspect of the project at an academic meeting, then the project involves research and should not be done without IRB approval. At some institutions, project investigators are told that if a project is or was done without IRB approval, then institutional policy prohibits them from publishing project results, as this would document noncompliance with federal research regulations. An information document from the Food and Drug Administration on Humanitarian Use Devices suggests that this approach to identifying research intent is not unique to the IRB community.[2]

The assumption that academic publication or presentation equals research is incorrect. Publication or presentation of results is clearly the goal of all research activity, but there are many situations in which academic forums are used to share the results of a nonresearch activity with interested colleagues in the hope that they will benefit from this information. Medical journals often contain articles that discuss information that is not the result of research activity, and the same is true with medical meeting agendas.[3,4,5] *Education*, not *research*, is the most accurate term for these kinds of activities. It is appropriate to inform project investigators that nonresearch activities can be published, but it is necessary to remind them that the word *research* cannot be contained within the publication. If *research* is used to describe the project, IRB review is required, and journal editors may inquire about the status of IRB review.

Would you conduct this project as planned if you knew you would never receive any form of academic recognition for it?

To classify projects accurately as either research or nonresearch, a critical factor may be the extent to which the project is being conducted to benefit people other than those who will participate directly in the activity. In our experience, questions about the publication or presentation of results in an academic forum are the most useful way to evaluate research intent, but the focus of the question should be different than as described previously here.

The important question is not whether the project investigator might want to publish or present results in the future, but rather if the project would be done as planned if academic recognition is definitely not a possibility. Our recommendation is that the IRB use the following question to determine whether a project that involves a systematic investigation and is likely to develop generalizable knowledge should be classified as research from the regulatory standpoint:

Would this project be conducted as proposed if the project investigator knew that he or she would never receive any form of academic recognition for the project, including publication of results in a medical journal or presentation of the project at an academic meeting?

If prohibition from receiving any form of academic recognition for the project would affect the conduct of the project in any way, then research is a motive for the activity to a degree that the project should be classified as research from the regulatory standpoint.

Quality Improvement (QI) Is Not Research

A variety of nonresearch methods (described later here) exist; however, the distinction between QI and research is most often at the forefront of discussions of "intent." When an activity is specifically initiated with a goal of improving the performance of institutional practice in relationship to an established standard, the activity is called QI.

If a project is originally initiated as a local QI project but the findings are of interest and the project investigator chooses to expand the findings into a research study, IRB review is required at that time. The project investigator turned researcher should clearly indicate to the IRB that the data were originally collected as part of a QI project. The IRB should be prepared to handle this type of review and take the next steps as required of all research projects (e.g., designation of exempt, expedited or full-committee-review, level of consent required).

At our site, after the institutional discussion was commenced related to the definition of research, the IRB developed a close working relationship with the institutional QI committee. The goals for the QI evaluators and the IRB are similar. The QI evaluators want QI projects to be performed with a high standard to protect confidentiality and to ensure that results are applicable. It is important for both entities to know when their review is applicable to a project.

In order to distinguish research from QI, we use the following criteria:

- Primary intent—the intent should be clear in the purpose/aim statement for the specific project. In general, QI projects are aimed at improving local systems of care (nongeneralizable). If the intent is to promote "betterment" of a process of care, clinical outcome, etc., then the project may be considered quality improvement.

If any of the following criteria are met, then the project receives consideration as to whether IRB review is required:

- Generalizability—if the primary intent of the project is to generate generalizable results
- Additional risk or burden—if the project will impose risks or burdens beyond the standard of practice to make the results generalizable
- Design—if a project involves randomization or an element that may be considered less than standard of care

Additional Notes
   a. Federal regulators have made it clear that any publication describing a project as "research" must have received prior IRB review and approval. Therefore, projects determined to be QI initiatives should not be published as "research."
   b. Projects considered QI must also maintain the highest integrity of confidentiality possible.
   c. Characterizing a project as QI does not necessarily negate the need for informed consent.

Informed Consent
HIPAA allows projects conducted within a covered entity with the intent of obtaining information related to treatment, payment, or health care operations to be conducted without additional patient authorization. Patients should be made aware of these uses of their data via the privacy notice required by HIPAA. A QI project may be appropriately initiated without patient authorization or consent; however, consideration must be given to whether or not health care workers should be aware of and possibly required to consent to the project. These are decisions that must be well thought out by the initiators of the quality improvement teams at the institution.

Research is not covered under the HIPAA "treatment, payment, or health care operations" exemptions, and

therefore, if research is being conducted, the requirements for waiving informed consent and/or waiving the requirements for documentation of informed consent must be met. These regulations are described in more detail in other chapters of this book.

Other Activities That Are Not Research
To understand when a project should be classified as research, it is important to understand the major categories of activities that may be appropriately classified as something other than research.

Quality Assessment
Activities that are designed to determine whether aspects of medical practice are being performed in line with established standards are called QA.

Quality Assurance
In New Hampshire, this term is used for the specific instance of the process of reviewing, analyzing, or evaluating *patient and/or provider specific data* that may indicate (the need for) changes in systems or procedures that would improve the quality of care. The analysis is protected from legal discoverability, and the review is often triggered by predetermined "thresholds/criteria." This analysis must be conducted with a specific committee structure. The knowledge generated is typically for local, immediate application.

The Case Report or Case Series
A physician requests access to her patient's medical record to prepare a "case report" for publication in a medical journal. The first step is to determine whether the project contains both of the elements from the regulatory definition of research (a systematic investigation and the intent to contribute to generalizable knowledge). In our opinion, it is not reasonable to suggest that the organization of information for a case report constitutes a systematic investigation to the extent that would be expected of a research project. Because the first element of the regulatory definition of research is not present, this project is not research and, therefore, is beyond the regulatory authority of the IRB. In our opinion, this kind of case report project is most appropriately classified as an educational activity. Care should be taken, however, to distinguish a case report from an "N-of-1" research study in which there is systematic manipulation of an intervention to produce generalizable results.

When discussing the classification of case-report projects, many people ask whether the inclusion of more than one patient requires that the project be classified as research. In our opinion, the number of patients is not a defining factor. Educational activities often involve discussion of the course of a group of patients. It is the use of statistical method such as subgroup comparisons and test for prognostic factors that are the distinguishing features of a systematic investigation. In the absence of the basic elements of a systematic investigation of a scientific question, the case-report project should be classified as an educational activity rather than research, regardless of the number of patients that form the basis for the discussion.

In the event a case report or case series cannot be published or presented without the potential for identifying the patients, permission from the patient(s) must be obtained before use of the data.

Medical Practice and Innovative Therapy
A commonly cited definition of medical practice describes an activity that is designed solely to enhance the well-being of an individual patient.[6] A type of medical practice that is often confused with research is a class of activities that has been called "innovative therapy."[7] Basically, innovative therapy describes an activity that is designed solely to benefit individual patient(s) but in which the ability of the activity to result in the desired outcome is to some degree unproven. Levine has explained that a better term for this class of activity is *nonvalidated practice*.[6]

Medical Practice for the Benefit of Others
In some situations, the goal of medical practice is to benefit people other than those directly affected by the health care intervention. Examples of medical practice for the benefit of others include blood donation and some vaccination programs. In terms of the research/nonresearch issue, the critical feature of this form of medical practice is that the goal of the activity is to benefit a well-defined group of people in a predictable way.

Public Health Practice
Public health practice is similar to medical practice for the benefit of others in that the activity involves people who do not directly benefit from the intervention. The most common situation in which there is confusion about the distinction between a public health practice and research is with public health practices that require the review of private, identifiable information about health status. Examples of public health practices that often do not involve research include surveillance (e.g., monitoring of diseases) and program evaluation (e.g., immunization coverage or use of clinical preventive services such as mammography).

Outcome Analysis
Outcome analysis is a nonspecific term that may be used to describe a variety of projects in which medical records are reviewed to evaluate the outcome of medical treatment or the course of patients with a specific medical condition.[3,8,9] Because medical research usually involves a formal analysis of outcome, use of the term *outcome analysis* to describe a nonresearch activity is confusing. Nevertheless, it is common practice for health care providers to perform descriptive analyses of medical outcomes that are appropriately described as something other than research but do not clearly fall into a better defined category. Recognizing that there is no accepted definition of outcome analysis in the context of health care evaluation, the main difference between a nonresearch outcome analysis and a quality-assessment project is that comparison of results to an established standard is not a defining feature of outcome analysis.

Resource Utilization Review
Medical record review is often conducted to evaluate the use of resources in a specific health care activity. Terms such as *cost control* are used to describe this class of activity,[10] but the terms *utilization review* or *resource utilization review* are more general and often more accurately reflect the fundamental goal of projects in this category. Although a research project may involve review of resource utilization, the term *resource utilization review* usually refers to a nonresearch activity.

Education
The transferring of information from one group of people to another is a common activity in all aspects of society. As we explain later in this chapter, the regulatory definition of research focuses on the desire to develop or contribute to "generalizable knowledge." The reason to mention education in the context of a discussion about the definition of research is that it is important to recognize that the goal of most educational activities is to spread or "generalize" knowledge. The fact that an activity is undertaken for the specific purpose of teaching somebody something does not mean that the activity involves research.

Conclusion

To determine whether a project should be classified as research, it is important to understand that nonresearch activities may use scientific methods and produce results that are suitable for publication in a medical journal. The defining characteristic of research is that a fundamental goal of the activity is to learn something that will benefit future patients (not the subjects enrolled in the research study). The following questions facilitate the evaluation of research intent: What is the primary intent of the project? Would the project be conducted as planned if the project director knew that he or she would never receive any form of academic recognition for the project, including publication of results in a medical journal or presentation of the project at an academic meeting?

References
1. Code of Federal Regulations. Title 45A—Department of Health and Human Services; Part 46—Protection of Human Subjects. Updated 1 October, 1997. Access date 18 April, 2001. http://www4.law.cornell.edu/cfr/45p46.htm
2. Center for Devices and Radiological Health. Humanitarian device exemption regulation questions and answers. Updated 4 January, 2000. Access date 26 March, 2001. http://www.fda.gov/cdrh/ode/hdeqna.html
3. Bull AR. Audit and research: Complementary but distinct. *Ann R Coll Surg Engl* 75(5):308–311, 1993.
4. Amdur RJ, Biddle C. Institutional review board approval and publication of human research results. *JAMA* 277(11):909–914, 1997.
5. Choo V. Thin line between research and audit. *Lancet* 352(9125):337–338, 1998.
6. Levine RJ. *Ethics and Regulation of Clinical Research*, 2nd ed. Baltimore, MD: Urban and Schwarzenberg; 1986.

7. Levine RJ. The impact on fetal research of the report of the National Commission for the Protection of Human Subjects of Biomedical and Behavioral Research. *Villanova Law Rev* 22:367–383, 1977.

8. Lynn J, Johnson J, Levine RJ. The ethical conduct of health services research: A case study of 55 institutions' applications to the SUPPORT project. *Clin Res* 42(1):3–10, 1994.

9. Casarett D, Karlawish JH, Sugarman J. Determining when quality improvement initiatives should be considered research: Proposed criteria and potential implications. *JAMA* 283(17):2275–2280, 2000.

10. Etzioni A. Medical records: Enhancing privacy, preserving the common good. *Hastings Cent Rep* 29(2):14–23, 1999.

Compassionate Use and Emergency Use Exemption

Elizabeth A. Bankert and Robert J. Amdur

INTRODUCTION

Institutional review boards (IRBs) that review biomedical research may be asked to approve the use of an investigational drug on a so-called compassionate-use basis. There is no way to know what an investigator means by *compassionate use* without evaluating the details of each individual request. It may be surprising for some IRBs or investigators to learn that there is no such thing as compassionate use from the standpoint of research regulation. The term *compassionate use* does not appear in either the Department of Health and Human Services (DHHS) or the Food and Drug Administration (FDA) regulations. The *IRB Guidebook*[1] states that the research community should not use this term because it serves to confuse discussions of access mechanisms. The purpose of this chapter is to clarify the role of the IRB in situations in which the IRB may encounter the terms *compassionate use* or *emergency use exemption*.

The Term *Compassionate Use*

Historically, *compassionate use* has been used to describe a situation in which an investigational drug is being used outside the setting of a clinical trial. The use is in a small number of extremely ill patients for whom standard therapy is unlikely to be effective. There are research studies that include the words *compassionate use* within the study title. For the most part, these projects require full IRB review (unless being used in the scenario described later here). The following scenario describes a situation that leads to a request for IRB approval of research on a compassionate-use basis.

Example
A physician has a patient with a condition for which an investigational drug may offer an advantage to all current FDA-approved treatments. The investigational drug is currently available only to patients enrolled in a clinical trial. The patient cannot receive the drug as part of a clinical trial because the trial is not being conducted in the medical system where the patient is being cared for or because the patient is ineligible for the trial. To treat the patient with the investigational drug, the physician must have the sponsor's permission to use the drug outside the setting of a clinical trial. The physician asks the IRB to approve the use of the investigational agent on a compassionate-use basis.

The sponsor will be violating FDA regulations and/or federal law if it releases the investigational drug under circumstances that are not specifically approved by the FDA. FDA regulations provide for the use of investigational drugs in research that is approved by an appropriately constituted IRB. Otherwise, FDA regulations provide for the use of investigational drugs outside the standard research setting in three circumstances: emergency use exemption from prospective IRB approval, treatment investigational new drug application, and the parallel track mechanism. Treatment investigational new drugs and parallel track programs are discussed in the *IRB Guidebook*.[1] The rest of this chapter focuses on the FDA's emergency use exemption option.

FDA

Federal regulations related to emergency use exemption from prospective IRB approval include 21 CFR 56,[2[Sec.102(d),104(c)]] 21 CFR 50,[3(Sec.23)] and 21 CFR 312.[4(Sec.36)] A description of the process can also be found in the FDA Information Sheets.[5] The FDA definition of *emergency use* makes reference to two essential components: (1) a life-threatening situation in which no standard acceptable treatment is available and (2) insufficient time to convene a quorum for full-board IRB approval. In an emergency situation as described previously here, prior IRB approval is not required for provision of the test article to one patient. Rather, the FDA requirement is that the IRB is notified before or within 5 days of the emergency use of the test article. It is important to understand that there is no type of expedited or subcommittee process allowed for IRB review and approval of the emergency use of a test article according to federal regulations.

Processing a Request for Compassionate Use—FDA Rules

This algorithm may help you when you receive the next phone call from an investigator at your institution requesting compassionate-use approval:

1. First, determine whether the compassionate-use request fulfills the FDA criteria for emergency use. Do not assume the investigator knows the FDA definition of emergency use: (1) a life-threatening situation exists in which no standard acceptable treatment is available, and (2) there is not sufficient time to convene a quorum for full-board IRB review and approval.

2. If the situation satisfies the FDA criteria for emergency use, the next step is to determine whether an IRB acknowledgment letter (versus an IRB approval letter) is what the sponsor requires. In some cases, the investigator misunderstands the sponsor's requirements for access to the test article. Explain to the investigator that the sponsor may actually be requesting IRB acknowledgment of emergency use before or within 5 days of use of the test article. It is unusual for a sponsor to require full-board IRB approval to release medication for emergency use in a single patient.

3. If the situation fits the criteria for emergency use and the sponsor requires an acknowledgment letter, follow the procedures for an emergency-use exemption described later here.

4. If the situation does not meet FDA criteria for emergency use, a convened full-board IRB review and approval of the protocol and consent form per standard IRB review procedure must be completed before release of the test article.

5. If the sponsor requires IRB approval before release of the test article, an IRB approval letter may only be written after a convened full-board review and approval of the protocol and the consent form according to standard IRB procedure. Remember, there is no type of expedited or subcommittee process allowed for IRB review and approval of the emergency use of a test article, according to federal regulations.

IRB Procedure for FDA Emergency Exemption

Instruct the investigator to generate a letter to the IRB chair describing the emergency-use situation. The letter must document compliance with specific FDA requirements for emergency use, indicating (1) a life-threatening situation exists in which no standard acceptable treatment is available, and (2) the test article must be used expeditiously, meaning insufficient time is available to convene a quorum for full-board IRB approval. The notification to the IRB must occur before or within 5 days of use of the test article. The IRB chair or appropriate designee (IRB member with appropriate medical knowledge) reviews the investigator's letter and confirms that (1) an emergency situation exists and that (2) there is not sufficient time to convene a full-board IRB meeting.

The IRB office generates a letter to be signed by the IRB chair acknowledging notification of emergency use of the test article.

The IRB letter should indicate only knowledge of, acknowledgment of, or appropriate notification of the use of the test article. The IRB letter should not indicate IRB review or approval.

All subsequent uses of the test article should be reviewed using the standard full-board IRB review process. If an investigator believes another request for the use of this test article is forthcoming, the full IRB review process should be initiated. The FDA acknowledges that subsequent uses should not be denied because the IRB could not convene in a timely manner. The IRB letter to the investigator should also describe the FDA subsequent-use requirement.

Informed Consent

The patient must understand the investigational nature of the test article. Informed consent must be obtained; however, the consent form is not a standard research consent form. In most cases, the sponsor will supply a consent form. The IRB is not involved in the review or approval of the consent form if the situation meets the criteria for emergency use. The FDA describes the "Exception from informed consent requirements" in 21 CFR 50.[3][Sec.24(a)]

Sample Letter Templates

[Department letterhead]

Date

Dear Dr. IRB chair name,

*Please regard this notice as a request for an IRB Emergency-Use Exemption for the use of the **drug xxx** for one patient (**initials**).*

According to FDA regulations, in order to qualify for an emergency-use exemption, the situation must involve a "life-threatening situation in which no acceptable standard treatment is available and in which there is not sufficient time to obtain full IRB approval."

*This situation complies with the definition because the **patient** [describe why the patient needs the drug in a timely manner]...*

Consent from the patient will be obtained ... [explain the process so that the patient understands that the drug is not FDA approved for this use and if a consent form will be used state so and include with this memo].

The data for this patient will not be used as part of a prospective research protocol.

Sincerely,

Dr. XYZ

Template letter from IRB to physician:
Dear Dr. Smith,

*The office of the institutional review board (IRB) has received your written notification of the request for the one-time emergency-use exemption of the investigational drug, **xxxx**, for one patient, **initials**.*

Prior IRB review and approval are not required for the emergency use of a test article as described in 21 CFR 56.102(d) and 21 CFR 56.104(c). This memo is not a notification of IRB review or approval.

The notification you have provided to the IRB meets the requirements of our IRB office and federal regulations. Please note, if subsequent use of drug xxxx is anticipated, please submit an application for review by the full IRB before its next use. The data from this use should not be used for prospective research purposes.

Thank you,

IRB chair signature

Written Policy and Procedures

There should be a description of the policy for emergency exemption from IRB approval. This should be located in the IRB internal procedure manual at your IRB office. The information in this chapter is sufficient to write this section. We also recommend that your office create an internal procedure document for emergency use that can readily be sent to an investigator on request. Again, this chapter contains the necessary information for this document. The requesting physician can send the document describing your emergency-use procedure to the sponsor, which ensures that all interested parties are aware of the appropriate procedures. Because time is often of the essence in these situations, having a description of the process ready to send out is very useful.

DHHS Rules

The procedures described in this chapter pertain only to FDA-regulated research. The FDA elected to make some changes in the DHHS federal policy (Common Rule). DHHS does not provide for an emergency exception to IRB review. However, DHHS allows physicians to provide emergency medical treatment to their patients.[6[Sec.116(f)]] The difference between research conducted through the DHHS and research regulated through the FDA is that in an emergency-use situation, the DHHS does not consider the patient a research participant. Thus, the data are not allowed as part of a prospective research study. The FDA does allow the data from an emergency-use situation to be used as part of a research study.

If the research is funded by the DHHS and/or your organization has agreed to abide by DHHS regulations and the research involves the use of a drug, biologic, or device, the research also falls under the jurisdiction of the FDA. Consequently, both sets of regulations must be followed.

In this instance, a sentence may be added to the IRB acknowledgment letter: *The data obtained from the emergency use of this investigational drug may not be used as part of a prospective research study.*

Conclusion

Guidance from federal regulatory authorities makes it clear that *compassionate use* is a term that should not be used to direct the process of research regulation. From the standpoint of IRB review of research, the term *compassionate use* has no meaning. This chapter has explained the situations in which the IRB will be asked to approve a study on a compassionate-use basis. Federal regulations related to approval of research by an expedited process and FDA rules related to emergency use of an investigational agent will direct the IRB in this setting. A step-by-step explanation of how an IRB should manage the compassionate use situation is presented.

References

1. Penslar RL, Porter JP, Office for Human Research Protections (DHHS). Chapter II, Part A, Section ii, Question 22. In: *Institutional Review Board Guidebook*, 2nd ed. Updated 27 June, 2000. Access date 9 August, 2001. http://ohrp.osophs.dhhs.gov/irb/irb_chapter2.htm

2. Code of Federal Regulations. Title 21, Chapter 1—Food and Drug Administration, DHHS; Part 56—Institutional Review Boards. Updated 1 April, 1999. Access date 27 March, 2001. http://www4.law.cornell.edu/cfr/21p56.htm

3. Code of Federal Regulations. Title 21, Chapter 1—Food and Drug Administration, DHHS; Part 50—Protection of Human Subjects. Updated 1 April, 1999. Access date 18 April, 2001. http://www4.law.cornell.edu/cfr/21p50.htm

4. Code of Federal Regulations. Title 21, Chapter 1—Food and Drug Administration, DHHS; Part 312—Investigational New Drug Application. Updated 1 April, 1999. Access date 18 April, 2001. http://www4.law.cornell.edu/cfr/21p312.htm

5. Food and Drug Administration. Information sheets: Guidance for Institutional Review Boards and clinical investigators, September 1998. Access date 9 April, 2001. http://www.fda.gov/oc/oha/IRB/toc.html

6. Code of Federal Regulations. Title 45A—Department of Health and Human Services; Part 46—Protection of Human Subjects. Updated 1 October, 1997. Access date 18 April, 2001. http://www4.law.cornell.edu/cfr/45p46.htm

Waiver of Consent in Emergency Medicine Research

Helen McGough

INTRODUCTION

In 1996, both the Food and Drug Administration (FDA) and the Office for Protection from Research Risks (OPRR) (now the Office for Human Research Protections) issued regulations permitting a waiver of the general requirements for informed consent for certain research settings involving risks to subjects that are greater than minimal. The intent of the regulations is to allow research on life-threatening conditions for which available treatments are unproven or unsatisfactory in situations in which it is not possible to obtain informed consent. The regulations establish additional protections to make sure the studies are as safe and ethical as possible. The situations to which the regulations apply are limited to cases in which subjects cannot give consent and for whom a legally authorized representative cannot be located by the time the intervention must be used to be effective. The underlying assumption is that these subjects, because they cannot either consent or refuse to consent, are a vulnerable population necessitating the additional protections provided by the regulations. The complete text of this regulation is included as the appendix to this chapter. Sufficient controversy surrounds the ethics of these regulations that an institutional review board (IRB) should be cautious about venturing into this arena.[1] The IRB should discuss the issues in the abstract before an actual case is presented to it for consideration. The intent of this chapter is not to debate the ethics of the regulation, but to assist the IRB in implementation, should it choose to allow the waiver of consent.

Applicability

The regulations allowing waiver of consent in emergency medicine research are limited to two kinds of situations. The first is when the research involves an investigational intervention that comes under FDA regulation. This includes drugs, devices, and biologics that are not approved for marketing at all, or are not approved for the emergency situations in which the researcher proposes to use them. For example, a researcher may wish to test an investigational drug to reduce brain swelling after closed head injury or to test an investigational defibrillator to resuscitate people who suffer cardiac arrest. The second is when the emergency research is either sponsored by a federal agency or conducted by an institution that has chosen to apply the federal regulations to all of its research activities. Examples of this second area of applicability might include research that evaluates an innovative emergency surgical procedure or evaluates approved treatments in an emergency research setting.

Implementing the Regulations

Implementing these regulations requires extensive time and effort by the IRB, the researchers, and the research sponsors. The remainder of this chapter breaks down the regulation (97-01[2]) into sections and addresses the points to consider from each section.

Section 1

> The human subjects are in a life-threatening situation; available treatments are unproven or unsatisfactory. In addition, the collection of valid scientific evidence, which may include evidence obtained through randomized placebo-controlled investigations, is necessary to determine the safety and effectiveness of particular interventions.

The points to be considered through the IRB review process include the following:

1. Are the potential subjects in a life-threatening condition? To answer this question, the IRB must have a clear notion of

how it defines "life threatening." Generally speaking, the determination is made within the context of the research protocol. The question to be asked and answered is: "Are the potential subjects in an emergent situation in which survival without the intervention is in question?"

2. Are there other treatments that could be used to save the lives of these subjects? The IRB must require the researchers to demonstrate (usually through a literature review) that no acceptable treatments are available for the condition under consideration or that the relative benefits of the proposed intervention, as compared with standard therapy, are thought to be equivalent ("clinical equipoise") or better.

3. Is a placebo control allowed? An algorithm for evaluating the ethics of placebo control is presented in Chapter 10-11 of this book. The IRB should ensure that when a placebo is used, standard care, if any exists, will be provided to all subjects. Subjects would then be randomized to receive, in addition to standard care, the study intervention or placebo. The IRB should use the same standards that it uses with nonemergency research to determine whether the use of placebo is ethically acceptable.

4. Is it necessary to experiment on human subjects to test the safety and effectiveness of the proposed intervention? The IRB may answer this question by requesting the researcher to describe research on the intervention already conducted using animal or other models or on consenting subjects who had a less serious condition.

Section 2

Obtaining informed consent is not feasible because: (i) the subjects will not be able to give their informed consent as a result of their medical condition, (ii) the intervention involved in the research must be administered before consent from the subjects' legally authorized representatives is feasible, and (iii) there is no reasonable way to identify prospectively the individuals likely to become eligible for participation in the research.

The IRB must ask the following questions:

1. Are the subjects incompetent to provide informed consent? The researcher must describe the general condition of the prospective subjects and describe why they are not in a position to provide consent.

2. Must the experimental intervention be initiated before it is possible to obtain consent from the subjects' legally authorized guardians? Generally, the experimental intervention should be one that must be implemented within a narrow window of time, making it impossible to either wait until the subjects become able to provide consent or to obtain proxy consent from a legally authorized representative. The researcher should document to the IRB's satisfaction that this is the case.

3. Is it possible to identify (and somehow obtain prospective consent from) the people who are likely to become subjects in this research? The researchers must document that it would not be possible to identify the proposed subject population beforehand and get prospective consent from them. For example, if a group of patients is at high risk for developing a condition for which no standard treatment is available, could the researcher obtain consent from the subjects to undergo the experimental intervention if they develop that condition? If the answer is yes, then a waiver of consent may not be necessary. However, the use of

prospective consent involves its own ethical dilemmas. Unless the community of interest and the IRB are willing to accept the concept of a "Ulysses contract," the concept of prospective consent may be difficult to justify. Basically, a Ulysses contract is one in which a subject contracts with a researcher to ignore any future objections the subject might have to the terms of the contract.[3]

Section 3

Participation in the research holds out the prospect of direct benefit to the subjects because (i) subjects are facing a life-threatening situation that necessitates intervention; (ii) appropriate animal and other preclinical studies have been conducted, and the information derived from those studies, and related evidence, supports the potential for the intervention to provide a direct benefit to the individual subjects; (iii) risks associated with the research are reasonable in relationship to what is known about the medical condition of the potential class of subjects, and the risks and benefits of standard therapy, if any, and of what is known about the risks and benefits of the proposed intervention or activity.

This criterion requires the IRB to ask the following questions:

1. Is there no other effective treatment available for the condition without which the subjects will die or will be seriously disabled? Most IRBs will rely on either the researchers themselves or special consultants to the IRB to answer this question. One of the difficult parts of making this determination is that the request for a an emergency waiver of consent often involves situations in which the study intervention may save the person's life. However, it is difficult for the researcher to determine what the subject's quality of life will be after the intervention. Second, there is usually no way of determining, in these kinds of situations, whether the subject has a "living will" or a "do not resuscitate" order that might prohibit life saving efforts.

2. Is there good scientific evidence that the study intervention will have a beneficial effect on the proposed subject population? IRBs should request documentation from the researcher that there is some evidence that the intervention will be effective.

3. Are the known risks of the study intervention reasonable when the IRB considers the risks the subjects face as a result of their life-threatening condition and the risks of available standard treatments? This is a difficult determination for the IRB in that the risks of the study intervention are often not well known and the risks of the condition are not known for individual subjects. IRBs should use expert consultants if their membership does not have the expertise to make these decisions.

Section 4

The research could not practicably be carried out without the waiver.

IRBs are often asked to consider the practicability of obtaining consent, particularly in research eligible for the expedited review procedure. In the case of emergency research, practicability usually means determining that the research goals could not be met if the study population was limited to those able to provide consent, either personally or through a legally authorized representative. If the IRB cannot make this determination, there is no need to allow a waiver. The IRB may wish to consider the following:

1. Would it take an unreasonable length of time to accrue a sufficient number of subjects who could give consent?

2. Does the context of the research (e.g., head trauma from vehicle crashes) make it highly unlikely that consent can be obtained from the subjects or that a legally authorized representative will be available?

3. Is the window of opportunity so short that the possibility of identifying or contacting legal representatives is small?

Section 5

The proposed research protocol defines the length of the potential therapeutic window based on scientific evidence. The investigator has committed to attempting to contact a legally authorized representative for each subject within that window of time and, if feasible, to asking the legally authorized representative contacted for consent within that window rather than proceeding without consent. The investigator will summarize efforts made to contact representatives and make this information available to the IRB at the time of continuing review.

This criterion requires the IRB to document the following:

1. Has the researcher presented solid scientific evidence to document the period of time within which the experimental intervention must be used? The IRB may wish to use the services of a consultant to assist in evaluating this information.

2. Has the researcher outlined what steps will be taken to learn the subjects' identity and to contact their legal representatives before implementing a waiver? For subjects who are already in a medical setting at the time they are considered to be eligible as potential research subjects, identities are usually known and legal representatives are available, making a waiver unnecessary. However, when subjects are brought to a medical setting *in extremis* or are treated by emergency personnel away from their homes, it may be impossible to get consent or to identify a legally authorized representative (LAR). The researchers must document to the IRB that they are prepared to take all steps necessary to obtain consent from the subject or from a subject's LAR. This may include locating LARs by telephone and obtaining oral consent or consent by facsimile if the LAR is not available to read and sign a consent form. The researchers should present the IRB with a written protocol documenting the steps they will take to identify the subject, identify the subject's LAR, contact and identify the LAR, and obtain oral or facsimile consent from the LAR.

3. At the time of continuing review, has the researcher summarized, on a case-by-case basis, the efforts that have been made to identify the subject and locate a legally authorized representative? The IRB has an obligation to make sure that the researcher is aware of this requirement at the time of initial approval. This permits the data to be collected in a systematic way that is easy for the IRB to evaluate at the time of continuing review or audit.

Section 6

The IRB has reviewed and approved informed consent procedures and an informed consent document in accord with Sections 46.116 and 46.117 of 45 CFR Part 46. These procedures and the informed consent document are to be used with subjects or their legally authorized representatives in situations where use of such procedures and documents is feasible. The IRB has reviewed and approved procedures and information to be used when providing an opportunity for a family member to object to a subject's participation in the research consistent with paragraph (b)(7)(v) of this waiver.

This criterion emphasizes that consent must be obtained from the subject or the subject's LAR whenever possible, even if the IRB has approved a waiver of consent. This means that the IRB must review and approve the following:

1. Written consent documents for the subject or the subject's LAR

2. Oral consent scripts for the subject or the subject's legal LAR

3. The researcher's protocol for identifying the subject and locating the subject's LAR

4. The researcher's protocol for contacting family members to obtain their permission for the subject to be in the research when it is not possible to contact the LAR

The IRB must be familiar with the laws pertaining to consent in the location where the study will take place. In some jurisdictions the laws that determine who may provide consent for health care treatment may be used to determine who may provide consent for participation in medical research. However, if an IRB has questions about this, it should consult an expert in the governing statutes.

Section 7

Additional protections of the rights and welfare of the subjects will be provided, including, at least: (i) consultation (including, where appropriate, consultation carried out by the IRB) with representatives of the communities in which the research will be conducted, as well as communities from which the subjects will be drawn; (ii) public disclosure to the communities in which the research will be conducted and from which the subjects will be drawn before initiation of the research, in addition to the plans for the research and its risks and expected benefits; (iii) public disclosure of sufficient information after completion of the research to apprise the community and researchers of the study, including the demographic characteristics of the research population and its results; (iv) establishment of an independent data monitoring committee to exercise oversight of the research; and (v) if obtaining informed consent is not feasible and a legally authorized representative is not reasonably available, the investigator has committed, if feasible, to attempting to contact within the therapeutic window the subject's family member who is not a legally authorized representative and asking whether he or she objects to the subject's participation in the research. The investigator will summarize efforts made to contact family members and make this information available to the IRB at the time of continuing review.

This criterion is perhaps the most difficult for an IRB to interpret and implement.[4] To meet this criterion, the IRB must ensure the following:

Community Consultation
The IRB must consult with, or have the investigator consult with, representatives of the communities in which the

research will be conducted and from which the subjects will be drawn. Typically, IRBs request researchers to conduct and document this consultation process in accord with directions from the IRB.[5]

1. The researchers and the IRB must first define the "community" in which the research will be conducted. Then it must determine whether there is a "community" of research subjects. For example, if the research is to be conducted by emergency medical personnel within a certain geographic catchment area, the IRB may define that area as the community. Likewise, if the research is to provide an experimental intervention to scuba divers who experience decompression, the community may be defined as "scuba divers."

2. The researchers and the IRB must determine the best way of "consulting" with these communities. In the examples given previously here, consulting with the geographic catchment area of a hospital might include conducting random surveys of residents with area codes within the area or consulting with local political organizations (city, town, or neighborhood councils, legislatures) and civic groups (business, church, or advocacy organizations). Consulting with the community of subjects in the case of scuba divers might include meeting with scuba diving organizations and schools and conducting surveys with divers at popular scuba diving sites. Care must be taken to consider the special community's characteristics (age, gender, ethnicity, cultural values, etc.) in designing and implementing community consultation. As with any information-gathering effort, the questions to be asked must be framed in a way that is value neutral and sensitive to community norms and expectations.

3. The researchers and the IRB must agree about the goals of community consultation and how the results of the consultation efforts are to be used. The regulation does not include an explanation of the purpose of consulting with the community. There are at least two possibilities: allowing the community to determine whether a study should be conducted and gathering information from the community on how to design and implement the study. The regulation also does not state how the consultation effort should be used. For example, suppose the researcher conducts a survey of community residents to ask their opinions about the conduct of a study. The results show that 45% of respondents reply that the study is ethical and should be conducted, 45% respond that the study is not ethical and should not be conducted, and 10% are undecided. The IRB and the researcher will have to agree on how the survey will be designed and implemented and how the results will be used before the survey is conducted.

Public Disclosure Before the Research Is Conducted

The IRB must work with the investigators to make the communities aware of the purpose of the research and its possible risks and benefits before the research begins. A wide range of possibilities may be considered in meeting this obligation, ranging from radio and television announcements, newspaper articles, press releases from the research site, announcements on billboards and public transportation to holding public meetings in a variety of locations. Disclosure of the study should also offer an opportunity to provide comments on the proposed study. This may be achieved by use of a toll-free telephone number, mailing address, public meeting, or website.

Public Disclosure After the Research Is Completed

The IRB must work with the investigators to make the communities aware of the results of the research (including the characteristics of the subject population) after the research has been completed. The same kinds of mechanisms that were used to notify the communities about the research before it was undertaken may also be used to publicize the results of the study. In addition, if the results of the study were positive, there is an ethical obligation on the part of the researchers to make sure that the study interventions are implemented as standard care when this is reasonable and appropriate.

Independent Data-Monitoring Committee

The IRB must require that the research protocol include a data safety and monitoring board (DSMB) that is independent of the research to provide oversight and to make sure that the study continues to be conducted as safely and ethically as possible. The DSMB has the authority to stop the study if the risks are greater than the anticipated benefits or if the study design must be changed to minimize risks. The DSMB may also stop the study if the benefits of the intervention are clear. Membership on the DSMB should not include representatives from the research team and should include experts in the field, ethicists, and statisticians experienced in research data analysis. Often the research sponsor establishes the independent DSMB. The IRB must request that the results of the DSMB meetings are forwarded to the IRB in a timely fashion.

Authorization From Family Members

The IRB should request from the researcher a protocol for identifying and contacting family members in the event that the subject cannot consent and the subject's legally authorized representative cannot be located. The protocol should include a script that requests identification of the family members, explains the study to the family members, and asks whether the family members object to the subject's participation in the research. At the time of each continuing review, the researcher should summarize these attempts to contact family members.[6]

Section 8

The IRB is responsible for ensuring that procedures are in place to inform, at the earliest feasible opportunity, each subject, or if the subject remains incapacitated, a legally authorized representative of the subject, or if such a representative is not reasonably available, a family member, of the subject's inclusion in the clinical investigation, the details of the investigation, and other information contained in the informed consent document. The IRB shall also ensure that there is a procedure to inform the subject, or if the subject remains incapacitated, a legally authorized representative of the subject, or if such a representative is not reasonably available, a family member, that he or she may discontinue the subject's participation at any time without penalty or loss of benefits to which the subject is otherwise entitled. If a legally authorized representative or family member is told about the clinical investigation and the subject's condition improves, the subject is also to be informed as soon as feasible. If a subject is entered into a clinical investigation with waived consent and the subject dies before a legally authorized representative or family member can be contacted, information about the clinical investigation is to be provided to the subject's legally authorized representative or family member, if feasible.

The IRB should request the following from the investigator:

1. A procedure for informing the subject at the earliest possible opportunity that they have been included in a research activity. This procedure should include as many of the elements of informed consent as are appropriate for consent to continue participation in the study.

2. A procedure for informing the subject's legally authorized representative or family member—whoever becomes available soonest—that the subject has been included in a research activity. The information must provide a description of the research activity, a request to allow the subject to continue to participate in the research activity, and an opportunity to discontinue participation in the research activity without penalty or loss of benefits to which the subject might otherwise be entitled. The regulation does not determine whether permission to continue or authorization to discontinue participation should be obtained in writing. It may be difficult for the researcher to develop a written template for the consent process. This is because it may not be possible to determine in advance at what point in the protocol the subject or the subject's legal representative or family member will be available to provide consent.

3. A procedure for documenting, on a case-by-case basis at continuing review (or whenever requested by the IRB), that these protocols were followed.

This procedure does not constitute requesting permission for what has already happened to the subject but only permission to either continue or discontinue participation.

Additional FDA Requirements

If the research involves a test article (drug, device, or biologic) regulated by the FDA, additional requirements must be met before the IRB may approve a waiver of consent. The IRB must determine that the researcher or the research sponsor has completed an investigational new drug (IND) application or obtained an investigational device exemption (IDE) from the FDA before implementing the research. The application to the FDA must include a protocol that clearly states that it will include subjects who are unable to consent. This requirement must be met even if there is an existing IND or IDE for the use of the test article in a protocol not requiring a waiver of consent.[7]

The IRB must document that a licensed physician "who is a member of or consultant to the IRB and who is not otherwise participating in the clinical investigation" concurs that the waiver of consent is allowable. IRBs should ensure that meeting minutes specifically record this concurrence.

If the IRB determines that it cannot approve a protocol involving a waiver of consent either because it does not meet the requirements of the regulations or because of other relevant ethical concerns, it must provide documentation of this decision promptly to the researcher and to the sponsor of the research. The sponsor must promptly disclose this information to the FDA and to other researchers who are conducting or have been asked to conduct this or similar protocols and to other IRBs that have been, or are, asked to review this or similar protocols by that sponsor.

Important Exceptions to the Waiver for Emergency Research

The waiver is explicitly excluded when the research involves certain protected research populations. These include fetuses, pregnant women, and human in vitro fertilization (Subpart B of 45 CFR 46) and prisoners (Subpart C of 45 CFR 46).

Conclusion

This chapter has reviewed the criteria for waiver of consent in emergency medicine research. This is a set of regulations that requires a list of specific activities on the part of the IRB and research team. It is important that the IRB understands that these regulations are applicable to only a narrow class of research activities. This chapter discusses each section of the regulations with the goal of clarifying the actions that researchers and the IRB must take to protect the rights and welfare of this extremely vulnerable research population.

References

1. Adams JG, Wegener J. Acting without asking: An ethical analysis of the Food and Drug Administration waiver of informed consent for emergency research. *Ann Emerg Med* 33(2):218–223, 1999.

2. Office for Human Research Protections. Human Subject—Dear Colleague Letters, 31 October, 1996 (No. 97-01). Access date 9 August, 2001. http://ohrp.osophs.dhhs.gov/humansubjects/guidance/hsdc97-01.htm

3. Annas GJ. Ulysses and the fate of frozen embryos—reproduction, research, or destruction? *N Engl J Med* 343(5):373–376, 2000.

4. Biros MH, Fish SS, Lewis RJ. Implementing the Food and Drug Administration's final rule for waiver of informed consent in certain emergency research circumstances. *Acad Emerg Med* 6(12):1272–1282, 1999.

5. Baren JM, Anicetti JP, Ledesma S, Biros MH, Mahabee-Gittens M, Lewis RJ. An approach to community consultation prior to initiating an emergency research study incorporating a waiver of informed consent. *Acad Emerg Med* 6(12):1210–1215, 1999.

6. Smithline HA, Gerstle ML. Waiver of informed consent: A survey of emergency medicine patients. *Am J Emerg Med* 16(1):90–91, 1998.

7. Kremers MS, Whisnant DR, Lowder LS, Gregg L. Initial experience using the Food and Drug Administration guidelines for emergency research without consent. *Ann Emerg Med* 33(2):224–229, 1999.

Appendix

OPRR Reports

October 31, 1996

Subject: Informed Consent Requirements in Emergency Research

Dear Colleague:

This letter advises Institutional Officials and Institutional Review Board (IRB) chairs of responsibilities related to informed consent when research subjects are enrolled in emergent circumstances.

As in the past, the regulations for protection of human subjects of the Department of Health and Human Services (DHHS) at 45 CFR Part 46 stipulate requirements for obtaining (Section 46.116) and documenting (Section 46.117) informed consent. The regulations give IRBs authority to alter or waive the required consent in certain circumstances (Sections 46.116(c)–(d)).[1] These provisions of DHHS regulations remain unchanged and in full force.

On October 2, 1996 (Federal Register, Vol. 61, pp. 51531–51533), the Secretary, DHHS, announced under Section 46.101(i) a waiver of the applicability of the 45 CFR Part 46 requirement for obtaining and documenting informed consent for a strictly limited class of research, involving research activities that may be carried out in human subjects who are in need of emergency therapy and for whom, because of the subjects' medical condition and the unavailability of legally authorized representatives of the subjects, no legally effective informed consent can be obtained. This waiver, which provides a third route through which IRBs may approve research in this class, takes effect November 1, 1996.

This waiver applies to the Basic DHHS Policy for Protection of Human Research Subjects (Subpart A of 45 CFR Part 46) and to research involving children (Subpart D of 45 CFR Part 46). However, because of special regulatory limitations relating to research involving fetuses, pregnant women, and human in vitro fertilization (Subpart B of 45 CFR 46), and research involving prisoners (Subpart C of 45 CFR Part 46), this waiver is inapplicable to these categories of research.

Emergency Research Consent Waiver

Pursuant to Section 46.101(i), the Secretary, DHHS, has waived the general requirements for informed consent at 45 CFR46.116(a) and (b) and 46.408, to be referred to as the "Emergency Research Consent Waiver" for a class of research consisting of activities, each of which has met the following strictly limited conditions detailed under either A or B below:

a. Research subject to FDA regulations
   The IRB responsible for the review, approval, and continuing review of the research activity has approved both the activity and a waiver of informed consent and found and documented:
   1. That the research activity is subject to regulations codified by the Food and Drug Administration (FDA) (see Federal Register, Vol. 61, pp. 51498–51531) at Title 21 CFR Part 50 and will be carried out under an FDA IND or an FDA IDE, the application for which has clearly identified the protocols that would include subjects who are unable to consent and
   2. That the requirements for exception from informed consent for emergency research detailed in 21 CFR Section 50.24 have been met relative to those protocols or

b. Research not subject to FDA regulations
   The IRB responsible for the review, approval, and continuing review of the research has approved both the research and a waiver of informed consent and has (i) found and documented that the research is not subject to regulations codified by the FDA at 21 CFR Part 50 and (ii) found and documented and reported to the OPRR that the following conditions have been met relative to the research:
   1. The human subjects are in a life-threatening situation, available treatments are unproven or unsatisfactory. In addition, the collection of valid scientific evidence, which may include evidence obtained through randomized placebo-controlled investigations, is necessary to determine the safety and effectiveness of particular interventions.
   2. Obtaining informed consent is not feasible because:

i. The subjects will not be able to give their informed consent as a result of their medical condition.

ii. The intervention involved in the research must be administered before consent from the subjects' legally authorized representatives is feasible.

iii. There is no reasonable way to identify prospectively the individuals likely to become eligible for participation in the research.

3. Participation in the research holds out the prospect of direct benefit to the subjects because:

   i. Subjects are facing a life-threatening situation that necessitates intervention.

   ii. Appropriate animal and other preclinical studies have been conducted, and the information derived from those studies and related evidence support the potential for the intervention to provide a direct benefit to the individual subjects.

   iii. Risks associated with the research are reasonable in relation to what is known about the medical condition of the potential class of subjects, the risks and benefits of standard therapy, if any, and what is known about the risks and benefits of the proposed intervention or activity.

4. The research could not practicably be carried out without the waiver.

5. The proposed research protocol defines the length of the potential therapeutic window based on scientific evidence, and the investigator has committed to attempting to contact a legally authorized representative for each subject within that window of time and, if feasible, to the asking of the legally authorized representative contacted for consent within that window rather than proceeding without consent. The investigator will summarize efforts made to contact representatives and make this information available to the IRB at the time of continuing review.

6. The IRB has reviewed and approved informed consent procedures and an informed consent document in accord with Sections 46.116 and 46.117 of 45 CFR Part 46. These procedures and the informed consent document are to be used with subjects or their legally authorized representatives in situations where use of such procedures and documents is feasible. The IRB has reviewed and approved procedures and information to be used when providing an opportunity for a family member to object to a subject's participation in the research consistent with paragraph (b)(7)(v) of this waiver.

7. Additional protections of the rights and welfare of the subjects will be provided, including, at least:

   i. Consultation (including, where appropriate, consultation carried out by the IRB) with representatives of the communities in which the research will be conducted and from which the subjects will be drawn.

   ii. Public disclosure to the communities in which the research will be conducted and from which the subjects will be drawn, prior to initiation of the research, of plans for the research and its risks and expected benefits.

   iii. Public disclosure of sufficient information following completion of the research to apprise the community and researchers of the study, including the demographic characteristics of the research population, and its results.

   iv. Establishment of an independent data monitoring committee to exercise oversight of the research.

   v. If obtaining informed consent is not feasible and a legally authorized representative is not reasonably available, the investigator has committed, if feasible, to attempting to contact within the therapeutic window the subject's family member who is not a legally authorized representative, and asking whether he or she objects to the subject's participation in the research. The investigator will summarize efforts made to contact family members and make this information available to the IRB at the time of continuing review.

In addition, the IRB is responsible for ensuring that procedures are in place to inform, at the earliest feasible opportunity, each subject, or if the subject remains incapacitated, a legally authorized representative of the subject, or if such a representative is not reasonably available, a family member, of the subject's inclusion in the research, the details of the research and other information contained in the informed consent document. The IRB shall also ensure that there is a procedure to inform the subject, or if the subject remains incapacitated, a legally authorized representative of the subject, or if such a representative is not reasonably available, a family member, that he or she may discontinue the subject's participation at any time without penalty or loss of benefits to which the subject is otherwise entitled. If a legally authorized representative or family member is told about the research and the subject's condition improves, the subject is also to be informed as soon as feasible. If a subject is entered into research with waived consent and the subject dies before a legally authorized representative or family member can be contacted, information about the research is to be provided to the subject's legally authorized representative or family member, if feasible.

For the purposes of this waiver, "family member" means any one of the following legally competent persons: spouses; parents; children (including adopted children); brothers, sisters, and spouses of brothers and sisters; and any individual related by blood or affinity whose close association with the subject is the equivalent of a family relationship.

On October 2, 1996 (*Federal Register*, Vol. 61, pp. 51498–51531), the FDA published a final rule that amends FDA regulations to authorize a waiver of informed consent in research that is regulated by the FDA. The joint publication of these actions permits harmonization of the DHHS and FDA regulations regarding research in emergency circumstances. The DHHS waiver, just as the FDA regulatory change, provides a narrow exception to the requirement for obtaining and documenting informed consent from each human subject or his or her legally authorized representative before initiation of research if the waiver of informed consent is approved by an IRB. The waiver authorization applies to a limited class of research activities involving human subjects who are in need of emergency medical intervention but who cannot give informed consent because of their life-threatening medical condition and who do not have available a legally authorized person to represent them. The secretary of the DHHS is authorizing this waiver in response to growing concerns that current regulations, absent this waiver, are making high-quality research in emergency circumstances difficult or impossible to carry out at a time when the need for such research is increasingly recognized.

Sincerely,

Gary B. Ellis, Ph.D.
Director
Office for Protection
from Research Risks

Melody H. Lin, Ph.D.
Deputy Director
Office for Protection from
Research Risks

PART 5

Initial Protocol Review and the Full-Committee Meeting

Overview of Initial Protocol Review

Sarah T. Khan and Susan Z. Kornetsky

INTRODUCTION

The purpose of this chapter is to provide an overview of the process of initial review of human subject protocols submitted to the institutional review board (IRB). We focus on the administrative procedures for performing a thorough initial IRB review, such as methods to ensure receipt of a complete protocol application. We also provide criteria for the administrative staff and IRB members to use when reviewing protocols. The last half of this chapter is devoted to issues for IRB administrators to consider when establishing policies and procedures, and for reviewers to think about during initial review.

The Protocol Application

To evaluate each human subject protocol fully in accordance with federally mandated criteria,[1(Sec.111),2] and local institutional policies, IRBs must receive well-organized information about the study. This should be accomplished using IRB-developed protocol forms, which allow investigators the opportunity to address both federal and institutional requirements.

Often, it is necessary to modify the protocol application form because new regulatory and ethical issues arise. For example, in recent years, the use of biological specimens for genetic research has raised ethical concerns. Questions can be incorporated into the protocol application to ensure that investigators address these concerns.

Information Required in Applications

IRBs may receive applications from cooperative group programs such as Eastern Cooperative Oncology Group (ECOG), industry or federally sponsored, or "home grown" investigator initiated studies. The following information must be included in each protocol application: background information, discussion of preliminary studies results, specific aims and hypotheses, recruitment practices, eligibility criteria, the proposed plan of research, plans for data analysis, adverse event reporting and monitoring, risks and benefits, and alternatives.

Unless a waiver of consent is requested, each application must also contain an informed consent form and an assent form if appropriate. If a waiver is requested, the investigator must satisfy the four federal criteria for obtaining a waiver. IRBs require additional information such as advertisements and flyers if these are to be used to recruit participants. Chapter 5-7 discusses these advertisements further. Some IRBs also request copies of actual assessment tools, case report forms, surveys, and questionnaires.

The Submission Process

The receipt of a complete protocol is the first step in IRB review. The timing of meetings and deadlines and ancillary review and signature requirements needs to be carefully considered and planned. The IRB must receive all materials that it needs to perform a meaningful and comprehensive initial review.

IRB Issues to Consider

Is there an established deadline for protocol application submissions? IRB members need ample time to review protocols. The timing of protocol submission will depend on the number of protocols, the number of committee members reviewing the protocols, and the IRB meeting dates. The time required for preparation of protocol materials before distribution to members will determine how far in advance applications need to be received in the IRB administrative office. Submission deadlines are helpful when there are set meeting dates. However, before setting deadlines, consideration should be given to whether all protocols and materials submitted by a deadline are *guaranteed* review at the meeting for which the deadline was set. IRBs at smaller institutions, specialized IRBs, or IRBs that meet very frequently may be able to work with deadline-oriented schedules. Another approach is a "first come, first served." In this case, the maximum number of protocols accepted for review at each meeting is set beforehand. Extra protocols are triaged to the next meeting that has available review slots. We recommend that protocols be distributed to IRB members at least 1 week in advance of the meeting.

How often and for how long does the IRB meet? This will influence how many protocols can be reviewed at each meeting. Many IRBs have moved to limit the number of protocols reviewed at each meeting because of past criticism for reviewing protocols too quickly or cursorily. IRBs want to allow ample time for thoughtful discussion during meetings. The ability to limit the number of protocols per meeting depends on the frequency of meetings. Limiting the number of reviews should be an individual decision for each IRB based on its resources.

Is a staff member available at all times to answer questions about protocol submissions? An IRB administrator should always be available during regular business hours to answer questions regarding protocol submissions.

How many copies of a protocol application should an investigator submit? What documents should each member receive? The answers to these questions depend on whether all members are to receive a full copy of every protocol or if only selected reviewers receive complete copies of each protocol. In addition, whether the IRB office has a budget sufficient to copy protocols will determine whether copying is a responsibility of the investigator or of the IRB. Electronic submissions make the full protocol accessible to all members.

Ancillary Review

Prior to IRB review, the institution may require multiple ancillary reviews depending on the nature of the study (e.g., nursing, institutional biosafety committee (IBC), radiation safety, pharmacy, resource management). Every institution should have a clear plan for investigators in order to efficiently allow these reviews to proceed (e.g., a unified application could be developed so that researchers are not required to complete multiple forms). The IRB should be aware of the results and the reviews should be appropriately documented as applicable.

Prereview and Distribution of Applications

Expedited versus Full Review
Determination of which protocols require full-committee review and which may be reviewed via the expedited process is an important task and therefore should be the responsibility of either the IRB chair or a designated IRB member who is familiar with the federal regulations pertaining to expedited review requirements (Federal Regulations 1 and 2, Section 110). Details about expedited review and the criteria for allowing such review can be found in Chapter 4-2.

Prereview Mechanisms
If a protocol requires full IRB review, there should be a process by which the protocol undergoes preliminary review before formal review by the IRB. Any preliminary review should help investigators focus on problem areas in the research protocol. Some examples and discussion of the pros and cons of different mechanisms for prereview follow.

Limited or No Prereview by Administrative Staff
The protocol materials are received, immediately copied, and distributed to IRB members or selected individuals for review. Although this method is the quickest, the potential for distributing incomplete or poorly constructed protocols to IRB members exists, and this will most definitely require significantly more time after the meeting to address the problem.

Prereview by a Designated IRB Member
The IRB designates an IRB member to perform a prereview of the protocol and question the investigator directly on any concern before the meeting. The investigator must respond to the comments before the protocol is distributed and reviewed by IRB members. The breadth of this type of review depends on the definition of the role of the previewer, including the assigned members' area of expertise.

Prereview by Administrative Staff
Depending on the educational background, experience, and training of the IRB administrative staff, preliminary review by the administrative staff members may be possible. Administrative staff can sufficiently review issues related to human subject protection, such as recruitment practices and informed consent methods and carry out the preparation of the protocol materials. However, they may not be able to review scientific issues such as significance of preliminary data, feasibility of specific aims, and data analysis plans.

Continuing Prereview or Consultative Discussions
Prereview or consultative discussions may occur at any time before submission to the IRB. At Children's Hospital in Boston, investigators are encouraged to seek advice and consultation from the IRB administrative staff in planning their research protocol. A preliminary review of the protocol application helps investigators strengthen the protocol application. Early consultation at the earliest time may provide investigators with guidance about what human subject issues are likely to be of concern and suggestions for addressing them in the protocol application.

Being able to offer this type of service within an IRB office requires adequate staffing and resources as well as a staff that has in-depth knowledge and experience. At its best, this consultative system works well and is well appreciated by investigators. It also helps promote the customer-service oriented and proactive image of the IRB by showing investigators that the IRB office is willing to work with them, as opposed to policing them. The experience of the staff at Children's Hospital in Boston has been that when the IRB works with investigators in trying to address human subject concerns, the investigators are more forthcoming with the issues that need addressing. This creates a positive feedback loop that helps the IRB accomplish its charge. This process may also save time during the review process.

An institution will need to ask several questions in determining what type of prereview to offer including the following: (1) How should protocols be tracked once they are received in an administrative office? (2) Does the IRB find value in a prereview process? If so, who is the appropriate person to perform this prereview? (3) At what level should a prereview occur? (4) How long does it take to perform a preliminary review, and how does this affect an IRB's time schedule? (5) Does the institution have appropriate staffing to perform prereview?

Assignment of Primary and Secondary Reviewers

All IRB members must receive a complete description of the study protocol and the consent form and be prepared to discuss the project at the IRB meeting. Many IRBs, however, have implemented a primary and secondary reviewer system whereby one to two members are expected to complete a detailed, thorough review of their assigned study. The primary reviewer presents a summary of the protocol and potential issues to the IRB at the convened meeting. The secondary reviewer may or may not have additional comments. After discussion a vote is recorded.

It is important for the IRB administrative staff and/or chair to be aware of the following points when considering primary and secondary reviewer assignments: (1) Area of expertise: An IRB member's area of expertise should be the first criterion considered when determining which protocol(s) he or she is assigned. (2) Potential conflicts of interest (COI).

Initial Review and the Reviewer Worksheet

The regulations specify criteria for IRB review and approval of 45 CFR 46.[1] [(Sec.111)] IRB members must apply these criteria during the review process and have appropriate knowledge and understanding of the regulations. A tool to assist investigators in performing an in-depth and thorough review is the reviewer worksheet. In some institutions, the use of a worksheet may be only suggested; at others, it may be mandatory. At Children's Hospital in Boston, primary and secondary reviewers must complete a worksheet for each assigned protocol.

The Children's Hospital Reviewer Worksheet incorporates ideas taken from many other institutions. The remainder of this chapter describes this worksheet as a model for the development of such a tool for any IRB. Children's Hospital in Boston has pledged to maintain review standards consistent with federal requirements for all clinical trials being conducted at the institution regardless of the agency funding the trials. The worksheet contains 12 sections (1–12 later here). Each addresses with specific questions one of the criteria for IRB approval as specified in the regulations. Additional space is provided so that reviewers can write questions that an investigator needs to address. A completed worksheet highlights the questions that an investigator needs to answer.

1. Introduction, Specific Aims, Background, and Significance

Review of any research protocol must begin with the IRB member asking and answering these questions: "Why is this research important to conduct?" and "What will be learned from the proposed study?" IRB members should be provided with adequate data regarding earlier related studies and associated references. Applications must include a clear description of the objectives of the research and a statement of the study hypothesis and should adequately address how data will be obtained.

Worksheet Questions

1. Are the study aims/objectives clearly specified?
2. Are there adequate preliminary data to justify the research?
3. Are adequate references provided?
4. Is there appropriate justification for this research protocol?

2. Drugs, Devices, and Biologics

When considering research protocols that include the use of drugs, devices, and biologics, IRB reviewers must apply the regulations of the FDA. If drugs or biologics are to be administered as part of a research protocol, investigators must specify their IND or IDE status. Information including the dose, route of administration, previous use, and safety and efficacy data need to be evaluated. Reviewers must consider the phase of drug/biologic testing as it relates to risks and benefits of participation. For the proposed use of investigational devices, reviewers must consider the classification of the investigational device as posing a nonsignificant risk or significant risk, as the definition applies to devices. This determination has implications for the sponsor/manufacturer of the device and their obligations for filing with the FDA. Details regarding the determination of significant risk versus nonsignificant risk are discussed elsewhere in this book. The following questions are helpful to include in the reviewer worksheet.

Worksheet Questions

1. Is the status of the drug or device described and appropriate (investigational, new use of an FDA-approved drug, or an FDA-approved drug with approved indications)?
2. Are the drug dose and route of administration appropriate?
3. Are the drug or device safety and efficacy data sufficient to warrant the proposed phase of testing?
4. Is the significant risk or nonsignificant risk status of the device described and appropriate? And do you, the reviewer, agree with this determination?
5. Does the protocol describe acceptable accountability, storage, access, and control of the devices?

3. Scientific Design

Institutions have varying policies and practices for reviewing and approving the scientific design and merit of a research protocol. Some institutions have a scientific review committee separate from the IRB; at others, the IRB assumes full responsibility for scientific review. At some institutions, scientific review is conducted at the departmental level, whereas others employ a combination of departmental and institutional services depending on the protocol. Even when scientific review is not designated as an institutional IRB responsibility, IRBs must feel confident that the scientific merit of a protocol justifies its risk/benefit ratio. IRBs are required to evaluate whether the study procedures are consistent with sound research design that minimizes risks to the subject.

Worksheet Questions

1. Is the scientific design adequate to answer the question(s)?
2. Are the aims/objectives likely to be achievable within a given time period?
3. Is the scientific design (i.e., randomization; placebo controls; Phase I, II, or III) described and adequately justified?

4. Research Procedures

IRB reviewers must fully consider the procedures involved in research. Reviewers should ask this: "What procedures will the subject undergo for the purpose of this research? How is this different from what is done as part of standard clinical care?" Reviewers must differentiate those procedures that are performed for research purposes from those that are performed for routine care or evaluation and determine whether the research is going to be conducted in a way that minimizes risks to subjects by employing procedures that are already being performed for diagnostic or treatment purposes (45 CFR 46 Section 111.a1). Reviewers are also responsible for understanding the actual studies, including the timing, the setting, and the qualifications of those conducting the research. If there are flow charts or schemas, it is important that they be consistent with the text of the protocol and the informed consent document. Procedures for monitoring the subject during the research must also be evaluated. When questionnaires and behavioral or psychologic assessments are included as part of the research evaluation, the reviewer should review these instruments. A description of what will happen to study data and to results should also be provided. The following questions are helpful in evaluating study procedures:

Worksheet Questions

1. Are the rationale and details of the research procedures accurately described and acceptable?
2. Is there a clear differentiation between research procedures and standard care and evaluation?
3. Are there adequate plans to inform subjects about specific research results that might affect the subject's health and/or decision to continue participation?

5. Inclusion/Exclusion Criteria for Subjects

Appropriate inclusion and exclusion criteria for research participants are essential in order to justify human subject research ethically. Selection of subjects must be equitable. Criteria for inclusion may consist of any combination of biomedical and behavioral characteristics. Poorly specified inclusion/exclusion criteria may result in inadvertent exclusion of eligible research subjects and an imbalance of or inappropriate enrollment of research subjects. IRBs are mandated to assure that special classes of subjects, especially vulnerable populations (i.e., women, minorities, and children), are included when appropriate. If for some reason inclusion criteria are not equitable, justification must be provided. Reviewer questions to consider include the following:

Worksheet Questions

1. Are inclusion and exclusion criteria clearly stated and reasonable?
2. Is the principle of distributive justice adequately incorporated into the inclusion and exclusion criteria for the research protocol? Is subject selection equitable?
3. Are minorities, women, children, or other vulnerable populations included in the study design? Is the inclusion or exclusion of special populations justified?
4. For subjects vulnerable to coercion or undue influence, are additional safeguards included to protect the rights and welfare of these subjects (e.g., prisoners, mentally ill, economically/educationally disadvantaged, employees)?

6. Statistical Analysis and Data Monitoring

Research protocols must contain well-conceived, well-formulated, and appropriate plans for interpretation of data and statistical analyses. The interpretation of data section should provide enough evidence to convince a reviewer that the proposed design has a reasonable chance of achieving the principal objectives of the research. IRB members should be given enough information to determine that the sample size and statistical power or precision associated with the sample size is adequate. In addition, forethought must be given to developing a sound method of data and statistical analysis, with adequate stratification factors and treatment allocation plans for the study design after study completion. IRB members must be adequately informed about plans for ongoing monitoring of the data.

Worksheet Questions

1. Is the rationale for the proposed number of subjects reasonable? Were formal sample size calculations performed and are they available for review?
2. Are the plans for data and statistical analysis defined and justified, including the use of stopping rules and endpoints?
3. Are there adequate provisions for monitoring data (Data and Safety Monitoring Board/Plan)?

7. Subject Privacy and Confidentiality

Reviewers must consider the extent to which research procedures could potentially invade privacy or breach patient confidentiality. These possibilities present a risk of harm to the subject. IRBs must consider the type and sensitivity of the information sought, how the information will be recorded, precautions taken to protect confidentiality, and who has access to the research records. Precautions can and should be taken, depending on the nature of the research. This may include the possibility of applying for a Certificate of Confidentiality.

Worksheet Questions

1. Are there adequate provisions to protect the privacy and assure the confidentiality of the research subject?
2. Are there adequate plans and provisions to protect the confidentiality of data during and after research?

3. Is the use of identifiers or links to identifiers necessary, and how is this information protected? Are these measures adequate?

4. Does the PI specify in the protocol and consent form whether research data and information (including informed consent) will be placed in the medical records?

8. Recruitment of Subjects

IRB members must consider how, when, and by whom participants are to be identified and approached for recruitment. Reviewers must consider methods for recruiting subjects (traditional paper or Internet advertisements, databases, newsletters, recruitment by sending letters, from physician referrals, medical record reviews, etc.). It is important to consider what study staff member is best suited to approach potential research subjects, when and where subjects should be contacted, and the amount of time provided for potential subjects to consider participation. All recruitment materials and practices must be reviewed and approved by the IRB. The IRB must be assured that the recruitment process promotes voluntary participation and is not coercive in any way.

Worksheet Questions

1. Are the methods for recruiting potential subjects well defined?

2. Are the location and timing of the recruitment process acceptable?

3. Is the individual performing the recruitment appropriate for the process?

4. Are all recruitment materials submitted and appropriate?

5. Are there acceptable methods for screening subjects before recruitment (e.g., mailings, record reviews)?

9. Subject Compensation and Costs

IRB members are charged with the responsibility of reviewing and approving compensation and/or reimbursement of costs to research subjects. Reimbursements may take the form of reimbursement for expenses associated with research participation such as travel expenses, lost wages, and parking costs. Compensation may be provided to participants for their time and effort. The IRB must be certain that the compensation or reimbursement offered is not so large as to be coercive. The compensation plan must be clearly described in the consent form.

Worksheet Questions

1. Is the amount or type of compensation or reimbursement reasonable and noncoercive?

2. Are there adequate provisions to avoid out-of-pocket expenses and costs by the research subject if insurance denies payment? If not, is there sufficient justification to allow subjects to pay for these expenses?

10. Potential Risks/Discomforts and Benefits for Subjects

IRB members are charged with the responsibility of reviewing the potential risks, discomforts, hazards, or inconveniences of participating in a research protocol.

This responsibility also includes evaluating the probability, magnitude, and duration of the risks involved. IRB members must identify the physical pain or discomfort as well as the psychologic, emotional, or sociological harm, including invasion of privacy, loss of confidentiality, harassment, and lessening of an individual's dignity. Inconveniences such as loss of time or pay are also included in this category. Risk to a community or a group of individuals must also be considered. The initial reviewer must consider the potential risks as well as the precautions that will be taken to avoid or minimize potential risks.

Potential benefits can apply directly to the subject or to the advancement of scientific knowledge. IRBs must consider the magnitude and probability of direct benefit to a subject to be certain the research protocol does not overstate the benefits or potentially raise false expectations of benefit for the participants. It is important for the IRB to evaluate the risk/benefit ratio and to understand the rationale for believing the risk/benefit ratio is acceptable.

The IRB must give special consideration to risks and benefits for research involving children, pregnant women, and other vulnerable populations such as the mentally impaired and prisoners. It is strongly recommended that the reviewer worksheet include specific questions about the special assessments to be made if vulnerable populations are part of the research population. Institution-specific questions should also be listed. For example, most protocols reviewed by the IRB at Children's Hospital in Boston are pediatric studies. When it is determined that a pediatric protocol poses greater than minimal risk, the reviewers must determine whether the increased risk is a slight increase over minimal risk. If in addition to being greater than minimal risk, no potential for direct benefit to the subject is expected, protocols must meet four criteria in order to be approved: (1) the risks of the study must represent a minor increase over minimal risk, (2) intervention/procedures must present experiences commensurate with those inherent in actual care, (3) intervention/procedures must be likely to yield generalizable knowledge about the subject's disorder of vital important for the understanding or amelioration of the subject's disorder, and (4) there must be adequate provisions for soliciting assent and permission of parents/guardians. These requirements are included in the standard Children's Hospital in Boston Reviewer Worksheet. A few additional questions are provided later here.

Worksheet Questions

1. Are the risks and benefits adequately identified, evaluated, and described?

2. Are the risks reasonable in relation to the benefits to be gained? Are the risks reasonable in relationship to importance of the knowledge to be gained?

3. Are the risks minimized to the greatest extent possible?

   a. This study uses procedures that are consistent with sound research design.

   b. This study uses procedures that do not unnecessarily expose subjects to risk.

c. When possible, study uses procedures already being performed on subjects for diagnostic/treatment purposes.

4. Example of more specific questions for a vulnerable population: If children are involved, within which category of risk/benefit does the protocol fall? Are all criteria within the category adequately addressed? Please refer to Chapter 9-7 for more information on the risk/benefit determination for protocols involving children.

11. Informed Consent/Assent

The consent and assent sections of the reviewer worksheet are divided into three sections: the consent/assent document(s), which includes a list of required elements; the consent/assent process; and any waivers or alterations of informed consent requirements.

11a. The Consent/Assent Document

General federal requirements for informed consent are provided in 45 CFR 46 Section 116. The checklist provided below combines the informed consent requirements of the Department of Health and Human Services and the FDA. Each element listed must be included in the informed consent, unless it is not applicable.

Assent and Witness Requirement

Unlike the consent document, no federal regulations exist for assent documents. However, many institutions still require separate assent documentation, whereas others require a child's co-signature on a parental permission form. For protocols that involve children, each IRB must determine whether the obtainment of assent is required and, if so, an appropriate mechanism for obtaining and documenting assent. The IRB must also determine whether the permission or one or both parents should be obtained. Assent obtainment and documentation requirements need to be considered on a per-protocol basis. The following reviewer worksheet questions prompt the IRB members to make this special determination when required.

Worksheet Questions

1. Is assent required?

2. If yes, is a separate assent form required? Is a witness signature or an attestation to the assent required?

3. For parental consent, if the subject is unable to consent, is the signature of one or both parents/guardians required?

Checklist of Informed Consent Required Elements

1. Consent/assent form checklist
2. Statement that the study involves research
3. Purpose of research stated in lay language
4. Reason subject is asked to participate
5. Expected duration of study
6. Study design described in lay language (number of groups, randomization, use of placebo)
7. Study procedures or treatments
8. Description of drug or device (if applicable); state whether it is investigational
9. Compensation or reimbursement

10. Number of subjects in the trial
11. Potential risks or discomforts to the subject
12. Potential direct benefits or benefits to society
13. Alternatives available (indicate if none)
14. Statement that participation is voluntary and subject may withdraw
15. Additional costs associated with participating—who will pay for what
16. How confidentiality will be protected; who has access to the data

Elements required only if applicable to study:

17. Anticipated circumstances under which a subject's participation may be terminated
18. Statement that significant new findings will be disclosed
19. Consequences of withdrawal
20. If greater than minimal risk, statement included regarding compensation in event of injury

11b. Process of Obtaining Informed Consent/Assent

Although the regulations require the inclusion of certain elements in the informed consent document, they do not provide rules or requirements for the process of obtaining informed consent. At Children's Hospital in Boston, investigators and reviewers are urged to consider the following general recommendations and suggestions when proposing or reviewing a method of obtaining consent.

Who?

It is important to consider what type of relationship exists between the patient and the person approaching the patient for consent.

When?

When potential subjects are being educated or informed about the research opportunity available to them, timing is very important. The IRB should consider when subjects would be approached regarding participation in a research study.

Where and How?

The IRB should consider where the informed consent process will take place and how it will be conducted.

Worksheet Questions

1. Is the process well defined?
2. Does the process provide sufficient time, privacy, and an adequate setting for the subject to consider participation?
3. Does this process minimize the possibility of coercion or undue influence?
4. Is the individual obtaining consent/assent appropriate to do so?
5. Are the issues of subject's comprehension and autonomy considered?

11c. Waiver or Modification of Informed Consent

Federal regulations permit the waiver or alteration of the informed consent document if a protocol meets very specific criteria. These are provided in other sections of this book. In order for the IRB to determine whether a protocol meets the criteria, it is essential that investigators seeking the waiver or alteration provide adequate justification for the request. The worksheet questions later here help IRB reviewers to look for the appropriate justification if a waiver or alteration is requested.

Worksheet Questions
Consider when appropriate:

1. Have the criteria for waiver/modification of informed consent documentation been met?
   a. The consent form would be the only record linking the subject with the research, *and* a potential risk would be a breach in confidentiality. In such case, it is up to the subject when asked if they want documentation.
   b. Study is no more than minimal risk of harm to subjects and involves no procedures for which written consent is normally required outside the research context.
2. If informed consent documentation is waived, should the investigator be required to provide subjects with a written statement regarding the research?
3. If children are included, have the criteria for waiver of parental/guardian consent been met?
   a. IRB must determine parental/guardian permission is not a reasonable requirement to protect subjects.
   b. Appropriate mechanisms must be implemented to protect children as subjects.
4. If *waiver or modification* to required consent elements was proposed, have all the criteria been met?
   a. The research involves no more than minimal risk to the subjects.
   b. The waiver/alteration will not adversely affect the rights and welfare of the subjects.
   c. The research could not practicably be carried out without the waiver or alteration, and when appropriate, the subject will be provided with pertinent information after participation.

12. Other Issues and Considerations

Other issues discussed previously in this chapter may be useful to question in this section of the reviewer worksheet (e.g., allocation of resources, continuing review, potential conflicts of interest, and the need for additional ancillary review). The interval between reviews must be determined on an individualized, per-protocol basis and must consider the degree of risk associated with the protocol. 45 CFR 46[1(Sec.109)] states that IRBs are required to conduct continuing review of research at intervals appropriate to the degree of risk and at a minimum, review must occur once annually. More frequent review may be necessary and is recommended for high-risk protocols.

Worksheet Questions

1. When should the next review occur? Should it occur before the required annual review of the study? If frequent reviews are necessary, how should the interval be determined?
2. Are there any notable conflicts of interest?
3. Institution-specific questions should also be listed here.
4. Are there appropriate resources (such as equipment, space, funding, staff) to conduct this research safely?
5. Has the investigator assured appropriate monitoring of subjects during and after the research? If applicable, will counseling, referrals, or other support services be provided?

6. If applicable, are there provisions included for research-related injuries?

Advantages of Using a Reviewer Worksheet

It is important to emphasize that a comprehensive initial review of a research protocol is essential to a smoothly functioning IRB. Depending on IRB policies and practices for initial review of research protocols, the reviewer worksheet may be used at different times during the initial review process. The time of use is not important, as long as the criteria listed on the worksheet are considered during the review process. In general, the earlier in the review process these criteria are evaluated, the better and more thorough the review will be.

There are several major advantages to using a reviewer worksheet during the initial review process. At Children's Hospital in Boston, completion and submission of the worksheet is mandatory for both the primary and secondary reviewers. Although all IRB members receive a copy of the protocol application and are encouraged to comment on each protocol, it is the responsibility of the primary and secondary reviewers to make certain that the issues included in the reviewer worksheet are addressed in each protocol they review. The reviewer worksheet serves the purpose of a reminder checklist of the mandated criteria they must consider before approving a protocol. It is also a convenient and organized way to assist the reviewers in discussing their critique of the protocol during a meeting.

The worksheet is also the basis for further discussion and dialogue between the IRB and investigators. The worksheet helps the IRB administrative staff to document comments and report the IRB's findings back to the investigator after the meeting, and prepare minutes of the IRB meeting. Additional advantages are as follows:

1. The reviewer worksheet is a quality-control mechanism that ensures that reviewers have considered all of the regulatory and institutional criteria for review and approval.
2. The reviewer worksheet encourages and provides a level of consistency in the IRB review process.
3. The reviewer worksheet can serve as written documentation that the initial review process occurred.

Conclusion

The purpose of this chapter is to provide an overview of the process of initial review of human subject protocols. Mechanisms such as those described here provide guidance for IRB offices to establish a process for initial protocol review.

References

1. Code of Federal Regulations. Title 45A—Department of Health and Human Services; Part 46—Protection of Human Subjects. Updated 1 October, 1997. Access date 18 April, 2001.
2. Code of Federal Regulations. Title 21, Chapter 1—Food and Drug Administration, DHHS; Part 56—Institutional Review Boards. Updated 1 April, 1999. Access date 27 March, 2001.

Evaluating Study Design and Quality

Robert J. Amdur

INTRODUCTION

It is not unusual for institutional review board (IRB) members, institutional officials, and researchers to debate the role of the IRB in evaluating study design or other aspects that affect the fundamental quality of the science of research. For example, is it appropriate for IRB members to vote not to approve a study because they believe study results would be more persuasive if a different control group were used or because previously completed research has already answered the study question? Is it appropriate for the IRB to question the validity of the statistical power calculation used to determine the number of subjects in a study? Some members of the research community are under the impression that it is not the role of the IRB to evaluate the quality of the science of a protocol. Many IRB chairs have been confronted with statements such as this: "The IRB's job is to evaluate ethics. The IRB has no business commenting on the science of a study." In most cases, this view will be presented by a researcher who has been criticized by the IRB, but in some situations, the argument will come from IRB members or institutional officials.

The purpose of this chapter is to explain the role of the IRB in evaluating study design and the other features of a study that may affect scientific quality. There is no question that the IRB not only has the authority to evaluate scientific quality, but also has the obligation to do so if it is to function in compliance with accepted ethical codes and federal research regulations.

Ethical Codes

Nuremberg Code (1949)

Several sections of the Nuremberg code address scientific quality and the risk/benefit profile. Point 3 is representative: "The experiment should be so designed and based on the results of animal experimentation and a knowledge of the natural history of the disease or other problem under study that the anticipated results will justify the performance of the experiment."

Declaration of Helsinki (2000)

Multiple sections of the latest version of this ethical code address specific aspects of study design. Sections 11, 18, and 29 are especially relevant to the question of IRB review of scientific quality.

> 11. Medical research involving human subjects must conform to generally accepted scientific principles and be based on a thorough knowledge of the scientific literature, other relevant sources of information, and adequate laboratory and, where appropriate, animal experimentation.
>
> 18. Medical research involving human subjects should only be conducted if the importance of the objective outweighs the inherent risks and burdens to the subject. This is especially important when the human subjects are healthy volunteers.
>
> 29. The benefits, risks, burdens, and effectiveness of a new method should be tested against those of the best current prophylactic, diagnostic, and therapeutic methods. This does not exclude the use of placebo, or no treatment, in studies where no proven prophylactic, diagnostic, or therapeutic method exists.

Federal Research Regulations

Department of Health and Human Services and corresponding Food and Drug Administration regulations require the IRB to determine that the study is designed so that risks to subjects are minimized and justified by potential benefits. This excerpt is from 45 CFR 46.[1][Sec.111(a)]

(a) Criteria for IRB approval of Research
  1. Risks to subjects are minimized by using procedures that are consistent with sound research design and that do not unnecessarily expose subjects to risk.
  2. Risks to subjects are reasonable in relation to anticipated benefits, if any, to subjects, and the importance of the knowledge that may reasonably be expected to result. In evaluating risks and benefits, the IRB should consider only those risks and benefits that may result from the research (as distinguished from risks and benefits of therapies subjects would receive even if not participating in the research).

The IRB's Responsibility to Evaluate Scientific Quality

The IRB reviews protocols to act in compliance with federal research regulations and makes decisions that support the ethical principles in accepted ethical codes such as the Nuremberg Code and the Declaration of Helsinki. The sections from these guidance documents reproduced previously emphasize that a characteristic of ethical research is that (1) the study is designed so that the risks to subjects are minimized and (2) the potential benefits of the research justify the potential risks. It is these two directives that establish the obligation of the IRB to consider carefully the study design and overall scientific quality of each study.

The Study Design
If revising the study design will meaningfully decrease the risk to subjects without a major compromise in the persuasiveness of the study results, then the IRB should not approve the protocol. There are also situations where the IRB should not approve research because the study design is so flawed that the value of the study results will be almost zero. In this setting, risks may be low, but the potential benefit is zero; thus, the overall risk/benefit profile of the study is unacceptable. Similarly, when a study that involves risk is designed to ask a question that is not important or has already been answered by previous research, the risk/benefit profile is likely to be unfavorable. The IRB is obligated to evaluate the study design and other aspects of scientific quality because these are ethical issues that affect the rights and welfare of research participants.

Having stressed the importance of evaluating the scientific quality of research, it is important to remember that, as with all ethical principles, the IRB should use individual judgment and common sense when considering not approving a study because of the study design. In organizations in which a large volume of social science research is done by students, it is not unusual for the IRB to review protocols in which the scientific design is not optimal but the risk to subjects is virtually zero. An example would be a survey study that attempts to correlate the attitudes of college students about globalization of the economy with their decision to apply to graduate school.

Although one could argue that many of these student projects could legitimately be classified as educational exercises rather than research, that is a separate issue. The point is that there are projects where the study design is flawed, but the risk is basically zero. Certainly, it makes sense for IRB members who are knowledgeable in this type of research to recommend revisions to the study plan. However, in the absence of meaningful risk, there is really no ethical justification for the IRB to make such revisions a condition for IRB approval. Each case must be evaluated independently.

Departmental Scientific Review Before IRB Review
Given that scientific quality is a criterion for IRB approval of research, the next question is the process of IRB review of scientific aspects of specific studies. Tasks such as evaluating the details of study design, the qualifications of the investigator, and the value of a proposed study in the context of what is already known require specialized expertise in the area that is being evaluated in the study. Many IRBs will find that the background of their membership is such that it is difficult for the committee to effectively evaluate scientific issues for the wide range of protocols that the committee reviews. One solution is to request a consultant who is expert in the area in question to comment on scientific issues. However, when scientific evaluations outside the IRB are needed on a regular basis, asking for consultant opinions on a case-by-case basis is likely to be awkward and inefficient.

To facilitate the evaluation of scientific quality in research, some organizations establish policy that requires a formal review of scientific issues by a representative of the investigator's department (or other relevant group) before the protocol is forwarded to the IRB. A system that works well for both researchers and the IRB has been in place for over 10 years at Dartmouth College and Dartmouth Medical School. The requirement for review of scientific quality before IRB review was established at the level of the Office of the Dean of the School of Medicine and is called "departmental scientific review." In most departments, a committee—usually consisting of three to six individuals with research experience—reviews each protocol that is to be submitted to the IRB from a member of that department. In small departments or departments with limited research experience, the departmental scientific review is handled by a single individual (possibly from another department) who is not a collaborator on the research under review. As the system has evolved, the IRB has found it useful to use an issue-specific form to guide and document evaluation of the scientific issues that are especially important to the IRB. The Dartmouth IRB asks for the name of a representative from the group conducting the scientific review who will be available to attend an IRB meeting to explain the protocol if this is considered necessary. This is a unique aspect of the Dartmouth system compared with that used at most other centers. Because the review form emphasizes that a member of the reviewing team may be expected to defend the science of the study to the IRB, there is a level of accountability that is not present when the scientific review committee knows that it is the principal investigator who will be discussing any contentious issues.

Conclusion

This chapter has explained the role of the IRB in evaluating study design and the other features of a study that may affect scientific quality. There is no question that the IRB not only has the authority to evaluate scientific quality, but it has the obligation to do so if it is to function in compliance with accepted ethical codes and federal research regulations. The Nuremberg Code, the Declaration of Helsinki, and federal research regulations contain sections that highlight the importance of study design and scientific quality as standards for ethical research. In most organizations, it will be useful to establish scientific review committees to comment on study design and scientific quality before the proposal goes to the IRB. A sample "Departmental Scientific Review Form" may be found on the Dartmouth College IRB website: http://www.dartmouth.edu/~cphs.

Reference

1. Code of Federal Regulations. Title 45A—Department of Health and Human Services; Part 46—Protection of Human Subjects. Updated 1 October, 1997. Access date 18 April, 2001. http:www4.law.cornell.edu/cfr/45p46.htm

The Study Population: Women, Minorities, and Children

Amy L. Davis

INTRODUCTION

This chapter introduces the ethical issues related to the selection of human research populations for behavioral/biomedical research studies. Federal regulations require the equitable selection of research subjects. To meet this mandate requires consideration of several questions: What constitutes equitable selection? Who is included in the study cohort? What are the inclusion/exclusion criteria? Do any of the criteria relate to sex, race, or age? Are the inclusion/exclusion criteria reasonably related to the purpose of the research? Are the criteria related to the study issue, or are they based on the convenience of the researcher? These are some critical questions an institutional review board (IRB) must consider at the outset of the protocol review.

The purpose of this chapter should be distinguished from that of other chapters in this book that discuss specific regulatory requirements for IRB review of protocols involving special populations. The questions answered in this chapter precede those addressed in later chapters. This chapter relates to study design and the ethics of initial subject selection. Initially, the IRB must determine that the target population is appropriate for the research project under the guidelines discussed in this chapter. If the target population is considered vulnerable, the IRB must then consider the additional protections, discussed in later chapters, applicable to the special population that is the subject of the research protocol. This chapter reviews the current regulations and related policy on the selection of human subjects. It covers the historical bases for the policy, its practical application, and finally, implementation issues that arise in the equitable selection of human research subjects.

The Regulations

Federal regulations set forth at 45 CFR 46[1][Sec.111(a)(3)] and at 21 CFR 56[2][Sec.111(a)(3)] state simply that "in order to approve research covered by this policy, the IRB shall determine that . . . selection of subjects is equitable." The regulation specifies three criteria that the IRB should consider in making this assessment:

1. The purpose of the research
2. The setting in which the research will be conducted
3. The special problems of research involving vulnerable populations

The regulation is based on *The Belmont Report's* principle of justice, which requires the fair distribution of both the benefits and risks of research.[3] The *IRB Guidebook*[4(Chap.III)] explains the purpose and application of this requirement as follows: "The requirement for an equitable selection of subjects helps ensure that the burdens and benefits of research will be fairly distributed." In evaluating the potential *benefits* of proposed research, the IRB must consider the purpose of the research and whether the subjects selected to participate are members of the population most likely to benefit from the research. In considering the *burdens* associated with the research, the IRB must consider whether the selected group of subjects is already burdened by poverty, illness, or institutionalization. If so, the IRB must consider whether the additional burdens associated with participating in research are justified. Accordingly, the equitable-selection-of-subjects criterion requires a preliminary assessment of risks and benefits of research in the context of the particular characteristics of the research subjects.

Historical Basis

The National Commission for the Protection of Human Subjects, which developed *The Belmont Report*, was created to identify the basic ethical principles that should be followed in conducting human subjects research.[3] In establishing the principle of justice and its corollary doctrine of equitable selection of human subjects, the commission was responding to certain historical examples of discriminatory practices in human subjects research.[3] The most egregious examples are the Nazi experiments with concentration camp victims. The Tuskegee experiments, where poor, black men from the rural South were recruited to participate in a study of the course of syphilis as it progressed untreated, form another example. Researchers have even exploited children confined to mental hospitals. In experiments conducted during the mid-1950s at the Willowbrook State Institution for "mentally defective children" in New York, for example, researchers deliberately infected newly admitted patients with the hepatitis virus to watch the course of the disease. At the Fernald School in Massachusetts, children with mental impairments confined to an institution were given cereal containing minute amounts of radioactive materials. The purpose of the study was to examine mineral uptake in the body. In this example, there was no scientific reason related to the purpose of the research that would justify the selection of this group of subjects. The only reason for selecting this group of children was for the convenience of the researchers.[5] These were the kinds of abuses that *The Belmont Report* aimed at preventing.

This history demonstrates that before the writing of *The Belmont Report* the burdens of human subjects research fell largely on poor and vulnerable populations, whereas the benefits of such research were enjoyed by the wealthy and powerful segments of societies. Today, such blatant examples of unjust research practices are rare. Nevertheless, inequities in subject selection can occur, and IRBs must be sensitive to the more subtle variations.

Recent Policy Developments: Inclusion of Women, Minorities, and Children

Since the publication of *The Belmont Report* and the human subjects protection regulations in the early 1970s, there have been several refinements to the general principle that research subjects be equitably selected. These developments reflect the intrinsic conflict between ensuring that research benefits are equitably distributed and protecting vulnerable populations. The *IRB Guidebook* instructs IRBs not to overprotect vulnerable populations to the extent that they are systematically excluded from the benefits of research.[4(Chap.III)] The challenge is determining the level of risk to which vulnerable subjects may be exposed.

The struggle to balance the interest in fairly distributing the benefits of research with the interest in protecting the vulnerable is particularly evident in the development of regulations pertaining to the inclusion of women and children in research studies. In 1977, the Food and Drug Administration (FDA) issued guidance that excluded women of childbearing potential from participation in early studies of new drugs.[6] The rationale was to protect the fetus from unknown risks of unapproved experimental drugs. This policy was developed in part in response to the tragic effects associated with two drugs: thalidomide and diethylstilbestrol.[7] Thalidomide, used to treat nausea in pregnant women, was found to cause deformed limbs in newborns.[7] Diethylstilbestrol, prescribed to prevent miscarriage, was later associated with a rare form of cancer of the vagina in the daughters of women who had taken the drug.[7]

As a result of the 1977 regulation, little scientific information was collected about the effect of many therapies and drugs in women. For example, studies done to evaluate the effect of aspirin on cardiovascular disease excluded women, thereby excluding women from any benefit that would have resulted from the research.[6]

In 1993, the FDA revised its policy to restrict the participation of women of childbearing age in early clinical trials, including pharmacology studies.[6] The revised policy was based on the expectation that women could be relied on to take appropriate measures against becoming pregnant while enrolled in a research trial. In addition, testing could be done to ensure that pregnant women were not enrolled in a drug trial.[6]

Less than a year later, the National Institutes of Health (NIH) issued a new policy requiring the inclusion of women and minorities in clinical research.[8] The new policy prohibited the routine exclusion of women of childbearing potential from NIH-funded research. Specifically, the policy states this:

> Women and members of minority groups and their subpopulations must be included in all NIH-supported biomedical and behavioral research projects involving human subjects, unless a clear and compelling rationale and justification establishes to the satisfaction of the relevant Institute/Center Director that inclusion is inappropriate with respect to the health of the subjects or the purpose of the research.[8]

Policy development related to the inclusion of children in research reflects a similar debate. In response to what policy makers perceived to be overprotective research practices in connection with children, NIH issued a new policy in 1998 to encourage the enrollment of children in research studies.[9] The NIH policy was a deliberate application of the regulation to select subjects equitably and addressed the potential risks of treating children with medications that receive FDA approval based on research done on adults.[9] Like the policies requiring the inclusion of women and minority groups in research studies, this policy is based on the assumption that children may experience discrete biologic responses to new treatments or drugs. Notwithstanding these regulations, the wisdom of including children in clinical trials is still vigorously debated among research professionals. This history of human subjects protection policy reflects a shift in advocacy from protecting subjects from the risks of research to ensuring the inclusion of subjects in research.[10]

IRB Review and the Principle of Equitable Subject Selection

The goal of the equitable selection policy is to distribute fairly the risks and benefits of research among the populations that stand to benefit from it. The IRB has the authority and the responsibility to examine the extent to which this goal is achieved or impeded in each protocol it reviews. Obviously, the goal cannot be achieved or impeded by any individual protocol, but every protocol has an impact on the ultimate distribution of benefits and risks.

The IRB is in the best position in any given institution to assess that institution's overall performance on this criterion of ethical research. This section outlines a strategy for conducting IRB review of compliance with the equitable selection criterion. It is intended to break down the IRB analysis of equitable selection into the following discrete questions.

What Is the Study Population?

First, the IRB must review a description of the study population. Every study should provide a thorough description of the study population in terms of sex, race, ethnicity, and age. Is the study limited to a certain sex, a certain age group, certain racial or ethnic categories, or certain socioeconomic categories? If some of this information is missing, the IRB must request and evaluate it before approving the protocol.

To answer some of these questions, it may not be sufficient merely to examine the protocol description of the target population. It may also be necessary to examine the methods and manner of recruitment. If, for example, the study intends to target a representative population of men and women of multiple races and ethnic backgrounds but recruitment will only take place through suburban hospitals located in mostly white neighborhoods, the IRB may be justified in challenging the recruitment methodology as inadequate to meet the goal of enrolling a representative group of human subjects.

Is the Description of the Study Population Reasonably Related to the Purpose of the Research?

The IRB should be sure that criteria for selecting certain groups or individuals to participate in a study are scientifically related to the goals of the research and not based merely on criteria of convenience, such as where the researchers or the subjects live or work. For example, an IRB should question the ethics of a study in which the researcher from a medical school targets medical students to study the efficacy and safety of a new drug to treat diabetes. In such a case, there would be no research-related reason for targeting medical students. Medical students do not share unique biologic characteristics that might affect the pharmacokinetics of the new drug. Moreover, the

convenience of recruiting human subjects from the same institution in which the researcher works is not sufficient justification for selecting this group. In addition, there may be a risk that the medical students could feel some pressure to enroll in a study conducted by a person of authority and influence over them.

Similarly, it would probably be unethical to conduct a clinical study of a new drug to treat AIDS using a prison population because prisoners do not share biologic characteristics that differ from other populations. Therefore, the selection of prisoner subjects would have no scientific relevance to the drug's effects.

What Are the Inclusion/Exclusion Criteria for the Study Population?

A related principle is that the target population should be representative of the population that stands to benefit potentially from the research. Research that has the potential to benefit men, women, and children or different races should target study subjects that reflect this diversity in sufficient numbers to distinguish differing effects, risks, and benefits.[8] No group or individual should be categorically *excluded* from the research without a good scientific reason to do so.[11]

An example of unethical exclusion may be a study of the effectiveness of a new drug for hypertension using a male-only cohort. It may be difficult to justify such a study because women also suffer from hypertension and, therefore, could potentially benefit from a new drug for treating the condition. In such a case, both men and women should either be represented in a single study cohort or be represented in two separate studies of the same drug. In this manner, data are collected on the efficacy and safety of the drug in men and women.

Fair representation in the study cohorts of the populations that could benefit from the research, may not be sufficient to meet the federal standards. Researchers must be sensitive to the possibility that variations in data may be based on sex, race, or ethnicity. The 1994 NIH Guidelines specifically require investigators planning Phase III clinical trials to examine data from prior studies to determine whether significant differences exist in intervention effect among sexual or ethnic groups.[8] If such differences are detected, then the Phase III trial must be designed to study the effect separately for each group.[8] In evaluating a Phase III trial protocol, the IRB must assess whether the investigator has met this obligation.

IRBs should also be sensitive to the potential for indirect exclusion of certain groups. A study that includes men and women may still enroll a disproportionate number of one sex. For example, a study of cardiovascular disease that has an exclusion criterion related to age could indirectly exclude women, who contract heart diseases at older ages than men.[12]

The requirement that the study population be representative of the population that may benefit from the research does not mean that it is unethical to study the effect of a drug or intervention on one sex. Because there is less research information on the effects of certain drugs or treatments in women, it may be ethical to conduct "catch-up" research with an all-female cohort. Moreover, there may be gender-specific research questions that might justify a single-sex research study. For example, a study of a drug's effect in menopausal women would most likely satisfy this ethical standard.[6]

What Is the Rationale for Inclusion/Exclusion Criteria?

Since the early 1990s, awareness has grown that research findings ought to be generalizable to individuals outside the study population and that IRBs should not overprotect vulnerable populations. Routine exclusion of certain populations based on sex, race, or age results in a disparity of information about treatment options for the excluded groups and unequal distribution of the risks and benefits of research.[12]

An IRB should review the inclusion/exclusion criteria for the study population and determine whether any group that could be affected by the research is excluded. If such a group is excluded, the IRB should determine whether there is a justification in the proposal for the exclusion and whether that justification is reasonable in relationship to the risks, benefits, and purpose of the research. For example, a study of risk factors for breast cancer could justifiably exclude men, and probably children, but most likely could not justify the exclusion of minority women.

This requirement, that groups not be excluded without adequate justification, does not mean that it is never appropriate for exclusion criteria to be based on race, sex, or age. If there is evidence from prior research that men and women, for example, experience a particular condition disproportionately, then it may be appropriate to conduct separate studies of a particular treatment for that condition using different study populations. For example, because women are affected by osteoporosis in far greater numbers than men, it would be appropriate to study the effects of a new treatment for the condition using an all-female study population.[7(p.89)] In another, less obvious example, it may be appropriate to study the effectiveness of an intervention to prevent HIV infection in a study population of women only. Such a study may be justified by data produced in previous studies that demonstrate that unprotected, heterosexual intercourse poses greater risk to women than men.

To assess the rationale for selecting certain subject groups, IRBs will need to review information on the distribution of the health condition in the general population.[13] If the IRB is not satisfied with the justification for excluding a certain group, the IRB may decide to ask for additional justification from the investigator, condition its approval on the removal of the exclusion criterion, or disapprove the research.

Conclusion

IRBs may be reluctant to demand additional information on the justification for subject selection. Limited resources and excessive demands force IRBs to focus on other approval criteria, such as the balance of risks and benefits

and the effectiveness of the informed consent document. Moreover, IRBs are often concerned about maintaining positive relationships with the researchers with whom they work.[13]

In assuming the awesome responsibility for assessing equity in subject selection, IRBs should be aware that the responsibility is shared with research sponsors. The distribution of research funds nationally determines the ultimate justice of subject selection. An individual study is unlikely to affect the overall equality of the distribution of research risks and benefits.[7(p.89)] Researchers and IRBs should also remember that the equitable selection of research subjects is directly linked to the generalizability of research. Research that is broadly generalizable has greater value than other research.[13]

As with so many challenges of human subjects research, the most effective solution may be training. Education of researchers that heightens sensitivity to the equitable selection of subjects may be the most effective method of realizing the goal.

References

1. Code of Federal Regulations. Title 45A—Department of Health and Human Services; Part 46—Protection of Human Subjects. Updated 1 October, 1997. Access date 18 April, 2001. http://www4.law.cornell.edu/cfr/45p46.htm

2. Code of Federal Regulations. Title 21, Chapter 1—Food and Drug Administration, DHHS; Part 56—Institutional Review Boards. Updated 1 April, 1999. Access date 27 March, 2001. http://www4.law.cornell.edu/cfr/21p56.htm

3. National Commission for the Protection of Human Subjects of Biomedical and Behavioral Research. *The Belmont Report: Ethical principles and guidelines for the protection of human subjects of research*. Updated 1979. Access date 22 March, 2001. http://ohsr.od.nih.gov/mpa/ belmont.php3

4. Penslar RL, Porter JP, Office for Human Research Protections. *Institutional Review Board Guidebook.* Updated 6 February, 2001. Access date 29 March, 2001. http://ohrp.osophs.dhhs.gov/irb/irb_guidebook.htm

5. Advisory Committee on Human Radiation Experiments. *The Human Radiation Experiments: Final Report.* New York: Oxford University Press; 1996. http://tis.eh.doe.gov/ ohre/roadmap/achre/report.html (DOE 061-000-00-848-9)

6. Food and Drug Administration. Guidelines for the study and evaluation of gender differences in the clinical evaluation of drugs. *Fed Regist* 58(139):39406–39416, 1993.

7. Mastroianni AC, Faden R, Federman D (eds.). Committee on the Ethical and Legal Issues Relating to the Inclusion of Women in Clinical Studies, Division of Health Sciences Policy, Institute of Medicine. *Women and Health Research: Ethical and Legal Issues of Including Women in Clinical Studies,* Vol. 1. Washington, DC: National Academy Press; 1994. http://search.nap.edu/books/ 030904992X/html/

8. National Institutes of Health. NIH Guidelines on the Inclusion of Women and Minorities as Subjects in Clinical Research (RIN 0905-ZA18). *Fed Regist* 59:14508–14513, 1994.

9. National Institutes of Health. NIH Policy and Guidelines on the Inclusion of Children as Participants in Research Involving Human Subjects, 6 March, 1998. Access date 13 August, 2001. http://grants.nih.gov/grants/guide/notice-files/not98-024.html

10. Accountability in Clinical Research: Balancing Risk & Benefit Forum Report; National Patient Safety Foundation; April 24–26, 2002. University Place Conference Center; Indiana University, Purdue University Indianapolis, Indiana; http://www.researchsafety.org/download/2002ForumReport.pdf, pp. 4–5.

11. Emanuel EJ, Wendler D, Grady C. What makes clinical research ethical? *JAMA* 283:2701–2711, 2000.

12. Weijer C. The IRB's role in assessing the generalizability of non-NIH-funded clinical trials. *IRB: A Review of Human Subjects Research* 20(2,3):1–5, 1998.

13. Rothenberg KH. The Institute of Medicine's report on women and health research: Implications for IRBs and the research community. *IRB: A Review of Human Subjects Research* 18(2):1–3, 1996.

Community Consultation to Assess and Minimize Group Harms

William L. Freeman, Francine C. Romero, and Sayaka Kanade

INTRODUCTION

The primary goals of this chapter are, first, to explain group harms and, second, to show the importance of community consultation by researchers to minimize group harms in research that focuses on a vulnerable population. The recommendations in this chapter are a "best practice" for human research protection programs.

A Hypothetical Research Protocol

Consider the following hypothetical research protocol: an Indian reservation that has two distinct subgroups derived from tribes that had been enemies in the 19th century. One subgroup has a more traditional lifestyle and lives primarily in an eastern enclave of the reservation; the other has a more acculturated lifestyle and lives primarily in a western enclave. The research hypotheses are that the average stress level will be less in the group with a more traditional lifestyle, but the expression of genes that have been linked to the stress response will be similar in each group. The methods include qualitative ethnography, quantitative surveys of traditional beliefs and of likely confounding factors (alcoholism, substance abuse, history of being sexually or physically abused in childhood or as a spouse), and blood tests for both levels of stress-related hormones and variants of stress-related genes.

In research ethics, the term *risk* is defined as the magnitude of the potential harm or discomfort and the probability of the harm or discomfort occurring.[1] In this chapter, however, we discuss the *types* of harms, that is, the nature or content of potential harms.

When evaluating the ethics of this hypothetical protocol, the IRB should consider the harms not just to individual participants but also to *groups*: to the community (group) itself and to the community's subgroups. For example, what are potential harms of this research to the reservation population that is the focus of the research, to subgroups currently living on the reservation, and even to people from other tribes?

At this point, please *stop reading*. Please *write* on a sheet of paper all potential group harms that you think are important to consider with this kind of research. After you have completed your list, please continue reading the chapter.

Individual and Group Harms

Research that caused great harm to individual participants are well known and frequently cited.[2] Many such projects involved research participants who were ethnic minorities, women, or economically impoverished, for example, the Public Health Service Syphilis Study.[3] An example of ethically questionable research that involved American Indian or Alaska Native (AI/AN) people was the Public Health Service longitudinal study of the health of uranium miners.[4] A large percentage of the miners were Navajo or Pueblo. The purpose of the research was to document the deaths caused by lung cancer. Although it was well known at the time of the study that uranium mining caused lung cancer, the researchers did not inform the participants of that risk.

In those two examples, the primary physical harm was to the research participants themselves. Some members of the immediate families of the participants may have suffered secondary physical harm: being infected with syphilis in the syphilis study and inhaling radioactive dust from the clothes of the miners in the uranium miners' study. However, the entire ethnic group (African Americans or Native Americans) did not suffer the same physical harm.

In the past few years, the National Bioethics Advisory Commission (NBAC) in the United States, the Canadian research establishment,[5] and bioethicists[6] have discussed another kind of harm: harms to groups, sometimes labeled "group-related harms." In its report on research with human tissues, the NBAC stated, "Research that is designed to study a group or that retrospectively implicates a group may . . . result in members of the group facing, among other things, stigmatization and discrimination in insurance and employment whether or not they contributed samples to the study."[7]

In "group harm," then, the group is the focus of the harm. All or most members of the group are potentially harmed, even those far removed from the research itself and from the research participants. Many observers have seen group harms in especially biomedical research with tissues.[8] However, group harms can occur in all types of research.

Historical Examples of Group Harms

The potential harms of research to groups of people other than the individual research participants is often overlooked by IRBs and researchers. Examples of research that caused group harm were the many studies comparing the average IQ of various racial groups, especially of African-American people. Culturally biased IQ tests plus unscientific stereotypes allegedly proved the mental inferiority of African Americans and thus reinforced the prevailing discrimination.[9] Most IQ research and reports of results did not attempt to minimize the group harms to all African Americans.

Some AI/AN tribes have also experienced group harms due to research. The following examples have had more than one public report.

Example A.
Researchers announced the bleak results of their study on alcoholism in an identified far-northwestern small Native city at a news conference in Pennsylvania.[10] The publicity immediately affected that community adversely by making it difficult to raise investment capital on Wall Street[11] and producing feelings of shame and being stigmatized by community members, even those living away from the city. Those feelings are still felt strongly and expressed decades later.

Example B.
Epidemiologists studied an outbreak of syphilis, including congenital syphilis, in a southwestern Indian tribe.[12] The report gave its exact population in the 1980 U.S. Census, and the State Health Department named the tribe. After local newspapers publicized it, reservation children were called derogatory names in off-reservation schools, and Indians were prohibited from using restrooms in nearby gas stations.[13]

Example C.
A possible example of group harm is a lawsuit at the time of this writing.[14] Arizona State University researchers conducted a study about the genetics of diabetes among the Havasupai tribe. The researchers asked for and obtained the approval of the tribal government, and more than 200 Havasupai individuals consented and participated. Without seeking additional tribal approval or individual consent, researchers then used the specimens and data for several other sensitive studies, including population migration, schizophrenia, and inter-relatedness,[15] in spite of the tribe's cultural and religious beliefs and concerns.[16]

Example D.
A researcher used specimens from the Nuu-chah-nulth First Nations people in Canada to do a population migra-

tion study, instead of completing the original study on their severe atypical arthritis.[17] The Nuu-chah-nulth wanted the specimens returned so that other researchers could complete the original research; the dispute was recently resolved without a lawsuit.[18]

If you have thought of new potential group harms for the hypothetical research protocol, please *add* them to your list, then read the rest of the chapter.

Vulnerability of Groups

In its final report, the NBAC discussed types of vulnerability: cognitive or communicative, institutional, deferential, medical, economic, and social.[19] The NBAC defined social vulnerability as "a function of the social perception of certain groups, which includes stereotyping and can lead to discrimination. . . . [These] perceptions devalue members of such groups, their interests, their welfare, or their contributions to society."

This definition may imply a negative intent by researchers or IRB members. In our experience, however, most researchers and IRBs try not to stereotype and discriminate; if stereotyping occurs, it is usually unintentional. Vulnerability more often is not that of being disvalued, but of being *dissimilar*. The vulnerability is due to the group having values, concerns, life experiences, and problems dissimilar from those of most researchers and IRB members and, thus, not well known or understood by them. The vulnerability in research of the Amish, of parents of children with a rare genetic disease, and of ethnic groups who are discriminated against and stereotyped by society is often due to ignorance by researchers and IRBs, not to negative intent. Community consultation can reduce that ignorance.

Potential Group Harms to Consider

In the same final report, the NBAC listed six broad categories of harms that research may cause: physical, psychologic, social, economic, legal, and dignitary.[20] ("Dignitary harms" are moral wrongs in which people are not respected as persons, such as violation of privacy or being enrolled without consent in research for which consent should be obtained.) We have also seen a seventh harm: *relational vis-a-vis research or health care*, that is, disrupting the relationship with important research or trusted researcher or with health care.

All seven broad categories of harms may occur to not just individual research participants, but also to groups as well. We compiled the following list of group harms from recent articles or public or private reports to IRBs about actual experiences in research of vulnerable groups (defining vulnerable as "dissimilar").

1. *Physical*
   Distrust of health care. Tribal members grew to distrust not just the type of research (e.g., genetic research) but also all research and even that type of health care (e.g., genetic services), resulting in an adverse impact on physical health (also example C [Havasupai] mentioned previously).

2. *Psychological (for Group)*
   Internal genetic determinism and self-stigmatization of the group. "We Jews are defective because our genes make us prone to cancer," or "We American Indians are defective because our genes make us prone to alcoholism" (also examples A [alcoholism study] and B [syphilis study] previously here). *Disruption of the tribe's values.* The research made public to the outside world what should remain private tribal knowledge.

3. *Social*
   External genetic determinism and stigmatization of the group. Stereotypic conclusions in which genes predict outcomes and absolutist statements based on a partial statistical association such that they are actually value statements, for example, "Ashkenazi Jews are genetically prone to cancer," or "American/Canadian Native peoples are genetically prone to alcoholism."
   Fostering discrimination and stigmatization by others. Reporting socially undesirable and stigmatizing conditions about the group (examples A [alcoholism study] and B [syphilis study] previously here).

4. *Economic*
   Loss of economic status by the community (example A [alcoholism study]). *Loss of status in the majority society.* A newspaper editorial asserted that because science proved that Indians are immigrants to the North American continent, just like Europeans, the treaties with Indians should no longer be observed.

5. *Legal*
   Public policy genetic determinism. A federal agency or state or tribal government determines group membership by presence or absence of genetic markers for being a Native person or tribal/band member.[21]

6. *Dignitary*
   Violate group privacy.[22] Revealing the identity of the tribe in socially undesirable and stigmatizing situations (examples A [alcoholism study] and B [syphilis study]). *Disruption of the tribe's self-understanding.* Having one's origin stories attacked by a study using tribal specimens without the permission of the tribe or participants (example C [Havasupai]). *Disruption of the tribe's values.* The research made private tribal knowledge public, without the tribe's permission. *Violate the community's control.* A study recruited tribal members living in a city distant from the reservation, even though the researchers had first asked for tribal approval and the tribe had said no. *Violate the community's norms.* A nontribal researcher had a public affair with a married community person.

7. *Relational (vis-a-vis Research or Health Care)*
   Not completing the original research intended to help the group (example D [arthritis study]). *Researcher breaking relationship with community.* Researcher, someone who the community trusted and with whom it was working intensively on a major problem, left to take a position at a distant university. *Raising expectations, then disappointing.* Services that were started by the research program were discontinued when the research was completed, or funding was not continued or was discontinued prematurely.

If you know of other group harms from research not listed previously here, please e-mail them to us.

Some people interpret Section .111(a)(2) of the Common Rule to prohibit IRBs from considering group harms.

> The IRB should not consider possible long-range effects of applying knowledge gained in the research (for example, the possible effects of the research on public policy) as among those research risks that fall within the purview of its responsibility.[23]

We disagree with that interpretation for two reasons. First, NBAC did not interpret that section to prohibit consideration of group harms. The Office for Human Research Protections (OHRP) publicly states that minimizing group harms is an important part of IRB responsibility. Second, all seven categories of group harms listed previously here occurred soon after the research; they were not "long-range effects." With the possible exception of loss of status in dominant society, none involved "effects of the research on public policy."

Community Consultation Can Prevent Group Harms

Section 46.107(a) of the Common Rule states that "if an IRB regularly reviews research that involves a vulnerable category of subjects, consideration shall be given to the inclusion of one or more individuals who are knowledgeable about and experienced in working with these subjects."[24] Although such inclusion is necessary and important, it may not be sufficient to minimize harms. NBAC and many observers believe that "community consultation" by the researcher is often also necessary. Thus, a key recommendation by NBAC in 1999 stated that "investigators should to the extent possible plan their research so as to minimize such harms and should consult, when appropriate, representatives of the relevant groups regarding study design."[25]

The major purpose of community consultation is to make the researchers more knowledgeable about the vulnerable group (i.e., its values, concerns, life experiences, and problems that are dissimilar to those of most researchers and IRBs), the potential group harms of the research, and how to minimize those harms.

NBAC made its recommendation even as it recognized that community consultation may be difficult because most communities are not homogenous. Allen Buchanan noted for the NBAC that researchers and IRBs may not know what is the relevant "community," especially when community members have differing opinions about the proposed research or "authentic" community values, may not know who "speaks" for "the community," and may not see that leaders in some communities may coerce other community members concerning the consultation process or research itself, or may hold views not representative of the entire community.[26]

A major reason that the NBAC recommended community consultation was the success of that approach in HIV/AIDS clinical trials,[27] genetic research,[28] and efforts to improve health disparities by the Centers for Disease Control and Prevention (CDC)[29] and several other health agencies.[30] NBAC repeated its recommendation in its final report in 2001. "[S]ocial perceptions are pervasive and often insidious and can affect persons' conceptions of certain groups. Thus, investigators, IRB members, and research sponsors should be sensitive to such social perceptions and their effects, and efforts should be made to allow members of such groups to participate in decision making and oversight processes. *Involving the community in the various stages of the research process, especially in study planning, can be helpful in reducing stereotyping and stigmatization*" [emphasis added].[31]

The OHRP, National Institutes of Health, Food and Drug Administration, CDC, and the other members of the DHHS Working Group agreed with the NBAC's recommendation on community consultation.

Notwithstanding the silence of federal regulations on this point, the Working Group agrees that investigators should plan research in a manner that minimizes potential harm to groups. Consultation with representatives of relevant groups may identify potential harms and other problems as well as benefits and opportunities in the proposed research that may not have been evident to the investigator. Appropriate consultation may thus minimize harms, maximize benefits, and increase the likelihood that the research will be carried out successfully.[32]

Many authorities and officials around the world have also recommended community consultation to minimize potential harm to vulnerable groups. For example, official reports in Canada[33] and Australia[34] require community consultation with "collectivities," including aboriginal or indigenous groups. Several other research codes require or recommend community consultation.[35]

Community Consultation Will Improve Human Research Protection

Can your IRB and researchers fully recognize and minimize potential harms involving vulnerable groups in research without community consultation? Our experiences as chair and co-chair of the IHS IRB are relevant to that question. Although the membership of both scientists and nonscientists was more than 70% Native American, the IRB sometimes did not recognize important group harms in specific research proposals. Community consultation outside of the IRB sometimes identified a group harm that the IRB had missed. Even with 70% AI/AN membership, the IHS IRB relied on community consultation with the tribe(s) involved to supplement its own reviews.

Community consultation can identify not only potential harms but also potential benefits. For instance, Fisher consulted with teenagers concerning confidentiality when a researcher finds a teenager is a victim or is behaving in ways teens themselves perceive as serious problems.[36] Teens did not want researchers to maintain absolute confidentiality, but preferred that researchers inform a concerned parent or adult about problematic behavior. Teens thus wanted the researchers to be proactive and paternalistic rather than to observe confidentiality as usually defined by researchers and IRBs. Fisher concluded, "Failure to consider prospective participants' point of view . . . can lead to acceptance of research procedures causing significant participant distress or to rejection of potentially

worthwhile scientific procedures that subjects and their families would perceive as benign and/or worthwhile."

How Researchers Can "Consult the Community"

Many researchers are intimidated by community consultation. Many vulnerable groups are heterogeneous and do not have a recognized spokesperson. We recommend that researchers consider the community as "stakeholders." For instance, as one of the authors personally knows, the Jewish community is fractionated, with multiple leaders with different perspectives. Yet the National Human Genome Research Institute officials consulted with the Jewish community at a meeting organized by Hadassah that included leaders of most national Jewish organizations. Even though differences were expressed, the National Human Genome Research Institute officials heard widespread concern about possible economic and social discrimination that could result from the genetic research being considered.[37] Similarly, HIV/AIDS clinical trial researchers routinely engage in community consultation by having discussions with the many local HIV/AIDS advocacy groups.[38] An Institute of Medicine committee recommended that "even if there are multiple overlapping groups involved, the IRB could ensure that the investigator had consulted several representatives and at least had some input even if it is not possible to have a definitive or comprehensive statement."[39]

Community consultation thus is quite similar to stakeholder consultation. If researchers already have an ongoing relationship with subgroups and leaders in a community, community consultation means discussing the research with individuals, in groups, and in other ways that will become apparent from these initial discussions (such as public meetings in the community). If researchers do not have an ongoing relationship, they can start the process by asking people from or knowledgeable about the community for names of people with whom to discuss the research. Researchers need not shy away from community consultation because it may be unfamiliar or because there is no standard way of obtaining this kind of input.

Community consultation with AI/AN and Canadian First Nations and Inuit tribes, bands, and communities includes an aspect additional to the usual process of community consultation, namely, that they have recognized governments. Community consultation in that setting thus includes formal approval by the government or council for the tribe or band. If you, your researcher, or your IRB/REB is considering research in that setting and would like more information, please contact the authors via e-mail.

Conclusion

When research targets a vulnerable, dissimilar, population, it is important for researchers and IRBs to consider potential harms of the research to that group, not just to individual research participants. This chapter presented seven categories of group harms to vulnerable populations. Community consultation by the researcher is necessary to supplement the IRB's assessment of group harms and how best to minimize them. Community consultation is practicable in most research with potential group harms. IRBs, therefore, should encourage researchers to consult with communities in a wide range of research.

Acknowledgments

The authors thank the members of the IRBs we have served on and many other Native and non-Native people who gave us wise teachings. They also thank Elizabeth Bankert for her review. The authors can be contacted at the following e-mail addresses: williamlfreeman@att.net, epiromero@aatchb.org, epikanade@aatchb.org.

References

1. Code of Federal Regulations. Title 45—Department of Health and Human Services; Part 46—Protection of Human Subjects. Section 46.102(i). Revised 13 November, 2001. Effective 13 December, 2001. Access date 28 January, 2005. http://www.hhs.gov/ohrp/humansubjects/guidance/45cfr46.htm

2. Levine RJ. *Ethics and Regulation of Clinical Research*, 2nd ed. Baltimore, MD: Urban and Schwarzenberg; 1986.

3. Jones JH. *Bad Blood: The Tuskegee Syphilis Experiment*. New York; Simon & Schuster; 1992.

4. Advisory Committee on Human Radiation Experiments. *The Human Radiation Experiments: Final Report*. New York: Oxford University Press; 1996.

5. Tri-Council Policy Statement: Ethical Conduct for Research Involving Humans, 1998, (Updated 2000, 2002). Access date 28 January, 2005. http://www.pre.ethics.gc.ca/english/policystatement/introduction.cfm

6. Weijer C. Protecting communities in research: Philosophical and pragmatic challenges. *Camb Q Health Ethics* 8:501–513, 1999.

7. National Bioethics Advisory Commission. Research Involving Human Biological Materials: Ethical Issues and Policy Guidance. Volume 1: Report and Recommendations of the National Bioethics Advisory Commission. Rockville, MD: NBAC; 1999. Access date 28 January, 2005. http://www.georgetown.edu/research/nrcbl/nbac/hbm.pdf

8. Weir RF, Olick RS. *The Stored Tissue Issue: Biomedical Research, Ethics, and Law in the Era of Genomic Medicine*. New York City: Oxford University Press; 2004.

9. Tyack D. Schooling and social diversity: Historical reflections. In: Hawley WD, Jackson AW (eds.). *Toward a Common Destiny*. San Francisco: Jossey-Bass; 1995:3–38.

10. Klausner S, Foulks E. *Eskimo Capitalists: Oil, Alcohol and Social Change*. Montclair, NJ: Allenheld and Osmun; 1982.

11. *American Indian and Alaskan Native Mental Health Research* 3(2, Spring); 1989.

12. Gerber AR, King LC, Dunleavy GJ, Novick LF. An outbreak of syphilis on an Indian reservation: Descriptive epidemiology and disease-control measures. *Am J Public Health* 79:83–85; 1989.

13. Freeman WL. The role of community in research with stored tissue samples. In: Weir RF (ed.). *Stored Tissue Samples: Ethical, Legal, and Public Policy Implications*. Iowa City, IA: University Iowa Press; 1998:267–301.

14. Hendricks L. Havasupai tribe files $50M suit against ASU. *Arizona Daily Sun* Flagstaff, AZ, 16 March, 2004.

15. Dalton R. When two tribes go to war. *Nature* 430:500–502, 2004. Access date 28 January, 2005. http://www.nature.com/news/2004/040726/pf/430500a_pf.html

16. Rubin P. Indian givers. *Phoenix New Times* Phoenix, AZ. 27 May, 2004. Access date 28 January, 2005. http://www.phoenixnewtimes.com/issues/2004-05-27/news/feature.html

17. Tymchuk M. Bad blood. Quirks & Quarks CBC Radio. October 7, 2000. Access date 28 January, 2005. http://radio.cbc.ca/programs/quirks/archives/00-01/oct0700.htm

18. Wiwchar D. Nuu-chah-nulth blood returns to West coast. Ha-Shilth-Sa Port Alberni, BC, Canada. 16 December, 2004. Access date 28 January, 2005. http://www.nuuchahnulth.org/hashilthsa/dec1604.pdf

19. National Bioethics Advisory Commission. Ethical and Policy Issues in Research Involving Human Participants. Volume 1: Report and Recommendations of the National Bioethics Advisory Commission. Rockville, MD: NBAC; 2001:88–90. Access date 28 January, 2005. http://www.georgetown.edu/research/nrcbl/nbac/human/overvol1.html

20. National Bioethics Advisory Commission. Ethical and Policy Issues in Research Involving Human Participants. Volume 1: Report and Recommendations of the National Bioethics Advisory Commission. Rockville, MD: NBAC; 2001;71–72. Access date 28 January, 2005. http://www.georgetown.edu/research/nrcbl/nbac/human/overvol1.html

21. Vermont General Assembly Committee on Health and Welfare. An Act Relating to DNA Testing and Native Americans. Proposed bill H-809. 2000.

22. Alpert S. Privacy and the analysis of stored tissues. In: National Bioethics Advisory Commission. *Research Involving Human Biological Materials: Ethical Issues and Policy Guidance. Volume II: Commissioned Papers*. Rockville, MD: NBAC; 2000;A1–A36. Access date 28 January, 2005. http://www.georgetown.edu/research/nrcbl/nbac/hbmII.pdf

23. Code of Federal Regulations. Title 45—Department of Health and Human Services; Part 46—Protection of Human Subjects. Section 46.111(a)(2). Revised 13 November, 2001. Effective 13 December, 2001. Access date 28 January, 2005. http://www.hhs.gov/ohrp/humansubjects/guidance/45cfr46.htm

24. Code of Federal Regulations. Title 45—Department of Health and Human Services; Part 46—Protection of Human Subjects. Revised 13 November, 2001. Effective 13 December, 2001. Access date 28 January, 2005. http://www.hhs.gov/ ohrp/humansubjects/guidance/45cfr46.htm

25. National Bioethics Advisory Commission. Research Involving Human Biological Materials: Ethical Issues and Policy Guidance. Volume 1: Report and Recommendations of the National Bioethics Advisory Commission. Rockville, MD: NBAC; 1999:vii, 73. Access date 28 January, 2005. http://www.georgetown.edu/research/nrcbl/nbac/hbm.pdf

26. Buchanan A. An ethical framework for biological samples policy. In: National Bioethics Advisory Commission. *Research Involving Human Biological Materials: Ethical Issues and Policy Guidance. Volume II: Commissioned Papers.* Rockville, MD: NBAC; 2000:B-27. Access date 28 January, 2005. http://www.georgetown.edu/research/nrcbl/nbac/hbmII.pdf

27. Committee on the Role of Institutional Review Boards in Health Services Research Data Privacy Protection, Institute of Medicine. *Protecting Data Privacy in Health Services Research.* Washington, DC: National Academy Press; 2000. Access date 28 January, 2005. http://www.nap.edu/ html/data_privacy/

28. Foster MW, Sharp RR, Freeman WL, Chino M, Bernsten D, Carter TH. The role of community review in evaluating the risks of human genetic variation research. *Am J Hum Genet* 64(6):1719–1727, 1999.

29. Public Health Practice Program Office, Centers for Disease Control and Prevention. *Principles of Community Engagement.* Atlanta, GA: CDC; 1997. Access date 28 January, 2005. http://www.cdc.gov/phppo/pce/index.htm

30. *Building Community Partnerships in Research: Recommendations and Strategies.* Washington, DC: U.S. Department of Health and Human Services; 1998.

31. National Bioethics Advisory Commission. Ethical and Policy Issues in Research Involving Human Participants. Volume 1: Report and Recommendations of the National Bioethics Advisory Commission. Rockville, MD: NBAC; 2001:91. Access date 28 January, 2005. http://www.georgetown.edu/research/nrcbl/nbac/human/overvol1.html

32. Response of the Department of Health and Human Services to NBAC's Report "Research Involving Human Biological Materials: Ethical Issues and Policy Guidance," 2001. Access date 28 January, 2005. http://www.aspe.hhs.gov/sp/hbm/index.htm

33. Tri-Council Policy Statement: Ethical Conduct for Research Involving Humans, 1998, (Updated 2000, 2002). Access date 28 January, 2005. http://www.pre.ethics.gc.ca/english/policystatement/introduction.cfm

34. Chalmers D. Research ethics in Australia. In: National Bioethics Advisory Commission. *Ethical and Policy Issues in Research Involving Human Participants. Volume 2: Commissioned Papers and Staff Analysis.* Rockville, MD: NBAC; 2001. Access date 28 January, 2005. http://www.georgetown.edu/research/nrcbl/nbac/human/overvol2.html

35. Weijer C, Goldsand G, Emanuel EJ. Protecting communities in research: Current guidelines and limits of extrapolation. *Nat Genet* 23:275–280, 1999.

36. Fisher CB. A relational perspective on ethics-in-science decision making for research with vulnerable populations. *IRB* 19(5):1–4, 1997.

37. Stolberg SG. Concern among Jews is heightened as scientists deepen gene studies. *New York Times,* Section A Ed. A:24, 1998.

38. Levine C, Dubler NN, Levine RJ. Building a new consensus: Ethical principles and policies for clinical research on HIV/AIDS. *IRB* 13(1–2):1–17, 1991.

39. Committee on the Role of Institutional Review Boards in Health Services Research Data Privacy Protection, Institute of Medicine. *Protecting Data Privacy in Health Services Research.* Washington, DC: National Academy Press; 2000. Access date 28 January, 2005. http://www.nap.edu/html/data_privacy/

Privacy and Confidentiality

David G. Forster

INTRODUCTION

This chapter addresses the role of privacy and confidentiality in the institutional review board (IRB) review of human subject research. Subjects benefit from having privacy and confidentiality protected when appropriate, and subjects need to be informed of the extent to which they can expect that their privacy and the confidentiality of information identifying them will be maintained.

Both privacy and confidentiality are complex concepts with a multitude of facets and potential definitions. For the purposes of this chapter, the definitions of *privacy* and *confidentiality* presented in the 1993 Office for Protection From Research Risks *IRB Guidebook*[1] will be used:

> Privacy can be defined in terms of having control over the extent, timing, and circumstances of sharing oneself (physically, behaviorally, or intellectually) with others. Confidentiality pertains to the treatment of information that an individual has disclosed in a relationship of trust and with the expectation that it will not be divulged to others in ways that are inconsistent with the understanding of the original disclosure without permission.

Relationship of Privacy and Confidentiality to the Belmont Principles

Privacy and confidentiality are supported by two of the three principles of research ethics identified by the National Commission for the Protection of Human Subjects of Biomedical and Behavioral Research in *The Belmont Report*:[2] respect for persons and beneficence. Respect for persons requires that subjects be allowed to exercise their autonomy to the fullest extent possible, including the autonomy to maintain their privacy and to have private information identifying them kept confidential. Beneficence requires that risks to subjects are minimized, benefits are maximized, and risks to subjects do not outweigh the benefits to subjects and others. The maintenance of privacy and confidentiality helps to protect subjects from a variety of potential harms, including psychological distress, loss of insurance, loss of employment, or damage to social standing, that could occur as the result of an invasion of privacy or a breach of confidentiality.

Federal Guidance and Regulations

The Common Rule and the Food and Drug Administration (FDA) regulations address the issues of privacy and confidentiality in several places. Furthermore, both the Office for Human Research Protections (OHRP) (formerly the Office for Protection from Research Risks) and the FDA have issued valuable guidance on the topic. This section reviews human subject protection regulations and guidance that require the IRB to consider privacy and confidentiality and discuss issues on which there is disagreement among IRBs.

Criteria for Approval of Research

Both the Common Rule and the FDA regulations require the IRB to determine, as part of the IRB review of research, that privacy and confidentiality are protected when appropriate. The wording used in the two regulations is slightly different but identical in meaning.

Common Rule, 45 CFR § 46.111, Criteria for IRB approval of Research

> **(a)** In order to approve research covered by this policy the IRB shall determine that all of the following requirements are satisfied. . . . (7) When appropriate, there are adequate provisions to protect the privacy of subjects and to maintain the confidentiality of data.

FDA, 21 CFR § 56.111, Criteria for IRB approval of research

> **(a)** In order to approve research covered by these regulations, the IRB shall determine that all of the following requirements are satisfied. . . . (7) Where appropriate, there are adequate provisions to protect the privacy of subjects and to maintain the confidentiality of data.

In fulfilling the regulatory requirements,[3][Sec.111(a)(7)], [4][Sec.111(a)(7)] the IRB should consider the degree of privacy of the information being collected and the measures that have been established to protect the confidentiality of the information. In determining the degree of privacy of the information, the IRB should use the standard of a reasonable member of the research population and consider whether such a reasonable member would consider the information collected in the research to be private. In addition, the IRB should consider whether the reasonable member would consider the release of the information without permission to be an invasion of privacy. However, views on privacy vary greatly within and across cultures and research populations, and information that is not considered particularly sensitive by one individual may be very sensitive to another individual. For research involving unique cultures, the IRB should consider having a representative of the culture on the IRB or consulting with individuals knowledgeable of feelings about privacy within the culture.

The IRB should require the investigator or other relevant parties to explain how privacy and the confidentiality of the information obtained in the course of the study will be maintained. This is most easily accomplished by requiring investigators to provide this information on the IRB submission form. Investigators may employ several methods to protect privacy, particularly in research involving questionnaires. In a face-to-face interview, investigators can allow subjects to provide information in writing or by using a computer keyboard, instead of orally. With the availability of laptop computers, the investigator can allow subjects to provide answers to some or all questions on the computer in a field setting. For research conducted by telephone, subjects can answer using the touch tones. For clinical research, the IRB may wish to consider privacy protections that go beyond those available in traditional clinical care.

Common measures employed by investigators to protect confidentiality include storage of records in locked file cabinets, in locked offices, on computers protected by a password, or on computers that are not linked into a network. Another common protection is to code the data with an identifier and to keep the key to the code located in another physical location or on a separate computer. Destruction of the research records also provides protection by eliminating the potential for inadvertent disclosure. Many IRBs require the investigator to state on the submission form how long the records will be kept. Some IRBs require the data to be destroyed after the research is finished unless the investigator provides a compelling reason for maintaining the records.

Subject Recruitment and Long-Term Follow-Up

The IRB must also consider the protection of privacy and confidentiality during the subject recruitment process. The manner in which subjects are identified and approached for participation in research may constitute an invasion of privacy or confidentiality. For instance, it has not been uncommon in the past for research staff to search medical records to which they do not have clinical access. This constitutes a breach of confidentiality of the patients' medical records. If potential subjects are identified in this manner and the individuals are contacted by research staff

with whom they have had no previous contact, these individuals may rightly feel that their privacy has been violated. Similar concerns arise with any search of a database conducted to identify potential subjects. Examples of databases include disease registries, nonpublic state records, insurance records, and pharmacy records.

Issues of confidentiality should be particularly scrutinized in research conducted over an extended period of time. Some longitudinal studies extend for periods of 10 or more years. Likewise, many cancer studies can include subject follow-up until death. During the course of such a study, the subjects' values and circumstances can change greatly, causing changes in the importance of privacy and the confidentiality of the records. For instance, subjects may not have informed spouses or other family members of their past participation in research. A poorly conducted follow-up call could create severe family disruption and psychological harm in such a case.

Another potential breach of privacy is the collection of sensitive information during the screening period and subsequent retention of the information without consent from the subject. This is particularly troubling if the information is maintained even though the potential subject declines to participate in or does not qualify for the research. Some pharmaceutical sponsors and contract research organizations have created databases of potential subjects based on these recruitment procedures. The FDA offers the following guidance on privacy and confidentiality during the screening process in the FDA Information Sheet, "Recruiting Study Subjects."[5]

The first contact prospective study subjects make is often with a receptionist who follows a script to determine basic eligibility for the specific study. The IRB should assure that the procedures followed adequately protect the rights and welfare of the prospective subjects. In some cases, personal and sensitive information is gathered about the individual. The IRB should have assurance that the information will be appropriately handled. A simple statement such as "confidentiality will be maintained" does not adequately inform the IRB of the procedures that will be used.

The following issues are appropriate for IRB review: What happens to personal information if the caller ends the interview or simply hangs up? Are the data gathered by a marketing company? If so, are names, etc., sold to others? Are names of noneligibles maintained in case they would qualify for another study? Are paper copies of records shredded, or are readable copies put out as trash? The acceptability of the procedures would depend on the sensitivity of the data gathered, including personal, medical, and financial.[5]

IRBs can ask for this information on the IRB submission form. If IRBs do not ask, they may not receive the information in the submitted study documents such as the protocol. This is particularly true for large, multisite research projects that often have centralized subject recruitment procedures.

For research involving particularly sensitive information, such as drug abuse, the IRB may also require that the investigator obtains a Federal Certificate of Confidentiality to protect the research records from release in any federal, state, or local civil, criminal, administrative, legislative, or other proceeding. The subject of Chapter 8-10 is Certificates of Confidentiality.

The IRB must decide on a case-by-case basis whether there are adequate provisions to protect the privacy of subjects and to maintain the confidentiality of data. The committee must take into account the degree of sensitivity of the information obtained in the research and the protections offered. As with other aspects of IRB review, these determinations will be dependent on the factual circumstances.

Confidentiality in the Consent Form

After the IRB has decided that there are adequate provisions in the research plan to protect the privacy and confidentiality of the subjects, it must also ensure that the consent form accurately provides the subject with information concerning the confidentiality of the research records. This allows the subject to make his or her own determination of whether the provisions for protecting privacy and confidentiality are adequate. The Common Rule and the FDA regulations differ in regard to the requirements for the consent form.

Common Rule, 45 CFR § 46.116, General requirements for informed consent

(a) Basic elements of informed consent. Except as provided in paragraph (c) or (d) of this section, in seeking informed consent the following information shall be provided to each subject. . . . (5) A statement describing the extent, if any, to which confidentiality of records identifying the subject will be maintained.

FDA, 21 CFR § 50.25, Elements of informed consent

(a) Basic elements of informed consent. In seeking informed consent, the following information shall be provided to each subject. . . . (5) A statement describing the extent, if any, to which confidentiality of records identifying the subject will be maintained and that notes the possibility that the Food and Drug Administration may inspect the records.

The essential difference between the Common Rule[3][Sec.116(a)] and the FDA regulations[6][Sec.25(a)] is that the FDA regulations require that subjects are informed of the possibility that the FDA may inspect the records of the study. The Common Rule regulations do not impose a similar requirement for the consent form. However, many of the agencies that have adopted the Common Rule do have the authority to investigate the misconduct of research and/or human subject protection violations, and in the process, confidential subject records could be reviewed.

IRBs across the country have taken very different approaches to satisfying the requirements of these regulations. At one end of the spectrum, some IRBs have adopted a standard statement to the effect that "research records will be kept confidential" and also include a statement that "the FDA may inspect the research records" for research under FDA jurisdiction. At the other end of the spectrum, some

IRBs have taken the position that it is overly reassuring to subjects to promise confidentiality. Instead, they state that confidentiality cannot be guaranteed and then list the parties who may have access to research records, including government agencies, sponsors, sponsor contractors, the IRB, and the institution.

The best practice is to address both sides of the issue in two paragraphs. First, the consent form should present the procedures that are in place to protect the confidentiality of data, such as the use of coding systems and locked file cabinets. Second, the form should disclose those parties who could potentially have access to the research data. This dual approach provides the subjects with the material information about the confidentiality of their research records, allowing them to make their own choice about the adequacy of the protections and the acceptability of the possible release of private information to the listed parties.

The FDA has issued the following guidance to clarify its interpretation of 21 CFR 50[6][Sec.(a)(5)] in the FDA Information Sheet, "Informed Consent."[5]

Study subjects should be informed of the extent to which the institution intends to maintain confidentiality of records identifying the subjects. In addition, they should be informed that the FDA may inspect study records (which include individual medical records). If any other entity, such as the sponsor of the study, may gain access to the study records, the subjects should be so informed. The consent document may, at the option of the IRB, state that subjects' names are not routinely required to be divulged to the FDA. When the FDA requires subject names, it will treat such information as confidential, but on rare occasions, disclosure to third parties may be required. Therefore, absolute protection of confidentiality by the FDA should not be promised or implied. Also, consent documents should not state or imply that the FDA needs clearance or permission from the subject for access. When clinical investigators conduct a study for submission to the FDA, they agree to allow FDA access to the study records. Informed consent documents should make it clear that when a subject participates in research, the subject's records automatically become part of the research database. Subjects do not have the option to keep their records from being audited/reviewed by the FDA.[5]

In addition, the FDA has issued the guidance to clarify its interpretation of access by other third parties to research records in the FDA Information Sheet, "Sponsor—Investigator—IRB Relationship."[5]

Sponsor–Investigator–IRB Relationship

The IRB is responsible for ensuring that informed consent documents include the extent to which the confidentiality of medical records will be maintained.[6][Sec.25(a)(5)] The FDA requires sponsors (or research monitors hired by them) to monitor the accuracy of the data submitted to the FDA in accordance with regulatory requirements. These data are generally in the possession of the clinical investigator. Each subject must be advised during the informed consent process of the extent to which confidentiality of records identifying the subject will be maintained and of the possibility that the FDA may inspect the records. Although FDA access to medical records is a regulatory requirement, subject names are not usually requested by the FDA unless the records of particular individuals require a more detailed study of the cases or unless there is reason to believe that the records do not represent actual cases studied or actual results obtained. The consent document should list all other entities (e.g., the sponsor) that will have access to records identifying the subject. The extent to which confidentiality will be maintained may affect a subject's decision to participate in a clinical investigation.[5]

Privacy Considerations in the Definition of Human Subject

Under the Common Rule, the definition of human subject involves as one of the criteria an analysis of whether information is private.[3[Sec.102(f)]]

Human subject means a living individual about whom an investigator (whether professional or student) conducting research obtains (1) data through intervention or interaction with the individual or (2) identifiable private information.

When an IRB is considering whether an individual is a subject because of the collection of information about that individual (without direct intervention or interaction), it must necessarily consider whether the information obtained is private or not. One situation in which this regulatory definition[3[Sec.102(f)(2)]] applies is the collection of information about "secondary subjects." Secondary subjects exist when an investigator asks a primary subject, with whom the investigator is directly interacting, to provide information about other individuals, often family members. For example, in a well-publicized case, a father reviewed a research questionnaire sent to his daughter. The questionnaire contained several very personal questions to be asked of the daughter about her father and other family members, covering topics such as abnormal genitalia, mental illness, and substance abuse. In reviewing such research, the IRB must consider whether the information collected about the secondary subjects is private.

An important factor in this consideration is the relationship between privacy and confidentiality. If the information is clearly private in nature but the confidentiality protections are adequate to ensure against all but the most unlikely sources of improper breach, is this information still private? Some have argued that the protection of the confidentiality of the information lessens the private nature of the information. However, many individuals will feel that the release of this type of information without their consent is an invasion of privacy, regardless of whether there are confidentiality protections in place. If privacy is defined as "having control over the extent, timing, and circumstances of sharing oneself (physically, behaviorally, or intellectually) with others,"[1] then the collection of sensitive information about secondary subjects without their consent clearly involves a breach of privacy.

Confidentiality Requirements for Research Exempt From IRB Review

Confidentiality is explicitly addressed in the Common Rule,[3[Sec.101(b)(3)(ii)]] which allows certain research to be exempt from IRB review if there are federal statutes that require that the confidentiality of the personally identifiable information will be maintained. However, this is not an exemption that is used on a regular basis by most IRBs.

Title §46.101, To what does this policy apply?

(b) Unless otherwise required by Department or Agency heads, research activities in which the only involvement of human subjects will be in one or more of the following categories are exempt from this policy. . . . (2) Research involving the use of educational tests (cognitive, diagnostic, aptitude, achievement), survey procedures, interview procedures, or observation of public behavior, unless:

(i) information obtained is recorded in such a manner that human subjects can be identified, directly or through identifiers linked to the subjects; and

(ii) any disclosure of the human subjects' responses outside the research could reasonably place the subjects at risk of criminal or civil liability or be damaging to the subjects' financial standing, employability, or reputation.

(3) Research involving the use of educational tests (cognitive, diagnostic, aptitude, achievement), survey procedures, interview procedures, or observation of public behavior that is not exempt under paragraph (b)(2) of this section, if:

(i) the human subjects are elected or appointed public officials or candidates for public office; or

(ii) Federal statute(s) require(s) without exception that the confidentiality of the personally identifiable information will be maintained throughout the research and thereafter.[3Sec.(101)]

The fourth category of exempt research also brings up questions about privacy and confidentiality. The following class of research is exempt from IRB review:[3[Sec.101(b)(4)]]

Research involving the collection or study of existing data, documents, records, pathologic specimens, or diagnostic specimens. If these sources are publicly available or if the information is recorded by the investigator in such a manner that subjects cannot be identified, directly or through identifiers linked to the subjects.

In August 2004, the OHRP released guidance describing the application of this exemption criteria and its interaction with the definition of human subject at 45 CFR 46 Sec. 102(f)(2). This new guidance cleared up many of the questions that had existed before its release and was a welcome release from the OHRP. Because of its extensive detail, it is recommended that the reader directly review the guidance itself. The guidance is entitled "Guidance on Research Involving Coded Private Information or Biological Specimens" and is available online at http://www.hhs.gov/ohrp/humansubjects/guidance/cdebiol.pdf.

Confidentiality in the Waiver of Documentation of Informed Consent

Another regulatory section specifically requiring the IRB to address the issue of confidentiality is 45 CFR 46,[3[Sec.117(c)(1)]] which allows for a waiver of documentation of consent.

Title §46.117 Documentation of informed consent

> **(c)** An IRB may waive the requirement for the investigator to obtain a signed consent form for some or all subjects if it finds either:
>
> **(1)** That the only record linking the subject and the research would be the consent document and the principal risk would be potential harm resulting from a breach of confidentiality. Each subject will be asked whether the subject wants documentation linking the subject with the research and the subject's wishes will govern or
>
> **(2)** That the research presents no more than minimal risk of harm to subjects and involves no procedures for which written consent is normally required outside of the research context. In cases in which the documentation requirement is waived, the IRB may require the investigator to provide subjects with a written statement regarding the research.

An example of research that fits under the waiver of documentation of consent would be an anonymous questionnaire on risk factors for HIV conducted at a public free-needle-exchange table. Because the questionnaire is anonymous and does not include names, the only way to link subjects to the research would be the name on the consent form. In this case, the main risk of harm is the breach of confidentiality that could occur if individual subjects were linked to receiving free needles, indicating that they are using illegal drugs. The subjects must be asked whether they want to be linked to the information, and the subjects' wishes govern. This waiver from documentation of consent does not exist under the FDA regulations and cannot be used for any research falling under FDA oversight.

Waiver of Consent Under Common Rule

Under the Common Rule, an IRB may allow an investigator to conduct research without consent of the subjects if four criteria are met.[3[Sec.116(d)]]

An IRB may approve a consent procedure which does not include, or which alters, some or all of the elements of informed consent set forth in this section or waive the requirements to obtain informed consent provided the IRB finds and documents that:

1. The research involves no more than minimal risk to the subjects
2. The waiver or alteration will not adversely affect the rights and welfare of the subjects
3. The research could not practicably be carried out without the waiver or alteration
4. Whenever appropriate, the subjects will be provided with additional pertinent information after participation

The IRB must consider privacy and confidentiality in its analysis of criteria 1 and 2. Under criterion 1, the IRB must decide whether the research under consideration represents a minimal risk to the study subjects. Some research that involves no physical risk may still represent more than minimal risk because of potential breaches of privacy and confidentiality. For example, genetic research concerning a chronic or fatal disease could lead to loss of insurance, employment, or social standing or to psychological distress if there were a breach of identifiable information. This type of harm is more likely if the research records are kept with medical records and are thereby accessible to insurers or employers, whether intentionally or accidentally. There have been reported cases of genetic discrimination in the past few years, making this a very real concern.

Under criterion 2, the IRB must consider whether the waiver or alteration will adversely affect the rights and welfare of the subjects. One of the central rights to be considered in this analysis is privacy. Subjects should not have their reasonable expectations about privacy violated without their permission. Even if the release of identifiable information is not likely to cause economic or other harm to the subjects, such as loss of insurance, an IRB should still consider whether the collection of the information, even with reasonable protections on confidentiality, may still constitute an invasion of privacy.

The International Conference on Harmonisation Consent Form Requirements Regarding Confidentiality

The International Conference on Harmonisation (ICH) is an international agreement allowing drug research results to be submitted to drug-approval agencies of many countries if the research is conducted in accordance with ICH requirements. The ICH is discussed in detail in Chapter 8-3. The ICH has been adopted by the FDA only as guidance in the United States, and therefore, compliance is not mandatory for IRBs in the United States. However, many sponsors request that IRBs state that they are compliant with ICH. In comparison with FDA and Common Rule requirements, compliance with ICH requires that the subject is informed of and authorizes much broader access to research records by third parties. The relevant sections of the ICH regarding the information presented in the consent form are as follows.

> ICH § 4.8.10 Both the informed consent discussion and the written informed consent form and any other written information to be provided to subjects should include explanations of the following:
>
> That the monitor(s), the auditor(s), the IRB/IEC, and the regulatory authority(s) will be granted direct access to the subject's original medical records for verification of clinical trial procedures and/or data, without violating the confidentiality of the subject, to the extent permitted by the applicable laws and regulations and that, by signing a written informed consent form, the subject or the subject's legally acceptable representative is authorizing such access.
>
> That records identifying the subject will be kept confidential and, to the extent permitted by the applicable laws and/or

regulations, will not be made publicly available. If the results of the trial are published, the subject's identity will remain confidential.

The ICH also requires the sponsors to ensure that there is access to identifiable subject information.

ICH § 5.15.1 The sponsor should ensure that it is specified in the protocol or other written agreement that the investigator(s)/institution(s) provide direct access to source data/documents for trial-related monitoring, audits, IRB/IEC review, and regulatory inspection.

ICH § 5.15.2 The sponsor should verify that each subject has consented, in writing, to direct access to his or her original medical records for trial-related monitoring, audit, IRB/IEC review, and regulatory inspection.

Because the ICH is an international agreement, "regulatory inspection" as used in §§ 5.15.1 and 5.15.2 covers the drug-approval agencies of many countries. Subjects who enroll in research complying with ICH need to be clearly told about the ramifications to confidentiality and privacy. Several IRBs have received complaints from subjects regarding the consent form sections regarding potential access of personal medical records by agencies of other countries. Some subjects have refused to participate in research being conducted in compliance with ICH requirements because of this confidentiality issue. Similarly, many IRB members are uncomfortable with this international access to identifiable research data. Each IRB, investigator, and institution must decide whether it truly wishes to comply with ICH requirements, including the broad potential access to identifiable research data.

Other Federal Regulations and Laws Addressing Privacy and Confidentiality

A variety of federal regulations and laws address privacy and confidentiality in addition to those previously described that are not specific to research but could affect the conduct of research. The Health Insurance Portability and Accountability Act of 1996 required the passage of regulations providing privacy and confidentiality protections for electronic medical records. If, or when, Health Insurance Portability and Accountability Act of 1996 regulations are activated, IRBs will need to be aware of these regulations and the institution's procedures for their implementation.

The Freedom of Information Act of 1966[7] allows public access to many records maintained or created by the federal government. One of the categories of records exempt from disclosure under the Freedom of Information Act is "personnel and medical files, and similar files the disclosure of which would constitute a clearly unwarranted invasion of personal privacy."[7[Sec.(b)(6)]] The Federal Privacy Act of 1974[8] provides individuals with some control over personal information maintained or created by the federal government. Both DHHS and FDA have enacted regulations implementing the Freedom of Information Act and the Federal Privacy Act.

Two public health service acts also deal with the protection of confidential information regarding patients in drug and alcohol treatment programs at federally funded clinics.[9[Sec.dd-3, ee-3]] Many additional federal laws exist that could affect privacy and confidentiality of research subjects, but an inclusion of all of them is beyond the scope of this work.

State Laws Addressing Privacy and Confidentiality

IRBs must consider state laws concerning privacy and confidentiality when reviewing research. These may take the form of either statute or case law. The Common Rule and FDA regulations[3[Sec.107(a)],4[Sec.107(a)]] require the IRB to be able to ascertain the acceptability of proposed research in terms of "applicable law," which includes state law. The Common Rule and FDA regulations also clearly state that other laws are not preempted by the federal regulations and continue to apply.[3[Sec.101(f)],4[Sec.103(c)]] Therefore, any state laws that require greater protections for subjects than the Common Rule and FDA regulations continue to apply.

A variety of state laws address privacy and confidentiality. These laws generally can be grouped under broad categories. The first category is laws allowing patients to have access to their own medical records. Many states provide detailed requirements for patient access to their medical records, but many states do not have statutes addressing this issue.

The second category is laws that require various third parties, such as physicians, hospitals, and HMOs, to maintain the confidentiality of patient medical records. These laws do not exist in all states, and where they do exist, they vary greatly in scope and the identity of the restricted parties. Often, states have different laws addressing specific medical conditions. For instance, there are often stricter confidentiality protections in place for drug abuse or mental health records than for other types of medical records.

The third category is laws that require informed consent from patients before medical information is released to third parties. Again, these do not exist in all states and vary greatly in those states where they do exist.

A fourth category is laws that allow the disclosure of patient records for research purposes. Such laws have not been adopted in all states. Sometimes they require patient consent; other times they do not. Many of them are limited to certain types of records, such as cancer or mental health.

A fifth category of state laws comprises mandatory reporting laws of various types. Many types of medical conditions must be reported to the state, such as sexually transmitted diseases and cancer. Evidence suggesting child abuse, and often older-person or other-population abuse, must also be reported by physicians and other professionals. IRBs across the country are very inconsistent in their approach to child-abuse reporting requirements. Some IRBs require that information regarding this requirement be included in every consent form involving a medical procedure or an interview that could elicit information regarding child abuse. Other IRBs only require such consent form disclosure when the research is very likely to elicit this type of information. Many IRBs rarely or never disclose the existence of these laws.

Finally, many state laws affecting medical privacy and confidentiality do not fit into neat categories. For instance, some states such as Arizona prohibit genetic testing without specific, written informed consent. This would potentially affect the conduct of research involving genetic testing on stored tissue samples in Arizona and would be important for IRB consideration.

In addition, many state laws potentially could affect research but do not specifically address medicine or research. These include privacy provisions of state constitutions, state freedom of information acts (often known as sunshine laws) that control access to records maintained or created by the state government, and common law actions regarding the right to privacy.

Conclusion

IRBs must consider the protection of privacy and confidentiality as part of their ethical and regulatory duty to protect the rights and welfare of human subjects. Although privacy and confidentiality are difficult to define and are viewed differently by different individuals, IRBs can successfully apply them to research projects on a case-by-case basis. The IRB must consider both privacy and confidentiality for each segment of the research, from subject recruitment through follow-up and maintenance of the research records after the study has finished. Often, particularly in behavioral research, the main risk to subjects will be the possibility of an invasion of privacy or a breach of confidentiality. In the consent process, subjects must be informed of the precautions that will be taken to protect the confidentiality of the subjects' information and also be informed of the parties who will or may have ac-

cess to the information. This will allow the subjects to decide whether they agree with the IRB's assessment that the human subjects protections are adequate.

References

1. Office for Protection From Research Risks. *OPRR Guidebook* (1993). Updated 23 June, 2000. Access date 3 April, 2001. http://ohrp.osophs.dhhs.gov/irb/irb_guidebook.htm
2. National Commission for the Protection of Human Subjects of Biomedical and Behavioral Research. *The Belmont Report: Ethical principles and guidelines for the protection of human subjects of research.* 1979. Access date 22 March, 2001. http://ohsr.od.nih.gov/mpa/belmont.php3
3. Code of Federal Regulations. Title 45A—Department of Health and Human Services; Part 46—Protection of Human Subjects. Updated 1 October, 1997. Access date 18 April, 2001. http://www4.law.cornell.edu/cfr/45p46.htm
4. Code of Federal Regulations. Title 21, Chapter 1—Food and Drug Administration, DHHS; Part 56—Institutional Review Boards. Updated 1 April, 1999. Access date 27 March, 2001. http://www4.law.cornell.edu/cfr/21p56.htm
5. Food and Drug Administration. Information Sheets: Guidance for Institutional Review Boards and Clinical Investigators. September 1998. Access date 9 April, 2001. http://www.fda.gov/oc/oha/IRB/toc.html
6. Code of Federal Regulations. Title 21, Chapter 1—Food and Drug Administration, DHHS; Part 50—Protection of Human Subjects. Updated 1 April, 1999. Access date 18 April, 2001. http://www4.law.cornell.edu/cfr/21p50.htm
7. 104th Congress. The Freedom of Information Act. 5 U.S.C. § 552. 1996. Amended by public law No. 104-231, 110 Stat. 3048. http://www.usdoj.gov/oip/foia_updates/Vol_XVII_4/page2.htm
8. 104th Congress. The Federal Privacy Act of 1974. 5 U.S.C. § 552a. 1996.
9. 103rd Congress. Public Health Service Act (§290)—Title 42 U.S.C., 1 January, 2001. http://frwebgate2.access.gpo. gov/cgi-bin/waisgate.cgi?waisdocid=2637221675101010& waisaction=retrieve

Recruitment of Research Subjects

Matthew D. Whalen and Felix A. Khin-Maung-Gyi

INTRODUCTION

Certain critical topics related to human participant recruitment in clinical trials serve as focal points for this chapter, including the following:

1. Recruitment of subjects as the beginning of the informed consent process
2. Principles of information, comprehension, and voluntariness: what the institutional review board (IRB) will especially attend to in the course of its deliberations, which also provides the underpinning of this discussion
3. The Office of the Inspector General (OIG) reports of June 2000; what the OIG is, what their reports are, and why they are still important for those involved in clinical research
4. Facing the reality of recruitment in a world of e-trials and e-IRBs; emerging technologies and their impact on the recruitment process

Recruitment of Subjects

The sponsor of the research, the sponsor's agents involved in implementing certain aspects of a trial (such as a contract research organization), the investigator, the study coordinator, and the IRB are all intimately involved in the recruitment of subjects. Their interactions ought to be as proactive and collaborative as possible because each brings a different perspective and set of concerns in developing, reviewing, and/or implementing recruitment efforts. For some trials and sites, recruitment efforts are centralized. For others, they are highly localized, and for yet others, there is a mix of both approaches.

Regardless, one of the most fundamental issues is: Is information that is clear and accurate also sufficient? The answer is no, as re-emphasized by OIG reports on patient recruitment. Informed consent is a process—a communications process. Possibilities for misinforming or disinforming potential subjects abound, whether in overly enthusiastic public relations material or by an overly zealous study coordinator. Indeed, the possibilities for inadvertent, unintentional coercion, or undue influence are also high. Solutions such as separating the investigator from the potential subject's physician and having third-party auditing of the process have been offered as remedies. Their usefulness in most cases is unclear. Certainly, IRB review authority over recruitment efforts, from fundamental advertising through screening scripts and websites, appears to be a meaningful step in the right direction. When more elaborate public relations/communications firm-based campaigns are used, having IRB or ethics consultations as early as possible can maximize both impact and human research protections.

The OIG Reports of June 2000: Information, Comprehension, and Voluntariness

The OIG of the Department of Health and Human Services has released reports of great interest to IRB participants and professionals since June 1998 in particular. Three OIG reports released in June 2000 are of particular interest relating to subject recruitment.

The first report is entitled "Recruiting Human Subjects: Pressures in Industry-Sponsored Clinical Research."[1] It noted that reviewing recruitment methods provides "additional opportunity for oversight bodies to monitor the actual content of the consent process." Herein lies the importance of recruitment. For IRBs, the significance of their involvement with subject recruitment, whether in e-commerce or paper-flyer media, is because recruitment is tied intimately to the consent process itself.

From an ethical and regulatory perspective, the OIG reports specifically refer to issues of information, comprehension, and voluntariness. Dr. Bert Spilker, at the time with the trade association of major drug manufacturers (PhRMA), simplifies what these practices are in his commentary on the draft of the first report. He suggests that there are three primary means of recruiting:

1. An investigator's own patients
2. A physician referring patients to an investigator

3. Advertising to recruit subjects not previously known to investigators or their colleagues

When IRBs attend to recruitment, one method is to consider the ethics-inclusive issues of information, comprehension, and voluntariness in each setting of recruitment (the investigator's own patients, the referring physician, and advertising). Information focuses on possible disinformation or misinformation as much as on accurate information. Comprehension concerns presentation and communication. Voluntariness means a lack of coercion and undue influence as well as freedom of choice.

Recruitment in a World of E-Trials and E-IRBs

Contemporary subject recruitment is an industry unto itself. In an age of multimedia and technology, the range of avenues for recruiting has expanded exponentially. Major public relations, marketing, and advertising firms construct mass-media campaigns to support clinical research studies. The point of intersection of both business and ethical issues is the conference table of the IRB.

There are two basic issues in regard to the IRB itself: *Who* is deliberating around the table and *what* are they deliberating when it comes to reviewing recruitment?

The OIG reports on recruitment offer unambiguous statements in regard to who is deliberating. The recommendations are to "require more extensive representation on IRBs of nonscientific and noninstitutional members" and to acknowledge that "the perspectives of independent lay members are of particular importance." Clearly, whether the issues are subject protection or otherwise, lay and unaffiliated representation is essential. This representation emphasizes that the voice of the IRB is a social and cultural one and not exclusively one of technical (scientific, public policy, legal, public relations, political, or economic) expertise.

As to *what* is being deliberated, it has already been suggested: creating a matrix to consider the ethical issues of information, comprehension, and voluntariness in each setting of recruitment (the investigator's own patients, the referring physician, and advertising). However, another issue for deliberation is *how much* the IRB should know, ranging from reviewing advertising budgets and plans for nationwide public relations campaigns to wire frames of websites, in order to assure lack of coercion and maintenance of confidentiality.

The Four Cs of Recruitment From an IRB Perspective

The issues of greatest concern for IRBs and for IRB staffs relating to recruitment campaigns may be summarized in terms of four Cs:

1. Consent (ongoing or continuing)

2. Coercion (of medium and message)

3. Confidentiality and privacy

4. Completeness (accuracy as well as truthfulness versus deception)

To address each briefly:

Consent is an ongoing process and an opportunity to retain subjects in trials. In an era of sound and sight "bites," the potential for subtle *coercion* abounds. That the public and the clinical research enterprise as a whole have become highly sensitive to issues of *confidentiality*, thanks to the Privacy Act (most familiarly known by the acronym HIPAA), is of great benefit to IRBs who well may need to assist investigators in interpreting the implications, but have less of an uphill battle in defending their concerns. Finally, with recent and ongoing investigative journalism coverage of clinical research, the value of *completeness* is becoming more and more self-evident throughout clinical research, beginning with sponsors.

Assuring Research Subject Protection: Closing Communication Loops

Sites and sponsors need to communicate directly and fully to each other and to the IRB, indicating any and all forms of recruitment, from mining databases through centralized media campaigns, that are either going to be used or may be used. Discussions between sites and sponsors result in what the IRB will review.

The IRB must oversee both sponsor and site by way of direct communications. That is to say the IRB needs to receive full documentation on all aspects of the recruitment campaign as planned or envisioned by the investigator or site as well as the sponsor. Such disclosure needs to be thorough permitting the IRB to extract the size, scope, and dimensions of how subjects will be enlisted, and to confirm that the IRB, sponsor, and site have the exact same information by copying communications to each.

Reference

1. Office of Inspector General D. Recruiting Human Subjects: Pressures in Industry-Sponsored Clinical Research (OEI-01-97-00195). Department of Health and Human Services, June 2000. Access date 12 April, 2001. http://www.hhs. gov/oig/oei/reports/a459.pdf

Advertisements for Research

Rachel Hepp, Rachel Krebs, Linda Medwar, Christina Di Tomasso, and Anne Dyson

INTRODUCTION

The purpose of this chapter is to explain the role of the institutional review board (IRB) in evaluating the practices used to recruit subjects for research participation. Federal Regulations (45 CFR 46.111) state that selection of subjects must be equitable. In making this assessment, the IRB should take into account the purposes of the research and the setting in which the study will be conducted. The IRB should be particularly cognizant of the special challenges of research involving vulnerable populations, such as children, prisoners, pregnant women, mentally disabled persons, or economically or educationally disadvantaged persons. The IRB must determine that the procedure for recruitment is not coercive and that it accurately describes the likely risks and benefits of study participation.

Recruitment of subjects is considered the start of the consent/assent process. It is important for investigators to consider how study subjects will be recruited both before a study is initiated as well as throughout the course of the study.[1] In order to fulfill its responsibility in protecting the rights and welfare of human subjects, the IRB must review the methods, materials, procedures, and tools used to recruit potential research subjects before they are implemented. Direct advertising refers to any activity that solicits research participation directly from potential subjects. All direct advertising must have IRB approval before being used. Some of the more commonly used types of direct advertising include flyers, posters, brochures, media advertisements, recruitment letters, and word-of-mouth recruiting. Each of these recruitment methods presents different ethical issues for an IRB to consider and is discussed in the following sections.

Direct Advertising

During its review of advertisements, the IRB should consider both the information contained in the advertisement and the mode of communication by which the information is delivered. Before approving an advertisement, the IRB should determine that it is not coercive and that it accurately describes the potential risks and benefits of study participation. A 1998 update of the Food and Drug Administration (FDA) Information Sheet: Recruiting Study Subjects presents guidelines for the format of study advertisement.[2]

1. Name and address of the investigator and/or research facility
2. Condition under study and/or the purpose of the research
3. In summary form, the criteria that will be used to determine eligibility for the study
4. A brief list of participation benefits, if any (e.g., a no-cost health examination)
5. The time or other commitment required of the subjects
6. The location of research and the person or office to contact for further information

Flyers, Posters, Brochures

Flyers, posters, and brochures are often used to solicit potential research subjects. These types of advertisements are typically placed in strategic locations in hopes of targeting the population being studied. Some of these locations may include bulletin boards, professional offices/businesses, schools, public transportation (buses, subways, trains), and other public areas such as restaurants. In addition to obtaining IRB approval for use of such advertisements, it may also be necessary for an investigator to obtain approval from the various sites where the flyer, poster, and/or brochure will be placed. Ancillary approval should be obtained before posting or distributing the advertisement, and evidence of this approval may be required by the IRB. Because these types of advertisements are visible tools of recruitment, they must present information that is adequate, accurate, and balanced so that potential subjects can make an informed decision about possible participation. The decision to include compensation and/or reimbursement in the advertisement may be made on a case-by-case basis, depending on the study itself and the particular policies and guidelines of the IRB. Although compensation or reimbursement may factor into one's decision to participate in a study, the offer must be carefully thought out and worded appropriately so as not to coerce a subject to participate. Examples of acceptable and unacceptable research advertisements will clarify these issues.

Example 1: Unapproved advertisement
Lose Weight Fast and Receive Cash!!!
Join an Exciting Weight-Loss Study

- *Are you a teenager?*
- *Are you fat and want to lose weight?*

If you answered YES to these questions, you may qualify to participate in a weight-loss study.

You will receive a free medical evaluation and participate in a cutting-edge nutrition program.

You will also receive $$$ money $$$ and parking vouchers. No medications will be given.

Call (213) 456–9870 for more information.

This advertisement should not be approved by the IRB for several reasons.

1. There is an emphasis on monetary compensation.
2. The advertisement uses catchy words such as *exciting*, *fast*, *cutting-edge*, and *free*.
3. Ages for eligibility are not specified.
4. The purpose of the study is not specified.
5. No mention is made about the study being "research."
6. Terms such as *fat* may be insulting.
7. The name of the contact person is not included.
8. The study location is not included.
9. The advertisement is misleading concerning its purpose.

Example 2: Revised advertisement
Weight-Loss and Diabetes-Prevention Study
Be part of an important Nutrition Research Study

- *Are you between 13 and 21 years of age?*
- *Do you want to change your eating habits in order to lose weight?*

If you answered YES to these questions, you may be eligible to participate in a nutrition research study.

The purpose of this research study is to compare the effectiveness of different diets in preventing type 2 diabetes. Benefits include a comprehensive medical evaluation and nutrition program. Participants will also receive monetary compensation and parking vouchers. No medications will be given.

Both adolescents (13 years of age and older) and adults (21 years of age and younger) are eligible. The study is being conducted at Central Hospital.

Please call John Smith at (555) 123–4567 for more information.

This is an example of an advertisement that meets the basic guidelines for IRB approval.

1. The approach is straightforward and honest.
2. "Research" is specified.

3. The ages for eligibility are included.
4. The purpose is clearly stated.
5. The benefits are included.
6. The contact person's name is included.
7. The institution is identified.

Media Advertisements (Newspaper, Television, Radio, Internet)

As a result of the increasing complexity and number of research studies, investigators are often interested in the use of recruitment tools that have the capability to reach a large number of potential research subjects. Media advertisements serve this role, as newspapers, television and radio communication, and Internet advertisements allow for the dissemination of research information to many people over the course of their daily lives. In these situations, individuals are not necessarily searching for such advertisements, but an individual who is interested in an advertised research study may nonetheless pursue contacting the research site for further information. All media research advertisements must be reviewed and approved by the IRB before use.

Coercion in Media Advertising

One of the key issues an IRB will focus on in reviewing media advertisements is the elimination of coercion. Subtle forms of coercion may appear in media advertisements without an investigator's awareness. Coercion that is subtle could be apparent in the tone of voice used, the speed of speech, and/or the inclusion of soothing background music. The guidelines for the development of flyers, posters, and brochures, as discussed earlier in this chapter, should be adhered to in creating media advertisements. In general, media advertisements should be straightforward and honest in order to target the appropriate audience and elicit the desired response from potential research subjects.

IRB Approval of Media Advertisements

A recording of all potential radio advertisements must be approved by the IRB before broadcasting. It is recommended that the advertisement text be submitted for review before the final taping occurs, as the IRB may require changes to the wording. The final tape should then be submitted to the IRB so that the delivery of the text can be reviewed for potential coercion. This process is also recommended for the development and implementation of television advertisements. An institutional policy may be developed in which the IRB chair reviews television and radio advertisements and then determines whether the entire IRB should review the advertisement before approval. The final version of newspaper advertisements must also be approved by the IRB before publication.[1]

Internet Advertising

The use of the Internet as a recruitment tool presents unique challenges to the IRB. As the Internet has become more widely used by patients and patient advocacy groups, it has also become a popular method for recruiting research subjects. The Internet may be used as a recruitment tool by adding a study to a listing of research studies or by posting research advertisements. For example, clinical trials are listed on http://www.clinicaltrials.gov, a website maintained by the National Institutes of Health (NIH) that lists both federally and privately sponsored (industry, foundation, etc.) clinical trials. The NIH requires evidence of IRB approval before listing a clinical trial on this website, as does the commercial site Centerwatch, http://www.centerwatch.com. Institutional policies may indicate that advertisements and listings of research studies require IRB approval, even though this is not a federal regulatory requirement.

The FDA has provided guidance regarding the use of the Internet for recruiting research subjects. As stated in the FDA Information Sheets, "IRB review and approval of listings of clinical trials on the Internet would provide no additional safeguard and is not required when the system format limits the information provided to basic trial information, such as the title; purpose of the study; protocol summary; basic eligibility criteria; study site location(s); and how to contact the site for further information."[2] However, if Internet postings extend beyond the realm of what is considered to be basic factual information, the FDA recommends IRB review and approval.

An additional issue to consider regarding Internet listings of research studies is the method by which interested individuals should contact a research site. Certain populations may prefer calling a research center instead of sending an e-mail response, as their anonymity may not be assured with an e-mail response.

Another electronic method for advertising research studies is the use of an internal intranet system within an institution. This method may be used for two purposes: to inform employees of studies they may consider for participation, such as occupational health studies, or to inform employees of studies for particular patient populations. In an effort to minimize coercion and allow employees to decide whether they would like to view the research studies, it is preferred to have the option of clicking into a listing of research studies as opposed to sending a broadcast e-mail message to all employees. An internal intranet system also allows research investigators to become familiar with studies being conducted by other physicians and researchers at their institution. Additionally, some institutions now also use external research Internet sites that allow patients and patrons to search a listing of the institution's active research studies.

Recruitment Letters

Many investigators use recruitment letters as the first step in the recruitment process. Depending on the nature of the research, the recruitment letter may or may not need to include all of the elements normally disclosed in an informed consent document. The investigator may choose to explain the purpose of the research, what participation will involve, the risks and benefits associated with subject participation, whether any compensation will be offered, and the fact that participation is voluntary. On the other hand, if the research study involves sensitive material, the investigator may choose to keep the recruitment letter vague. For example, in an effort to protect the privacy of a potential subject, an investigator may decide not to disclose many details of the study in case the letter gets into the hands of someone other than the potential subject for whom it was intended. Regardless of what the research involves, the recruitment letter should explain how the investigator obtained the potential subjects' names.

The intended audience is a key factor in influencing the content of a recruitment letter. The following sections will outline some of the issues that investigators must consider when they wish to send recruitment letters to potential subjects who are patients, students in schools, and employers/employees.

Patients

Additional factors must be considered when the research involves recruiting a population of patients. Some research studies will seek the enrollment of patients who were previously seen by the investigator, whereas other studies will seek new patients for the research. If an investigator has received a list of potential research subjects from another investigator, this should be disclosed in the recruitment letter.

The provisions set forth in the Privacy Rule may impact an investigator's plans for patient recruitment. As stated in the NIH guide "Institutional Review Boards and the HIPAA Privacy Board," the

"Privacy Rule permits, under section 164.512(i)(1)(ii), a covered entity to provide investigators with access to PHI for purposes preparatory to research, such as for identifying potential human subjects to aid in study recruitment, among other things. Such access is permitted provided that the covered entity receives certain required representations from the researcher and the researcher does not remove any PHI from the covered entity during the course of the review."

Activities in which an investigator obtains and records individually identifiable health information for purposes of identifying potential human subjects to aid in study recruitment, among other things, involve human subjects research under the Department of Health and Human Services (DHHS) regulations at 45 CFR part 46 and would not satisfy the criteria for any exemption under DHHS regulations at 45 CFR 46.101(b). As a result, if such activities are conducted or supported by DHHS or conducted under an applicable Office for Human Research Protections (OHRP) approved assurance, the research activities must be reviewed and approved by an IRB in accordance with DHHS regulations at 45 CFR 46.109(a). In addition, informed consent of the subjects, about whom identifiable private information (e.g., health information) is being obtained, must be sought and documented in accordance with and to the extent required by DHHS regulations at 45 CFR 46.116 and 46.117, respectively."[3]

Other points to consider mentioning in the recruitment letter include whether the subjects' participation will affect their current or future care and whether the research results will be released to the subjects. It is especially important to consider these points because the risk of the subject confusing research with clinical care is increased.

Schools/Students

Investigators who wish to recruit potential subjects from schools should be aware of federal laws that govern the conduct of these research studies and disclosure of information. The Family Educational Rights and Privacy Act and the Protection of Pupil Rights Amendment are two laws that directly address the conduct of research involving school children. The Family Educational Rights and Privacy Act defines the rights of students and parents concerning reviewing, amending, and disclosing education records and requires written permission to disclose personally identifiable information from a student's education record, except under certain circumstances such as an order of subpoena. The Protection of Pupil Rights Amendment applies to survey research conducted in schools and states that parents and/or guardians have the right to inspect surveys and questionnaires distributed within schools. This amendment also specifies that parental permission must be obtained to have minors participate in surveys that disclose certain types of sensitive information.

Employers/Employees

When research studies are intended for businesses and their employees or employers, the investigator should consider the following factors when sending recruitment letters to such businesses. The potential subject (employer/employee) should not be pressured into participating in the research for fear of job loss, delayed promotion, or other influences from the supervisor or superior. An investigator should make it clear that information disclosed will remain confidential. Employees would likely be reluctant to participate in a research study if they have not been made aware that their confidentiality is guaranteed. The investigator should consider whether the employer needs to be aware that employees are being recruited for research. If the research is to be conducted at the place of employment during the course of a regular business day, the employer may need to be notified. It is important to remember that the investigator may need to obtain permission from the employer before approaching or sending a recruitment letter to the employees.

Postcards and Phone Calls

Aside from considering the types of subjects that will be recruited and the timing for sending the recruitment letter to potential subjects, an investigator should consider what the next course of action will be if subjects do not respond to the recruitment letter. Many investigators choose to resend the recruitment letter and questionnaire or survey to those individuals who did not respond to the initial mailing. If the investigator plans to send a second mailing, he or she may wish to state this in the initial recruitment letter. Some investigators choose to include return postcards with the mailing of their recruitment letters on which subjects may indicate their desire to participate in the research

or not. In this case, the investigator will know whom to contact for further discussion and clarification about the research study. If the study involves a sensitive subject, the investigator may opt to have the postcard be vague in its identification of the study, or the investigator may include an envelope in which subjects can return the postcard so as to secure privacy and confidentiality. It is important that the investigator state the appropriate response instructions in the recruitment letter in order to generate the greatest response rate, as well as protect the privacy of potential subjects.

If an investigator wishes to contact potential subjects by telephone, a recruitment letter stating this should first be sent to the potential subject. Several considerations should be kept in mind during the development of this type of recruitment letter. The recruitment letter should state that the investigator will be telephoning potential subjects. A postcard can be included with the recruitment letter asking interested subjects to include their telephone number and the appropriate times that the investigator may reach them. On this postcard, subjects may also have the choice to indicate that they do not want to participate in the research. An investigator who will be contacting subjects by telephone should be conscious of the privacy and confidentiality of these subjects and should only call during the times indicated by potential subjects.

Certainly, individual IRBs may have their own requirements regarding the use of recruitment letters. The previously mentioned information should serve merely as a guide for what investigators should consider when developing recruitment letters. An investigator should consult with the IRB office to inquire about specific guidelines and policies relevant to the particular study in mind.

Advertising and Recruiting Through Word of Mouth

Subjects may be drawn to participation in a research study simply through word of mouth. Information about research studies is often disseminated to appropriate target audiences at organized meetings such as advocacy groups and business workshops. For example, physicians often inform their peers about their need for research subjects within the peer's community or area of expertise. Word-of-mouth recruitment can also occur through the formation of social networks of individuals who share a common concern or interest. Through these social networks, people will exchange information pertinent to their needs, including their health. For example, if an individual with a rare form of cancer chooses to participate in an investigational treatment protocol, he or she may inform others with the same cancer about this research protocol. If investigators consider information disclosed through word of mouth to be among their recruitment tools, then this should be acknowledged and mentioned in the written protocol. The investigator should submit any written materials that may be discussed or given out at such advocacy groups, business workshops, or peer meetings to the IRB for review and approval.

In-Person Recruitment

The first step of the recruitment process often occurs through the efforts of research personnel approaching potential research subjects in person. There are many issues that those who are involved in directly approaching individuals for possible inclusion in a research study must consider. The time at which an individual is approached is of particular importance; it should be a time that is convenient for the potential subject and should not occur at a time that would likely increase a person's anxiety level (i.e., right before major surgery). Sometimes it is helpful to present a research study to individuals in advance so that they can take the consent form and other recruitment materials home to review with family members. This approach would provide potential research subjects with ample time to consider whether or not participation is of interest to them.

The location of recruitment should also be considered. Research studies of a more sensitive nature, such as some survey questionnaires, may require privacy, in which case an individual examination room or office may be the most appropriate environment for discussing and/or completing the questionnaire, rather than in a busy waiting room.

It is important to note that the investigator may not always be the best person to recruit, as he or she may unduly influence the potential research subject.[4] For example, if the investigator is also the potential subject's physician, the patient may confuse the physician's role as a clinician with the role as a researcher. Potential coercion could also occur if a researcher attempts to recruit individuals from his/her own staff. It is important to keep in mind individual institutions' policies on recruiting one's own patients and colleagues/employees.

Conclusion

IRB members and staff play an important role in ensuring that investigators are informed of the process for the review and approval of recruitment materials. Educational sessions provide an opportunity for teaching investigators about the review process. Additionally, within the protocol application itself, it may be helpful to include information about the materials that must be submitted to the IRB along with specific application questions about recruitment. Such questions may inquire as to how potential research subject names are obtained before contact is made, who recruits potential subjects for the study, where potential subjects will be recruited from, and what process will be used to recruit potential subjects.

Direct advertising represents the majority of recruitment tools used by investigators to identify potential research subjects. It is important to remain mindful of the fact that recruitment methods are the first step in the consent process. Every aspect of research, including recruitment, should adhere to the guidelines set forth in *The Belmont Report* and the Code of Federal Regulations. Furthermore, individual IRBs can establish more rigorous guidelines for the review and approval of recruitment materials than those contained in the federal regulations. Individual institutional policies should outline the circumstances under which recruitment tools require expedited or full IRB review and approval. With increased awareness of human subject protection issues, the interpretation and implementation of the federal regulations and institutional policies have evolved to ensure more appropriate protection of research subjects. As better protection methods are developed and secured, better recruitment methods will evolve. Potential subjects need to be given sufficient information that is accurate and balanced in order to make an informed decision about their participation in a research study.[5]

We end with a final list of recommendations regarding the recruitment of subjects for research.

1. Clearly state that the project is research.
2. Err on the side of underestimating benefits and overestimating risks.
3. Do not make claims of safety, equivalence, or superiority.
4. Avoid phrases such as "new treatment," "new medicine," or "new drug."
5. Avoid using the term *free* in reference to treatment procedures.
6. Do not emphasize compensation.
7. Obtain approval to post advertisements from all applicable groups.

References

1. Dunn C, Chadwick G, Allen W (eds.). *Protecting Study Volunteers in Clinical Research*. Boston, MA: Center Watch; September 1999.
2. Food and Drug Administration Information Sheets: Guidance for Institutional Review Boards and Clinical Investigators. September 1998. Access date 6 January, 2005. http://www.fda.gov/oc/ohrt/irbs/toc4.html#recruiting
3. U.S. Department of Health and Human Services, National Institutes of Health. Institutional Review Boards and the HIPAA Privacy Rule: NIH Fact Sheet. Access date 15 August, 2003. http://privacyruleandresearch.nih.gov/irbandprivacyrule.asp
4. Office of Inspector General. Recruiting Human Subjects: Pressures in Industry-Sponsored Clinical Research (OEI-01-97-00195). June 2000. Access date 6 January, 2005. http://oig.hhs.gov/oei/reports/oei-01-97-00195.pdf
5. Office of Inspector General. Recruiting Human Subjects: Sample Guidelines for Practice (OEI-01-97-00196). June 2000. Access date 6 January, 2005. http://oig.hhs.gov/oei/ reports/oei-01-97-00196.pdf

Paying Research Subjects

*Bruce G. Gordon, Joseph S. Brown, Christopher J. Kratochvil, Toby L. Schonfeld,
and Ernest D. Prentice*

INTRODUCTION

Payment of human subjects to participate in research remains one of the more contentious ethical problems facing institutional review boards (IRBs). Although concerns over this practice have existed for many years, there are few regulatory guidelines or indeed any consensus to shape institutional and individual IRB policy. In this chapter, we briefly review the ethical arguments pertaining to this practice, the federal regulations and guidance, as well as some of the models proposed to standardize the practice.

In this chapter, we have deliberately avoided providing the opinion of the authors regarding the "optimal" compensation scheme or specific recommendations addressing the other issues described later here. This is a conscious decision that is grounded in the understanding that the relative weight of ethical arguments may vary from institution to institution and from IRB to IRB.

Ethical Arguments

It has been suggested that the payment of subjects represents "undue inducement," which influences a potential subject to do something he would not ordinarily have done.[1-4] One may argue that research participation should be based on a risk/benefit relationship in which the benefits are those inherently present in the research itself. For "therapeutic research," these potential benefits may include relief from disease, diminished suffering, or the provision of diagnostic information. For nontherapeutic research, subjects ideally participate for entirely altruistic reasons, to benefit society. In exchange for these benefits, subjects accept a certain degree of risk, the acceptability of which reflects each subject's goals and values. In the case of either therapeutic or nontherapeutic research, but more obviously in the latter case, payment may influence this calculation. Now risk is balanced against health or societal benefit and financial reward, and the scale is shifted, however slightly. Hence, the subject no longer acts solely for the benefit of his health, or for altruism, but for some other reason (i.e., money).

On the other hand, it may be just as cogently argued that financial reward is a benefit no less valid than altruism or relief from illness, and there is no *a priori* reason to exclude it from the risk–benefit analysis. Indeed, for an IRB to do so may represent excessive paternalism in presuming that it can determine what benefits ought to be important to a person. The ethical principle of autonomy might be invoked to allow an informed, reasoning person to decide for himself or herself what value he or she places on money and what risks he or she is willing to undertake in exchange for that value.

A second argument against payment of research subjects is that such payment may result in economically disadvantaged persons bearing a disproportionately large share of the risks of research.[1,4] Such a policy would thus appear to contravene the principle of justice. However, it has been asserted that this view is rather one sided: it considers research solely as a "burden."

To the extent that the benefits of research are distributed primarily to participants, one might argue that any procedure such as payment of subjects that encourages recruitment of populations that have traditionally not participated in clinical research, such as African Americans, is ethically acceptable and appropriate. Of course, this argument is based on the assumption that participation in the research is undoubtedly beneficial. Members of minority populations clearly disagree with that assumption in many cases, or they would participate without inducement. Certainly, historical abuses such as the Tuskegee Study suggest that a certain suspicion of the research community is not without foundation.

In addition, this counterargument is not compelling from a utilitarian standpoint. Certainly, if there are features of the underserved population that can only be assessed by their direct participation in research, benefits to that population as a whole may outweigh risks to the individuals participating in the research. In a drug study, for example, different physiologic populations such as children, pregnant women, or the older population may require participation from these groups to assess how a specific medication is metabolized in that subgroup. However, in the absence of a reason to believe economically disadvantaged persons metabolize a drug differently than more affluent persons do, the "benefit" of enrolling those economically disadvantaged persons accrue only to the subjects themselves (not the population) and only if the subjects have the disease being treated by the drug, only to the subjects randomized to receive the drug, and only for the duration of the trial. Moreover, if the eventual cost of the new drug under study will be significant, as is often the case, the population who undertook the risks to test the drug may not be able to afford the benefits of its use. Taken together, the limited benefits make it unlikely that the assumption that research participation is "undoubtedly beneficial" would be met.

A third argument against paying research subjects is that payment dehumanizes the subject and, by making him a "salaried worker," potentially alters the relationship between the subject and the investigator. Wartofsky asserted that "payment for participation in research amounts to selling the services of one's body, often at some significant risk."[4]

However, payment for labor is not fundamentally unethical: a person's services or capacities are commodities that are regularly exchanged for wages. It would generally not be considered unethical to pay wages for work that is inherently risky (police, firefighters, and commercial fisherman regularly experience risk in their jobs). However, we are not paying for the risk *per se*. That is, although the job is risky, we pay for someone to perform the work, not specifically for someone to undertake the risk.

Wartofsky eloquently compared the extent to which prostitution is like wage labor, "involving, as it were, the sale of a disposition over one's body for a certain purpose, at a certain rate and for a certain time. The relevance of the inquiry lies in the fact that what is being bought and sold in prostitution, just as in participation in research, is something which is so intimate to one's person that there is something disturbing in the notion that it is alienable, as a commodity."[4] In his view, "The ethical objections to prostitution, and to being a paid research subject, derive from the translation of relations which are supposed to express fundamental aspects of humanity into an economic exchange. In the paid research context, both the investigator and the subject are reducing an essential human capacity (putting oneself at risk for others) to a commodity; so doing, they may dehumanize each other."[4]

Empiric Data

Data regarding the importance of payment in the decision of research subjects to participate supports the notion that financial compensation is an important motivator, at least among healthy volunteers. Payment was sited as the most important reason to participate in subjects undergoing pharmacologic studies[5,6] or physiology studies,[7] among participants in private or university-based research projects[5] and among new participants and experienced volunteers.[8,9]

There are less data regarding participants in so-called therapeutic research because payment is less common in these trials. Among patients with asthma and allergies enrolled in therapy trials, health improvement was the primary motivator, but financial reward was still cited as a reason, especially among experienced participants.[10]

Halpern and coworkers surveyed 126 patients with hypertension to determine how payment affected their perception of risk and likelihood of participating in a hypothetical placebo-controlled Phase III trial of an antihypertensive drug.[11] They found a decreased willingness to participate with higher risk of the trial and with lower payment level. They acknowledge the influence of payment level on willingness to participate. However, they found it "of greater ethical import" that higher payments did not alter the subjects' perception of risk, and therefore, they concluded that payment was neither undue nor unjust.

Bentley and Thacker published very similar results.[12] They found that, among pharmacy students asked about a hypothetical nontherapeutic research study, monetary payment influenced willingness to participate regardless of level of risk, but higher monetary payments did not blind subjects to risks. The authors conclude that "monetary payments appear to do what they were intended to do: make subjects more willing to participate in research." Interestingly, they also noted that higher payments did influence subjects' behaviors regarding concealing restricted activities (such as consumption of alcohol or caffeine that would have made them ineligible for the research) and raise concern that payments may lead to reduction in the integrity of the study's findings.

Russell and colleagues took a different approach, surveying a group of unpaid participants in a vaccine trial, seeking information not on why they participated, but on their opinions as to whether compensation was ethical.[13] A majority of respondents disagreed with the payment of research subjects regardless of whether the subjects were healthy volunteers (76%) or patients (73%). In their comments, respondents identified potential problems with payment, including undue pressure to participate and impact on costs.

Respondents recognized that payment could improve recruitment, and many thought it appropriate if recruitment was a problem. Also of interest, some commented that payment might be justified in order to obtain more equitable representation across social strata so that poorer persons could have a chance to benefit from the research. This is in contrast to most traditional ethical arguments that focus on the burdens of research rather than on the potential benefits. Respondents distinguished between payment as incentive, payment of expenses, compensation for injury, and payment as recognition for time and effort. The latter three were judged more acceptable than the first.

Although these data are interesting, it is important to consider that the respondents were already self-selected as being, perhaps, more altruistic than others because they had all agreed to participate in a trial with some risk, no direct benefit to them, and no monetary compensation. Therefore, results from this study may be difficult to extrapolate to other populations.

Regulations and Guidelines

Neither the Department of Health and Human Services (DHHS) (45 CFR 46) nor the Food and Administration (FDA) (21 CFR 50, 56) regulations offer specific limitations on the payment of research subjects. DHHS regulations state only that "an investigator shall seek such consent only under circumstances . . . that minimize the possibility of coercion or undue influence" (45 CFR 46.116). The Office for Human Research Protections (OHRP) has issued no guidance on the definition of "undue influence," and it has been widely and variously interpreted. As described previously here, some have argued that any financial remuneration, over and above reimbursement of direct costs to the subject, represents "undue inducement." A more temperate interpretation would require examination of the amount of payment, in relationship to the risks and burdens of the research, before deciding whether influence is "undue."

FDA guidance on payment of research subjects is no more informative.[14] The FDA Information Sheets stated, "It is not uncommon for subjects to be paid for their participation in research, especially in the early phases of investigational drug, biologic or device development." The FDA neither endorses nor prohibits payment to subjects, but charges IRBs with the responsibility to "review both the amount of payment and the proposed method and timing of disbursement to assure that neither are coercive or present undue influence [21 CFR 50.20]." The FDA does, however, assert that "payment to research subjects for participation in studies is not considered a benefit; it is a recruitment incentive." In other words, IRBs should not consider payment in their assessment of the risk benefit relationship of the research (although subjects may).

The OHRP *IRB Guidebook* acknowledges the differing opinions regarding the ethics of payment of research subjects, but neither endorses nor condemns the practice.[15] It does point out appropriately that "free health care for persons with limited resources and major medical problems may be a significant inducement to participate in research (even if the research activity is non-therapeutic)" but goes on to say that "there is no consensus as to whether this kind of inducement is unacceptable." The guidebook offers several models for payment, including compensation "according to an established fee schedule, based upon the complexity of the study, the type and number of procedures to be performed, the time involved, and the anticipated discomfort or inconvenience," or "an hourly rate or a fixed amount, depending on the duration of the study and whether the study requires admission to research ward [with] extra payments . . . provided for a variety of additional inconveniences."

Most international codes, likewise, provide no firm guidance. The International Conference on Harmonization (ICH) does not address the issue at all, and the 2000 revision of the World Medical Association Declaration of Helsinki states only that "the researcher should also submit to the [ethical review] committee . . . information regarding . . . incentives for subjects."[16] Only the Council for International Organizations of Medical Sciences (CIOMS) offers a more definitive answer. Guideline 4 (Inducement to Participate) of the "International Ethical Guidelines for Biomedical Research Involving Human Subjects," states this:

> Subjects may be paid for inconvenience and time spent, and should be reimbursed for expenses incurred, in connection with their participation in research; they may also receive free medical services. However, the payments should not be so large or the medical services so extensive as to induce prospective subjects to consent to participate in the research against their better judgment ("undue inducement").[17]

Thus, it would appear that CIOMS is of the opinion that at least reimbursement is not only ethical, but also an obligation to the subject.

Models for Payment

IRBs that ultimately decide to allow payment to research subjects must decide what level of compensation is appropriate. Dickert and Grady[18] have proposed various models of payment that we describe later here.

Market Model

In this model, the laws of supply and demand determine how much a subject should be paid for participating in a given trial. Payment is a "benefit" to offset risks associated with a particular trial. Studies that involve greater risk (or have no other benefit) would likely have the highest rate of compensation. Studies in which subjects stand to gain a significant health benefit (i.e., therapeutic studies) would likely have minimal or no monetary payment. This model also allows for higher compensation to speed recruitment and bonuses to assure subjects complete the study.

The advantages of the market model are obvious: recruitment for high-risk (or low-benefit) studies would be augmented, and completion bonuses would help to ensure that subjects finish the research. The market model is not unlike wage payment for a dangerous job: the laborer is compensated for services despite risk.

The major disadvantage of the market model is that payment may be so high that potential subjects enroll and remain on the study against their own best interests. Potential subjects may also conceal important health information in order to remain eligible and thus place themselves (and the research protocol) at even higher risk. Finally, economically vulnerable groups are most likely to be attracted by this model, thereby inequitably distributing risks of research.

Wage Payment Model

In this second model proposed by Dickert and Grady, and based on previous work by Ackerman,[1] payment is made based on the premise that participation in research is unskilled labor that requires little training and some risk. Thus, subjects are compensated "on a scale commensurate with that of other unskilled but essential jobs,"[18] that is, a fairly low, standardized hourly wage, with bonuses for hazardous procedures.

The wage payment model appears less likely to present undue inducement to subjects because the "wages" they would earn from participation would be no more than they could earn in other unskilled labor. Furthermore, the standardization of payment would reduce competition for subjects between studies (which would be expected to drive up "prices" on the market model).

On the other hand, the wage payment model reduces but does not eliminate the potential for inequitable distribution of the risks of research to economically vulnerable groups. Although there is less undue incentive than with the market model, the wage payment model still presents a source of income to persons who may be unemployed and having difficulty finding jobs. Potential subjects with higher income are more likely to avoid studies that compensate using this model because participation may entail a loss of income (if time has to taken off from work). This is particularly problematic, as the bonuses for hazardous procedures will once again place the risks of research predominantly on the backs of the economically disadvantaged. Finally, from a more philosophic point of view, as Dickert and Grady, and others[19,20] suggested, "Treating the subject's role as an unskilled job may be seen as inappropriately commercializing participation in research."[18]

Reimbursement Model

In this model, payment is provided to cover a subject's expenses (travel, food, gasoline). The definition of "expenses" may be somewhat flexible and can, at one end of the spectrum, be considered to include lost wages because of time taken off from work without pay. This model is based on the view that "research participation should not require financial sacrifice, but should be revenue neutral for participants."[18]

The reimbursement model notably eliminates the risk of undue inducement to participate in research. It also reduces the likelihood that potential subjects will withhold medical information so as not be to excluded from a study, although it does not eliminate the possibility that subjects will withhold information for some other benefit like access to a new treatment or free medical exams. Finally, it is not likely that financially disadvantaged potential subjects will be attracted inappropriately to these studies.

On the other hand, studies that reimburse using this model will be more apt to accrue subjects slowly (particularly if other competing studies utilize a different model). Accrual will be slower still if compensation does not include lost wages. For those studies that do include compensation for lost wages, the reimbursement model could paradoxically lead to targeting low-income populations by the sponsors in order to reduce costs.

Prorating Payment

The FDA clearly requires prorating payments based on the duration of participation of the subject in the research. The FDA Information Sheets stated, "Any credit for payment should accrue as the study progresses and not be contingent upon the subject completing the entire study."[14] Prorated payment should be made regardless of whether withdrawal was voluntarily or involuntarily, that is, whether the withdrawal was based on the decision of the subject to discontinue or based on some withdrawal criteria of the research protocol.

Protocols submitted to the IRB should clearly define the scheme for payment of subjects who withdraw from a study and this scheme should be described in the consent documents. Often, payment is awarded based on a fixed fee per clinic visit or per intervention. The amount paid for each visit or intervention needs to be examined by the IRB in consideration of the ethical issues raised previously, such that subjects are not unduly induced to continue when they would otherwise not have done so. The FDA does allow for the payment of "a small proportion as an incentive for completion of the study," providing that such an incentive is not coercive.[14]

Payment to Minors

The ethical concerns raised previously here regarding payment of subjects are magnified when the subjects are minors. The literature offers minimal and sometimes conflicting guidance regarding compensation of minors involved in research. In their position paper on ethical conduct of studies involving children, the American Academy of Pediatrics (AAP) noted that the practice of payment is consistent with "the traditions and ethics of society."[21] The European Union, in contrast, has prohibited all "incentives or financial inducements" for research involving minors.[22] Weise and coworkers found that the majority (66%) of IRBs allow payment of children who participate in research, although the specifics of the practice vary widely.[23] Borzekowski and colleagues similarly found that 55% of studies involving adolescent subjects involved payment for participation.[24]

Children and adolescents may be more or less prone to being unduly influenced by financial reward, depending on their age and maturity. To a 10-year-old, a $5 payment is a fortune; to a 3-year-old, it may be irrelevant. Although the (monetary) benefits may appear especially clear, children and younger adolescents often have limited capability to understand the risks and, therefore, are not likely to perform an adequate assessment of the risk/benefit relationship. This may be especially true for adolescents, who feel invulnerable and indestructible, and therefore may be especially prey to monetary inducements. It may be difficult to determine "appropriate" compensation, even based on the models described previously here.

If payment to the child is concerning, payment to the parent is also ethically problematic. The AAP notes that "serious ethical questions arise when payment is offered to adults acting on behalf of minors in return for allowing minors to participate as research subjects."[21] However, in consideration of Dickert and Grady's reimbursement model, it could be argued that payment to the parent is preferable because the parent (rather than the child) incurs the financial costs of participating in research (e.g., loss of wages, car expenses, food).

The best compromise may be a combination of payments: compensation for financial costs to the parents associated with participation (as per reimbursement model), as well as some remuneration to the child who is bearing the burden of research.[22] Wendler suggested payment of teenagers based on minimum wage.[22] The AAP, in contrast, states "remuneration should not be beyond a token gesture of appreciation."[21]

Payment in Kind

Certain populations may be at higher risk of being unduly induced by monetary payment. As discussed previously here, children may overvalue cash. Subjects of low socioeconomic status (including the homeless) may be particularly vulnerable because of their economic situation and their need for financial resources. It has been argued that such need may overwhelm the potential subject's ability to make reasoned decisions about the risks and benefits of participating in the venture.[25] For this reason, these populations are often offered payments "in kind": an item of value equivalent to the amount of money that is appropriate for the study but is in fact not money itself.[23]

For various reasons, we find payment in kind (at least for subjects of low socioeconomic status) to be ethically problematic.[26] Despite attempts at equalization, a payment in kind is, almost without exception, of lesser value than a cash payment.[27] This is because cash can be converted into any of a number of products: $50 cash can purchase $50 worth of product X or $50 of product Y. The payment in kind, on the other hand, is only one thing: $50 worth of product X, whether that product is wanted or not. Because payment in kind is worth less than cash, to offer it to some populations and not others seems inequitable.[26]

Perhaps more importantly, the restriction of options inherently restricts the autonomy of subjects. An individual's autonomy lies in the choice. To act autonomously, an individual must be able to make a meaningful choice according to his or her own life plan, and limitations on the range of options may require a significant compromise to the subject's autonomy. There is significant value in the choice itself, and payment in kind limits a participant's choice. As respect for a person's autonomy is a fundamental requirement for participation in research, the restriction of such rights requires considerable justification.[26]

IRB Responsibilities

As the proportion of studies offering payment for participation shows no evidence of decreasing, it is essential that IRBs develop guidelines to judge appropriateness of payment schemes. Few institutions have coherent policies.[28] Such guidelines require consensus within the board and within the community of stake holders. This is made especially difficult considering the multiplicity of ethical arguments for and against each payment model (and, indeed, for and against payment per se).

Nonetheless, at a minimum, guidelines developed by IRBs should require that compensation is not of a nature that it interferes with the ability of the potential subject to give informed consent, without the possibility of coercion

or undue influence (understanding, of course, that the meaning of this is nebulous at best). IRB guidelines should also stress the need for prorating compensation and define the limited situations under which such proration is not needed. Finally, guidelines should address the particularly sensitive issues related to direct compensation of minors.

Acknowledgments

Much of the material in the section "Payment in Kind" is drawn from an earlier paper, "Research involving the homeless: Arguments against payment-in-kind (PinK)," published in *IRB Ethics and Human Research* as cited later here.

References

1. Ackerman T. An ethical framework for the practice of paying research subjects. *IRB* 11(4):1–4, 1989.
2. McGee G. Subject to payment? *JAMA* 278:199–200, 1997.
3. Macklin R. "Due" and "undue" inducements: On paying money to research subjects. *IRB* 3(5):1–6, 1981.
4. Wartofsky M. On doing it for money. In: *Research involving prisoners: Report and recommendations.* Washington, DC: National Commission for the Protection of Human Subjects of Biomedical and Behavioral Research; 1976.
5. Hassar M, Pocelinko R, Weintraub M, Nelson D, Thomas G, Lasagna L. Free-living volunteer's motivations and attitudes toward pharmacologic studies in man. *Clin Pharmacol Ther* 21(5):515, 1977.
6. van Gelderen C, Savelkoul T, van Dokkum W, Meulenbelt J. Motives and perception of healthy volunteers who participate in experiments. *Eur J Clin Pharmacol* 45(1):15–21, 1993.
7. Whinnery J. Motivational analysis of human volunteers for centrifuge acceleration research. *Aviat Space Environ Med* 53(10):1017–1020, 1982.
8. Bigorra J, Banos J. Weight of financial reward in the decision by medical students and experienced healthy volunteers to participate in clinical trials. *Eur J Clin Pharmacol* 38(5):443–446, 1990.
9. Novak E, Seckman CE, Stewart RD. Motivations for volunteering as research subjects. *J Clin Pharmacol* 17(7):365–371, 1977.
10. Aby J, Pheley A, Steinberg P. Motivation for participation in clinical trials of drugs for the treatment of asthma, seasonal allergic rhinitis, and perennial nonallergic rhinitis. *Ann Allergy Asthma Immunol* 76:348–354, 1996.
11. Halpern SD, Karlawish JH, Casarett D, Berlin JA, Asch DA. Empiric assessment of whether moderate payments are undue or unjust inducements for participation in clinical trials. *Arch Intern Med* 164:801–803, 2004.
12. Bentley JP, Thacker PG. The influence of risk and monetary payment on the research participation decision making process. *J Med Ethics* 30:293–298, 2004.
13. Russell M, Moralejo D, Burgess E. Paying research subjects: Participants' perspectives. *J Med Ethics* 26:126–130, 2000.
14. Food and Drug Administration. *Information Sheets: Guidelines for Institutional Review Boards and Clinical Investigators.* Rockville, MD: U.S. Government Printing Office, 1998.

15. Office for Human Research Protections. *IRB Guidebook.* http://ohrp.osophs.dhhs.gov/irb/irb_chapter3.htm

16. World Medical Association Declaration of Helsinki. Ethical Principles for Medical Research Involving Human Subjects. Revised October 2000. http://www.wma.net/ e/policy/17-c_e.html

17. Council for International Organizations of Medical Sciences. *International Ethical Guidelines for Biomedical Research Involving Human Subjects.* Geneva: CIOMS, 1993.

18. Dickert N, Grady C. What's the price of a research subject? Approaches to payment for research participation. *N Engl J Med* 341(3):198–203, 1999.

19. Titmuss R: *The Gift Relationship: From Human Blood to Social Change.* New York: New Press; 1997.

20. Murray T. Gifts of the body and needs of strangers. *Hastings Cent Rep* 17(2):30–38, 1987.

21. American Academy of Pediatrics. Guidelines for the ethical conduct of studies to evaluate drugs in pediatric populations (RE9503). *Pediatrics* 95:286–294, 1995.

22. Wendler D, Rackoff JE, Emanuel EJ, Grady C. The ethics of paying for children's participation in research. *J Pediatrics* 141(2):166–171, 2002.

23. Weise KL, Smith ML, Maschke KJ, Copeland HL. National practices regarding payment to research subjects for participating in pediatric research. *Pediatrics* 110(3):577–582, 2002.

24. Borzekowski DL, Rickert VI, Ipp L, Fortenberry JD. At what price? The current state of subject payment in adolescent research. *J Adolesc Health* 33:378–384, 2003.

25. Grady C. Money for research participation: Does it jeopardize informed consent? *Am J Bioethics* 1:40, 2001.

26. Schonfeld TL, Brown JS, Weniger M, Gordon B. Research involving the homeless: Arguments against payment-in-kind (PinK). *IRB Ethics and Human Res* 25(5):17–20, 2003.

27. Giuffrida A, Torgerson DJ. Should we pay the patient? Review of financial incentives to enhance patient compliance. *Br Med J* 315:703–707, 1997.

28. Dickert N, Emanuel E, Grady C. Paying research subjects: An analysis of current policies. *Ann Intern Med* 136:368–373, 2002.

Provisions for Data Monitoring

Robert J. Amdur

INTRODUCTION

Issues surrounding provisions for data safety monitoring remain one of most difficult areas with which IRBs need to contend. The FDA held a public hearing in March 2005 Docket No. 2005N-0038: Reporting of Adverse Events to Institutional Review Boards. Please check current FDA guidance for up-to-date information. One criterion for institutional review board (IRB) approval of research at the time of initial protocol review is that the study plan makes adequate provisions for the ongoing monitoring of data throughout the life of the study. Ongoing data monitoring is important because study results may differ from what was predicted before starting the study. The purpose of this chapter is to explain the responsibilities of the IRB at the time of initial protocol review related to the plan for data monitoring. As data-monitoring procedures are important to the IRB throughout the course of a study, there is overlap of this chapter with those in the continuing review section of this book.

Federal Regulations

Federal regulations and guidance documents make it clear that the IRB has a responsibility to determine that the research plan provides for the ongoing monitoring of data in a way that is sufficient to protect the welfare of research participants: Department of Health and Human Services (DHHS) regulations[1][Sec.111(a)(6)] and Food and Drug Administration (FDA) regulations[2][Sec.111(a)(6)] state a criterion for IRB approval of research is that "when appropriate, the research plan makes adequate provisions for monitoring the data collected to ensure the safety of subjects."

The Office for Human Research Protections (OHRP) *IRB Guidebook*[3(pp.3–9)] states, "At the time of initial review, the IRB should determine whether an independent data and safety monitoring board or committee is required, and should also set a date for reevaluating the research."

Limitations of the IRB

In many situations, it will be appropriate to have an individual or group other than the IRB take primary responsibility for data and safety monitoring throughout the course of a study. The three main options that the IRB will need to consider in this regard are discussed in the next section. First, however, it is important to understand a basic controversy that may affect the standards that the IRB should use to approve a data-monitoring plan at the time of initial protocol review. This controversy concerns the role of the IRB in analyzing individual adverse data events, particularly adverse events from multicenter trials.[4] Basically, an IRB must decide whether it is going to take responsibility for analyzing individual event reports from the standpoint of making aggregate comparisons.

The role of the IRB in evaluating individual serious adverse event reports (SAERs) is discussed in detail in several other sections of this book. The IRB's job is to protect the rights and welfare of research participants. Theoretically, IRB review of SAERs from an ongoing clinical trial might result in study modification or the notification of participants about new findings that may affect their decision to continue research participation. However, for review to be meaningful, the IRB must be able to recognize when an event is in some way unexpected for the study population. When the study population is small and the adverse event is exotic in nature or being reported at an extremely high frequency, a local IRB might be able to recognize an important pattern simply by reviewing SAERs that are forwarded from the investigator. However, when the study population is large and diverse, as is the case with most multicenter clinical trials, a local IRB does not have access to the information that it needs to evaluate the importance of SAERs in the overall context of the trial. The problem is best illustrated with an example.

Example
An IRB receives four SAERs of fatal stroke from a large multicenter trial of a new chemotherapy regimen for breast cancer. To make a decision about the importance of these SAERs, the IRB

needs to know whether the observed incidence of stroke exceeds what is expected to occur in this study population independent of research participation. This type of evaluation requires sophisticated information about the number of participants at risk for stroke and the distribution of stroke risk factors in the study population. If the observed exceeds the expected incidence of stroke, the IRB will need to know whether this difference is statistically significant and clinically meaningful in the context of the other medical problems in this population. As the IRB does not have the database, administrative support, or expertise to evaluate these parameters, it is impossible for the IRB to make even a rough estimate about how these or other SAERs might affect the rights and welfare of study participants.

For many kinds of studies, meaningful evaluation of study events requires a group of experts with the resources to monitor data in an ongoing fashion and to compare event data with predetermined stopping or modification rules. Sophisticated statistical analyses are often essential for meaningful ongoing monitoring from the standpoint of protecting research participants. The IRB cannot function as a data-monitoring committee for studies when sophisticated data monitoring is required.[4] A panel of experts convened to evaluate the issue of data monitoring in clinical research concluded this: "Institutional review boards should not be forced to function as data-monitoring committees, and there should be no overlap of their functions."[5]

Federal Policy Statements

It is reasonable to interpret federal regulations to mean that the IRB is responsible for being sure that there is a mechanism in place to perform a high-quality evaluation of study data throughout the course of the study, but the IRB need not be that mechanism. In the past few years, multiple federal policy statements have supported this view.

1998 National Institutes of Health (NIH) Policy Statement

"Data and safety monitoring is required for all types of clinical trials, including physiologic, toxicity, and dose finding studies (Phase I); efficacy studies (Phase II); efficacy, effectiveness and comparative trials (Phase III); etc. . . . The data and safety monitoring functions and oversight of such activities are distinct from the requirement for study review and approval by an Institutional Review Board."[6]

2000 NIH Policy Statement

This statement discusses data monitoring requirements in Phase I and Phase II trials.

For Phase I and Phase II clinical trials, investigators must submit a general description of the data and safety monitoring plan as part of the research application. A detailed monitoring plan . . . must be included as part of the protocol and submitted to the local IRB and reviewed and approved by the funding Institute and Center (IC) before the trial begins. We strongly encourage the IRB to review the plan. Each IC should have a system for appropriate oversight and monitoring of the conduct of clinical trials to ensure the safety of participants and validity and integrity of the data. IC oversight of the monitoring activities is distinct from the monitoring itself. . . . ICs have the flexibility to determine the reporting requirements of adverse events.[7]

2000 OPRR Clarification Letter

OPRR guidance in the form of a letter dated May 22, 2000, indicated the following:

. . . continuing review of research by the IRB should include consideration of adverse events, interim findings, and any recent literature that may be relevant to the research. OPRR recognizes that such information may not be readily available to local investigators participating in multicenter clinical trials or their local IRBs. However, OPRR (now OHRP) notes that such trials are often subject to oversight by a Data Safety and Monitoring Board (DSMB) . . . operating in accordance with the National Cancer Institute (NCI) policy. . . . In such circumstances, IRBs conducting continuing review of research may rely on a current statement from the DSMB indicating that it has reviewed study-wide adverse events, interim findings, and any recent literature that may be relevant to the research, in lieu of requiring that this information be submitted directly to the IRB.[8]

Three Basic Options for Data Monitoring

As previously explained, federal regulations require that the IRB determine that "the research plan makes adequate provisions for monitoring the data collected to ensure the safety of subjects."[1[Sec.111(a)(6)]] When evaluating provisions for data monitoring, the first thing that the IRB should do is to determine whether the formal process of data and safety monitoring will be performed by an individual investigator, an internal monitoring group employed by the study sponsor, or an independent DSMB.

An Individual Investigator

When the study population is small and the range of study events that could have an important impact on the risks and benefits of research participation is narrow, it may be appropriate for the principal investigator to manage the data and safety monitoring. As stated in the 1998 NIH policy statement, "Every clinical trial should have provision for data and safety monitoring. A variety of types of monitoring may be anticipated depending on the nature, size, and complexity of the clinical trial. In many cases, the principal investigator would be expected to perform the monitoring function."[6] Subsequent guidance from the NIH discusses data monitoring by an individual investigator based on study design and risk level: "For many Phase I and Phase II trials, independent DSMBs may not be necessary or appropriate when the intervention is low risk. Continuous, close monitoring by the study investigator may be an adequate and appropriate format for monitoring, with prompt reporting of toxicity to the IRB, FDA, and/or NIH. In studies of small numbers of subjects, toxicity may more readily become apparent through close monitoring of individual patients, while in larger studies risk may better be assessed through statistical comparisons of treatment groups."[7]

A Group Representing the Study Sponsor

There is no formal term for this class of programs for data and safety monitoring. Some discussions simply refer to a "data-monitoring committee." The reason to define this general category is that with industry-sponsored research, the research plan may explain that data and safety monitoring will be performed "by the sponsor." What this usually means is that employees of the organization that is funding or directing the study will be responsible for analyzing study information to evaluate data integrity and the risk/benefit profile of research participation for current and future subjects. There are no federal standards that describe the composition of, or procedures for, monitoring groups other than DSMBs (discussed later here). Conflict of interest is an important consideration when employees of the study sponsor have the primary responsibility for monitoring data from the standpoint of scientific integrity and participant safety.

Federal guidance statements do not directly explain when it is or is not acceptable for data monitoring to be done by the study sponsor. Guidance documents exist that explain the general conditions under which it is acceptable for an individual investigator to monitor study data and others that suggest criteria for requiring an independent DSMB. However, there is no federal guidance that provides definitive advice for the IRB when data and safety monitoring is too complex for a single investigator but may not meet the criteria that demand an independent DSMB. This middle ground is a confusing area for the IRB because it describes many industry-sponsored multicenter trials.

In the absence of published guidance, it is appropriate to consider oral recommendations that have been made in national forums. For example, at the October 30, 2000, meeting sponsored by the Public Responsibility in Medicine and Research (San Diego, CA), FDA representative Susan Ellenberg, MD, directed a workshop on data monitoring in clinical research. In this forum, Dr. Ellenberg explained that the types of sponsor-controlled monitoring systems that are routinely used in industry-sponsored multicenter trials are appropriate for studies in which death or severe disability is not a major risk of research participation. Dr. Ellenberg also explained that requiring independent DSMBs for such studies would have a negative impact on the progress of research in this country. She urged the IRB community to approve low- and moderate-risk research based on a plan whereby the study sponsor is responsible for data and safety monitoring. The 1998 NIH policy statement supports this message: "All clinical trials require monitoring. Monitoring should be commensurate with risks. Monitoring may be conducted in various ways or by various individuals or groups. These exist on a continuum from monitoring by the principal investigator . . . to the establishment of an independent data and safety monitoring board for a large Phase III clinical trial."[6]

A DSMB

In a discussion of clinical trial monitoring, the terms *DSMB* and *independent DSMB* are used interchangeably. A DSMB is a committee that is established specifically to monitor data throughout the life of a study to determine whether it is appropriate, from both scientific and ethical standpoints, to continue the study as planned. In 1999, the National Cancer Institute established formal standards for DSMB composition and procedures.[9] Other federal agencies have referred to these standards when discussing criteria for IRB approval of research.

Basically, a DSMB is made up of an eclectic group of experts in the fields of medicine and science that are applicable to the study, individuals with statistical expertise, lay representatives, often administrators, and people from other backgrounds that are likely to help the committee make an unbiased assessment of study progress. In most cases, the DSMB is funded by the study sponsor, but the funding is independent of committee determinations, and DSMB members are not permitted to have affiliations or interests that could be affected by study outcome. DSMBs usually meet several times a year, but the frequency of discussion depends on the nature of the study. It is both complex and expensive to use a DSMB to monitor a study; therefore, a DSMB should only be required when it is unreasonable to consider other options.

Guidance Documents

Three federal guidance documents and one panel statement describe situations when data should be monitored by a DSMB. The statements differ in their recommendations. Several statements suggest that study design (Phase III versus I or II) is the critical factor for requiring a DSMB. Other statements suggest that risk level and the number of study sites should determine the need for a DSMB, independent of study design. The latest NIH statement introduces additional factors such as blinding and the vulnerability of the study population.

The Duke Working Group
"In definitive Phase III trials, we recommend that the sponsor allocate responsibility for safety evaluation to an independent data monitoring committee to minimize conflicts of interest among those making the necessary judgments during the trial."[5]

1998 NIH Policy Statement
"The establishment of data safety monitoring boards (DSMBs) is required for multisite clinical trials involving interventions that entail potential risk to the participants."[6] However, a later statement in this document suggests that DSMBs should be required in all Phase III trials, regardless of risk: "In 1994 the Committee on Clinical Trial Monitoring [presented] a strong recommendation that all [Phase III] clinical trials, even those that pose little likelihood of harm, should consider an external monitoring body. This policy affirms the Committee's recommendations concerning DSMBs."[6]

1999 NCI Policy Statement
"Phase I and Phase II studies may be monitored by the principal investigator/project manager, by NCI program staff or designee, or jointly. . . . All phase III randomized clinical trials supported by NCI require monitoring by a DSMB."[9]

2000 NIH Policy Statement
"The NIH already requires data and safety monitoring, generally in the form of DSMBs for Phase III clinical trials. For earlier trials (Phases I and II), a DSMB may be

appropriate if the studies have multiple clinical sites, are blinded (masked), or employ particularly high-risk interventions or vulnerable populations."[7]

Communication Between the IRB and DSMBs

At the time of initial protocol review, the IRB should evaluate not only the provisions for data and safety monitoring, but also the plan to communicate the findings of the monitoring activity to the IRB. Several reports from the Office of the Inspector General have explained that a major problem with current monitoring programs is that IRB review of the activities of DSMBs and other monitoring groups is neither timely nor substantive.[10] Many IRBs are unable to get access to DSMB or sponsor-run monitoring committee reports even when they formally request them.

Federal Policy Statements
To respond to this problem, several federal agencies have released policy statements that address the issue of IRB access to information about data and safety monitoring activities. These statements are presented later here. The bottom line is that the 1999 NIH policy statement makes it clear that the IRB is expected to review a detailed plan for data and safety monitoring at the time of initial protocol review and to review interim reports from the DSMB during continuing review. The main focus of these statements is to require the study directors to make DSMB summary reports related to toxicity available to the IRB.

It is also important to note that these policy documents show that federal authorities expect the line of communication to be between the IRB and local investigators. It appears that the IRB is not supposed to speak directly to study directors or to the DSMB. This is spelled out most clearly by NCI policy in which the DSMB is instructed to send reports to the study leadership, who are in turn instructed to forward it to local investigators, who are then supposed to share it with the IRB. The DSMB does not release outcome data before the general dissemination of final recommendations except under specific conditions, none of which involve the IRB. None of the statements specify how long an IRB should expect to wait to receive a DSMB report after a DSMB meeting.

1999 NIH Policy Statement
Effective July 1, 1999, all multisite trials with DSMBs are expected to forward summary reports of adverse events to each IRB involved in the study. . . . After a DSMB is established, each IRB should be informed of the operating procedures with regard to data and safety monitoring (e.g., who, what, when, where, and how monitoring will take place). If the IRB is not satisfied with the monitoring procedures, it should request modifications. . . . The DSMB's summary report should provide feedback at regular and defined intervals to the IRBs. The institutes and centers should assure that there is a mechanism in place to distribute the report to all participating investigators for submission to their local IRB. For example, after each meeting of the DSMB, the executive secretary should send a brief summary report to each investigator. The report should . . . summarize the board's review of the cumulative toxicities reported from all participating sites without specific disclosure by treatment arm. It should also inform investigators of the board's conclusion with respect to progress or need for modifications of the protocol. The investigator is required to transmit the report to the local IRB.[9]

1999 NCI Policy Statement: Responsibilities of the DSMB
After each DSMB meeting, provide the study leadership with written information concerning findings for the trial as a whole related to cumulative toxicities observed and any relevant recommendations related to continuing, changing, or terminating the trial. The study leadership will provide information on cumulative toxicities and relevant recommendations to the local principal investigators to be shared with their IRBs. . . . In general, outcome data should not be made available to individuals outside the DSMB until accrual has been completed and all patients have completed their treatment. At this time, the DSMB may approve the release of outcome data on a confidential basis to the trial principal investigator for planning the preparation of manuscripts or to a small number of other investigators for purposes of planning future trials.[11]

Stopping Rules

This chapter began by reviewing federal regulations at §46.111(a)(6) that require the IRB to determine that "the research plan makes adequate provision for monitoring the data collected to ensure the safety of subjects." The first step in responding to this directive is to decide who—meaning what individual or group—should take primary responsibility for analyzing individual events to determine whether the study should be modified to minimize risk to current or future research subjects. The basic options of an individual investigator, a group representing the study sponsor, or an independent DSMB are discussed previously here along with published guidance on standards the IRB should consider when making this decision. A level of detail that is not addressed in any of the regulations or guidance documents pertaining to this subject is the question of stopping rules. *Stopping rules* is the general term for specific and predetermined parameters that guide the data monitoring process. These parameters specify when and how research is revised, including the criteria for terminating the study, in response to interim data analysis. Some people may prefer to call these guidelines "revision rules." However, to simplify this discussion, the term *stopping rules* will be used to refer to any guideline that is established for the specific purpose of forcing a revision of the study protocol based on review of events that occur during the conduct of the study. Stopping rules are presented in a variety of ways depending on the nature of the study. Stopping rules should be specific about the endpoints that will be used and the decisions that will be made. The following example is instructive.

Example

A multicenter, industry-sponsored, single-arm Phase II study of an investigational antifungal agent in patients with serious fungal infections that are refractory to first line standard therapy is proposed. The IRB application explains that the sponsor will perform the data and safety monitoring. The data-monitoring section of the protocol contains a detailed list of stopping rules based on statistical evaluation of aggregate data: "This multicenter trial will be monitored after every 12th patient, with a recommendation for termination if the accumulating data provide evidence that the conventional response rate does not exceed the 17% rate observed in historical experience by at least 13%, that is, an increase to a 30% conventional response rate. A Bayesian monitoring scheme will be used, comparing data to the prior response experience of 192 patients treated on a variety of protocols at MDACC. The trial will be recommended for termination if the probability is less than 5% that the new target response level of 30% is achieved, based on data accumulated after every 12th patient."

The reason to discuss stopping rules in this chapter is that these guidelines establish the critical parameters of the data-monitoring process. Every study that involves significant risk to the participants should include a clear description of the endpoints that are going to be evaluated as part of the data-monitoring process and the decisions that are going to be made if these endpoints are reached. Stopping rules are a fundamental part of the research methods. These guidelines should be presented as part of the research plan at the time of initial protocol review.

When the protocol application describes stopping rules, then, clearly, IRB approval of the study requires that the IRB approve these guidelines. However, many study applications do not describe stopping rules, or at least do not describe them in much detail. In this situation, the IRB must operate without guidance from federal authorities. Is it acceptable for the IRB to approve a study application that explains that data will be monitored by an investigator, the sponsor, or a DSMB, but does not describe the stopping rules that will guide protocol revision? In my opinion, the answer is no. Stopping rules are an essential feature of ethical research. A study plan that does not describe guidelines that are appropriate in detail and content does not give the IRB the information it needs to conclude that the research plan makes "adequate provision for monitoring the data collected to ensure the safety of subjects" as required by federal regulations. IRB policy should require a careful review and approval of stopping rules at the time of initial protocol review.

Conclusion

1. The research plan should provide for data and safety monitoring. The IRB should understand that federal regulations require that the IRB determine that the research plan makes provisions for data and safety monitoring that are sufficient to protect the rights and welfare of research participants.
2. The IRB should not be the primary mechanism for data and safety monitoring. The IRB should interpret federal research regulations to mean that the IRB is required to

determine that an appropriate monitoring mechanism is in place before starting the study, but the IRB need not be that mechanism.

3. The IRB should not attempt to function as a data monitoring committee. When a study involves a large number of subjects and multiple study sites, the IRB will not be capable of performing the type of data comparisons and analyses that are required to make the data-monitoring process meaningful from the standpoint of protecting research subjects.

4. The research plan should describe the basic parameters of the data-monitoring process. All IRB applications should include a section that describes a plan for data and safety monitoring. The information in this section should permit the IRB to determine that the plan is adequate to protect research participants.

   a. The IRB should be told whether the plan is to assign the responsibility for data and safety monitoring to an individual investigator, the sponsor, or a DSMB.

   b. If the study sponsor will be responsible for data and safety monitoring, the IRB application should explain the number of people who will be responsible for this task and their qualifications to function in this capacity.

   c. The IRB application should describe the planned frequency of data analysis. Will data be analyzed on a per time basis (e.g., every 6 months), on a per-subject basis (e.g., after every 10 subjects), or in response to specific events (e.g., after any fatality)?

   d. The IRB should require a description of stopping rules regarding the potential outcomes of the study that are likely to have a major impact on the rights or welfare of research participants.

5. The IRB should establish criteria for requiring a DSMB. The IRB should understand that federal guidance statements do not establish unambiguous criteria that the IRB can use to determine when an independent DSMB should be a requirement for approval of research. The following guidelines may be useful when evaluating a plan for data and safety monitoring.

   a. Do not require a DSMB if it is reasonable to accept an alternative option. An independent DSMB is complicated and expensive to assemble. The IRB should require a DSMB only in those situations where there is no other reasonable alternative.

   b. First, decide whether data monitoring requires sophisticated capabilities. The first thing to decide is whether a committee with the resources to perform sophisticated statistical comparisons or aggregate data analyses is required to make data monitoring meaningful from the standpoint of protecting research participants. If this is the case, then it is not acceptable for data monitoring to be done by an individual investigator, and it is unlikely that it would be acceptable to approve a plan where data monitoring would be done by a small group of employees of the sponsor. When data monitoring requires sophisticated capabilities, then the IRB should require an independent DSMB or an appropriately constructed data-monitoring committee that is employed by the study sponsor. The IRB should understand that commercial sponsors have a long track record of administering complex data-monitoring programs with good results in terms of the protection of research participants.

   c. Decide whether conflict of interest is likely to bias the data-monitoring process. Conflict of interest is discussed in other chapters in this book. There are no absolute guidelines for making this determination. The NIH, NCI, and Duke Working Group statements presented previously all require DSMBs for Phase III trials. IRBs should follow this recommendation with the understanding that a Phase III trial refers to a large multicenter trial that is being done to make a definitive determination about the efficacy of a study agent, usually to support an application for FDA approval. There are prospective, randomized trials that do not present the same issues regarding potential bias and conflict of interest. These trials would not be considered Phase III by FDA criteria and may not require DSMBs.

   With single-arm studies (including FDA categories Phase I and II), the IRB must evaluate the potential for bias on a case-by-case basis. It is appropriate for an individual investigator or the study sponsor to monitor data in many of the trials in this category. The most recent NIH policy statement implies that multiple clinical sites, blinding, high-risk interventions, or vulnerable populations should be considered as absolute indicators for the need for data monitoring by an independent DSMB. The IRB should consider these factors carefully when evaluating the potential for bias that might result from a sponsor-directed monitoring system.

References

1. Code of Federal Regulations. Title 45A—Department of Health and Human Services; Part 46—Protection of Human Subjects. Updated 1 October, 1997. Access date 18 April, 2001. http://www4.law.cornell.edu/cfr/45p46.htm

2. Code of Federal Regulations. Title 21, Chapter 1—Food and Drug Administration. Part 56—Institutional Review Boards. Updated 1 April, 1999. Access date 27 March, 2001. http://www4.law.cornell.edu/cfr/21p56.htm

3. Penslar RL, Porter JP, Office for Human Research Protections. *Institutional Review Board Guidebook.* Updated 6 February, 2001. Access date 29 March, 2001. http://ohrp.osophs.dhhs.gov/irb/irb_guidebook.htm

4. Bankert E, Amdur RJ. The IRB is not a data and safety monitoring committee. *IRB: A Review of Human Subjects Research* 22(6):9–10, 2000.

5. Morse MA, Califf RM, Sugarman J. Monitoring and ensuring safety during clinical research. *JAMA* 285(9):1201–1205, 2001.

6. National Institutes of Health. NIH Policy for Data and Safety Monitoring. Updated 10 June, 1998. Access date 29 March, 2001. http://www.nih.gov/grants/guide/notice-files/not98-084.html

7. National Institutes of Health. Further Guidance on a Data and Safety Monitoring for Phase I and Phase II Trials. Updated 5 June, 2000. Access date 29 March, 2001. http://grants.nih.gov/grants/guide/notice-files/NOT-OD-00-038.html

8. Director Division of Human Subjects Protection, DHHS. Continuing Review of DSMB-Monitored Clinical Trials. Updated 22 May, 2000. Access date 18 April, 2001. http://ohrp.osophs.dhhs.gov/humansubjects/guidance/dsmb.htm

9. National Institutes of Health. Guidance on Reporting Adverse Events to Institutional Review Boards for NIH-Supported Multicenter Clinical Trials (from NIH Guide for June 11, 1999). Access date 29 March, 2001. http://grants.nih.gov/grants/guide/notice-files/not99-107.html

10. Office of Inspector General D. Protecting Human Research Subjects: Status of Recommendations (OEI-01-97-00197). Department of Health and Human Services. April 2000. Access date 9 April, 2001. http://oig.hhs.gov/oei/reports/ a447.pdf

11. National Cancer Institute. Policy of the National Cancer Institute for Data and Safety Monitoring of Clinical Trials, 22 June, 1999. Access date 9 April, 2001. http://deainfo/ nci/nih.gov/grantspolicies/datasafety.htm

Conflict of Interest: Researchers

Daniel K. Nelson

If you have no conflict of interest, then you would stand out like a sore thumb.
—Clinical trials investigator, 1999

INTRODUCTION

Conflicts of interest are inherent to the conduct of research. This was recognized in 1978 by the National Commission for the Protection of Human Subjects of Biomedical and Behavioral Research, which wrote that "investigators are always in positions of potential conflict by virtue of their concern with the pursuit of knowledge as well as the welfare of the human subjects of their research."[1] The Commission echoed earlier reports by the National Institutes of Health (NIH) and the Surgeon General in viewing investigators as poorly positioned to reconcile these competing interests on their own and in calling for a shared responsibility that incorporated independent review (e.g., the institutional review board [IRB]). The National Bioethics Advisory Commission reiterated this fundamental observation over 20 years later, noting that research "necessarily creates a conflict of interest for investigators" through their use of fellow humans to obtain knowledge.[2] Neither commission held these conflicts to be irreconcilable, nor did they link conflict of interest to character flaws of investigators as individuals or as a class.

Notwithstanding this prior recognition, several factors have converged to propel conflict of interest to the forefront as one of the major concerns facing IRBs and the research community. These factors include increased funding of research, increased competition, greater involvement of commercial interests, larger payoffs for successful outcomes, more direct participation of investigators and institutions in those rewards, and a shift in the settings where research is performed. Against that background, several recent events have lent credence to the growing sense of concern. The tragic death of Jesse Gelsinger in a gene transfer study in 1999 prompted a reexamination of many aspects of human subjects research, but perhaps no single aspect more than conflict of interest.[3-7] The goals of this chapter are to define conflict of interest and provide examples, to describe how the research environment has evolved in ways that increase the opportunity for conflicts, to review existing regulations, and to discuss management strategies.

Definitions

Before considering conflicts of interest as they relate to research involving human subjects, it is important to establish a working definition. Explaining what we mean by conflict of interest is not straightforward, partly because the topic is emotionally charged and frequently misunderstood.[8,9] The problem that we are trying to avoid is bias in judgment. We are looking for a term to describe situations where the potential for bias is such that decisions may be called into question. This is of particular concern in relationship to professional roles or obligations, especially those that come with positions of trust.

One of the most misunderstood aspects of conflict of interest is that the problem may exist in the absence of documented bias or improper decisions. Saying that a conflict of interest exists does not mean that somebody made the wrong decision. It means that people who evaluate the situation may reasonably conclude that the potential for bias is such that improper decisions are possible. Thus, it is the people who evaluate the decision who determine whether a conflict of interest exists, not the person making the decisions. As Friedman explains, "A conflict exists whether or not decisions are affected by the personal interest; a conflict of interest implies only the potential for bias or wrongdoing, not a certainty or likelihood."[9]

With regard to financial relationships, Angell[5] has defined conflict of interest as "any financial association that would cause an investigator to prefer one outcome . . . to another." Both Angell and Friedman argued that terms like "potential" conflict of interest are misleading and misused because conflict is a function of the situation and not of the investigator's response to that situation.[5,9] The opportunity need not be acted on to represent a conflict of interest and a situation worthy of concern.

For the purposes of this chapter, a conflict of interest can be defined[5,8–12] as a *set of conditions in which an investigator's judgment concerning a primary interest (e.g., subject welfare, integrity of research) could be biased by a secondary interest (e.g., personal or financial gain).*

Sources of Conflict of Interest in Research

Although the following discussion largely focuses on financial incentives, it is important to recognize that there are many rewards associated with research that are not directly linked to money.[5,6,13–15] Admirably, many investigators are driven by pursuit of knowledge in its purest sense. The altruistic desires to advance scientific frontiers, contribute to society, alleviate suffering, and improve lives are powerful motivators, as are more personal goals that become important to many investigators, including respect of peers, appointments, promotions, tenure, grants, fame, prizes, and the publications that support all of these. Some have argued that these academic pressures present greater conflicts than the prospect for material gain. Anyone who has observed the battles that can be waged over authorship or tenure may be hard pressed to disagree. However, these academic incentives are embedded within the fabric of research. They are widely recognized and broadly shared and, therefore, tend to be viewed with less concern.

Most recently, attention has been focused on financial conflict of interest in clinical research, where both the risks and the rewards are potentially the greatest. Examples of such interests include equity holdings in commercial sponsors, consulting fees, royalties, patent rights, and honoraria for serving on advisory boards or for giving lectures. Any of these may be problematic if linked to the sponsor of research or the product under study. Also of concern are scenarios in which faculty may assign students or trainees to work on projects from which the investigator stands to benefit. Even the negotiated budgets to compensate investigators and institutions for conducting research may represent sizable conflicts of interest, depending on how they are structured and how the resulting revenues are handled.[16–19]

There is ample evidence that health care providers preferentially refer patients to facilities in which they hold

a personal financial stake.[5,8] Given incentive, investigators might similarly be inclined to enroll as many subjects as possible, push the limits on entry criteria, promote research participation when other alternatives might be preferable, or report positive findings when results are equivocal. At a minimum, even the appearance of conflict calls into question the judgment of the investigator and the integrity of the process. This is no small matter if it jeopardizes the trust and confidence of the public. At its worst, conflict of interest may endanger lives—not only those of the immediate subjects under study, but those of future patients treated on the basis of biased results.[5,16,20] To understand why conditions today create increased opportunities for conflict requires an understanding of how clinical research has evolved.

Evolution of the Clinical Research Enterprise

The modern investigator must be just as good a business person as a scientist.
—Inaugural issue of *Clinical Researcher,* 2001

Once upon a time, most biomedical research was funded by the government and conducted in academic centers. The rewards were primarily related to advancement of knowledge. To be sure, advancement of careers and reputations was also a motivator, albeit of a different nature than the current focus on advancement of wealth. Clinical studies tended to be small in scale, observational, investigator initiated, and relatively inexpensive.[8]

This began to change in the decades after World War II as both federal and industrial funding of research increased. The nature of clinical research also evolved, with large-scale, multicenter, randomized trials providing the safety and efficacy testing that society demanded before new products were brought to market.

This growth has continued to the present, with investments in research and development by pharmaceutical companies increasing from $2 to $30 billion over the past 20 years (see "Industry Serves Through Innovation" in the Annual Report 2001–2002 of the Pharmaceutical Research and Manufacturers of America at http://www.pharma.org /publications/publications/annual2001). The return on this investment is also considerable, with many drugs now exceeding $1 billion per year in sales. Total spending on clinical trials by government and industry reached $4.5 billion in 2000 in the United States alone, and rapid expansion is now occurring in the international arena. Of this amount, only 20% is now funded by the government, with 80% coming from industry.[21]

In the 1990s, managed care influenced the clinical trial environment at several levels. At the corporate level, the economics of drug development changed such that companies could no longer increase their prices, as they had previously, to recoup costs and generate profits. This brought pressure to cut costs, move more drugs through the pipeline, and reduce time to market in order to beat competitors and maximize their time under patent protections. These pressures forced sponsors to reevaluate every aspect of drug development, including the sites they used to conduct their clinical trials. Academic medical centers were traditionally a locale of choice for conducting clinical trials, owing to their expertise, prestige, and access to large numbers of patients. As pressures mounted, however, sponsors came to view academic centers as "slow, inefficient, expensive, not always top quality, and sometimes exasperating to work with."[22]

Although IRBs are often identified as a bottleneck in this process, other institution-based entities (e.g., contracts and grants, sponsored programs, other peer-review committees) contributed to this perception of a clogged bureaucracy. Faced with a competitive, market-driven environment, sponsors were free to take their business where they pleased, and they did this by actively avoiding academic centers when selecting sites to conduct their trials. Filling the niche were independent sites, private-practice or hospital-based physicians not affiliated with academic centers, perhaps gathered into networks by site management organizations. Contract research organizations (CROs) became a major force, allowing companies to outsource much of the work of managing their trials.[20,22]

As managed care exerted pressures on industry, it also created difficulties and opportunities for physicians at an individual level.[4,13,16,17,22,23] The difficulties came in the form of declining reimbursements by third-party payers as the costs of delivering care and maintaining practices continued to rise. However, as managed care closed the door on fee-for-service reimbursement on the clinical side, many saw the opportunity to replace lost revenues by conducting industry-sponsored research studies. Clinical trials are now reimbursed on what amounts to a fee-for-service basis, presenting lucrative alternatives for physicians who were frustrated with Health Maintenance Organizations (HMOs) and capitated payments. Although some physicians incorporated research as a supplement to clinical practice, others effectively transferred their focus to conducting clinical trials. Thus was born a new player in this enterprise: the independent, for-profit investigative site.

With physicians based outside of academic centers looking to increase their involvement, sponsors were happy to engage this emerging workforce, which came unencumbered with the unwieldy bureaucracies of more traditional sites. As the number of sites conducting studies tripled during the mid-1990s, most of that growth occurred in office-based settings. The number of private-practice physicians involved in drug studies increased by 60% over a 5-year span. Conversely, the proportion of trials conducted in academic medical centers dropped from 80% to 40% over the same period of time, during which the industry as a whole was enjoying steady growth. From a business perspective, academic centers lost market share.[12,16,22–25]

This migration of clinical trials away from academic medical centers has not gone unnoticed by those centers, which are facing many of the same financial pressures as community-based practices. A growing number have established clinical trials offices to centralize administrative processes, streamline IRB submissions and contract negotiations, and facilitate interactions with industrial sponsors.[22,23] Fewer than 10% of academic centers had such centralized structures as recently as 1997. Within 3 years, that number had increased to over 50% as academic sites regrouped to make themselves more competitive in the modern environment.[21] Some are also forming networks with community-based practices to provide broader access to potential subjects. This effort is having the desired effect, and industry has begun to return to this traditional base. Academic centers are again reporting increases in revenue from industry grants.[21]

As a backdrop to the economic pressures driving change at corporate, individual, and institutional levels, a change in federal law signaled a shift in the government's approach to the proceeds of research. In 1980, Congress passed the Bayh-Dole Act, which provided universities with incentives to move research results into commercial applications. Before Bayh-Dole, the government retained the intellectual property rights to technology developed through federal support. It was observed, however, that only a tiny fraction of publicly funded technology ever made it to the marketplace. The 1980 legislation encouraged academic institutions to patent new products, to license these products to industry, and to share resulting royalties with their faculty. This technology transfer paved the way for productive joint ventures between the nonprofit and for-profit sectors. It also, however, paralleled the evolution described previously in creating new and unanticipated opportunities for conflict of interest.[4,10,26,27]

The preceding discussion is neither to defend nor criticize the various players in this enterprise but to describe its evolution and current state for readers expected to oversee research conduct. That growth and restructuring are occurring and driven by real-world market forces is undeniable. Whether it can occur in a way that optimizes the safety and well-being of subjects is the question, and it represents a challenge for all involved.

Regulations and Guidance

Reflecting the increased attention to conflict of interest, the October 2000 revision of the Declaration of Helsinki contains guidance for physician–investigators and IRBs in this area.[28] Researchers are instructed to disclose "any possible conflicts of interest" (including sources of funding) to independent ethical review committees, to subjects, and in publications resulting from the research. There is no guidance as to what constitutes an inappropriate interest from the standpoint of IRB review.

With regard to U.S. federal regulations directed at IRBs, specific guidance is limited to removing members from review of projects in which they have a conflicting interest (e.g., as an investigator). Beyond that, there is little to guide IRBs in considering investigator conflict of interest. Conflict of interest for IRBs and their members is discussed in Chapter 5-12. The requirements for informed consent[29(Sec.116),30(Sec.20)] instruct that: "An investigator shall seek consent only under circumstances that . . . minimize the possibility of coercion or undue influence." One potential source for coercion to enroll is investigators themselves, if they hold a significant conflict of interest in relation to a given study.[13] Similarly, IRBs must determine that risks are minimized, reasonable in relationship to benefits and disclosed to subjects. Conflict of interest can be viewed as one such risk.[29(Sec.111),31(Sec.111)] Although federal regulations empower IRBs to act at their discretion, these readings require broad interpretations, and specific guidance is only recently forthcoming.[6,32]

Within the last decade, regulations have begun to address investigator conflicts of interest. In July 1995, the Public Health Service (which includes NIH) and the National Science Foundation issued guidelines that required disclosure and peer review of any "significant financial interests" held by investigators applying for federal funds.[3,4,33] The NIH had first proposed guidelines in 1989 suggesting that conflicts should be prohibited, but these were viewed as overly restrictive by the research community and were withdrawn. The final rule[34(Sec.604)] gave research institutions discretion in how they would manage conflicts at the local level, and they are not required to report details to the government. The threshold for disclosure is $10,000 in income, $10,000 in equity, or 5% ownership in a company, if these might be affected by the investigator's research. Institutions receiving federal funds were charged with establishing and enforcing policies to "manage, reduce, or eliminate" the conflict of interest, once disclosed. With much discretion given to institutions, it is not surprising that considerable variability exists in implementation of these policies.[10,35,36]

In February 1998, the Food and Drug Administration (FDA) issued a final rule[37] that required sponsors to certify the absence of financial interests of investigators who conducted their studies, or to disclose those interests. Such interests include patents, equity, or payments of $25,000 or more to support investigator activities outside of conducting the clinical study (e.g., equipment, honoraria, or consulting fees). This disclosure is tied to the submission of a marketing application to the FDA, and the intent is to protect the integrity of supporting data.

Beyond federal regulations, an increasing number of professional organizations have begun to establish policies to guide their members. For example, the American Society of Gene Therapy recommended that "investigators and team members directly responsible for patient selection, the informed consent process and/or clinical management in a trial must not have equity, stock options or comparable arrangements in companies sponsoring the trial."[38] Although this policy was prompted by problems in gene transfer trials, conflicts of interest are by no means limited to this small field, and it is hoped that other professional groups will take equally strong positions.

Managing Conflict of Interest

Publicity is justly commended as a remedy for social and industrial diseases. Sunlight is said to be the best of disinfectants...
—Supreme Court Justice Louis Brandeis, 1914

Disclosure

Disclosure to the Government
Identification of conflicts is an important first step in managing them, and disclosure might occur at one or more levels. As explained, disclosure to the government of investigator conflicts is required by federal agencies (e.g., FDA, Public Health Service, National Science Foundation). In the case of grant awards, institutions are expected to manage the conflicts, and reporting of details to the granting agency is not required. In the case of marketing applications to the FDA, disclosure of investigator interests that might affect the reliability of submissions is made through the sponsor. Disclosure occurs at the time of submission to the FDA, after the study is completed, and does not apply to practices that might affect subjects (e.g., recruitment incentives; see Chapter 5-11). For these reasons, disclosure to the government does not impact the protection of research subjects in a substantive way.

Disclosure to the Institution
Disclosure to the institution is mandatory for those investigators receiving federal funds, with their institutions given discretion in how they manage any conflicts. Predictably, there is considerable variability in how institutions handle this process.[10,35,36] Many, including the author's home institution, have established policies requiring disclosure by all faculty members. However, few institutions have linked this process to protection of human subjects, as suggested by the fact that none of 235 institutions recently surveyed incorporated disclosure to either IRBs or subjects as a management strategy in their conflict of interest policies.[36]

Several universities are currently working to strengthen the link between conflict of interest mechanisms and human subjects protections. A complete review of issues that institutions should address in their policies is outside the scope of this chapter and outside the scope of IRB purview, but several recent reports provide guidance.[2,5,6,10,14,32,35,36,39] With regard to the broader goal of protecting all subjects, however, we must remember that a majority of industry-sponsored studies are now conducted at sites where there may be no institutional policies. That is, there may be no "institution" beyond the investigator or research team and, therefore, no local oversight.

Disclosure to the IRB
Disclosure to the IRB is increasingly advocated as a routine part of protocol review. The Office for Human Research Protections (OHRP) has strongly recommended that financial relationships be described when investigators submit IRB applications and that IRBs should take into consideration the funding arrangements between

sponsor and investigator institution.[32] A survey of 200 IRBs that oversee clinical trials found that only 25% review such financial matters.[39] These arrangements have tended to be regarded by both investigators and IRBs as "none of our business." IRBs should be aware of any interests on the part of investigators that are likely to bias their judgment or actions in areas that affect the rights and welfare of research participants.

Disclosure to Subjects

Disclosure via the informed consent process[12] is at once the most direct and ethically intuitive route of disclosure, but also the most difficult to accomplish in a meaningful way. At the very least, subjects should be aware that the study is sponsored by outside entities, be they commercial or governmental. The consent form might include a lay definition of what this means (e.g., "investigators/institution are compensated for the costs of conducting this research"), as sponsorship may not be understood by the public in terms we take for granted. As to the level of detail provided, I must stop short of advocating that consent forms include dollar amounts from routine study budgets, even when paid on a per capita basis. Although there may be a temptation, in the spirit of full disclosure, to suggest language like "your study doctor will receive $7,800 for enrolling you in this study," this begs additional clarification and may only confuse what is already a complicated process. Placing this statement in perspective demands that subjects also understand that (from this seemingly large amount) X goes to pay for the extra MRI scan done for research purposes only, Y goes to hire the study nurse who is attending to their needs, Z goes to institutional overhead, and so on. Thus, dollar amounts may be misleading because many may represent legitimate expenses.

Subjects should certainly be made aware of any conflicts of interest on the part of investigators or institution that might affect their decision to participate. We should not take it on ourselves to make that decision for them. On the other hand, IRBs should avoid "passing the buck" to subjects who may not be in a position to fully integrate the information provided. An analogy might be drawn to disclosure of physical risks associated with the study. We routinely describe every possible adverse event, even though many are no more likely to occur than the chance that enrollment is swayed by financial incentives. Nevertheless, disclosure does not obviate the need for IRBs to assess risks. If we accept conflict of interest as yet another risk, it is relevant to inform subjects, but disclosure alone is not sufficient.[2,12,26]

Managing Beyond Disclosure

Management strategies should be aimed at removing or minimizing conflict of interest. Some have argued that the only acceptable solution is a complete prohibition of interests that could potentially influence the research in an adverse manner. These observers would ban any institution or investigator from conducting research from which they stood to benefit. Others view that as an unattainable—perhaps even undesirable—goal in the modern environment. They advocate mechanisms to manage the conflict while still permitting what they perceive to be vital relationships to exist. This debate is ongoing[3,5,14,26] and will not be resolved by this chapter. The Department of Health and Human Services (DHHS) has, however, issued guidance that provides useful questions to consider.[32] Although IRBs may not be well situated or equipped to directly oversee this process, they should establish open lines of communication with those institutional bodies that are (e.g., conflict of interest committee). IRBs should then consider the mechanisms proposed to manage the identified conflict, with a particular eye for aspects that could affect research subjects. This could include removing the conflicted investigator from designing the study, obtaining informed consent, performing procedures, monitoring or reporting adverse events, or analyzing data.[12] Readers may surmise that excluding investigators from any or all of these aspects of the study is tantamount to removing them altogether, and that remains an option if the IRB or institution determines that a given conflict is unmanageable.

Simply put, the conflicted person should not be involved in any aspect of the research that could be influenced by that conflict. In some cases, the only way to accomplish that may be for investigators to divest themselves of their conflicting interest or identify someone else to conduct the research. If the latter approach is taken, the IRB should ensure that the substituted investigator is not subordinate to the conflicted investigator or otherwise situated so that this becomes a meaningless exercise, with the "real" investigator still controlling the study. The same rationale may be extended to institutional interests in a given line of research. If institutional holdings (e.g., major ownership in a start-up company) are such that the integrity of the research can be called into question, it may be preferable to perform the study elsewhere.

Given that even the appearance of impropriety is enough to damage individual careers and institutional reputations, it can truly be said that a cautious approach to these issues is in everyone's mutual interest. IRBs may first need to overcome the perception that managing conflict of interest is reliant on their trust of the investigator in question. Management should not hinge on anyone's perception of an individual but on an objective assessment of situations in which people have placed themselves. All parties involved in this process should be clear that managing conflict of interest has everything to do with the situation, and nothing to do with the character or honesty of the individual. Here is another area where proactive education can be helpful by creating a culture of compliance that promotes self-identification and cooperative resolution of conflicts before they become problems.

Much of the foregoing presumes involvement of an institution, with institution-based mechanisms in place. Managing conflicts of interest in the extrainstitutional settings where the majority of clinical trials are now performed presents an even greater challenge for the central IRBs that oversee these sites, for sponsors (who are themselves conflicted, by definition), and for the public at large.

Conclusion

Since the first edition of this book, multiple initiatives are having a substantial impact on our thinking about and management of conflict of interest. Several groups, including the Association of American Universities, the Association of American Medical Colleges, the American Medical Association, the NIH, the National Bioethics Advisory Commission, the OHRP, and Congress have turned their attention to financial interests in research.[12,32,40–45] The recommendations and policies that are coming out of these deliberations are providing guidance more in keeping with the modern research environment.

For example, the Association of American Universities and the Association of American Medical Colleges have recommended[40,41] something approaching a "zero tolerance policy" that would prohibit investigators from conducting human subjects research in which they held financial interests, unless there are compelling circumstances (e.g., the conflicted investigator is the only person capable of conducting that research). Recommendations call for tighter links between conflict of interest management and the IRB review process. The same groups have also considered institutional conflict of interest, recognizing that arrangements and pressures frequently exist at levels beyond the individual so that the institutions in which they work may be equally conflicted. More recently, NIH policies in this area came under scrutiny after reports that top-ranking officials were receiving large sums in consulting fees from industry collaborations, including pharmaceutical and biotechnology companies in position to benefit from NIH decisions and programs.[42–45] The appearance of impropriety led to congressional hearings and, in relatively short order, much tighter restrictions on external arrangements by NIH employees. These many initiatives and reports have yet to translate into requirements that affect the entire research community but provide a clear signal of current thinking.

Whatever form evolving requirements take, they will represent a minimum floor, and IRBs are well advised to establish policies in anticipation. It is difficult to imagine that local efforts could be overprotective of subjects in addressing conflict of interest, whether that protection is grounded in ethics, regulations, or common sense.

References

1. National Commission for the Protection of Human Subjects of Biomedical and Behavioral Research. Report and recommendations: Institutional review boards (DHEW[OS]78-0008). Washington, DC: Department of Health, Education, and Welfare; 1978.

2. National Bioethics Advisory Commission. Ethical and policy issues in research involving human participants. Bethesda, MD: U.S. Government Printing Office, August 2001. Access date 20 March, 2001. http://bioethics.gov/pubs.html

3. Agnew B. Bioethics: Financial conflicts get more scrutiny in clinical trials. *Science* 289(5483):1266–1267, 2000.

4. Andrews LB. Money is putting people at risk in biomedical research. *The Chronicle of Higher Education*, Washington DC, 10 March, 2000, B4–B5.

5. National Institutes of Health. *Conference on Human Subject Protection and Financial Conflicts of Interest*, 15–16 Aug 2000 (transcript).

6. National Institutes of Health. Financial conflicts of interest and research objectivity: Issues for investigators and institutional review boards, June 2000. http://grants.nih.gov/grants/guide/notice-files/NOT-OD-00-040.html

7. Shalala DE. Protecting research subjects—What must be done. *N Engl J Med* 343(11):808–810, 2000.

8. Spece RG Jr, Shimm DS, Buchanan AE. *Conflicts of Interest in Clinical Practice and Research*. New York: Oxford University Press. 1996.

9. Friedman PJ. The troublesome semantics of conflict of interest. *Ethics and Behavior* 2(4):245–251, 1992.

10. Cho MK, Shohara R, Schissel A, Rennie D. Policies on faculty conflicts of interest at US universities. *JAMA* 284(17):2203–2208, 2000.

11. Thompson DF. Understanding financial conflicts of interest. *N Engl J Med* 329(8):573–576, 1993.

12. Morin K, Rakatansky H, Riddick FA, et al. Managing conflicts of interest in the conduct of clinical trials. *JAMA* 287(1):78–84, 2002.

13. DeRenzo EG. Coercion of the recruitment and retention of human research subjects, pharmaceutical industry payments to physician-investigators, and the moral courage of the IRB. *IRB: A Review of Human Subjects Research* 22(2):1–5, 2000.

14. Korn D. Conflicts of interest in biomedical research. *JAMA* 284(17):2234–2237, 2000.

15. Levinsky NG. Nonfinancial conflicts of interest in research. *N Engl J Med* 347(10):759–761, 2002.

16. Eichenwald K, Kolata G. Drug trials hide conflicts for doctors. *The New York Times*, May 16, 1999.

17. Eichenwald K, Kolata G. A doctor's drug studies turn into fraud. *The New York Times*, May 17, 1999.

18. LaPuma J, Kraut J. How much do you get paid if I volunteer? Suggested institutional policy on reward, consent, and research. *Hospital and Health Services Administration* 39(2):193–203, 1994.

19. Shimm DS, Spece RG Jr. Conflict of interest and informed consent in industry-sponsored clinical trials. *J Leg Med* 12(4):477–513, 1991.

20. Bodenheimer T. Uneasy alliance: Clinical investigators and the pharmaceutical industry. *N Engl J Med* 342(20):1539–1544, 2000.

21. CenterWatch Clinical Trials Listing Service. Home Page. Updated 2001. Access date 25 April, 2001. http://www.centerwatch.com/

22. Lightfoot G, Getz KA, Harwood F, Hovde M, Rauscher SM, Reilly P, Vogel JR. Faster Time to Market, 1998. Access date 20 April, 2001. Association of Clinical Research Professionals. http://www.acrpnet.org/whitepaper2/white_paper-home.html

23. Hovde M, Seskin R. Selecting U.S. clinical investigators. *Appl Clin Trials* 8:34–42, 1997.

24. Kowalczyk L. Drug trials branch from teaching hospitals: Suburban doctors answer call to help. *The Boston Globe*, August 16, 2000, C01.

25. Maguire P. Marriage of town and gown brings clinical research to busy practices. *ACP-ASIM Observer* 21(1):1,14–16, 2001.

26. Angell M. Is academic medicine for sale? *N Engl J Med* 342(20):1516–1518, 2000.

27. Boyd EA, Bero LA. Assessing faculty financial relationships with industry: A case study. *JAMA* 284(17):2209–2214, 2000.

28. World Medical Association. Declaration of Helsinki: Ethical Principles for Medical Research Involving Human Subjects. World Medical Association, Inc.: WMA Policy. First adopted in Helsinki, Finland, in 1964. Updated 10 July, 2000. Access date 20 March, 2001. http://www.wma. net/e/policy/17-c_e.html

29. Code of Federal Regulations. Title 45A—Department of Health and Human Services; Part 46—Protection of Human Subjects. Updated 1 October, 1997. Access date 18 April, 2001. http://www4.law.cornell.edu/cfr/45p46.htm

30. Code of Federal Regulations. Title 21, Chapter 1—Food and Drug Administration, DHHS; Part 50—Protection of Human Subjects. Updated 1 April, 1999. Access date 18 April, 2001. http://www4.law.cornell.edu/cfr/21p50.htm

31. Code of Federal Regulations. Title 21, Chapter 1—Food and Drug Administration, DHHS; Part 56—Institutional Review Boards. Updated 1 April, 1999. Access date 27 March, 2001. http://www4.law.cornell.edu/cfr/21p56.htm

32. Department of Health and Human Services. Final Guidance Document: Financial Relationships and interests in research involving human subjects: Guidance for human subject protection, 5 May, 2004. Date of access 31 Jan 2005. http://www.hhs.gov/ohrp/humansubjects/finreltn/fguid.pdf

33. Mervis J. Conflict of interest: Final rules put universities in charge. *Science* 269(5222):294, 1995.

34. Code of Federal Regulations. Title 42, Chapter 1—Public Health Service, DHHS; Part 50—Policies of General Applicability. Updated 2001. http://www4.law.cornell.edu/ cfr/42p50.htm

35. Lo B, Wolf L, Berkeley A. Conflict-of-interest policies for investigators in clinical trials. *N Engl J Med* 343(22): 1616–1620, 2000.

36. McCrary SV, Anderson CB, Jakovljevic J, Khan T, McCullough LB, Wray NP, Brody BA. A national survey of policies on disclosure of conflicts of interest in biomedical research. *N Engl J Med* 343(22):1621–1625, 2000.

37. Code of Federal Regulations. Title 21, Chapter 1—Food and Drug Administration, DHHS; Part 54—Financial Disclosure by Clinical Investigators. Updated 1 April, 1999. Access date 25 April, 2001. http://www4.law.cornell.edu/cfr/21p54.htm

38. American Society of Gene Therapy. Policy on financial conflict of interest in clinical research. Updated 5 April, 2000. Access date 25 April, 2001. http://www.asgt.org/ policy/index.html

39. Office of Inspector General. Recruiting human subjects: Pressures in industry-sponsored clinical research (OEI-01-97-00195), June 2000. Access date 12 April, 2001. http://www.hhs.gov/oig/oei/reports/a459.pdf

40. Association of American Universities. Report on individual and institutional financial conflict of interest. October 2001. www.aau.edu

41. Association of American Medical Colleges. *Protecting subjects, preserving trust, promoting progress: Policy and guidelines for the oversight of individual financial interests in human subjects research.* December 2001. Access date 7 June, 2005. http://www.aamc.org/members/coitf/

42. Steinbrook R. Financial conflicts of interest and the NIH. *N Engl J Med* 350(4):327–330, 2004.

43. Willman D. Stealth merger: Drug companies and government medical research. *The Los Angeles Times,* December 7, 2003.

44. Willman D. NIH to ban deals with drug firms. *The Los Angeles Times,* February 1, 2005.

45. NIH Office of the Director. NIH announces sweeping ethics reform. NIH News. 1 February, 2005. Access date 1 February, 2005. http://www.nih.gov/news

Conflict of Interest: Recruitment Incentives

Daniel K. Nelson

> *When there is a possibility that you are going to get a car, you're going to do whatever you can.*
> —A study coordinator who was offered a Honda Accord as an enrollment bonus

INTRODUCTION

This chapter focuses on the various incentives that are offered to promote enrollment of subjects in research. These include payments and other inducements to investigators, research staff, or referring physicians, but do not include payments to subjects themselves. Recruitment incentives may come in several forms, including enrollment bonuses, referral or finder's fees, and nonmonetary "perks" or rewards. For the purposes of this discussion, the distinguishing feature of these incentives is that they generally occur outside of the negotiated payments that represent compensation for work performed. Although budgeted payments may also represent considerable conflicts of interest, many observers find these additional incentives to be particularly troubling.

As discussed in the preceding chapter, the clinical research environment has changed dramatically, and the resulting competition has placed sponsors under pressure to move new drugs through the development pipeline and get them to market faster than ever before. This pressure has translated into increasingly aggressive practices to recruit subjects into clinical trials. Thus, another distinguishing feature of these incentives is their intended purpose of spurring investigators to enroll as many subjects as possible, as quickly as possible.

Financial Incentives

Enrollment Bonuses

In keeping with the competitive nature of the clinical trials environment, a reward system has developed so that faster-enrolling study sites are rewarded. Conversely, study sites that fall short of projected enrollment targets or proceed more slowly than anticipated are effectively penalized.[1-3] This also explains why investigators are often frustrated with the pace of institutional review board (IRB) review; they may be facing "competitive enrollment," which means that subjects are accepted on a first-come, first-served basis. Sites that are too slow in securing the necessary approvals from the IRB and other institutional entities (legal, sponsored programs, contracts and grants, etc.) may find all available slots filled and the

study completed before they enroll their first subject. After those approvals are obtained and enrollment begins, this time pressure remains as yet another source for conflict of interest in recruiting subjects.

Because sponsors typically reimburse sites on a per-capita basis, this reward system is, in one sense, embedded within the normal contractual process. However, it has now become commonplace that "bonuses" are offered outside of the negotiated budget. For example, investigators or study coordinators may receive a letter from the contract research organization (CRO) managing the study, urging them to find the last few subjects needed to meet the predetermined enrollment goals and offering additional payments for each subject. This typically occurs late in a trial when a deadline is looming and is meant to stimulate what may be flagging interest on the part of study staff to find those last few patients. Depending on the study, these bonuses may range from a few hundred to several thousand dollars per subject. The CRO may itself be eligible for a bonus if enrollment targets are met by sponsor-imposed deadlines; thus, it becomes natural in this market-driven environment for the CRO to provide "trickle-down" incentives to their study sites. These sites are, after all, helping them to achieve their goals. From the CRO and/or sponsor's perspective, this will be money well spent if it helps them retain the millions of dollars that may be lost with a delayed marketing approval.

Although it can be argued that extra costs will be incurred in identifying these last few subjects, the amounts offered often exceed those costs, even if advertising is involved. Moreover, the budget negotiated to cover the actual cost of conducting the research often includes amounts for advertising or recruitment efforts. Thus, enrollment bonuses are typically over and above actual costs and may represent something approaching pure profit for the investigator. Sponsors may also approach study coordinators directly with these offers, recognizing that these staff are often the first points of contact with potential subjects. Whether investigators or study coordinators can accept these bonus payments may depend on institutional policies. Remember, however, that clinical trials are increasingly conducted in more entrepreneurial settings where profit taking may not only be allowed but encouraged. This stands in contrast to more traditional settings in which investigators are more likely to be prohibited from profiting personally.

Implications for IRBs: Enrollment Bonuses

There are few empirical data to document the prevalence of this practice, but what there are suggest that the use of bonuses is on the rise, tracking with the heightened economic pressures surrounding clinical trials. Ironically, there is also some suggestion that these financial incentives may be ineffective in accomplishing their intended purpose.[2,3] Nevertheless, the offering of enrollment bonuses is a feature of many clinical trials, and IRBs should be aware of the practice.

As with any study-related payments to investigator and/or institution, enrollment bonuses represent a source for conflict of interest. However, because the costs of conducting the study have already been covered in the initial budget, it can be argued that enrollment bonuses constitute an even bigger conflict. There is inherent risk that such incentives might lead an investigator or study coordinator to influence inappropriately a potential subject's decision to participate. This might occur through downplaying the risks of a study, overselling the possible benefits, ignoring alternatives that might be available, overlooking medical history that might exclude a patient, or otherwise pushing the limits on entry criteria. The odds that members of the research team would consciously subvert the process in these ways may be quite small, but there is ample opportunity for subconscious influence. Recruitment, screening, and enrollment of subjects in a clinical trial are complex, multistep processes, involving subjective determinations that might be swayed by financial incentives.

At least two factors call into question the ability of IRBs to oversee this aspect of subject recruitment. First, IRBs have not traditionally had access to financial information regarding the studies they review, although this is now changing. Even when they do request budgetary information, IRBs may not be privy to bonuses offered after a trial is approved and running. Second, surveys suggest that the great majority of IRBs are uncertain about their authority to review financial incentives offered to investigators.[3] This may explain why so few IRBs evaluate this aspect of research in any detail.

This author's personal opinion is that IRBs hold regulatory and ethical imperatives to review any aspect of a clinical trial that might influence the enrollment or well-being of subjects and that recruitment incentives are one such aspect. IRBs are encouraged to develop policies that require the disclosure of enrollment bonuses, including those offered as a trial progresses, so that all incentives might be reviewed in the context of subject recruitment. As a general rule, IRBs should not approve a study in which investigators or their staff will receive an enrollment bonus.

Referral Fees

Referral fees, also called "finder's fees" or "bounties," are payments offered to physicians or other primary caregivers for identifying patients who may be eligible study subjects.[3,4] These might be offered at the suggestion of the sponsor or CRO but, unlike enrollment bonuses, would typically be offered indirectly, by or through the principal investigator. Like enrollment bonuses, referral fees are intended to promote identification and recruitment of subjects.

In one scenario, a specialist conducting a trial might send out "Dear Colleague" letters to primary care physicians who are likely to come across patients fitting a certain profile, offering them $100 for every patient referred to the study. In another scenario, residents at a hospital might be offered certificates for textbooks or meals at a fine restaurant for identifying potential subjects. At some level, it might be argued that these amount to token gestures, particularly if the referring party performs any work in screening patients for eligibility criteria. In this case, the referring physician may actually be serving as an extension of the research team, and compensation of some sort may be appropriate. At another level, however, the payment of referral fees interjects an influence that may run counter to the fiduciary obligation of a primary caregiver. That is, the health professional may be motivated by financial interests to refer a patient when such referral might not be of any benefit to the patient. There may, of course, be circumstances when research participation holds the potential for direct medical benefit and represents an option that the primary caregiver cannot offer. This might especially be true for patients with life-threatening illnesses such as cancer or AIDS, when trials are designed with therapeutic intent. These may also, however, be among the studies least likely to offer finder's fees to referring physicians.

The act of referring may also influence the potential subject's decision making if participation in research is perceived to be the recommendation of a trusted caregiver. Thus, referral could effectively translate into diminished autonomy for the patient considering participation. This is not an abstract possibility, given the difficulty many patients (and their caregivers) have in recognizing that research studies are not designed to treat each subject for his or her individual benefit (i.e., the "therapeutic misconception").

Implications for IRBs: Referral Fees
For the reasons discussed previously here, many institutions have taken a stand against the practice of referral fees. For example, this author's home institution established a policy in 1990 that the IRB should "not approve of finder's fees being paid to physicians, nurses, and others who have a treating and/or counseling relationship to the patient being referred for enrollment in a clinical trial." This policy has support from the American Medical Association's Code of Medical Ethics, which states that "a physician may not accept payment of any kind, in any form, from any source, such as a pharmaceutical company . . . for prescribing or referring a patient to said source" and that "offering or accepting payment for referring patients to research studies (finder's fees) is also unethical."[5(Sec.6.02,6.03,8.0315)] Indeed, other authors have equated referral or finder's fees with fee splitting by physicians, which is prohibited in the clinical practice setting. The American College of Physicians has also taken a stand against this practice, holding that "giving finder's fees to individual physicians for referring patients to a research project generates an unethical conflict of interest."[6]

There would not appear to be any federal guidelines that specifically address referral fees, other than what might be extrapolated from requirements that promote a subject's voluntary and informed choice in a setting free from undue influence.[7(Sec.20),8(Sec.116)] The Department of Health and Human Services (DHHS) Office of the Inspector General, in its recent report on recruitment practices, identified referral fees as one of several questionable practices,[3] but this has yet to translate into regulatory requirements. Nevertheless, IRBs may wish to draft local policies and should, at the very least, establish mechanisms to screen for referral fees being offered by or through investigators under their jurisdiction. The acceptability of such offers can then be assessed on a case-by-case basis, with a particular eye toward potentially negative influences on subject recruitment and consent.

Nonmonetary Perquisites or Rewards

A "bonus" of another kind involves nonfinancial incentives given as a study progresses or after its completion. As discussed in the preceding chapter, there are many rewards or outcomes associated with research that are not linked directly to money. Some have argued that concerns for promotions, tenure, publications, and grants provide motives more powerful than cash, but these tend to be linked to research productivity in a more global sense; that is, these rewards accrue to the study as a whole or, more likely, to a collective body of investigator-initiated work. In the present context, let us consider nonmonetary rewards that are linked more directly to the number of subjects enrolled, much like financial recruitment incentives.

Token Gifts
Token gifts might include lunches during sponsor site visits, gift certificates, baseball caps, coffee mugs, sweatshirts, or other articles of clothing. Emblazoned with the sponsor's logo, or perhaps even the study logo if the trial is large enough to warrant its own, these gifts may represent nothing more than token gestures of the sponsor's appreciation for the team's hard work. As such, they are often neither solicited nor offered but simply arrive after the first subject is enrolled, perhaps increasing in value with subsequent subjects. Sponsors doubtless view these as innocuous gifts and/or subliminal reminders to keep the study in mind, and few could argue that a sweatshirt is likely to unduly influence an investigator's behavior.

Poststudy Rewards
Of greater concern are goal-oriented awards intended to stoke competition and interest, again serving much the same purpose as monetary bonuses. One of the most extravagant vacations this author ever took was an all-expenses-paid trip to Cancun as a poststudy reward for having enrolled five subjects in a rather ordinary clinical trial. In return, the sponsor flew three members of our research team and spouses to a luxury resort, where we joined similar groups from other sites that had also hit their enrollment targets. Ostensibly at an "investigator's meeting," we spent 30 minutes reviewing the results of the trial, and 3 days on the beach. Was this enjoyable? Absolutely. Did the prospect of being rewarded in this manner, advertised through periodic newsletters showing our enrollment in relation to other sites, color our judgment in recruiting subjects? I don't think so and certainly hope not. However, we had already been adequately reimbursed for the costs of conducting the study through the negotiated budget, with some profit built in. Given that I was serving as an IRB chair at the time, should I have recognized the conflict of interest and rejected this perk? Perhaps so, but neither I nor my colleagues nor several hundred honorable investigators perceived this as inappropriate. Am I being hypocritical in telling this story now, as an example of conflict of interest? Again, perhaps so. However, I hope it illustrates the insidious nature of this reward system and the very human response we can expect when investigators are offered what might be judged in hindsight to be a conflict. For me, this personal experience confirms yet again the fundamental observation that investigators are not always in a position to assess their own circumstances critically, despite the best of intentions.

Authorships
For some investigators, poststudy rewards may also come in the form of authorship on publications reporting a clinical trial.[1,9,10] In the past, papers were authored by the lead investigators who designed and conducted the study,

analyzed the resulting data, and wrote the manuscript. This remains the case for "homegrown" protocols, but authorship on industry-sponsored research has evolved into yet another recruitment incentive. Manuscripts are increasingly drafted by the sponsor's medical writers, with authorship on the final publication offered to investigators who enrolled the most subjects, or to prominent scientists in the field who may not have been involved in the actual research. Such "gift authorships" lend credibility to the resulting publication and constitute another element in the evolving reward system. These rewards may be especially important to investigators from the academic sector, where publications represent a valuable form of compensation.

Future Participation

One final example in this category of rewards is the cultivation of high-enrolling sites as members of a pool from which the sponsor or CRO will draw in the future. Top-performing sites that meet (or exceed) their enrollment targets in a timely manner take on "most-favored site" status and will be invited to participate in future studies. Conversely, low-enrolling sites will be dropped. Again, this is a very logical approach in a market-driven environment, but the linkage to number of subjects enrolled makes this an indirect form of recruitment incentive.

Implications for IRBs: Nonmonetary Perks or Rewards

Of the types of incentives discussed in this chapter, nonmonetary rewards may be hardest for IRBs to identify or assess. As with monetary bonuses, they may arise as a study progresses or after a study is complete, at which point the IRB may be removed from the process. Even if review is ongoing, disclosure is unlikely. Few institutions and even fewer investigators or sponsors are likely to regard these incentives as legitimate causes for concern. At some level, however, these rewards hold enough intrinsic value (e.g., cars, vacations) that their nonmonetary nature becomes irrelevant. Something valued at several thousand dollars provides incentive as great as an equivalent amount of cash, perhaps greater if the cash is taxed in ways the gift is not. Tied as they are to number of subjects enrolled, these are recruitment incentives in their own right and warrant consideration as conflicts of interest.

Conclusion

Recruitment incentives are a particularly direct expression of the pressures inherent to the current research environment. For all intents and purposes, this phenomenon is limited to the setting of industry-sponsored clinical trials. Whether these incentives come in the form of financial bonuses or referral fees or as nonmonetary rewards that may include trips, gifts, or authorships, they represent sources for conflict of interest. As discussed in Chapter 5-10, such incentives need not impact negatively on subjects to be of legitimate concern. That is, the potential for bias in judgment exists, even if conflicting motivations are not acted on. IRBs should establish mechanisms to monitor recruitment incentives that may be offered in the studies under their purview.

References

1. Eichenwald K, Kolata G. Drug trials hide conflicts for doctors. *The New York Times,* 16 May, 1999.

2. Harper BD. The effectiveness of sponsor/CRO-site performance incentives. *The Monitor (Association of Clinical Research Professionals)*:9–18, 1997.

3. Office of Inspector General. Recruiting human subjects: Pressures in industry-sponsored clinical research (OEI-01-97-00195). Department of Health and Human Services, June 2000. Access date 12 April, 2001. http://www.hhs.gov/oig/oei/reports/a459.pdf

4. Lind SE. Financial issues and incentives related to clinical research and innovative therapies. In: Vanderpool H (ed.). *The Ethics of Research Involving Human Subjects.* Frederick, MD: University Publishing Group; 1996:185–202.

5. American Medical Association. American Medical Association's Code of Ethics. Access date 31 January, 2005. http://www.ama-assn.org/ama/pub/category/8288.html

6. American College of Physicians. *American College of Physicians Ethics Manual,* 4th ed. "The Ethics of Practice," and "The Changing Practice Environment." Access date 7 May, 2001. http://www.acponline.org/journals/annals/01apr98/ethicman.htm

7. Code of Federal Regulations. Title 21, Chapter 1—Food and Drug Administration, DHHS; Part 50—Protection of Human Subjects. Updated 1 April, 1999. Access date 18 April, 2001. http://www4.law.cornell.edu/cfr/21p50.htm

8. Code of Federal Regulations. Title 45A—Department of Health and Human Services; Part 46—Protection of Human Subjects. Updated 1 October, 1997. Access date 18 April, 2001. http://www4.law.cornell.edu/cfr/45p46.htm

9. Bodenheimer T. Uneasy alliance: Clinical investigators and the pharmaceutical industry. *N Engl J Med* 342(20):1539–1544, 2000.

10. Boseley S. Scandal of scientists who take money for papers ghostwritten by drug companies. *Guardian Unlimited.* 7 February, 2002. Access date 12 February, 2002. http://www.guardian.co.uk

Conflict of Interest: Institutional Review Boards

Daniel K. Nelson

INTRODUCTION

This chapter reviews conflicts of interest that may face either the institutional review board (IRB) as an entity or the individuals that contribute to the IRB's mission. Given the central role of IRBs in overseeing the ethical conduct of research involving human subjects, it is critical that they operate free from inappropriate influence. Accordingly, IRB members, chairs, and staff should follow policies and procedures similar to those of investigators to eliminate or minimize any conflicts of interest. In this context, a conflict of interest can be defined as *any situation or relationship that biases or has the potential to bias the conduct or outcome of IRB review.*

Possible sources of conflict of interest for IRBs are listed as an appendix to this chapter. These might originate or be experienced at individual or institutional levels. None of these scenarios or factors, in and of themselves, may represent unmanageable conflicts. However, any of these could exert inappropriate influence on the IRB and should be considered.

Sources of IRB Conflict of Interest: Individual Level

Research by Members

Perhaps the most widely recognized conflict of interest for IRBs is when research conducted by one of the members comes up for review. The investigator–member has an obvious interest in seeing the research approved for a number of personal and professional reasons. Because this type of conflict is usually apparent, proper management is largely a procedural matter. Beyond this direct conflict involving review of members' own research, there are multiple sources for indirect conflict of interest. These may be harder to discern and, therefore, harder to manage.

Members' Financial Interests

One example of these less apparent conflicts is the situation in which an IRB member or staff holds significant equity or other interests in the research itself or in the sponsors of research. These might include equity holdings, consulting arrangements, or patent rights—in short, the same types of financial conflicts that investigators might hold. Although the majority of academic research institutions have policies governing financial conflicts of interest,[1] these invariably focus on faculty serving as investigators and not as IRB members. The same concerns would apply, however, regarding the objectivity of individuals who stand to gain financially from research they are being asked to review and approve.

Loyalty to Colleagues

Another potential source of conflict is loyalty to colleagues submitting research for IRB review, be they peers, subordinates, or superiors. Members might logically be inclined to support the work of departmental colleagues with whom they interact every day (i.e., more directly than with other IRB members). Beyond mere camaraderie, members may sense a need to promote the work of subordinates or to avoid antagonizing their chief with a critical review. At a practical level, this conflict may be difficult to avoid because few institutions are large enough to assemble a panel of individuals with sufficient insight who do not also have overlapping interactions with colleagues submitting research.

Members' Areas of Expertise

Selection of members with sufficient expertise to comprehend the complexities of the research under review presents another potential problem. Members whose training or own area of research is closely tied to the studies under review may tend to show more leniency than they might to other areas with which they are less familiar. That is, it may be natural for them to take novel issues or procedures for granted. Conversely, this familiarity might work in the opposite direction if reviewers regard submitting investigators as competitors or rivals and are more critical than they might be otherwise. Members in this position might also find themselves with access to proprietary information when reviewing protocols, providing tempting insight to ongoing research in their personal area of interest (i.e., "insider trading"). Whether overly lenient or overly critical, neither tendency is conducive to the objective review that the IRB should strive to achieve.

As an aside, the potential for biased reviews may be something for institutions to consider before establishing "specialty boards" as a means of focusing expertise in a given area. The increased insight that comes with this structure must be viewed as a trade-off for decreased diversity of perspectives.

Impact of Decisions

IRB members might also be mindful of the possible impact of IRB decisions on their own work. For example, an IRB member who does clinical outcome studies may be reluctant to support IRB decisions that strengthen privacy protection if these lead to policies that restrict his or her own access to medical records for research.

Personal Agendas

Personal agendas of members may also interfere with the review process. For example, members of an advocacy group for a given disease or disorder can yield valuable insight as community representatives but can represent a negative influence if they see their role as promoting a certain agenda.

Non-IRB Roles

The institutional roles filled by members in their daily work outside the IRB may carry inherent conflicts of interest. For example, the director of a university contracts and grants office, whose primary duties revolve around bringing more research funding into the institution, may not be an appropriate individual to serve on the IRB. The same could be said for any institutional official charged with promoting or supporting the research enterprise if that obligation might run counter to a critical assessment of protocols. Indeed, reliance on individuals with these types of positional conflicts has been cited as an unacceptable situation in recent federal compliance actions.[2] Another institutional role that may exclude a person from IRB service is that of the legal counsel. Although legal counsel can be extremely helpful in an advisory capacity, a primary role of protecting the institution may run counter to the IRB's mission of protecting the subject. It can be argued that these goals are not incompatible to the extent that "a happy subject is a happy institution," but care must be exercised to avoid conflicting objectives.

The preceding discussion should not detract from the clear benefit of having IRB members with legal training, which is increasingly important for interpreting and applying regulations, interdigitating with state laws, and multiple other functions. Similarly, members with insight on the financing of research can provide valuable input to IRB deliberations. Nevertheless, care should be taken when appointing members who will be forced to wear too many institutional hats in serving the IRB.

Sources of IRB Conflict of Interest: Institutional Level

Protecting the Institution

Apart from any internal desire to protect the institution on the part of individual members, the institution must also avoid placing external pressure on the IRB to serve in this capacity. This may be a natural expectation for deans, provosts, presidents, and other officials and, as mentioned, is not necessarily incompatible with the role of the IRB, but should never be confused with its primary role. This separation of roles will be especially important as penalties for noncompliance continue to increase and institutions come to view their IRBs as a chief means of preventing regulatory sanctions.

Enhancing the Institution

In a more positive direction, a related source of conflict could arise from members' innate concerns for their institution's reputation or prestige, to the extent that this is enhanced through an active research portfolio. Once again, this desire is not incompatible with sound IRB review, but should never be an excuse for relaxing standards in the review of research.

Promoting Research

Yet another related concern is the desire on the part of individual members—and on the part of the IRB as an agent of the institution—to promote research in general. This is a laudable goal but should never be pursued to the extent that it detracts from the IRB's reason for being, which is to protect the rights and welfare of human subjects.

Undervalued Membership

Undervaluation of service to the IRB is another factor that could translate into a conflict of interest. If members do not believe that their work on the IRB is appreciated or valued by their superiors, they may not believe that they can or should devote the time necessary to do the job well. Department chairs, deans, and other institutional officials should send a clear signal that IRB membership is a necessary and important activity and recognize such service when considering promotions, tenure, and clinical work schedules. Some institutions are going beyond this by purchasing or "protecting" a percentage of faculty effort for IRB service.

Liability

The potential for legal liability is another factor that could influence an IRB's decision making. Although lawsuits implicating the IRB have been relatively few in number and most institutions are likely to indemnify IRB members in the performance of their professional duties, the threat of lawsuit is an ever-present possibility in our litigious society. Possible sources of lawsuits include not only subjects who have been injured in research, but also investigators who believe their research has been unfairly hindered by an IRB. Liability of IRB members is the subject of Chapter 8-9.

Institutional or Community Values

Institutional or community values are another source of possible conflict to the extent they may be reflected in reviews by individual members or the IRB as a whole. Clearly, there is a regulatory mandate[3(Sec.107(a)],4[Sec.107(a)] that the IRB do exactly that (reflect community attitudes), but there may be times when these values run counter to the mission of the IRB. For example, some institutions may be particularly sensitive to social or political issues (e.g., abortion) in ways that run counter to regulatory guidance that IRBs should not consider the long-range public policy implications of research under review.[3(Sec.111)] This separation from institutional values may admittedly be difficult to achieve when beliefs are deeply held.

Pressure for Speed

IRB members or staff often come under pressure from individual investigators or from the institution to conduct speedy review. Although it may be in everyone's best interest to establish systems for review that are both effective and efficient, the process should not be hastened to the point that important issues are overlooked.

Institutional Holdings or Interests

Institutions are increasingly entering agreements with industry that may create conflict of interest for the institution itself. These arrangements might include patent rights for new innovations, spin-off companies, technology licensing, or equity holdings (see Chapter 5-10). If an institution will be conducting research in which it bears a direct financial interest, appropriate firewalls should be in place to ensure that ethical oversight (i.e., the IRB) is not subject to influence from the institution. If the independence of the IRB cannot be assured, it may be preferable to solicit the services of another IRB or to conduct the research at other institutions.

Review Fees

Finally, the charging of review fees may create a conflict of interest that biases IRB review. Institutions that compete successfully for federal grant support receive a sizable percentage in the form of indirect costs, which are intended to support a variety of functions necessary to conduct research. Many institutions, perhaps now the majority, have begun charging review fees for industry-sponsored protocols as a means of generating additional support for the IRB. These fees, ranging from a few hundred to a few thousand dollars, are legitimate sources of revenue for work performed. All parties should be clear, however, that the fees are linked to protocol submissions and are not contingent on approval by the IRB. It is also highly advisable that the fees be administered through mechanisms separate from the IRB (e.g., contracts and grants office, billing department, or other administrative entities) so that the IRB is not placed in the position of bill collector. Ideally, the IRB should operate in complete ignorance of the billing status of any individual protocol.

This also presents a conflict for independent, for-profit IRBs, which may derive their entire revenue from such fees. There is nothing inherently improper in this arrangement, and many independent IRBs conduct credible, ethical review. They are, however, subject to an added element of conflict because they are businesses in their own right. This makes them dependent on the good will and satisfaction of their clients (e.g., pharmaceutical companies or contract research organizations), who are free to take their business elsewhere. This might logically occur if reviews were consistently perceived as being nitpicky, unfavorable, or slow. Thus, independent IRBs may be subject to conflict of interest pressures over and above those facing institution-based IRBs. Conversely, it can be argued that independent IRBs are free from many of the influences discussed previously because they are not subject to institutional expectations and pressures. By definition, each setting will have its own set of motivating factors, and neither is free from conflicts of interest.

Regulatory Guidance

If the IRB is to function in an independent, unbiased manner, it must not be subject to inappropriate pressures. Recognizing this, federal regulations specifically addressed IRB conflict of interest long before investigator conflict of interest became a focus of regulatory guidance. Both Department of Health and Human Services (DHHS)[3[Sec.107(e)]] and Food and Drug Administration (FDA)[4[Sec.107(e)]] regulations instruct that:

> No IRB may have a member participate in the IRB's initial or continuing review of any project in which the member has a conflicting interest, except to provide information requested by the IRB.

This means that each IRB should have clearly defined mechanisms for identifying conflicts among its members and for excluding conflicted members from a situation where review may be compromised.

Management of IRB Conflicts of Interest

In contrast to the enormous attention paid to investigator conflicts of interest in recent years, very little has been paid to similar conflicts on the part of IRBs. This may be partly because IRBs are not involved hands-on with the actual conduct of the study and partly because those involved with ethical review are seen as somehow immune to baser instincts. For whatever reason, few authors or policy makers have specifically addressed the conflicts that might be faced by IRBs or their resolution.[5] As with conflicts for investigators, the first (and perhaps most difficult) task is to recognize that a conflict exists. After this potential is identified and acknowledged, steps should be taken to eliminate or minimize its impact.

For the purpose of discussion, let us consider the fairly routine scenario where an IRB member is involved as an investigator on the research under review, recognizing that many of the conflicts described above might be addressed through similar mechanisms. As with identification of conflicts for the larger pool of investigators outside the

IRB, this process would typically rely on self-identification by the investigator–member. After this identification, written policies and procedures should describe how the conflicted member would be removed from deliberations on the protocol for which they hold the conflict.

Recusal of Members from Meetings

In the setting of a convened meeting, the most obvious solution is that the member in question should physically leave the room during consideration of that protocol. This approach minimizes two sources of influence, neither of them desirable. First, the investigator–member would naturally be inclined to give the protocol preferential treatment. Second, other members may not feel completely free to discuss openly or to criticize out of deference to their fellow board member. Thus, removal from the meeting is the clearest means by which to manage that member's conflict. Some IRBs, however, may wish the member to remain present for initial discussion to answer any questions, as they would any other investigator. As noted previously, this is expressly allowed by the regulations. If an IRB chooses to adopt this as local policy, remaining members should be given further opportunity for discussion once the conflicted member eventually does leave the meeting.

In some circumstances, the IRB may be placed in an untenable position if the physical absence of a conflicted member would force the loss of quorum, thereby halting the meeting. This creates a catch-22 of sorts if the IRB would prefer that any conflicted member leave the room, yet needs that member present in order to meet regulatory requirements for quorum. Under these circumstances, one would hope that the valid concept of having sufficient numbers present to conduct business (i.e., quorum) would give way to the intent behind these regulatory requirements, namely, to ensure that research undergoes review by an unbiased, independent body.

This author's personal opinion is that we may be missing the forest for the trees if it means compromising review by keeping a conflicted member present only to preserve an arbitrary quorum. This argument gains more credence when we remember that the minimum quorum under existing regulations only requires that three members be present (of the minimum five total members) and that most IRBs are much larger than that in practice, even at half strength. That is, one could envision a situation in which an IRB with 20 members had 11 members in attendance and wished to temporarily excuse a conflicted member. It is difficult to accept that the remaining 10 members are insufficient to conduct review, when 10 still represents thrice the number required for a duly constituted quorum under regulatory requirements.

All that said, the regulations do require the presence of a quorum,[3(Sec.108),4(Sec.108)] and the foregoing is not an argument to disregard that requirement. The best approach is to ensure that adequate numbers of members will be present so that quorum is never endangered. This can be accomplished through the use of alternates to cover absences, reminders on the days of meetings, and selection of members who will take seriously their commitment to attend.

Regulatory Guidance

Regulatory guidance on the question of conflicted members leaving the room is vague and subject to interpretation. As previously noted, the regulations themselves only state that the conflicted member should not "participate" in the review of a given project. The FDA has both clarified and reversed its position on this question. In the 1998 update of its Information Sheets, the FDA indicated that an IRB could lose quorum when members with a conflict of interest leave the room for deliberation and voting on a study.[6] In a subsequent addendum, published February 1999, the FDA clarified that

The quorum is the count of the number of [voting] members present. If the number present falls below majority, the quorum fails. The regulations only require that a member who is conflicted not participate in the deliberations and voting on a study on which he or she is conflicted. The IRB may decide whether an individual should remain in the room.

Through still further clarifications, the FDA took an interim position that members who abstain from the vote are still counted as present even if they are required to leave the room for voting so that an IRB would not lose quorum through conflicted members' abstentions. Most recently, however, the FDA has agreed with the Office for Human Research Protections (OHRP) that quorum may be lost through the recusal of conflicted members (Paul Goebel, personal communication, 2001), and OHRP has cited this as a finding of noncompliance.[2] In whatever way the recusal of conflicted members is handled, study files and minutes of IRB meetings should reflect the identity of members recused for deliberations or voting. Given the increasing attention to detail in minutes, it may be advisable to also note the nature of the member's conflict that led to recusal.

IRB Reporting Structure

Beyond the recusal of investigator–members for deliberations or voting on their own protocols, the more systemic forms of conflict may be more difficult to manage, but no less important. Attention should be paid to the placement of the IRB within the institution and resulting reporting relationships, as well as to institutional policies that might negate some of the influences already discussed. The reporting structure of the IRB is the subject of Chapter 2-1 in this book.

Selection of Members

One of the most effective mechanisms to manage IRB conflict of interest lies in the appointment of a diverse membership.[7] This would include, but not be limited to, recruitment of unaffiliated members not beholden to the host institution.[3(Sec.107(d)),4(Sec.107(d))] Consideration to potential conflict of interest should be given when selecting members from inside the institution. Involvement in research gives valuable and necessary insight and should not exclude a potential member from serving on an IRB. However, if circumstances would lead a member to be recused from a majority of protocols considered, he or she may not be a good choice. This might occur in settings where a single investigator or department accounts for a disproportionate amount of the institution's total research portfolio. This creates a dilemma in populating the IRB with sufficient expertise to review studies while simultaneously avoiding conflicts of interest, as the individuals with the greatest insight into scientific aspects of studies under review may also be conflicted. The potential for problems when institutional roles outside of service to the IRB run counter to a primary focus on protecting subjects has already been discussed. This may especially be true in smaller institutions, where individuals may be forced to wear multiple hats.

Education

As with every other aspect of human subjects protection, proactive education is another important component of an effective management strategy. Investigators, IRB members and staff, and institutional officials should all be made aware of existing policies and of potential for conflicts of interest in their own activities. This may be especially relevant for IRB chairs, members, and staff, who may be accustomed to looking for conflicts in the investigators they oversee but not in themselves. After initial draft guidance from OHRP in 2001, the DHHS has now issued final guidance on financial relationships and interests in human subjects research.[7] They included a section on IRB operations and members, providing perhaps the first federal guidance specifically directed at this group of individuals. Along with reiterating the need for education and training activities in this area, OHRP and DHHS added financial interests to the conflicts chairs and members should be mindful of during the review process. This guidance suggests that IRBs remind their members of policies at the outset of each meeting, providing members with the opportunity to consider any personal conflicts relating to the protocols they are about to review. They should then follow clear procedures for recusal from deliberations and voting, as previously discussed, and document these actions.

Conclusion

Any conflicts of interest on the part of the IRB undermine the credibility of the process and must be avoided at all costs. Whether a particular influence is real or perceived, originates from within or without, or is felt consciously or subconsciously, IRBs are not immune from conflicts of interest. No one doubts the integrity or motivation of those serving to protect human subjects, but we are no more or less human than the investigators we oversee and can only benefit from self-awareness in areas that might impact our effectiveness.

References

1. McCrary SV, Anderson CB, Jakovljevic J, Khan T, McCullough LB, Wray NP, Brody BA. A national survey of policies on disclosure of conflicts of interest in biomedical research. *N Engl J Med* 343(22):1621–1626, 2000.

2. Office for Human Research Protections COB. OHRP Compliance activities: Common findings and guidance; 2002. http://www.hhs.gov/ohrp/compliance/findings.pdf

3. Code of Federal Regulations. Title 45A—Department of Health and Human Services; Part 46—Protection of Human Subjects. Updated 1 October, 1997. Access date 18 April, 2001. http://www4.law.cornell.edu/cfr/45p46.htm

4. Code of Federal Regulations. Title 21, Chapter 1—Food and Drug Administration, DHHS; Part 56—Institutional Review Boards. Updated 1 April, 1999. Access date 27 March, 2001. http://www4.law.cornell.edu/cfr/21p56.htm

5. Spece RG Jr, Shimm DS, Buchanan AE. *Conflicts of Interest in Clinical Practice and Research*. New York: Oxford University Press; 1996.

6. Food and Drug Administration. Information sheets: Guidance for institutional review boards and clinical investigators, September 1998. Access date 9 April, 2001. http://www.fda.gov/oc/oha/IRB/toc.html

7. Department of Health and Human Services. Final Guidance Document: Financial Relationships and interests in research involving human subjects: Guidance for human subject protection, 5 May, 2004. Date of access 31 January, 2005. http://www.hhs.gov/ohrp/humansubjects/finreltn/fguid.pdf

Appendix

Individual Level

Member is investigator on research under review

Members or staff hold significant financial interest in sponsor of research

Loyalty to colleagues submitting for review

Members closely tied to area of research under review
    Familiar = too lenient
    Competitor = too critical

Possible impact of decisions on member's own work (e.g., policy changes)

Personal agendas or advocacy positions

Non-IRB roles of members
    Contracts and grants office
    Legal counsel

Institutional Level

Pressure or desire to protect institution

Concern for institution's reputation or prestige

Promoting research versus protecting subjects

Undervaluation of IRB service

Potential liability

Institutional or community values

Pressure for speedy reviews

Institutional equity or ownership

Review fees

Administrative Tasks Before the Meeting

Rebecca Carson Rogers

INTRODUCTION

A successful full-committee institutional review board (IRB) meeting is largely dependent on the comprehensiveness of the administrative details completed before the meeting. The variety and number of these tasks are considerable, and all are critical; however, when done efficiently, they will be virtually inconspicuous to committee members. The purpose of this chapter is to discuss the administrative tasks that should be done in preparation for the full-committee meeting.

General Administrative Tasks

A well-prepared meeting allows the IRB to have the information it needs:

1. To be compliant with regulations
2. To make a definitive determination regarding each agenda item the first time that it is discussed

The specific internal office processes that each organization develops will depend on many variables such as the number of IRBs, how often IRBs meet, and the number of IRB office staff. This chapter outlines a variety of processes and gives examples from the IRB office at Dartmouth College.

To start, we strongly endorse the development of good will and mutual respect with the research community. Time spent in reaching out to researchers in a comprehensive manner, before a study is even submitted, will save the IRB office time in the long run. Provide as much administrative assistance as possible to researchers and their staff. Names, e-mail addresses, and phone numbers of staff who can answer questions should be easily available. If the IRB office has resources to review all or parts of a protocol before submission, this should be communicated. Researchers may be directed to any other online examples of protocols or consent forms, as well as workshops that cover these topics.

Work with Your Researchers

Good communication with researchers about meeting submission requirements helps foster a good working relationship between the IRB and research teams.

Providing prereview and editing service for researchers before the meeting, particularly of consent forms, allows the IRB to focus on substantive ethical and regulatory concerns. Notify researchers of upcoming review dates, materials submission deadlines, and submission procedures.

New Study Submission

Establish a deadline policy for materials submission and communicate your policy to the research community in as many ways as possible (e.g., IRB website, newsletter, researcher guidance materials). A "rolling submission" policy for new studies allows only a certain number of new protocols to be reviewed at each IRB meeting, and submissions are dated as they are submitted. A set submission deadline date policy allows studies to be reviewed at the next IRB meeting if they are received in the office by a certain date.

Continuing Review (Renewal) Notifications

Protocol renewal is discussed in detail in Chapter 7-2. Researchers should be notified of the date that full IRB renewal of their study is required if they wish to proceed with uninterrupted participant enrollment. We provide renewal notification 6 weeks before the deadline of material submission and again 2 weeks before the deadline.

Revision Submission

Protocol revisions are discussed in detail in Chapter 7-1. Depending on the nature of the revision, a full-committee review may be required.

Collecting Submission Materials

IRB office preview of submitted materials can determine that a submission is complete, and thus, the IRB will be able to review as per the regulations and per institutional policies.

IRB offices use different material submission methods. These range from complete hard copy submission requirements to fully electronic web-based systems. There are both commercially and institutionally developed online systems available.

Using National Institutes of Health Enhancement Grant Funds, Dartmouth College in collaboration with Children's Hospital of Philadelphia has developed IRBNet. With this system

- Researchers can develop protocols and consent forms using educational guidance based on best practices, ethical principles, and federal regulations.

- Sponsors and researchers can distribute multisite studies to collaborating researchers and submit studies to their local IRBs.

- IRB administrators can share local IRB status and access real-time decisions of other IRBs in multisite trials.

More information is found at www.irbnet.org.

Materials Needed for Submission

Regardless of the method for collecting submission materials, researchers appreciate a checklist of required documents. Your list will depend on the type of study, the type of review, and institutional policy.

This list is for a new study submission. Many of these materials will also be submitted for continuing (renewal) review or study revision review.

1. Protocol—full sponsor protocol or National Institutes of Health protocol

2. Institutional "summary protocol" and attachments—We have spent a considerable amount of time developing our summary protocol, which guides the researcher and subsequently the IRB members through the project with a specific focus on human subject issues. Interested readers may access current Dartmouth College IRB forms at http://www.dartmouth.edu/~cphs. For example, if a project involves minors, the minors attachment is submitted with the summary protocol. Other examples include attachments required for medical devices, use of placebo, genetic research, employee and student participants, illiterate subjects, incompetent participants, waiver of participant consent, and waiver of signed consent form. This format has been very useful for IRB members, as it assists us in the review process by ensuring that all appropriate issues are covered.

3. Consent form/Health Insurance Portability and Accountability Act (HIPAA) authorization (if applicable)—When a research study involves Protected Health Information, HIPAA authorization is required unless waived per regulation. At Dartmouth, we use a single compound form for consent to participate in a research study that involves Protected Health Information. Editing the study consent form

by the IRB office before the meeting helps keep the meeting focused on substantive concerns rather than minor consent form edits needed.

4. Investigator brochure—required when a study involves an investigational new drug (IND)

5. Clinical trial agreements

6. Site agreements/federalwide assurance (FWA) information

7. Recruitment materials—These may include advertisements, posters, videos, radio scripts, website materials, and brochures. Editing these materials by the IRB office before the meeting helps keep the meeting focused on substantive concerns rather than minor edits needed.

8. Interview questions, copies of surveys, patient diaries

9. Approval notifications from other committees/agencies—Depending on the type of study and your institutional policies this may include the Food and Drug Administration, the Recombinant DNA Advisory Committee, the Institutional Scientific Review Committee, the Institutional Biosafety Committee, the Radiation Committee, Nursing, Pharmacy, other institutional review committees—for example, Dartmouth Brain Imaging Center. Dartmouth requires a scientific review of a study to be done before IRB submission. This is done by scientific review committees set up at the department or section level.

10. Institutionally required submission forms—for example, signed "cover sheet" Dartmouth Human Subject Review Form, financial disclosure/conflict of interest forms

11. IRB education certificate—This is required for all DHHS funded projects. At Dartmouth, we require all key research personnel to meet our IRB education requirement regardless of their study funding source.

12. IRB fees—Communicate your fee policy to researchers in your submission materials and establish a billing system to meet your institutional requirements.

Work with Your IRB Members

Determine Attendance for the Upcoming Meeting

Quorum is needed for all IRB meetings. IRB members and alternates must be canvassed regarding their attendance at the upcoming IRB meeting. Be sure a "majority of the members of the IRB are present, including at least one member whose primary concerns are in nonscientific areas."[1][Sec.108(b)] Five members is the minimal size for an IRB, as per federal regulations.[1][Sec.107(a)] For a five-member IRB, quorum is three.

Let IRB members know your deadline for committing to meeting attendance and determine a plan for when members cannot attend. Decide who invites alternates to attend a meeting. A strategy of rotating meeting attendance between a member and their alternates works well for some institutions.

Depending on the type of studies to be reviewed, a specialized member may be needed; for example, if studies involve prisoners or children. A consultant may be needed if the IRB does not have the expertise among members to properly review a study.

Distribution of Materials to Committee Members

Distribute meeting materials allowing adequate time for members to review studies before the meeting and for any follow-up they may be expected to do with the researcher before the meeting.

Along with study review materials, before every meeting, we distribute new continuing education materials to our IRB members. These may include copies of journal articles, local news articles, new federal guidance documents, or drafts of institutional policies to review and discuss at the meeting.

As with the collection of study materials, there are many different ways to get materials to IRB members from using hard copies to electronic formats. At Dartmouth, we prepare and deliver individual three-ring binders to each member before the meeting. Other institutions provide members with a laptop computer and distribute materials electronically via a web-based system.

Other IRB Office Tasks

Many institutions have more than one IRB, and an initial administrative task for meeting preparation is to determine which committee will review a study.

Preparing the Agenda

There are no federal regulations to guide us in the development of an IRB meeting agenda. We have found the order of items on the agenda plays an important role in the efficiency and effectiveness of the IRB meeting. After trying several different formats, we have settled on the following agenda outline.

1. Continuing education
2. Review of minutes from the previous month
3. Announcements
4. Studies to be reviewed, which are broken down into the following categories:
   a. Studies previously voted "not approved"
   b. Studies previously voted "conditionally approved"
      In most instances, a study voted "conditionally approved" is not required to be rereviewed by the full committee because the conditions of approval are such that simple concurrence by the researcher is all that is required to receive final approval. Usually this is accomplished by the review of revised materials by the IRB chair. However, on occasion, the researcher does not provide simple concurrence; in that case, the study is rereviewed by the full committee.
   c. New protocols
   d. Revisions to previously approved studies
      At our institution, the full committee must review all study revisions that increase the risk to participants.
   e. Renewals with revisions

This category is for studies that are being renewed and also have revision requests.
   f. Renewals
   g. Serious adverse events
      On occasion, we receive an adverse event report that merits a review by the full committee as per our adverse event reporting procedure.

After all studies are on the agenda, IRB reviewers are selected and their names added to the respective studies on the agenda.

Assigning Reviewers

The primary reviewer system used at Dartmouth requires the assignment of IRB members to specific studies. It is expected that all IRB members review all the studies. However, we rely on the primary reviewers to conduct a particularly detailed analysis of their assigned studies and to provide a verbal summary of potential issues at the IRB meeting. We assign IRB members who have expertise in the area of the study being reviewed. All members realize that their comments, whether as primary reviewer or not, are important and listened to at the meeting. Work with your IRB members to obtain feedback and establish an assignment system with which everyone is comfortable.

Schedule Guests

Some IRBs require each researcher to either attend the IRB meeting or be available for questions during the IRB meeting time. We have found it very effective to contact researchers with questions related to their study before the IRB meeting. All IRB members, particularly primary reviewers, are encouraged to either contact the researcher directly with questions before the meeting or to contact the IRB office with a request to obtain further information from the researcher. During the days immediately before the meeting, the IRB administrative staff at our institution expects to spend hours relaying information back and forth between reviewers and researchers. There is no substitute for trying to solve problems and clarify issues before the full committee is assembled. In most cases, questions that would have consumed considerable full-committee time are answered during the premeeting dialogue. When a reviewer thinks that there are likely to be questions for the researcher or objections to approving the protocol, then this perspective is relayed to the researcher by the IRB staff before the meeting. The researcher is asked either to attend the meeting or, more frequently, to be available by pager to answer questions by telephone or to come to the meeting on short notice.

Of course, there are times when important issues are not brought out until the discussions at the IRB meeting. However, the attempt to solve problems and clarify issues before the meeting promotes a positive rapport with researchers and dramatically improves the efficiency and effectiveness of the full-committee meeting. It is very satisfying when an IRB member says, "I had a question about aspect X of the study; however, I contacted the researcher, and she explained it to me. Thus, from my perspective on this issue, we just need 'simple concurrence' in a revised consent form."

Prepare for Meeting Minutes to Be Taken

The ability to take the minutes of the meeting directly on a computer is a great advantage. In this case, the meeting agenda can be used as the outline for the minutes. Many automated electronic IRB systems now include the ability for the minutes to be directly entered into the system.

IRB Meeting Space

After attendance is determined, meeting room reservations should be confirmed and refreshments ordered. We have morning IRB meetings and thus provide a buffet breakfast to our IRB members. We suggest a comfortable, quiet location, slightly removed from the hustle and bustle of daily work life for your IRB meetings. IRB members should feel relaxed and able to concentrate on the important task at hand.

Conclusion

For an IRB meeting to be productive and efficient, it is essential to complete a wide range of administrative tasks before the meeting begins. This chapter lists the tasks that are most important to perform and explains how IRB administrators should go about getting them done. In our experience, it is especially important to establish the practice of routinely contacting researchers before the meeting to discuss areas of confusion or potential problem issues. Whenever possible, the IRB staff should help IRB members and researchers prepare the research proposal so that the IRB will have the information it needs to make a definitive determination the first time the protocol is discussed.

Reference

1. Code of Federal Regulations. Title 45A—Department of Health and Human Services; Part 46—Protection of Human Subjects. Updated 1 October, 1997. Access date 18 April, 2001. http://www4.law.cornell.edu/cfr/45p46.htm

Guidelines for Review, Discussion, and Voting

Robert J. Amdur and Elizabeth A. Bankert

INTRODUCTION

Every institution needs to address the logistics and procedures for their unique site. However, as is a theme throughout this book, it is often helpful to know what procedures other sites have implemented. This chapter suggests guidelines regarding three aspects of the process of full committee review. These aspects are what institutional review board (IRB) members should do to prepare for the meeting, the format for presenting and discussing each study, and the voting options.

What IRB Members Should Do to Prepare for the Meeting

Conduct a Systematic Review of the Application Material

Many IRBs find that the primary reviewer system improves the quality and efficiency of IRB review. The primary reviewer system means that a limited number of IRB members, usually two or three, are assigned as special reviewers for each protocol to be reviewed at the full committee meeting. Although each IRB member must review all of the materials and be prepared for discussion, the primary reviewer(s) is often responsible for presenting a brief summary of the study and to have reviewed the study in detail with the intent of contacting the investigator with questions before the IRB meeting and/or responding to questions raised by other IRB members. Some experienced IRB reviewers favor the following approach as a primary reviewer:

- Consent document: Read the consent document first. The purpose of the document is to explain the important aspects of the study to potential subjects in lay language; it should give the reviewer a basic introduction to the protocol. The purpose of this reading is to orient the reviewer to the context of the study.

- Summary study plan: The next step is to review the IRB summary study plan. Most institutions require some type of summary of the project for the IRB members (in addition to a full biomedical protocol). This summary should contain the key aspects of the elements required for IRB approval. A sample study plan created by the Dartmouth IRB can be found at http://www.dartmouth.edu/~cphs/.

- Supporting material: Next read the supporting material that backs up the information presented in the study plan. For example, previous studies that relate to the study treatment or that validate study procedures, statistical power analysis, qualifications of the investigator, adequacy of research facilities, recruitment advertisements, etc.

- Read the consent document again: Record suggested corrections or questions for the investigator, and ensure that the consent form adequately describes the actual study design.

- Use a review template: Use a review template to take notes while reading the study plan, supporting material, and consent document. A template helps to organize the review, reminds the reviewer what issues have and have not been addressed, is useful for presenting the review at the full committee meeting, and can be kept in the IRB file as documentation that a detailed review was performed. Some reviewers make up their own templates according to the format that works best for them. Some IRBs ask every reviewer to use the same template. Some IRBs use review forms that are lengthy and extremely detailed. In organizations that view the primary purpose of the reviewer template as a mechanism for documenting compliance with federal regulations the template may contain legalistic wording.

Answer as Many Questions as Possible Before the Meeting

A hallmark of effective and efficient IRBs is the extent to which IRB reviewers and support staff work to prepare the protocol application, answer questions, and resolve controversial issues before the full committee meeting. Clearly, it is an enormous task to ask IRB members to conduct a thorough protocol review *and* to find answers to unresolved issues prior to the full committee meeting, but in the long run, this approach will pay large dividends for both the IRB and the research community.

There are multiple reasons why it is undesirable to use routinely the full committee meeting to clarify issues and identify questions to discuss with the investigator. It takes a considerable amount of resources to assemble the full committee, and thus, the IRB should use the meeting to accomplish things that could not be done in other settings. It is useful to structure the review process so that the full committee IRB meeting is primarily a place to make decisions rather than gather information.

It is important for the IRB to work closely with the research team before the full committee meeting to maximize the chance that the full committee will be able to make a definitive and informed decision the first time the protocol is reviewed. It is in the best interest of the research team, the IRB, research subjects, and the overall organization for the IRB review process to be as efficient as possible. Not approving a protocol at the full committee meeting because the IRB needs clarification on basic issues or revisions that could have been addressed before the meeting decreases the efficiency of IRB review. Efficiency and quality are related because anything that decreases respect for the IRB process compromises the ability of the IRB to protect the rights and welfare of research participants. Several other chapters in this book explain how the IRB administrative staff members should function as colleagues of the researcher before the meeting by helping the research team revise the consent document or application material to facilitate IRB review.

Specific Recommendations for IRB Reviewers

- Review study information before the meeting: Most IRB members receive materials at least a week in advance of the IRB meeting. Although the IRB office should ensure materials are complete, in some instances, a thorough evaluation of the IRB issues requires information that was not included in the application package. After reading the protocol application, the reviewer may need to discuss the protocol with a colleague, with IRB staff, or with the investigator. It is essential to give the evaluation process the time that it deserves in advance of the meeting.

- Try to get your questions answered *before* the meeting: This is a restatement of the fundamental message of this chapter.

- Do not hesitate to discuss the protocol with the investigator: Collegial interaction between the investigator and primary IRB reviewer will facilitate the IRB review and promote respect for the local IRB. The IRB chair or administrative director should encourage members to contact investigators for further information or clarification. However, the IRB office should also be willing to serve as an intermediary between IRB members and investigators.

- Decide whether the investigator should attend the meeting: When an investigator cannot be contacted or an issue cannot be resolved before the meeting, the reviewer should inform the IRB administrator or chair of the situation. Reviewers should indicate whether they think it will be important for the investigator to attend the IRB meeting. The most common reason that the IRB should ask an investigator to attend the IRB meeting is to discuss an important issue that could not be resolved before the meeting. There are, however, situations in which a reviewer identifies a situation that he or she thinks will be important for other IRB members to hear an investigator explain in his or her own words, rather than have the reviewer explain to the committee that there is no reason for concern.

Format for Discussion at the Meeting

Federal regulations and guidance documents do not discuss the format for discussion of protocols at the full committee meeting. Conversation with experienced IRB chairs around the country suggests that there are a variety of routines that work well. Again, each IRB should use the approach that fits best with the personalities and interpersonal styles of the committee. The important thing is to use a system that promotes an efficient discussion of important IRB issues in an atmosphere that encourages all members to express their views. Here is a basic routine that has worked well for several experienced IRBs:

1. The first primary reviewer presents the protocol. There are no questions or interruptions until this presentation is completed.

2. The first primary reviewer uses an organized format to summarize the important issues that the IRB should consider. The reviewer should not take a significant amount of time to discuss the details of the study because all IRB members are expected to have read the materials. It is important that the reviewer mention all of the issues that are important for the IRB to evaluate and not just the ones that are of particular concern in this specific protocol. A template like the one included at the end of this chapter will simplify both the processes of review and presentation. The presentation should end with a summary of any issues that are unresolved in the mind of the reviewer or issues that the reviewer thinks require revision. The reviewer should be encouraged to make a recommendation regarding how the committee should vote on the protocol.

3. The second primary reviewer comments on the protocol. The second reviewer does not repeat the information presented by the first reviewer, but rather indicates where he or she agrees or disagrees with the assessments of the first reviewer, with a brief explanation of the rationale for any disagreements. The second reviewer adds or clarifies information. The second reviewer ends with a voting recommendation that might or might not agree with the first reviewer's recommendation.

4. If there are three or more assigned reviewers, they present their comments according to the same guidelines as described for the second reviewer. The chair should discourage questions or comments until all of the assigned reviewers have had a chance to complete their initial presentations.

5. The chair opens the discussion up to the full committee. The chair should control the discussion by calling on people in turn. The chair should ask the primary reviewers to respond to the questions or comments by other IRB members, but in many cases, it will be more appropriate for the chair or a member other than one of the primary reviewers to respond.

Under the best of circumstances, it may be difficult to manage the full committee discussion of a controversial protocol. The goal is to discuss the protocol in a way that encourages all IRB members to express their views and identifies the issues that are important for the IRB to consider. There is no formula for this process, but it is essential that the chair be able to manage this aspect of the meeting if the IRB is to function effectively. There must be a mechanism to terminate the discussion so that the committee can turn its attention to the vote. Some IRBs let the discussion continue until an IRB member seconds a motion for a vote. In other committees, the chair determines when all of the important issues have been raised, declares the discussion over, and calls for the vote.

The Voting Options

The section of federal research regulations that addresses the different determinations that the IRB may make regarding a research protocol (voting options) is 45 CFR 46.109(a) and analogous FDA regulations that say this: "An IRB shall review and have authority to approve, require modifications in (to secure approval), or disapprove all research activities covered by this policy." As discussed in other chapters, federal regulation 45 CFR 46.108(b) requires a majority of IRB members to convene a full committee meeting. The second part of this regulation gives the requirement for an approval determination: "In order for the research to be approved, it shall receive the approval of the majority of those members present at the meeting." In other words, a majority of IRB members (or their alternates) must be present for a quorum, and a majority of the members at the meeting must agree to approve a study. Majority means more than half. Also, all votes are recorded in the minutes.

Every institution has developed their own set of voting options to best meet their needs. A few common voting options include "approved," "conditionally approved," "approved pending modifications," "table," "disapprove," "substantive revisions required," "not approved," "abstain," and "recuse."

Our suggested voting options are as follows: approved, minor revisions required, not approved, recuse, and abstain. Each option and the reason we chose it is briefly discussed in the following paragraphs:

Approved—The study has been approved as submitted. The investigator is not required to change any aspect of the protocol or consent document. The approval date is the date of the IRB meeting. The approval is valid for one year unless the committee designates a shorter period due to the risk of the study. An approval letter will be sent to the investigator.

Minor Revisions Required—There has been considerable discussion related to the "conditionally approved" and iterations thereof category. The consensus seems to be that in order to ensure the researcher is not confused when she or he sees the word *approved* in conjunction with another word, it is best not to use the word *approved* at all until there is indeed final approval of the study. For years, we have used the voting option "conditional approval." However, we will make the change to "Minor Revisions Required" after our new computer system is in place. A vote of "Minor Revisions Required" means that the full committee does not need to review the study again unless the researcher does not provide "simple concurrence" with the minor revisions requested. A letter describing the concerns of the committee will be sent to the investigator.

The letter will make it clear that the study may not begin until the IRB has issued a letter of approval.

As mentioned, simple concurrence of the listed items in the letter is required before final approval. Because the requests are "no more than minimal," the review can be completed via an "expedited" review by the chairperson or designee. The investigators' response will be reviewed for appropriateness and concurrence. If an investigator does not provide simple concurrence, the investigators' response needs review by the full committee. A final IRB approval letter will be sent to the investigator once the response has been approved. At that time, the study may begin. The approval date is the date of the *original* IRB meeting at which the "Minor Revisions Required" determination was made (even in the event that it may take several months to receive the minor revisions from the investigator). IRB approval is valid for one year unless the committee designates a shorter period due to the risks of the study.

Not Approved—The magnitude and/or number of concerns, questions, and/or problems are such that "Minor Revisions Required" is not appropriate. A letter describing reasons the study was not approved is sent to the investigator. The tone of this letter can set the stage for the relationship between the IRB and the investigator. We suggest this letter be written so as to educate the investigator as the issues the IRB encountered, and the reasons *why* the IRB considered the items problematic. At some institutions a copy of a not-approved letter is also sent to the department chairperson and departmental scientific reviewer in order to alert these individuals of the committee's decision. A designation of "Not Approved" indicates that resubmission of the study must be reviewed by the full committee. The investigator will be notified of the opportunity to respond to the IRB in writing or in person with regard to the IRB determination. Some institutions chose to use "disapproved" or "substantial revisions required" in place of not approved in order to send a message to the investigator that the committee believes the overall goals of the study may be worthwhile but that outstanding issues remain. If a study is resubmitted for full review and the study is approved at the second meeting, the date of approval is the date of the second meeting.

Recuse—If an IRB member has a conflict of interest with any part of the study, the IRB member may not participate in the initial or continuing review of the study except to provide information requested by the IRB. She or he must leave the room and not participate in the vote. This is considered a "recusal" and will not be counted as part of the voting quorum. Conflicts of interest include financial interest, active participation in the trial as principal investigator or co-principal investigator, or any other issue for which the member feels his or her vote could be considered potentially conflicted.

Abstain—If an IRB member does not have a "conflict" but feels unable to vote (e.g., left the room for discussion, does not comprehend the study or the issues) the member may "abstain" from voting. A vote to "abstain" will be included as part of the voting quorum.

Conclusion

IRB member preparation for a meeting, the format for presenting and discussing each study at the meeting, and the voting options are three important items to consider when striving to make the IRB meeting as efficient and effective as possible while also ensuring a respectful relationship with investigators. Whatever process an IRB chooses to implement should adequately address the importance of maintaining a positive connection with investigators and ensure that the time devoted by IRB members to this endeavor is used in a well organized and professional manner.

Administrative Tasks After Each Institutional Review Board Meeting

Jan Trott and Rebecca Carson Rogers

INTRODUCTION

Many of the administrative tasks that take place directly after the institutional review board (IRB) meeting are completed in order to comply with federal regulations that state, "The IRB shall prepare and maintain adequate documentation of IRB activities."[1(Sec.115),2(Sec.115)] These tasks also assure efficient and accurate tracking of the evolution of IRB-approved studies and communication with researchers. This chapter provides list of tasks that will help you with these tasks and the associated federal regulations. The individuals responsible for these administrative duties must have organized work habits that include attention to detail.

Communicating Meeting Results to the Researcher

Understandably, researchers are eager to learn the results of their study. This communication is required by regulation, and IRB offices are encouraged to implement systems to contact investigators promptly after the meeting.

Title 45 CFR 46.109(d)

An IRB shall notify investigators and the institution in writing of its decision to approve or disapprove the proposed research activity, or of modifications required to secure IRB approval of the research activity. If the IRB decides to disapprove a research activity, it shall include in its written notification, a statement of the reasons for its decision and give the investigator an opportunity to respond in person or in writing.

The letter to the researcher needs to state clearly the determination of the IRB, including any conditions that must be met before final approval. This applies to letters of approval for new proposals, full-board approval of revisions, and full-board approval of study renewals. We find that the content and tone of the letter to the researcher can help establish a culture of mutual respect. The letter should start with a description of the primary concerns of the IRB and end with requests for changes to the consent form.

After the researcher is notified that study modifications are required before final unconditional approval, the IRB office needs to follow up at specific time intervals. Many IRB offices will "close" a study if the researcher has not responded to modification requests within 90 days. On occasion, you may receive an inquiry from a researcher about a vote by a specific IRB member. The IRB functions and makes determinations as a committee. It is not appropriate for an IRB member or staff person to discuss votes by individual members of the committee.

Letters to Investigators

Include the following information when informing the principal investigator of the result of IRB review:

1. The identification number given to the study
2. The title of the study
3. If commercially sponsored, the version date of the protocol and consent document
4. The name of the IRB
5. The IRB determination: unconditional approval, conditional approval or minor modifications required, tabled, disapproved
6. The date of the determination
7. If approved, the duration of approval and date of rereview by the board
8. If conditionally approved or minor modification required, a list of conditions and a statement that the study should not begin until the investigator receives formal notification of IRB approval after review of the response to the approval conditions

9. If tabled or disapproved, the basis for the determination and a statement that the investigator is welcome to resubmit the proposal

Final approval letters provide an opportunity to remind researchers of proper conduct of their study. These may include the following, depending on the nature of the study:

1. Research is to be conducted according to the proposal that was approved by the IRB.

2. Changes to the protocol or its related consent document are to be approved by the IRB before implementation.

3. Adverse events are to be reported promptly to the IRB.

4. Subjects are to receive a copy of the consent document, if appropriate.

5. Regulations require records be retained for at least 3 years. Records of studies that collect protected health information are to be retained for 6 years.

6. Any future correspondence should include the IRB identification number provided and the study title.

Consent Document

The final draft of the consent document for an approved project should be stamped or somehow flagged as "IRB approved" with the date of final approval indicated. This documentation may be done with a "stamped" hard copy of the consent form sent to the investigator as an enclosure with the approval letter. Thanks to a variety of electronic methods, the IRB-approved consent document may be distributed to the investigator via e-mail or through an on-line system. Some sponsors require the expiration date on the form and the version date to appear on every page of the consent document.

Importance of Documentation

The two primary methods of "adequate documentation of IRB activities" are through the minutes of the IRB meeting and the maintenance of materials related to IRB-reviewed research studies. Audits conducted by sponsors and federal agencies rely exclusively on recorded information.

Preparation of Minutes

Title 45 CFR 46.115 (2)

Minutes of IRB meetings which shall be in sufficient detail to show attendance at the meetings; actions taken by the IRB; the vote on these actions including the number of members voting for, against, and abstaining; the basis for requiring changes in or disapproving research; and a written summary of the discussion of controverted issues and their resolution.

This regulation lists the items to be documented in the IRB minutes for every study reviewed. The template included as an appendix to this chapter is an example that allows each section to be completed with a few words that summarize the result of IRB deliberations. There is no reason to recount actual meeting conversations. We strongly advise against including information such as "Dr. Smith said, 'The study is unethical.'" In our opinion, it is a mistake to match any statement with a member's name in the minutes. As the regulation states, the minutes are to be a summary "of the discussion of controverted issues and their resolutions."

In other sections of the regulations, the words "the IRB finds and documents that…" or "the IRB finds…" or "… the IRB shall determine…" indicate specific issues to be addressed in the minutes or specifically documented elsewhere.

Examples (emphasis added)

Title 45 CFR 46.405

DHHS will conduct or fund research in which the IRB finds that more than minimal risk to children is presented by an intervention or procedure that holds out the prospect of direct benefit for the individual subject or by a monitoring procedure that is likely to contribute to the subject's well being, only if the IRB finds that…

45 CFR 46.111 Criteria for IRB Approval of Research

(a) In order to approve research covered by this policy the IRB shall determine that all of the following requirements are satisfied…

45 CFR 46.116(d)

An IRB may approve a consent procedure which does not include, or which alters, some or all of the elements of informed consent set forth in this section, or waive the requirements to obtain informed consent provided the IRB finds and documents that…

45 CFR 46.117(c)

An IRB may waive the requirement for the investigator to obtain a signed consent form for some or all subjects if it finds either…

In addition, if the research involves one of the special classes of subjects requiring additional protections (fetuses, pregnant women, human in vitro fertilization [subpart B], prisoners [subpart C], or children [subpart D]), a description that the appropriate regulations and requirements have been met, such as assent, should be recorded in the minutes and/or study file.

The ability to take the minutes of the meeting directly on a computer during the meeting proceedings is a great advantage. Even if that is not possible at your site, using the agenda outline for the preparation of the minutes is very helpful.

After the minutes have been reviewed and signed by the chair, the original should be filed in the IRB office. Copies of the minutes need to be distributed to IRB members and, in many cases, to other boards within your institution. IRB-member copies are often included with their materials for the next IRB meeting.

IRB Maintenance of Research Study Materials

Some IRBs use a primary reviewer checklist that documents the issues required for regulatory compliance. A potential problem with these checklist systems is that they rely on one reviewer to document all of the essential issues. Other IRBs require the submission of a protocol summary in which the investigator responds to a checklist similar to the one just described.

Regardless of the method of documentation about IRB meeting discussions, the IRB office is to maintain research study materials. This is still most often accomplished with files of hard copy documentation; however, electronic record maintenance is now possible.

What to Save for Each Study

1. The completed and signed application to the IRB
2. The IRB application form that summarizes the research plan
3. The stamped or dated approved consent document, if appropriate
4. Scientific reviews or opinions of consultants
5. Approval letters from other committees (e.g., the radiation safety committee)
6. Recruitment forms or advertisements for the study
7. The sponsor protocol or grant proposal
8. Attachments specific to the protocol (articles, surveys, questionnaires, investigator's brochures, etc.)
9. The IRB determination letter
10. Communications with the investigator

Throughout the life of a study, everything the IRB receives should be retained, preferably in chronologic order. This may include items such as adverse events reports, advertisements submitted for approval, changes or amendments submitted for approval, reapprovals granted, and so forth.

Tracking a Study
Tracking systems are discussed in detail in Chapter 2-3. Most institutions will track the status of each study with an electronic database system. After the IRB meeting, immediate updating of the database assures an accurate database.

The researcher is ultimately responsible for submitting timely renewal materials; however, most IRB offices have set up an "automatic" system of notification of upcoming study renewal reviews via an internal tracking system.

IRB Fee Invoicing

When IRBs charge for reviews, a system is needed to generate and track invoices. Details of this process will be specific to each institution. In some cases, a financial person or department will need the IRB office to provide a list of studies to generate the appropriate invoices. In most cases, generating a list of the studies according to review category (full board versus expedited) will be sufficient (see Chapter 2-6: *Charging for IRB Review*).

Conclusion

This chapter explained and provided tools for the administrative tasks to be accomplished after a full-committee IRB meeting. Although the need to document IRB activities in compliance with federal research regulation drives much of the process, prompt and clear communication with researchers also fosters a positive relationship with your research community.

References
1. Code of Federal Regulations. Title 45A—Department of Health and Human Services; Part 46—Protection of Human Subjects. Updated 1 October, 1997. Access date 18 April, 2001. http://www4.law.cornell.edu/cfr/45p46.htm
2. Code of Federal Regulations. Title 21, Chapter 1—Food and Drug Administration, DHHS; Part 56—Institutional Review Boards. Updated 1 April, 1999. Access date 27 March, 2001. http://www4.law.cornell.edu/cfr/21p56.htm

Appendix

IRB Full-Committee Minutes Template

Date:

Minutes from last month's meeting: The minutes from last month's meeting (or give date) were reviewed. There were no controversial entries or objections. The committee voted unanimously to approve the minutes.

Continuing education: The following items were distributed to all committee members before the meeting. The committee discussed these items with specific emphasis on the implications for future IRB practice.

Announcements:

Individual protocol reviews:
Protocol number and title
Type of review: Initial, Continuing, Revision, Adverse Event

For each initial protocol review:
Committee review included, but was not limited to, evaluation of the following issues:

The investigator: The investigator in charge of this project is qualified to conduct this study, and there are no conflicts of interest that would be expected to compromise the integrity of the study.

Vulnerable populations: The study does not specifically target people who have traditionally been considered "vulnerable" from the standpoint of needing additional protection from the risks associated with research participation.

The study specifically targets people who have traditionally been considered "vulnerable" from the standpoint of needing additional protection from the risks associated with research participation: children, adults who are not competent to give informed consent, pregnant women, prisoners, the mentally disabled, educationally or economically disadvantaged persons.

In this study, the investigator is sensitive to the ethical issues involved with research involving vulnerable subjects and is committed to conducting the research according to the highest of ethical standards. Specific safeguards include:

Informed consent: Written informed consent will be obtained from the subject.

This study may enroll children: Written informed consent will be obtained from the child's parent or guardian/both parents. When appropriate, verbal assent will be obtained from the subjects.

This study may enroll adult subjects who are not competent to give informed consent: Written informed consent will be obtained from the subjects legally authorized representative.

Birth control: Pregnancy is an exclusion criterion for this study. Women of childbearing potential may participate in this study. A pregnancy test is/is not required to participate in the study. Subjects are instructed not to become pregnant during this study. Birth control is recommended. This study may involve men who may be sexually active. Sexually active men are advised to use a condom during sexual intercourse.

Subject recruitment: Subjects will be recruited from the _____ (example: cardiology clinic). The person recruiting subjects may be/will not be the subject's health care provider. A research advertisement will/will not be used. The method and form of advertisement are acceptable.

Genetic testing: This study involves/does not involve testing for genetic markers that are known to predict for the development of disease.

Tissue repository: This study involves/does not involve the storage of tissue for future research. Tissue samples are/are not linked to personal identifiers. If yes, the procedures for collecting, storing, and controlling access to tissue samples appear to be adequate to protect the rights of research participants.

Cost of research participation relative to the nonresearch alternative: This study does/does not involve increased costs to participants relative to a research alternative. If yes, the increase in cost is ethical in this situation and adequately explained in the consent document.

Payment or reimbursements to research participants: This study does/does not reimburse or pay subjects for their participation in the study. If yes, the level and schedule of reimbursement/payment is reasonable in relation to study procedures. The investigators are sensitive to the issue of coercion and undue influence. Subjects for whom the payment is likely to be coercive will be excluded from the study.

Risks (relative to nonresearch alternative): The risks and discomforts of research participation were thoroughly evaluated. Risks are minimized by study design. The main risks of research participation are adequately summarized in the consent document.

Potential benefits: The committee determined that participation in this study:

- will not directly benefit research participants
- may directly benefit research participants

The study may benefit people in the future.

Altruism is the main reason that someone would participate in this study.

Risk/benefit ratio: Risks of research participation are reasonable in view of potential benefits.

Confidentiality: Provisions to protect the privacy of subjects and the confidentiality of data are adequate.

Data oversight: Study design provides for ongoing monitoring for the purpose of identifying unexpected results that would indicate a need for study revision. Data oversight will be performed by the principal investigator, the study sponsor, and a formal Data and Safety Monitoring Board.

Consent document: The consent document accurately describes the important aspects of this study. Recognizing that participants are expected to discuss the details of the study with members of the research team, the consent document is likely to be understood by study participants. Revisions in the consent document that are required before final study approval can be granted include:

Vote (quorum): approve, conditionally approve, not approve, abstain.

Interval of IRB approval: The study was approved for 12 months. The committee specifically addressed the issue of the degree of risk of the study when determining the approval interval.

PART 6

Informed Consent

The Institutional Review Board's Role in Editing the Consent Document

Robin L. Penslar

INTRODUCTION

Many institutional review board (IRB) critics have charged that IRBs spend an inordinate amount of their time and resources on the consent document. However, in my view, the time IRBs spend on consent documents is not misplaced. Consent documents are not more important than the assessment of risk and ensuring that risks are minimized, but the consent materials submitted to IRBs are often of such a poor quality that they require considerable time and effort to ensure that subjects are properly informed and that their consent is appropriately documented. The way IRBs go about ensuring that the final product is appropriate may vary, and I hope to offer here some advice about how they might do that. First, however, I want to provide IRBs support for their efforts.

Importance of the Consent Document

The fact that IRBs spend so much time on the informed consent document has drawn a certain amount of criticism, with critics implying that the IRB has become no more than a high-powered editing team. Nevertheless, because informed consent forms one of the cornerstones of the ethical conduct of research involving humans, it is imperative that IRBs ensure that participants are informed about and voluntarily consent to participation. That means that the study must not go forward until the IRB is assured that the consent process will take place in a way that ensures that prospective subjects' informed, voluntary decision to participate is not compromised and that the informed consent document communicates the necessary information in a meaningful, understandable way.

Document Versus Process

Although I am going to focus here on the consent document, I also want to stress that IRBs must insist that investigators[*] not refer to the consent document as "the consent." I am not saying that investigators do not, on some level, recognize the difference, but the language that is used is important, and IRBs must insist that the difference is acknowledged. Investigators must understand the difference between the presentation of information and even the signing of a consent document and bona fide consent as such. The document is not consent; it is only the record of what was supposed to have been communicated—something for participants or prospective participants to take home to help them remember what they have agreed to do or think about doing. (It is not, however, proof of what participants actually understood or proof that they

---

[*]I refer in the text to the investigator as the author of the consent document for the sake of simplicity. Readers whose experience with IRBs and human research is in the context of clinical trials may find references to the investigator rather than the sponsor misplaced. Although the investigator is responsible for obtaining IRB approval and is also responsible for obtaining informed consent, consent documents for clinical trials sponsored by pharmaceutical companies are prepared by the sponsor company and submitted for review and approval by each site investigator's local IRB. References in the text to "the investigator" should be understood to refer to either the sponsor, the investigator or both, as appropriate to the particular circumstances of the study under review. For example, in many large, multisite clinical trials, a central IRB reviews a template consent prepared by the sponsor. Either the same IRB or many local IRBs then review the individual investigators' local versions, which may be modified from the sponsor's template to account for issues relevant to the local context and which also contain additional site-specific information.

voluntarily consented, even it if says "I understand that . . ." and "I voluntarily consent. . . .") For many subjects, however, it is also the primary means through which they learn the details of the study. For many studies, the consent process is something like the following:

1. Tell the prospective subject that there is a study in which he or she might want to participate.
2. Give the prospective subject a consent form to read.
3. Ask the prospective subject whether he or she has any questions.
4. Ask the prospective subject to sign the form.

To be fair, I think that some of the confusion between process and document may have developed because the consent document has become the means through which investigators tell the IRB what it will tell subjects about the study, that is, the contents of the informed consent process. In that sense then, the consent document and the consent process overlap. However, they are conceptually distinct, and in my opinion, IRBs must be vigilant in ensuring that the distinction is recognized. With that being said, the consent document is the only means that IRBs have for determining what subjects will be told about the study and the language that will be used to provide that information.

The Importance of Grammar and Punctuation

Although they have to take care that the requested changes to consent documents are meaningful, IRBs must not blindly accept criticism that they are just nitpicking at the grammar or punctuation of the consent form. Consent documents often do not clearly communicate that the addressee is being invited to participate in research, what the study is trying to discover, what the procedures are, what the material risks are, and so forth. Even when all of the relevant information is in the document (comments regarding the length of consent documents will be left to another day), it may be scattered, use lingo, not make sense, have mistakes (e.g., information in the protocol does not match information in the consent document), or provide contradictory information. If the document is ungrammatical, it does not communicate; if it does not communicate, it cannot serve its purpose. If the investigator cannot produce a proper consent document, then either the study must be rejected or the IRB must redraft the consent; the investigator must wait for study approval until the document satisfies the IRB.

Education of Investigators

IRBs should not give up on investigators. They can learn to prepare proper consents—I have seen them. An IRB that invests time in an educational effort can train its investigators and sponsors, and this investment of time will reduce review time in the long run.

Although IRB members may be frustrated with the quality of consent materials, simply sending materials back with the directive to "rewrite this" is not helpful. A great deal of literature on consent and drafting consent

documents is not heeded; the question is how best to serve prospective subjects while providing timely reviews. I am arguing here that IRBs, who understand the issues the best, should accept the role of editor for projects submitted to them while working to improve the quality of consents-as-submitted for future projects. Investigators are so overwhelmed by the size of submission packets and instructional materials that they simply shut down, unable to absorb what they perceive as an unwarrantedly complex review process. They can benefit most from exemplary material for use in guiding the preparation of their submission together with the changes that are requested during the review. Often, subsequent submissions improve as the investigator implements in the first instance things that were changed in the earlier review. I would then suggest that educational efforts take place at two points in time: before the review and during the review.

As Part of the Presubmission Process

1. Prepare template consent materials, and make them available to investigators.
2. Distinguish between "required" language and "suggested" language.
3. If the IRB has decided that only certain language is acceptable, say so and provide it as part of the application packet.
4. If the IRB can provide suggested approaches to express various issues, provide several examples. Make it clear that the IRB will consider alternative language but that the examples provided have been determined to be acceptable ways to handle an issue.
5. Do not try to force investigators to use specific language unless it truly is necessary. However, at times, there are good reasons for insisting on certain language. Do not be intimidated by investigators who are anxious to begin the project and insist (for example) that the IRB is costing the university thousands of dollars by holding up their enrollments.
6. Remind investigators to review the consent before submitting it to the IRB to make sure that it addresses issues in the investigator's brochure or IRB application where risks, benefits, and procedures are described to make sure that there are not any contradictions and that all relevant risks are described. As a reviewer, I have often observed that the consent seems to be written from memory rather than from reference to the study documents.
7. Provide investigators a comprehensive list of the information that must go into a consent, with contingencies for various kinds of activities (e.g., videotaping, pregnancy testing, placebos).
8. Prepare advice for submitting investigators that addresses various issues that arise repeatedly. For example, warn investigators that if a study involves minors, they need to prepare an assent document as well as a parental permission document. Advise them to take care in the permission and assent documents' language regarding who is signing the document. Often, the language used in the parental permission confuses the parent's actions as opposed to the child's; keep clear what the parent is doing (allowing his child to do X if the child agrees, plus any activities that the parent is specifically required to do) and what the child is doing (the study procedures).

9. Prepare information about the consent issues in research in various settings (e.g., schools, workplaces) or when various relationships require special handling (e.g., a teacher who wants to do research in his or her own classroom).

10. Provide examples of what is meant by sixth- to eighth-grade reading level. One way to do this might be to provide an example of typical consent language describing a procedure alongside a second version written in simpler language.

In Response to the Investigator During the Review

1. Tell the investigator exactly what you want, and where possible, provide the exact language you want to be used or give sufficient, well-worded instructions about the issue and options for handling it. In most cases, it is unhelpful to say simply, "The risks are not clear" or "Include a statement about voluntariness." As advised earlier, be prepared to accept alternative wording if it satisfies the IRB's concerns.

2. Designate a single member of the IRB to be the primary consent editor. If your IRB charges for reviews, include a charge for consent editing, and pay a member a stipend for editing to cover the additional time editing takes.

3. Make clear to investigators that the final step before approval of the study will be a thorough edit of the consent document for readability. That way they will be forewarned that there will likely be more than one set of revisions to the consent document.

4. When communicating with the investigator about the approved consent document, suggest that he or she refer to the requested changes when preparing future submissions; this can reduce the review time that will be required. In other words, suggest that investigators use the approved consent as a kind of template for future submissions, taking into account differences in the study design and special aspects of the studies (e.g., involvement of children or persons of childbearing capacity, special confidentiality issues, etc.).

Conclusion

The time IRBs spend reviewing and editing consent documents is not misplaced. The consent document is one of the most important elements of the informed consent process. IRBs must be satisfied that informed consent documents communicate the necessary information in language that is likely to be understood by potential research subjects. In my opinion, it is the responsibility of the IRB to revise the consent document as needed when the researcher or sponsor is unable or unwilling to do so.

The Consent Document

Angela J. Bowen

INTRODUCTION

Institutional review board (IRB) members always hope that the consent document is only one step in the consent process. We know from experience, however, that it is not always so. The consent document should be clear and descriptive enough to stand alone in describing the essential elements of informed consent. This is not to say that the consent document should describe every event or potential risk that might be encountered by a study participant. Excessive detail may actually compromise the effectiveness of the consent document as an educational tool. As a basic guideline, the consent document should explain all of the information that a reasonable person would want to know to decide about research participation. The written format provides the subject with a continuing reference to the details of the research project and a historical reference, if needed. The review and processing of the document itself are often the most time-consuming parts of the entire review process. Although some of this is inevitable, there are economies of time that can be built into the system.

Processing the Document

As in most IRB staff work, there is no substitute for a well-trained staff member who knows the regulations and can write simple, declarative sentences. Most IRBs receive consent forms in a "finished" condition. That is to say, the sender thinks the document is finished. This is rarely the case. If the consent comes from the sponsor, it is likely to be too technical for the average reader. If the investigator has written it, expect the language to be on the reassuring side.

Have a seasoned staff member read the consent document before the full-committee meeting to be sure that it contains all of the required elements of informed consent. They are listed here:

1. Informed consent shall include the following elements.

   a. Statement that the study involves research (DHHS 45 CFR § 46.116(a)(1); FDA 21 CFR § 50.23(a)(1); ICH E6 § 4.8.10(a))

   b. Explanation of the purposes of the research (DHHS 45 CFR § 46.116(a)(1); FDA 21 CFR § 50.23(a)(1); ICH E6 § 4.8.10(b))

   c. Expected duration of the subject's participation in the research (DHHS 45 CFR § 46.116(a)(1); FDA 21 CFR § 50.23(a)(1); ICH E6 § 4.8.10(s))

   d. Description of the procedures to be followed (DHHS 45 CFR § 46.116(a)(1); FDA 21 CFR § 50.23(a)(1); ICH E6 § 4.8.10(d))

   e. Identification of any procedures that are experimental (DHHS 45 CFR § 46.116(a)(1); FDA 21 CFR § 50.25(a)(1); ICH E6 § 4.8.10(f))

   f. Description of any reasonably foreseeable risks or discomforts to the subject (DHHS 45 CFR § 46.116(a)(2); FDA 21 CFR § 50.25(a)(2); ICH E6 § 4.8.10(g))

   g. Description of any benefits to the subject or to others that may reasonably be expected from the research (DHHS 45 CFR § 46.116(a)(3); FDA 21 CFR § 50.25(a)(3); ICH E6 § 4.8.10(h))

   h. Disclosure of appropriate alternative procedures or courses of treatment, if any, that might be advantageous to the subject (DHHS 45 CFR § 46.116(a)(4); FDA 21 CFR § 50.25(a)(4); ICH E6 § 4.8.10(i))

   i. Statement describing the extent, if any, to which confidentiality of records identifying the subject will be maintained, and if applicable, a statement of the possibility that the Food and Drug Administration may inspect the records (DHHS 45 CFR § 46.116(a)(5); FDA 21 CFR § 50.25(a)(5); ICH E6 § 4.8.10(n) and (o))

   j. For research involving more than minimal risk, an explanation as to whether any compensation is available if injury occurs, whether any medical treatments are available if injury occurs, and if so, what they consist of or where further information can be obtained (DHHS 45 CFR § 46.116(a)(6); FDA 21 CFR § 50.25(a)(6); ICH E6 § 4.8.10(j))

   k. Explanation of whom to contact for answers to pertinent questions about the research, research subject's rights, and whom to contact in the event of a research-related injury to the subject (DHHS 45 CFR § 46.116(a)(7); FDA 21 CFR § 50.25(a)(7); ICH E6 § 4.8.10(q))

   l. Statement that participation is voluntary, that refusal to participate involves no penalty or loss of benefits to which the subject is otherwise entitled, and that the subject may discontinue participation at any time without penalty or loss of benefits to which the subject is otherwise entitled (DHHS 45 CFR § 46.116(a)(8); FDA 21 CFR § 50.25(a)(8); ICH E6 § 4.8.10(m))

2. When appropriate, one or more of the following elements of information shall also be provided to each subject:

a. A statement that the particular treatment or procedure may involve risks to the subject (or to the embryo or fetus if the subject is or may become pregnant) that are currently unforeseeable (DHHS 45 CFR § 46.116(b)(1); FDA 21 CFR § 50.25(b)(1))

b. Anticipated circumstances under which the subject's participation may be terminated by the investigator without regard to the subject's consent (DHHS 45 CFR § 46.116(b)(2); FDA 21 CFR § 50.25(b)(2); ICH E6 § 4.8.10(r))

c. Any additional costs to the subject that may result from participation in the research (DHHS 45 CFR § 46.116(b)(3); FDA 21 CFR § 50.25(b)(3); ICH E6 § 4.8.10(l))

d. Consequence of a subject's decision to withdraw from the research and procedures for orderly termination of participation by the subject (DHHS 45 CFR § 46.116(b)(4); FDA 21 CFR § 50.25(b)(4))

e. Statement that significant new findings developed during the course of the research, which may relate to the subject's willingness to continue, will be provided to the subject (DHHS 45 CFR § 46.116(b)(5); FDA 21 CFR § 50.25(b)(5); ICH E6 § 4.8.10(p))

f. Approximate number of subjects involved in the study (DHHS 45 CFR § 46.116(b)(6); FDA 21 CFR § 50.25(b)(6); ICH E6 § 4.8.10(t))

g. Study treatment(s) and the probability of random assignment to placebo or to each treatment (ICH E6 § 4.8.10(c))

h. The IRB may require that information, in addition to that required in Federal Regulations (DHHS 45 CFR Part 46; FDA 21 CFR Part 50) and ICH § 4.8 be given to research subjects when in its judgment the information would meaningfully add to the protection of the rights and welfare of subjects (DHHS 45 CFR § 46.109(b); FDA 21 CFR § 56.109(b); ICH E6 § 3.1.5).

If there are missing elements, staff can prepare a "redlined" version to go to the IRB, using autotext that has been previously approved by the IRB for use in such cases, or can request such language from the investigator. In no case should an incomplete document be sent to the IRB for review, as this only wastes precious IRB time. It cannot be emphasized enough that the use of a system whereby an experienced reviewer revises the consent document is needed before the full-committee meeting. The IRB system was not set up with the idea that the full committee would spend time polishing the wording of the consent document. Most institutions have drafted certain stock language for confidentiality, compensation for injury, etc. These are acceptable practices that save considerable time during review.

Reviewing the Document

The IRB as a whole may review the proposed consent document, or the primary reviewer system can be used. In the latter case, the consent document is assigned to a nonphysician IRB member who recommends to the IRB necessary changes to make the final version readable at an elementary level. IRB members may then comment and discuss until consensus is reached.

Some IRBs make the necessary changes and send the approved version to the investigator, along with notice of what changes have been made and why. If the investigator does not accept all of the changes made by the IRB, it will be necessary to resubmit and await further review. This system is preferred because it saves the IRB time and energy, improves the efficiency of the IRB process, and creates good will between the IRB and research community. However, some IRBs view this process as unacceptable because they do not like the idea of "doing work that the investigator should do." There are IRBs that use the full-board meeting to identify changes that should be made to the consent document. Then they send the submitted document back unapproved and request that the investigator try again. The belief, apparently, is that this exercise will provide engagement of the investigator into the consent process and provide needed instruction as well. This may be a useful approach in institutions where teaching young investigators is a part of the IRB's responsibility, but it certainly decreases IRB efficiency and is likely to compromise respect for the IRB process within the institution.

Whatever process is employed, careful review by a convened IRB must occur. After this review, the document must be approved and the pertinent discussions captured in the minutes. If the IRB has required additional changes, the reasons for these changes must be noted as well.

Finally, the document should be stamped "approved" on each page. This detail will prevent unauthorized changes, or at least render them easier to detect. The approval stamp should also include the date of approval and the designation of the approving IRB. Some boards include an expiration date, usually 1 year after initial approval.

If the board is making the required changes and sending out finished work, careful proofing must be included in the process. The chair, or designee, should assure that all IRB-directed changes were captured in the final version.

If the investigator is making the IRB-directed changes and preparing the final document, there must be included in the process some procedure for assuring that all of the IRB's directed changes have been carried out. This will require resubmission of the prepared final consent document for comparison with the original and the IRB-recommended changes. The final, complete version can then be stamped with the IRB's imprimatur as described previously here.

A copy of the final, approved version should be retained in the IRB's file for the study. The form, as submitted, should also be retained in the official study record.

Much has been written about the readability of consent forms. In the evaluation of this important element, the IRB should take into account the demographics of the population likely to be recruited into the research and make adjustments accordingly.

Conclusion

The consent document must be clear and descriptive enough to stand alone in describing the essential elements of informed consent. As a basic guideline, the consent document should contain all information that a reasonable person would want to know to decide about research participation. Information beyond this simple standard is likely to compromise the consent process. This chapter presents recommendations for processing the consent document before the IRB meeting and reviewing the document at the meeting.

Regulation Resources

Sections of several documents were cited in the text in abbreviated form.

DHHS 45 CFR 46

Code of Federal Regulations. Title 45A—Department of Health and Human Services; Part 46—Protection of Human Subjects. Updated 1 October, 1997. Access date 18 April, 2001. http://www4law.cornell.edu/cfr/45p46.htm

FDA 21 CFR 50

Code of Federal Regulations. Title 21, Chapter 1—Food and Drug Administration, DHHS; Part 50—Protection of Human Subjects. Updated 1 April, 1999. Access date 18 April, 2001. http://www4.law.cornell.edu/cfr/21p50.htm

FDA 21 CFR 56

Code of Federal Regulations. Title 21, Chapter 1—Food and Drug Administration, DHHS; Part 56—Institutional Review Boards. Updated 1 April, 1999. Access date 27 March, 2001. http://www4.law.cornell.edu/cfr/21p56.htm

ICH E6 Sections 3.1 and 4.8

Food and Drug Administration. International Conference on Harmonisation: Good clinical practice. Published in the *Federal Register*, Vol. 62, No. 90, May 9, 1997, pp. 25691–25709. http://www.ifpma.org/ich5e.html

Exculpatory Language in Informed Consent Documents

Michele Russell-Einhorn and Thomas Puglisi

INTRODUCTION

Investigators are frequently admonished by their institutional review boards (IRBs) to refrain from using exculpatory language in their informed consent documents (and, just as importantly, throughout the consent process). Almost as frequently, this admonishment comes with little or no explanation of what constitutes "exculpatory language." Indeed, many IRBs seem confused about where to draw the line in determining whether a proposed statement is exculpatory. The purpose of this chapter is to explain how IRB members and researchers can identify and avoid the use of exculpatory language in the consent.

Federal Regulations

Whenever there is doubt about a regulatory requirement, a careful reading of the regulatory language itself is an important starting point. Federal policy (the Common Rule) for the protection of human subjects in research sets forth the following prohibition.

> No informed consent, whether oral or written, may include any exculpatory language through which the subject or the representative is made to waive or appear to waive any of the subject's legal rights or releases or appears to release the investigator, the sponsor, the institution or its agents from liability for negligence.[1]

This prohibition is codified in exactly the same language in regulations of the Department of Health and Human Services (DHHS)[2(Sec.116)] and the Food and Drug Administration (FDA).[3(Sec.20)]

The Narrow (But Incorrect) Interpretation

A narrow interpretation of the regulatory language would limit the prohibition to statements involving a release from liability. Those who argue in favor of the narrow interpretation point out that in common usage (as verified by any current dictionary), the word *exculpatory* relates to lack of guilt. This is also the case relative to its usage in law. According to *Black's Law Dictionary*,[4] *exculpatory* involves clearing "from alleged fault or guilt" or releasing "from liability" for "wrongful acts."

The Broad (Correct) Interpretation

These arguments notwithstanding, the DHHS, through the Office for Protection from Research Risks (OPRR), its successor Office for Human Research Protections (OHRP), and the FDA, has a long history of applying a much broader interpretation of the exculpatory language

prohibition. A careful reading of the regulatory language reveals that, in this context, the meaning of the phrase *exculpatory language* is expanded to include any language "through which the subject or the representative is made to waive or *appear to waive* any of the subject's legal rights." Thus, any language waiving or appearing to waive any legal right (regardless of the nature of that right) is prohibited.

Practical Applications

In a practical sense, exculpatory statements tend to be statements in which a subject in a research protocol is asked to agree to or accept something, usually something unfavorable to the subject. A statement that sets forth simple facts, on the other hand, is usually not likely to be viewed as exculpatory.

In the following examples, the institution simply sets forth the facts describing the institution's intent and policy. These statements would not be considered exculpatory under the regulations, and would be permissible.

Examples
- The University Medical School has no policy or plan to pay for any injuries that you might receive as a result of participating in this research protocol.
- As part of the research protocol, the investigators will extract some cells from the blood you have donated. The university may commercialize some of these cells that derive from the research. The university does not plan to share any profits with the subject from whom the cells were obtained.

The following examples, however, would be considered exculpatory and are prohibited under the regulations. In these examples, subjects are being asked to make a statement that they agree with and accept the actions of the institution as a condition for participation in the research.

Examples

- I agree that the medical center will not pay me for any injuries that I might sustain as a result of participating in this research.
- I understand that the institution will not share with me any profits received from the sale or commercialization of any cells developed in this research.
- I agree that everything in this consent form is adequate and complies with the regulations.
- I understand that I will not sue the sponsor or the investigator for any negligence.
- Subjects agree to hold harmless all institutions, investigators, or sponsors affiliated with or in any way a part of this research protocol.

Again, a good rule of thumb is to state simply the factual situation and avoid any statement that requires the agreement or concurrence of the subject.

OHRP Guidance

The OHRP (formerly the OPRR) maintains a website that includes guidance on various topics relevant to the protection of human subjects in research. The OHRP's website includes the appended document on exculpatory language from the 1996 Cooperative Oncology Group Chairpersons Meeting.[5]

References

1. Federal Policy for Protection of Human Subjects (Common Rule). *Fed Regist* 56:28003, June 18, 1991 (Final Rule). Effective date August 19, 1991. Posted on University of Michigan IRB website. Access date 19 August, 2001. http://www.med.umich.edu/irbined/FederalDocuments/FedPolicy/FederalPolicy.html

2. Code of Federal Regulations. Title 45A—Department of Health and Human Services; Part 46—Protection of Human Subjects. Updated 1 October, 1997. Access date 18 April, 2001. http://www4.law.cornell.edu/cfr/45p46.htm

3. Code of Federal Regulations. Title 21, Chapter 1—Food and Drug Administration, DHHS; Part 50—Protection of Human Subjects. Updated 1 April, 1999. Access date 18 April, 2001. http://www4.law.cornell.edu/cfr/21p50.htm

4. Black HC. *Black's Law Dictionary: Definitions of the Terms and Phrases of American and English Jurisprudence, Ancient and Modern,* 6th ed. Nolan JR, Nolan-Haley JM (ed.). St. Paul, MN: West Publishing; 1990.

5. Office for Protection from Research Risks. "Exculpatory language" in informed consent. Cooperative Oncology Group Chairpersons Meeting, November 15, 1996. Access date 19 August, 2001. http://ohrp.osophs.dhhs.gov/humansubjects/guidance/exculp.htm

Appendix

Cooperative Oncology Group Chairpersons Meeting[5]
November 15, 1996

"Exculpatory Language" in Informed Consent

No informed consent, whether oral or written, may include any exculpatory language through which the subject is made to waive or appear to waive any of the subject's legal rights, or releases or appears to release the investigator, the sponsor, the institution, or its agents from liability for negligence (45 CFR 46.116).

Examples of Exculpatory Language

- By agreeing to this use, you should understand that you will give up all claim to personal benefit from commercial or other use of these substances.

- I voluntarily and freely donate any and all blood, urine, and tissue samples to the U.S. government and hereby relinquish all right, title, and interest to said items.

- By consent to participate in this research, I give up any property rights I may have in bodily fluids or tissue samples obtained in the course of the research.

- I waive any possibility of compensation for injuries that I may receive as a result of participation in this research.

Examples of Acceptable Language

- Tissue obtained from you in this research may be used to establish a cell line that could be patented and licensed. There are no plans to provide financial compensation to you should this occur.

- By consenting to participate, you authorize the use of your bodily fluids and tissue samples for the research described previously here.

- This hospital is not able to offer financial compensation nor to absorb the costs of medical treatment should you be injured as a result of participating in this research.

- This hospital makes no commitment to provide free medical care or payment for any unfavorable outcomes resulting from participation in this research. Medical services will be offered at the usual charge.

Requiring a Witness Signature on the Consent Form

Michele Russell-Einhorn and Thomas Puglisi

INTRODUCTION

Some institutional review boards (IRBs) require the signature of a witness on informed consent documents. The requirement for a witness signature could derive from four possible sources: (1) the Federal Policy (Common Rule) for the Protection of Human Subjects, (2) Food and Drug Administration (FDA) regulations, (3) state law, or (4) IRB or institutional policy.

Although specific situations—such as the use of a short form consent document—may require the use of the signature of a witness, there is no regulation that requires the signature on every informed consent document.

Federal Requirements

The Federal Policy (Common Rule) for the Protection of Human Subjects does not require a witness signature when the research uses a standard informed consent document that embodies all of the required elements of informed consent codified by the Department of Health and Human Services (DHHS) at 45 CFR 46.[1][Sec.116(a),(b)] Nor do the regulations require the investigator's signature when a standard consent document is used. In this situation, federal policy only requires that the consent document is signed by the subject or the subject's legally authorized representative.[1][Sec.117(b)(1)] FDA regulations add the requirement that the signature of the subject (or the legally authorized representative) must be dated.[2][Sec.50.27(a)]

The signature of a witness is required under federal policy only when the IRB authorizes the use of a "short-form written consent document."[1][Sec.117(b)(2)] In this situation, federal policy requires that the witness (1) observe the oral presentation of informed consent information to the subject, (2) sign the short-form written consent document, and (3) sign a copy of the summary of the oral presentation approved by the IRB. In addition, the summary must also be signed by the person obtaining consent, and the short-form consent document must also be signed by the subject or the subject's legally authorized representative. FDA regulations contain these same provisions.[2][Sec.27(b)(1),(2)]

State and Institutional Requirements

Although federal regulations require a witness signature on the informed consent document only in the circumstances described previously here, state laws regarding informed consent for research may require the signature of a witness in additional circumstances. It is important to understand that when state requirements provide protections for human subjects beyond those required under federal regulations, the more protective state requirements must be observed.

State laws vary widely as to the specificity of requirements for informed consent in research contexts. Consequently, IRBs have a responsibility to educate themselves thoroughly as to state law requirements.

In addition, an institution or an IRB may require the signature of a witness on informed consent documents as a matter of policy. Institutions and IRBs always have the authority to require protections for human subjects that exceed the minimum standards required under federal regulations.

The Purpose of Witness Signatures

It is important that investigators and IRBs understand the purpose of requiring witness signatures on informed consent documents. There are two key issues to be considered: (1) to what is the witness attesting, that is, what does the signature mean, and (2) under what circumstances should the witness refrain from signing the document?

Requiring that a witness merely observe the subject signing the consent document without witnessing any part of the consent process adds little or nothing to the goal of protecting human subjects. Such a requirement may serve to protect the investigator or the institution from liability, but it contributes nothing to the quality of the information exchange between investigator and subject.

On the other hand, a witness who observes the dialogue between the investigator and the human subject can qualitatively enhance the informed consent process. The mere presence of a witness–observer during the consent conference should motivate the investigator to ensure a complete and meaningful disclosure of information. The witness can then attest that the informed consent process included all required elements, that the subject appeared to be capable of making an informed decision, and that an opportunity was provided for the subject to ask questions of the investigator. In this situation, the witness signature means that the witness has observed a consent process that appeared to satisfy regulatory requirements.

Conclusion

To make the requirement for a witness signature meaningful, witnesses should be instructed about what to look for in observing the informed consent process and the circumstances under which they should decline to sign the informed consent document. If the witness observes any indication of coercion by the investigator or lack of understanding on the part of the subject, it would be appropriate for the witness to refrain from signing the informed consent document.

Finally, whether or not the signature of a witness is required, the fundamental purpose of informed consent must be honored. By whatever means, the subject must be provided with sufficient information to make a truly informed, voluntary decision free from coercion or undue influence. Regardless of the circumstances, any witness signature requirement should be made with the goal of serving this fundamental purpose.

References

1. Code of Federal Regulations. Title 45A—Department of Health and Human Services; Part 46—Protection of Human Subjects. Updated 1 October, 1997. Access date 18 April, 2001. http://www4.law.cornell.edu/cfr/45p46.htm
2. Code of Federal Regulations. Title 21, Chapter 1—Food and Drug Administration, DHHS; Part 50—Protection of Human Subjects. Updated 1 April, 1999. Access date 18 April, 2001. http://www4.law.cornell.edu/cfr/21p50.htm

Deception of Research Subjects

Laurie Slone and Jay Hull

INTRODUCTION

The purpose of this chapter is to discuss research in which the subject is intentionally deceived about research participation. Deception is common in studies that evaluate fundamental aspects of human behavior. The rationale for deception in this setting is that it is not possible to obtain accurate information about how people behave when they know that they are being observed or evaluated.

Despite its possible justification, the use of deception creates ethical problems for researchers. Although many would argue that some forms of deception can be justified, most would also argue that those who would use deception in their research must explicitly justify its use in their particular case. The very practice of deception may create harm, exacerbate harm created in other ways, and raise difficult issues regarding the nature and meaning of informed consent. Arguments against the use of deception are usually weighed against arguments in favor of the benefits of gaining knowledge about the causes of human behavior. This chapter explores both the costs and the benefits of the use of deception in psychological research for the purpose of outlining specific issues with which institutional review boards (IRBs) need to be concerned. The goal of this chapter is to describe when the use of deception may be considered justifiable as well as to indicate what forms of deception should not be tolerated.

Background

The use of deception in research on human behavior has been debated extensively over the past 40 years. Ironically, much of this debate was initially triggered by what many consider one of the most important sets of social psychological experiments ever conducted: research on obedience by Stanley Milgram (1963). In the Milgram studies, participants were recruited to participate in a "teacher–learner experiment." When they arrived, they were told that they were to play the role of the teacher. The other "participant" in the study was to play the role of the learner and was taken to a room next door. The "teacher" was told that the study concerned the effects of punishment on learning and that each time the "learner" made a mistake, he or she was to administer an electric shock. Shocks started at 15 volts, and for each mistake, the subsequent shock was to be increased by 15 volts. The maximum shock was labeled 450 volts and was two steps beyond the designation "Danger: Severe Shock." If at any time the "teacher" balked at administering the shocks, the experimenter adhered to a script that basically told the participant to continue and that the experimenter would

take responsibility for any consequences of the participant's action.

In actuality, (1) the study did not concern learning but rather concerned the causes of obedience; (2) the "student" was a confederate of the experimenter and did not receive any shocks, and (3) the behavior of interest was not the ability of the student to learn but rather the amount of shock that the participant would administer. As reported by Milgram,[1] independent judges estimated that very few people (1%) would go all of the way to the end of the shock scale. In fact, the majority of participants (65%) administered shocks up to and including the highest levels possible.

The Milgram experiment includes classic elements of many social psychological experiments that use deception: a "cover story" providing a plausible but inaccurate account of the purpose of the study, a "confederate" pretending to be another participant in the study, and misdirection regarding the particular behaviors of interest to the researchers. The Milgram experiments are also widely cited as some of the most important ever conducted in social psychology. This is because they provide striking insights into an aspect of human behavior held to be responsible for some of the worst atrocities of the twentieth century: unquestioned obedience to authority, as witnessed in the horrors of the Holocaust. As a consequence, these obedience studies place, in stark contrast, arguments for and against the use of deception in research on human behavior.

One of the most vocal early critics of the Milgram studies was Herbert Kelman. Kelman[2] argued that deception in psychological experimentation generally—and in the Milgram studies specifically—is unethical, potentially harmful to the research participant, harmful to the profession, and ultimately harmful to society. There is no denying that participants in Milgram's research were distressed by the experience. They were visibly upset during the experiment, and some were upset at the conclusion of the experiment when they realized the implications of their actions. They realized their own capacity to do harm to others—a lesson that was unaffected when they subsequently learned that no one was actually shocked. Kelman's other argument—that the use of deceptive research is harmful to the reputation of the profession and to society as a whole—appears to be less persuasive.

In counterpoint to Kelman's and others' critiques,[3] many have argued[4] that social psychological research often requires deceptive techniques. The argument for the selective use of deception in research is essentially twofold. First, it is important to understand the causes of human behavior (e.g., why and when people conform, what conditions facilitate and impede helping behavior, why people are aggressive, and the causes of prejudiced behavior). Second, to discern the true causes of such behavior, research at a minimum requires that the participant does not know the topic under investigation. Thus, for example, it is argued that one cannot study the dynamics of conformity by asking participants whether they would or would not go along with the majority when the latter was obviously wrong. Rather, one must lead a participant to believe that he or she is the only individual in a group to hold a particular opinion.[5] Similarly, one cannot study helping behavior by having people imagine how they would behave if they heard another person cry for help. Rather, one must lead them to believe that another person actually needs help, and observe what they do.[6] According to a review by Gross and Fleming,[7] 90% of the studies on compliance/conformity, altruism, and aggression use deceptive techniques. In addition, 50% or more of the studies on attribution processes, achievement motivation, attraction/affiliation, attitude formation/consistency/change, nonverbal communication, bargaining, self-disclosure, self-awareness, and interpersonal equity use deceptive techniques. In essence then, "experimenters often find themselves in the troublesome position of concealing the truth from their subjects in order to reveal a truth about human behavior."[8]

Milgram's research is itself a good example that a person's response to a hypothetical situation cannot be taken as representative of how that person would actually act. Although a small minority of individuals was thought to be capable of administering extreme shocks, in point of fact, a majority of people actually did. Multiple well-established lines of research provide support for the claim that individuals do not actually know why they do what they do, but this does not stop them from making up coherent accounts of their actions. These accounts are often at odds with the actual causes of their behavior in such circumstances.[9] Thus, simply asking participants to "role play" how they would act in a particular situation does not produce the same behavior as that actually observed by "naive" participants.[10] Some researchers are interested in studying such "as if" behaviors in the sense that the stories people tell about how they would act and the theories they have about themselves and others are themselves interesting objects of study. However, few would claim that these behaviors are governed by the same processes that yield spontaneous behavior when confronting actual situations.

Thus, the argument is made that to build a base of knowledge on what causes people to act certain ways, one must examine their behavior in situations they regard as "real." This often requires deception.

Guidelines for Research Involving Deception

If one grants that it is impossible to study certain aspects of human behavior without adopting deceptive techniques, then the justification of such research evolves into a question of costs and benefits: the benefits gained by knowledge relative to the potential harm caused by deception. To some extent, this is a question of personal values. However, it also suggests that specific codes of conduct should be developed that serve to minimize the negative impact of deceptive techniques. The American Psychological Association (APA) has developed just such a code.[11] The two sections relevant to deception in research are presented here.

8.07 Deception in Research

(a) Psychologists do not conduct a study involving deception unless they have determined that the use of deceptive techniques is justified by the study's significant prospective scientific, educational, or applied value and that equally effective nondeceptive alternative procedures are not feasible.

(b) Psychologists do not deceive prospective participants about research that is reasonably expected to cause physical pain or severe emotional distress.

(c) Psychologists explain any deception that is an integral feature of the design and conduct of an experiment to participants as early as is feasible, preferably at the conclusion of their participation, but no later than at the conclusion of the data collection, and permit participants to withdraw their data.

8.08 Providing Participants with Information About the Study

(a) Psychologists provide a prompt opportunity for participants to obtain appropriate information about the nature, results, and conclusions of the research, and they take reasonable steps to correct any misconceptions that participants may have of which the psychologists are aware.

(b) If scientific or humane values justify delaying or with-holding this information, psychologists take reasonable measures to reduce the risk of harm.

(c) When psychologists become aware that research proce-dures have harmed a participant they take reasonable steps to minimize harm.

Basically, according to the APA, deception in research requires that the researcher (1) apply a cost–benefit analy-sis that explicitly considers the potential for harm created and/or exacerbated by the use of deception, (2) consider alternative methods, and (3) fully explain the nature of the deception at the conclusion of the study or explicitly justify withholding such information. In all cases, the safety and comfort of the participant should be of paramount concern.

Issues When Evaluating the Use of Deception in Research

As we have seen in the Milgram study, deception in an ex-perimental setting can take many forms, as can subterfuge regarding the specific behaviors that are the subject of study. For example, a "cover story" can provide an al-ternate account of the true nature of the experiment, and experimental "confederates" can be used to enact a partic-ular role for the sake of the experimental design. A review by Gross and Fleming[7] found that, among studies using de-ceptive techniques, 82% of the deceptions involved a cover story or false statements regarding the purpose of the research. In addition, 42% involved incorrect infor-mation concerning the stimulus materials and 29% in-volved the use of a confederate or actor. Eighteen percent involved false feedback to the participant, and 14% in-volved unawareness on the part of the participant that he or she was even in a study. Additionally, 9% involved two related experiments being presented as if they were un-related. Five percent involved false feedback about a confederate or another person, and 4% involved un-awareness that the study was in progress at the time of the manipulation.

As implied in the APA code, when evaluating the use of any of these deceptive techniques, IRB members should consider the following:

1. The scientific value and validity of the research
2. The efficacy of alternative procedures
3. The certainty that deception does not extend to influence participants' willingness to participate
4. The possibility of experimentally induced harm and the ability of the proposed procedures to remove such harm through debriefing
5. The potential of deception to facilitate unwanted and inap-propriate invasions of privacy

Validity of the Research
Deciding that the proposed research is a valid and worth-while undertaking is a mainstay of the scientific review process. Thoughtful planning, solid empirical background research, precedent, and a determination of the potential benefits of the proposed research all need to be considered.

Alternative Methods
Having made the decision that an experimental design is valid and potentially worthwhile, the researcher must consider alternative procedures before concluding that the knowledge sought by the study requires the use of de-ception. From a methodological perspective, deception is used on the premise that it is important to keep partici-pants naive about the purpose of the study so that they can respond to experimental manipulations sponta-neously. According to this view, deception is an essential method because it enables researchers to obtain ade-quate experimental control and to observe behavior of participants that would be qualitatively altered if nonde-ceptive techniques were used. Researchers must make the case that these arguments are in fact applicable to their specific hypotheses.

Limits
As stated in the APA code, the researcher cannot deceive prospective participants regarding "research that is reason-ably expected to cause physical pain or severe emotional distress."[11[Sec.8.07(b)]] In assessing this restriction, the char-acteristics, values, and experiences of the experimental sample must be carefully considered. A group of rape vic-tims will undoubtedly have quite a different reaction to viewing a re-enactment of coerced sex than will a group of participants who have not been subject to such trauma. Deception on specific topics should be reviewed with the target group in mind.

Potential Harm
Deception is rarely used when physical harm is a possibil-ity. Deception is sometimes used when the experimental procedures may result in temporary psychological dis-comfort including stress, loss in self-esteem in response to experimental manipulations, embarrassment at being deceived, and guilt at having been induced to commit regretted acts. For example, false feedback about task performance is often intended to induce a temporary loss of self-esteem, and regret can occur when participants are induced to present themselves in a manner that is incon-sistent with their own personal beliefs. Negative responses can occur even when the deceptive techniques appear rel-atively innocuous. Imagine, for example, a case in which participants are told they are being recruited for partici-pation in a study in which they will receive electric shocks. Imagine further that they never receive any shocks but are simply observed for their anticipatory reaction. In this case, the participants obviously receive less physical pain than they expected and agreed to undergo. Yet once they are told of the ruse, they also may feel a sense of embar-rassment over allowing themselves to be duped by the experimenter.

Researchers conducting studies in which temporary psychological discomfort may be created often follow two guidelines. First, an attempt is made to limit such discomfort to a level that is normally encountered in everyday life. Second, at the end of the study an attempt is made to eliminate any discomfort through a thorough and sensitive "debriefing." As stated in the APA code, such postexperimental debriefings involve a complete disclosure as to any deceptions or misconceptions that the participant may have about the purpose of the experiment, the nature of the manipulations, the role of confederates, the fact that they were randomly assigned to receive particular forms of feedback, etc. In addition, the experimenter should make explicit attempts to relieve any negative reactions that the participant may have experienced. How this is accomplished obviously depends on the nature of the experimental procedures and the particular experiences of the participants. However, in most cases in which deception is used as a technique, the experimenter must make sure that the participant understands the nature of the deception, the care with which it was designed to ensure that all participants would actually be deceived, and the necessity of its use to properly test the hypotheses of interest. Experimenters should especially be aware of the possibility of embarrassment at having been deceived. Additionally, they must go to some lengths to emphasize that it is not the gullibility of the participant but rather the skill of the experimenter that is responsible for the success of the deception.

Privacy and Confidentiality

Finally, the use of deception raises potential issues regarding unwanted invasions of privacy. Particularly with the advent and widespread availability of sophisticated surveillance technology, care must be taken either to obtain in advance the participants' approval to record their behavior for research purposes or in cases where they believed that they were not being recorded to allow them the opportunity to deny the use of such information after it has been acquired. Specific procedures are often used by researchers that require a separate signature of the participant on the debriefing form giving explicit permission to use video- or audiotapes of the participant's behaviors. On a related issue, participants should never be deceived regarding the confidentiality of the information they provide. Experimental data and results should be kept confidential, and if possible, the participants' identity should be kept anonymous, especially if the acquired information is of a sensitive nature.

Informed Consent

By definition, deceptive procedures eliminate the possibility of fully informed consent. As a consequence, the APA code explicitly states this: Psychologists do not deceive prospective participants about research that is reasonably expected to cause physical pain or severe emotional distress.[11][Sec.8.07(b)] Obviously, this places the researcher and the IRB in the position of determining whether the procedures are potentially of a nature such that they would cause distress sufficient to cause a participant to withdraw from the study if they were known in advance. The fact that all participants are informed that they may choose to withdraw from a study at any time for any reason does not reduce the responsibilities of the researcher in this regard. Furthermore, as stated earlier, at the conclusion of

the experiment, it is the researcher's responsibility to institute explicit procedures to alleviate any discomfort that was experienced during the course of the study.

Although participants may not be fully informed, they should obviously be informed of as much as possible without threatening the ability of the researcher to test the true hypothesis of the study. Our recommendation is that the consent form (1) should *never* be used as part of the deception and thus should not include anything that is untrue and (2) should reveal as much as possible to the participant regarding the procedures in the study. Indeed, in some research, it may be advisable to reveal to participants the possibility of deception. For example, it is standard practice in medical research for participants to be informed in the consent of the possible use of placebo drugs and procedures. However, the consent form does not need to detail specific elements of the study if this will eliminate the capability of the study to inform the process under investigation. A useful guideline to keep in mind is that the experimenter–subject relationship is a real relationship "in which we have responsibility toward the subject as another human being whose dignity we must preserve."[12]

Research on Participants' Reactions to Experiments Involving Deception

The relative incidence and psychological consequences of deceptive research have actually been examined empirically. According to reviews by Gross and Fleming[7] and Sieber et al. (as cited by Cozby[13]), for selected years between 1959 and 1992, between one third (32%) and two thirds (69%) of the articles published in the premier social psychological journal (*Journal of Personality and Social Psychology*) have involved deception. In 1992, 47% of articles in this journal were observed to use some form of deception.

The fact that rates remained relatively stable for over 30 years despite the advent of IRBs and changes in the APA standards for research suggests that the typical use of deception is seen as warranted and justified. Most deception in social psychological research involves laboratory research in which a cover story is constructed to lead the participant to believe that a particular set of circumstances exists. The deceptions are relatively innocuous, do not involve harm to the subject, and are clearly justified given the nature of the processes the researchers are interested in investigating and the procedures adopted to circumvent any negative consequences that may be caused or worsened by the deception. Support for this point of view comes from research that has directly examined participants' responses to their experiences in deceptive research.

Multiple studies that have examined the effects of deception on participants' perceptions have found that the vast majority of participants (90%) perceive social psychological experiments as valuable and valid. In addition, the use of deception is seen as necessary to examine the behavior of interest.[14] In one study, Gerdes[15] randomly assigned participants to 1 of 15 different experiments that used a range of deceptive techniques. It was found that participants reported virtually no annoyance (0.42 on a 5-point [0–4] scale, "not at all" to "very much") and stated they did not mind being misled (0.61 on the same scale). Indeed, Smith and Richardson[16] actually found that participants in deception experiments found the experience more enjoyable and reported more educational benefit than those in nondeception experiments, presumably because the former were less boring.

As noted earlier, Kelman[2] expressed concern over the potential harm of deceptive research to the reputation of the profession ("our potential subjects will become increasingly distrustful of us and our future relations with them are likely to be undermined"). In fact, a study by Sharpe et al.[17] compared ratings from 1970 and 1990 of participants' favorability toward psychological research. They concluded that their results "do not support the proposition that introductory psychology students . . . have become more negative toward psychological research over the last two decades."

Although empirical evidence does seem to support the continued use of deception in psychological research, we should not use this evidence to lull us into the complacent belief that deception is an acceptable procedure for use in all studies. Christensen[18] reported that although subjects do not appear to object to the use of deception in general, if deception is used as a means of invading their privacy, it is viewed less positively. If nonprivate behaviors are being investigated (as is typical in laboratory studies), deception is viewed as a rather innocuous experimental procedure. If behaviors are investigated where participants had a reasonable expectation of privacy, however, the use of deception serves to enhance the participants' perception that their privacy has been invaded. A study by Tanke[19] made a related point. This study revealed that the inclusion of deception is not independently correlated with the perception of ethicality: as long as the experimental procedure itself runs little risk in harming the research participant, deception is viewed as innocuous. However, perceived harm is correlated with the perception of ethicality of the study and interacts with deception such that if the experimental procedure has a significant potential for harming the research participant, then deception is viewed as ethically less acceptable than a nondeceptive design.

Conclusion

As previously noted, most forms of deception encountered by IRB members involve the creation of plausible but inaccurate cover stories and procedures designed to misdirect the participant's attention for the sake of examining spontaneous behavior. As long as the main procedures used in the study are judged to be innocuous, such deception is not typically viewed as objectionable. If the main procedures do engender temporary negative reactions of a nature typically experienced in the course of everyday life, the use of deception need not be viewed as objectionable as long

as it is scientifically justified and the researcher uses procedures specifically designed to alleviate such reactions. If the procedures cause negative reactions that could plausibly affect the participant's willingness to take part in the study, that are outside the range of everyday experience, or that are not amenable to alleviation through debriefing, then deception is in all likelihood inappropriate. IRBs and researchers must continue to work together to ensure proper and appropriate research procedures that protect experimental participants while supporting the pursuit of scientific knowledge.

References

1. Milgram S. Behavioral study of obedience. *J Abnorm Soc Psychol* 67:371–378, 1963.
2. Kelman HC. Human use of human subjects: The problem of deception in social psychological experiments. *Psychol Bull* 67:1–11, 1967.
3. Baumrind D. Some thoughts on ethics research: After reading Milgram's "Behavioral Study of Obedience." *Am Psychol* 19:421–423, 1964.
4. Aronson E, Carlsmith JM. Experimentation in social psychology. In: Lindzey G, Aronson E (eds.). *The Handbook of Social Psychology*, 2nd ed. Reading, MA: Addison-Wesley; 1968:1–79.
5. Asch S. Effects of group pressure upon the modification and distortion of judgments. In: Swanson GE, Newcomb TM, Hartley EL (eds.). *Readings in Social Psychology*. New York: Holt, Rhinehart and Winston; 1952.
6. Latane B, Darley JM. Group inhibition of bystander intervention in emergencies. *J Person Soc Psychol* 10:215–221, 1968.
7. Gross AE, Fleming I. Twenty years of deception in social psychology. *Person Soc Psychol Bull* 8:402–408, 1982.
8. Aronson E, Ellsworth PC, Carlsmith JM, Gonzales MH. *Methods of Research in Social Psychology*. New York: McGraw-Hill; 1990.
9. Nisbett RE, Wilson TD. Telling more than we can know: Verbal reports on mental processes. *Psychol Rev* 84:231–259, 1977.
10. Freedman JL. Role playing: Psychology by consensus. *J Person Soc Psychol* 13:107–114, 1969.
11. American Psychological Association. Ethical principles of psychologists and code of conduct. Updated 2002. Effective June 1, 2003. http://www.apa.org/ethics/
12. Kelman HC. The rights of the subject in social research: An analysis in terms of relative power and legitimacy. *Am Psychol* 27:989–1016, 1972.
13. Cozby PC. *Methods in Behavioral Research*, 6th ed. Mountain View, CA: Mayfield Publishing; 1997.
14. Fisher CB, Fyrberg D. Participant partners: College students weigh the costs and benefits of deceptive research. *Am Psychol* 49:417–427, 1994.
15. Gerdes EP. College students' reactions to social psychological experiments involving deception. *J Soc Psychol* 107:99–110, 1979.
16. Smith SS, Richardson D. Amelioration of deception and harm in psychological research: The important role of debriefing. *J Person Soc Psychol* 44:1075–1082, 1983.

17. Sharpe D, Adair JG, Roese NJ. Twenty years of deception research: A decline in subjects' trust? *Person Soc Psychol Bull* 18:585–590, 1992.

18. Christensen L. Deception in psychological research: When is its use justified? *Person Soc Psychol Bull* 14:664–675, 1988.

19. Tanke ED. Perceptions of ethicality of psychological research: Effects of experiment status, experimenter outcome, and authoritarianism. *Person Soc Psychol Bull* 5:164–168, 1979.

Research Without Consent or Documentation Thereof

Marianne M. Elliott

INTRODUCTION

The purpose of this chapter is to explain the situations wherein federal regulations permit the institutional review board (IRB) to approve research and waive the requirement for informed consent or the requirement for documentation of informed consent. A special case of the waiver-of-consent issue is the situation wherein research is conducted in the setting of medical emergency. Emergency medical research without consent is discussed in Chapter 4-5.

Respect for Persons

The principle of respect for persons described in *The Belmont Report* notes that individuals must be autonomous in their decisions about whether to participate in research. For individuals to make an informed decision, the researcher must provide specific information about the research to potential subjects. The Department of Health and Human Services (DHHS) human subject protections regulations[1(Sec.116)] and the Food and Drug Administration regulations[2] describe the specific context of the consent process and the required elements of a consent. Researchers must present this information to individuals in language understandable to them and assess that individuals have comprehended the information for them to make an informed decision. Researchers must also ensure that the consent process and the consent document affirm that each individual's decision to participate in research is voluntary and free from undue influence. In general, the researcher documents the consent process, whereas the individuals who decide to participate document their agreement to participate in the research by signing and dating the consent document.

In some instances, the IRB has authority based on federal regulations to waive the requirement to obtain informed consent from subjects and/or the requirement to have subjects sign a consent document. In these instances, the IRB determines that, before his or her participation in the research, the individual's informed consent, or elements of the process and document, can be waived. The IRB may also decide that the documentation of the consent from the individual subject can be waived. The regulations provide specific criteria that the IRB must consider before making a decision to waive or alter either informed consent or documentation of informed consent (obtaining the individual's signature on a consent document).

These two types of waiver are separate and distinct, yet researchers, IRB members, and IRB administrators frequently confuse the two different types. Each type of waiver must satisfy specific criteria before the IRB can grant the waiver. The IRB and IRB administrators must be aware of the limited instances where the IRB may waive these requirements.

Risk Assessment

To grant a waiver of informed consent, an alteration of the consent elements or procedures, or the requirement to obtain a signed consent document, the IRB must assess and evaluate the potential risks and expected benefits associated with participation in the research and the consent process. In evaluating the risk, the IRB must assess the risk or harms inherent in the informed consent process or documentation of informed consent. In some circumstances, the consent process and existence of a signed consent document may involve more risk or potentially more harm to subjects than participating in the research itself. Thus, the first step in determining whether a waiver is appropriate is the IRB's evaluation of the risks.

When the IRB approves a waiver of the requirement for informed consent or a procedure that does not include or alters elements of informed consent, the IRB must determine that the research meets the definition of minimal risk. The determination that the research involves minimal risk allows the IRB, if appropriate, to waive the requirement for obtaining informed consent from subjects. In essence, the IRB has acted under the principles of respect for persons, as an autonomous committee, and provided informed consent on behalf of the subject for the research to be conducted. The waiver or alteration is based on the determination of minimal risk to subjects.

In contrast, when the IRB waives the documentation of informed consent (i.e., the requirement to obtain a signed consent form), the IRB must determine that the principal risk is the potential harm from a breach of confidentiality of the signed consent forms while held by the researcher. Both the risks associated with participating in the research and the risks associated with a breach of confidentiality may be greater than minimal risk. In this instance, the IRB demonstrates respect for persons and their autonomy in allowing subjects to decide whether or not they wish to sign a consent document that identifies them as research subjects. By granting the waiver of the documentation of consent, the IRB minimizes potential harm to subjects from a confidentiality breach.

Waiver of Informed Consent

DHHS regulations[1][Sec.116(d)] describe the criteria for waiving the requirement for informed consent. A form that guides the IRB through these criteria is appended to this chapter.

An IRB may approve a consent procedure that does not include, or that alters, some or all of the elements of informed consent set forth in this section or waive the requirement to obtain informed consent provided the IRB finds and documents that:

1. The research involves no more than minimal risk to the subjects.
2. The waiver or alteration will not adversely affect the rights and welfare of the subjects.
3. The research could not practically be carried out without the waiver or alteration.
4. Whenever appropriate, the subjects will be provided with additional pertinent information after participation.[1][Sec.116(d)]

Example
The researcher plans to determine how mood and perception of one's body image may be related. Initially, student subjects complete a series of written questionnaires and scales about their body image. After the subjects are presented with visual images intended to evoke a negative mood, the subjects are asked to complete the same questionnaires and scales. The effect of evoking a negative mood is evaluated.

Although the actual purpose of the research is to determine how mood may be related to body image, subjects are informed that the research is actually two separate research projects, one related to moods and how they may change and the other related to body image. This deception is part of the research design, and the student subjects are not fully informed about the purpose of the research.

In this example, the IRB may find that an alteration of informed consent is appropriate and that the criteria from 45 CFR 46[1][Sec.116(d)] have been met based on the following:

1. The research involves minimal risk. The visual images are similar to those that the subjects might see in magazines or films about health and exercise. There are no provocative images. The questionnaires and scales are valid and reliable and are used in standard psychosocial testing.

2. The rights and welfare of subjects are not adversely affected because subjects are informed about the actual procedures, questionnaires, scales, and visual images involved in the research; the risks of feeling uncomfortable or upset with the questions or visual images; that there are no anticipated benefits from participating in the research; and that they may choose not to answer any questions that may cause them to be uncomfortable and they may stop their participation at any time without affecting their status as a student or their grades. Subjects are not informed that the research actually has one purpose and that the data will be evaluated for that intent.

3. The research could not practicably be carried out without the alteration in the informed consent process. The research design is intended to minimize the subject's preconceived thoughts or feelings by presenting visual images and measuring subject's responses before and after being exposed to those specific visual images resulting in a mood change.

4. In this research, it is appropriate to provide subjects with additional pertinent information after participation. The researcher debriefs the subjects after their participation to explain the actual purpose of the research and why the research design was appropriate. The researcher also offers to be available for any questions subjects may have and provides information about appropriate services if subjects experience distress or anxiety about their participation in the research.

Example
The researcher plans to determine whether some specific blood chemistry values change in individuals undergoing clinically indicated abdominal surgery and if there is a correlation of changes with the increased incidence of complications after surgery. The researcher plans to review the medical records of all individuals who have undergone abdominal surgery in the past 2 years. From a preliminary estimate, there are about 5,000 abdominal surgeries performed per year at the hospital. The researcher will collect limited data for this research. The types of data to be collected include such items as the diagnosis before surgery, the type of abdominal surgery, specific blood chemistry values before the surgery, the same specific blood chemistry values after the surgery, a description of problems after surgery, and the age ranges of the individuals. The researcher will double code the data so that only the researcher knows the link in the unlikely event the data must be verified for accuracy. The results of the research will not affect the clinical care of the individuals because the information will not be examined until after subjects leave the hospital.

In this example, the IRB may find that a waiver of informed consent is appropriate and that the criteria from 45 CFR 46[1][Sec.116(d)] have been met based on the following:

1. The research involves minimal risk, as the review of subjects' medical records is for limited information. The information is not sensitive in nature, and the data are derived from clinically indicated procedures. There is an extremely low probability of harm to subjects' status, employment, or insurability. The precautions taken to limit the record review to specified data and the double coding of the data further minimize the major risk, which is a breach of confidentiality. Contacting subjects to obtain their consent could be considered an invasion of privacy and cause subjects undue anxiety.

2. The rights and welfare of the individual would not be adversely affected because the clinically indicated surgical

procedure and the associated blood chemistry values were already completed, or would be completed, regardless of the research. None of the results of the research would affect the clinical decisions about the individual's care because the results are analyzed after the fact. Subjects are not being deprived of clinical care to which they would normally be entitled.

3. The research could not be practicably carried out without the waiver. Identifying and contacting the thousands of potential subjects, although not impossible, would not be feasible for a review of their medical records for information that would not change the care they would already have received.

4. It would not be appropriate to provide these subjects with additional pertinent information about the results of the research as the results would have no effect on the subjects. The surgical procedure and care afterward have both been completed for these subjects. There is no anticipated benefit to subjects that would change what has already occurred.

Example
A researcher plans to review the medical records using the same procedures as previously described. However, in this research, the hypothesis is that there is a correlation between a particular drug intervention and development of neurologic problems several years later.

In this example, the IRB may find that a waiver of informed consent is appropriate and that the criteria 1, 2, and 3 from 45 CFR 46[1][Sec.116(d)] have been met based on the same basic reasons. There is one potential difference.

Under criterion 4, it may be appropriate to provide these subjects with additional pertinent information about the results of the research. In this case, the IRB may not be able to determine whether the results of the research would or would not provide information that may be pertinent to those subjects. To make this determination, the IRB may require the researcher to submit the results of the research, along with an assessment of whether subjects should be provided additional pertinent information, to the IRB for review. If the results of the research submitted to the IRB indicate that no additional pertinent information should be provided to subjects (e.g., there was no statistical significance to support the research question), the IRB may determine that it is not appropriate to provide these subjects with additional information. In contrast, if the results of the research submitted to the IRB indicate that there is additional pertinent information that should be provided to subjects (e.g., there is a high probability that subjects who received the drug may experience late negative effects), the IRB may determine that the researcher should provide subjects with this information.

The IRB should work with the researcher to determine what pertinent information should be provided to subjects and how this information would be provided. For example, the IRB may require the researcher to outline a process that would include how the information about results of the research would be communicated to subjects, what the results might mean to subjects, and what to do if there are any questions. The IRB would review the process and perhaps a document, such as an information letter to subjects, much the way the IRB reviews the informed consent process and the consent document to ensure that the pertinent information is communicated clearly and in language that is understandable to subjects. The IRB may require the researcher to include a statement noting that subjects should or may wish to share this information with their primary care physicians.

Waiver of the Requirement to Obtain Documentation of Consent

DHHS regulations[1][Sec.117(c)] describe two circumstances in which an IRB may waive the requirement to obtain a signed consent form. A form that guides the IRB through these criteria is appended to the end of this chapter.

An IRB may waive the requirement for the investigator to obtain a signed consent form for some or all subjects if it finds either:

(1) That the only record linking the subject and the research would be the consent document and the principal risk would be potential harm resulting from a breach of confidentiality. Each subject will be asked whether the subject wants documentation linking the subject with the research and the subject's wishes will govern or (2) that the research presents no more than minimal risk of harm to subjects and involves no procedures for which written consent is normally required outside of the research context.

In cases in which the documentation requirement is waived, the IRB may require the investigator to provide subjects with a written statement regarding the research.[1][Sec.117(c)]

Example
A researcher plans to evaluate the effectiveness of a smoking cessation program with women who are receiving prenatal care at the local health clinic. During a prenatal visit, any women who are already participating in the smoking cessation program will be asked to complete a written questionnaire about the program. The one-time written questionnaire includes questions about how well the women are complying with the program and how they feel about their progress. There is no identifying information about subjects on the questionnaire, and whether the subjects complete the questionnaire has no effect on the care they may receive at the clinic.

In this example, the IRB may waive the requirement to obtain a signed consent form because the research presents no more than minimal risk of harm to subjects. The questionnaire has no identifying information about the subject, and the purpose of the research is to evaluate the effectiveness of the program itself. Normally, there is no requirement for written consent for completion of written questionnaires outside the research context. By virtue of completing the questionnaire, subjects have consented to participate in the research. In this case, the IRB may require the researcher to provide subjects with a written summary or an information sheet about the research. The IRB may further require that the information contain all the relevant elements of informed consent outlined in 45 CFR 46.[1][Sec.116] At a minimum, the IRB may require that the information sheets include the purpose of the research, the procedure, how much time is involved, the assessment of minimal risk, a statement that there is no benefit to subjects for completing the questionnaire, who to contact for questions about the research, and who to contact for questions about their rights as research subjects.

Example
A researcher plans face-to-face interviews with university students who belong to a support group on campus for transgendered, gay, lesbian, and bisexual individuals. The purpose of the research is to evaluate the quality of health care services for these individuals. The researcher plans to recruit subjects through flyers and information distributed at support group meetings. Potential subjects will contact the researcher directly. The researcher plans to conduct two face-to-face interviews 6 months apart. The interviews will be audiotaped, and the researcher will ask subjects to use a pseudonym during the interviews. Also, each subject will be assigned a coded number on the audiotape.

In this example, the IRB determines that the only record linking the subject and the research would be the consent document. The principal risk would be potential harm resulting from a breach of confidentiality if the consent documents were disclosed, purposefully or inadvertently. To minimize the potential harm to subjects, the IRB may permit the informed consent process to be conducted orally and have the researcher document, perhaps in a research note, the circumstances of the consent process. The IRB may also require the researcher to provide each subject with a written summary or information sheet about the research. However, in this example, even having an information sheet about the research could be potentially harmful to subjects who may already suffer from social stigma, embarrassment, or ostracism. The IRB may suggest providing subjects with a card that lists only the name and phone number of the researcher in the event they have any questions or concerns.

The IRB may then request that the researcher ask subjects whether they want documentation linking them with the research, and each subject's wishes will be honored. The IRB may ask the researcher to inform each subject about the temporal aspects of the risks associated with the signed consent document as the only link between the subject and the research. Subjects, as students or activists, might believe that the immediate potential harm from having a document with their signature confirming their participation in the research is minimal and a potential breach of confidentiality is not relevant. In contrast, the same subjects may find that the harm caused by an inadvertent breach of confidentiality perhaps 5 to 10 years later during a job interview to be greater.

Documentation of Waiver Determinations by the IRB

When the IRB approves a consent procedure that does not include, or alters, some or all of the elements of informed consent or waives the requirement to obtain informed consent, the IRB must both make the specific findings required by the regulations and document those determinations.

If the IRB approves a waiver of informed consent or waiver of the requirement to obtain a signed consent form for research reviewed during a convened IRB meeting, the IRB meeting minutes must document the IRB's findings regarding their decision to grant the waiver.

However, when a research protocol meets the criteria for review under expedited procedures,[1][Sec.110(b)] the review is conducted by the IRB chair or designated IRB members outside of a convened meeting. In this case, the IRB member's review must document the decision. There is the same documentation requirement regardless of whether the waiver is granted by the convened IRB or by the IRB member–reviewers through expedited review procedures.

Appended to this chapter are examples from IRB member review guides for determining and documenting whether a waiver of informed consent or waiver of documentation of informed consent may be granted. The IRB member–reviewers use the review guide regardless of whether the review of the research protocol and determination of a waiver are granted by the convened IRB or by IRB member–reviewers through expedited review procedures. If the determinations and decisions are documented in the convened IRB's meeting minutes, the IRB member–reviewer guide serves as additional documentation for the determination. When the IRB member–reviewer grants a waiver for a research protocol reviewed under expedited procedures, the IRB member–reviewer guide is the only documentation for the determination and decision.

Conclusion

The IRB may waive or alter the requirement for informed consent or waive the requirement to document informed consent from subjects if certain criteria from the federal regulations[1][Secs. 116,117] are satisfied. The IRB must always consider the principle of respect for persons and allow individuals autonomy with regard to their decisions about research participation. In some instances, the IRB waives informed consent and provides consent on behalf of subjects for the research to be conducted. The IRB must always determine the risks and potential harms involved in the research and the consent process before granting a waiver. The same standard of documentation is required regardless of whether the waiver is granted by the convened IRB or by the IRB members reviewing research through expedited review procedures.

References
1. Code of Federal Regulations. Title 45A—Department of Health and Human Services; Part 46—Protection of Human Subjects. Updated 1 October, 1997. Access date 18 April, 2001. http://www4.law.cornell.edu/cfr/45p46.htm
2. Code of Federal Regulations. Title 21, Chapter 1—Food and Drug Administration, DHHS; Part 50—Protection of Human Subjects. Updated 1 April, 1999. Access date 18 April, 2001. http://www4.law.cornell.edu/cfr/21p50.htm

Appendix

IRB REVIEWER GUIDE: Waiver of Informed Consent

If you are granting (a) a waiver of informed consent or (b) a waiver of the consent procedure requirement to include all or alter some or all of the elements of informed consent [45 CFR46.116(d)], you must document the responses to each of the following four statements.

	Circle One	
1. The research in its entirety involves no greater than minimal risk.	Yes	No
2. The waiver of informed consent will not adversely affect the rights and welfare of the subjects.	Yes	No
3. It is not practicable to conduct the research without the waiver/alteration.	Yes	No
4. Whenever appropriate, subjects will be provided with additional pertinent information after their participation.	Yes	No

If you have circled the "yes" response to each of the four previous statements, in order to receive the waiver, you must (a) describe the reason(s) the waiver is necessary and (b) explain whether entire informed consent is being waived or only certain required elements are being waived. (If so, list which ones.) _____

_____

_____

If a waiver is granted under the previously mentioned conditions, documentation of informed consent (i.e., signed consent form) is also waived. Even if the waiver is granted, the IRB may require other conditions. The IRB may require the researcher to provide subjects with an information sheet (written summary) about the research.

Used with permission from the University of Illinois at Chicago Office for Protection of Research Subjects.

Appendix

IRB REVIEWER GUIDE: Waiver of Documentation of Consent

If you are granting a waiver of the requirement to obtain a signed consent form for some or all subjects [45 CFR 46.117(c)], you must document responses to each of the following statements.

	Circle One	
1. The entire consent (or elements thereof) was waived under 45 CFR 46.116(d).	Yes	No
2. The only record linking the subject and the research is the consent document, and the principal risk is potential harm resulting from a breach of confidentiality. Subjects are asked whether they want documentation linking them to the research, and their wishes will govern.	Yes	No
3. The research involves no more than minimal risk of harm and involves no procedure for which written consent is normally required outside of the research context.	Yes	No

If you have circled the "yes" response to at least one of the previous questions, in order to grant the waiver, you must describe the reason(s) the waiver is necessary. ——————————————————
——
——

Even if the waiver is granted, the IRB may require other conditions. The IRB may require the researcher to provide subjects with an information sheet (written summary) about the research.

Used with permission from the University of Illinois at Chicago Office for Protection of Research Subjects.

Selecting a Surrogate to Consent to Medical Research

Robert J. Amdur, Natalie Bachir, and Elizabeth Stanton

INTRODUCTION

A clinical investigator requested permission from the Dartmouth College Institutional Review Board (IRB) to initiate a research study to evaluate the safety and efficacy of a new medication for the treatment of patients with bacterial sepsis. To be effective, the study medication had to be administered within hours of the patient's eligibility. Only patients who were both critically ill from sepsis and who had failed to respond to standard therapies were eligible for the study. Historical evidence suggested that most eligible patients would die of sepsis-related problems unless a new treatment proved to be effective. Preliminary data indicated a favorable risk/benefit profile for the experimental medication in this setting. The problem: most subjects would not be clinically competent to give informed consent to medical treatment.

Under New Hampshire law, there are only two categories of people who have explicit statutory rights to make decisions on behalf of incompetent patients: court-appointed legal guardians and agents under a durable power of attorney for health care (DPAHC). Most patients have neither. Once a patient becomes incompetent, it is too late to execute a DPAHC and when time is a factor, as in this case, it is usually impractical, if not impossible, to obtain guardianship. To complicate matters, New Hampshire does not have a law delineating a hierarchy of surrogate decision-makers (usually next-of-kin) to fill in the gap when patients fail to make their own surrogate assignments. This kind of legal environment makes life difficult for IRB members.

When state law does not provide guidance on health care consent by a surrogate, research institutions should establish a policy and procedure to address this issue. As part of this process, institutions should (1) consider the principles underlying the informed consent doctrine; (2) examine existing state law for any limitations on the consent power of the legal guardian or health-care proxy decision-maker (such as a DPAHC); (3) identify other relevant surrogate decision-making laws within the state, and (4) review and consider public policy reasons for allowing surrogate decision-makers to consent to experimental treatment when there are no applicable state laws.

Informed Consent

The legal doctrine of informed consent embodies some of the most important ethical and legal principles guiding the conduct of research involving human subjects. In 1914, Justice Cardozo articulated the basic principle of informed consent in medical care when he wrote, "Every human being of adult years and sound mind has a right to determine what shall be done with his own body."[1] Today, the informed consent doctrine provides recognition of individual autonomy and imposes on the physician a duty to disclose information in such a way that the patient can make an informed decision about care.[2(Sec.6–9,6–11)]

This is true whether the care is therapeutic or experimental, although experimental treatment is more highly regulated by the federal government.

Experimental treatment requires more regulation because of inherent design differences between therapeutic practice and research practice. The physician designs a therapeutic practice to enhance the well-being of a particular patient whereas the physician-researcher designs a research practice to test a hypothesis for generalizable knowledge. Though the research subject may benefit from the research practice, the physician-researcher has a dual interest and thus, to some degree, a conflict of interest in regard to the patient. The National Commission for the

Protection of Human Subjects of Biomedical and Behavioral Research (Commission) was created, in part, to develop protections against this inherent conflict

In 1979, the Commission presented the ethical foundation for the federal rules on human subject research in *The Belmont Report*.[4(A6–8)] In this report, the Commission established "respect for persons" as a fundamental principle in human subject research and as the principle underlying the doctrine of informed consent.[4(A6–10)] Respect for persons, the Commission elaborated, requires (1) recognition of the individual as an autonomous agent and (2) protection of the individual with diminished autonomy.[4(A6–10)] To recognize the individual's autonomy is to recognize the individual's ability to deliberate choices and then to act on that deliberation.[4(A6–10)] To protect the individual with diminished autonomy is to assess both the risk of harm and the likelihood of benefit to the individual from the research and to afford protection accordingly.[4(A6–10)]

In addition to *respect*, the Commission identified *beneficence* as another fundamental principle of human subject research. Beneficence, the doing of good, obligates the researcher to secure the individual's well-being by maximizing benefits and minimizing harms *to the individual research subject*.[4(A6–10)] Beneficence requires that the researcher perform a risk/benefit analysis, examining the probability and magnitude of possible harms and anticipated benefits to the individual In the case of a research subject with diminished autonomy, beneficence is enhanced through protections proportional to risks and harms.

The Commission applied the principles of respect and beneficence to informed consent in the conduct of research and identified certain codes of conduct. First, the individual must be informed about the risks and benefits of the research.[4(A6–12)] Second, the information must be conveyed in a clear, understandable, and intelligible manner.[4(A6–12)] Third, the researcher may not use coercion or undue influence to induce the individual to consent to participation. Finally, if the individual has diminished autonomy, there must be additional protections that are reflective of the risk of harm and the likelihood of benefit.[4 (A6–12)]

The federal rules on human subject research reflect the Commission's principles with varying degrees of success. Although federal protections are reasonably straightforward for the competent research subject, they are less well-defined when it comes to the incompetent research subject and are therefore more open to interpretation. Because the principles and guidelines defined by the Commission remain the foundation for legal analysis today,[5(pp.88–90),6(n.2)] states and research institutions should incorporate them into the laws and policies on surrogate decision making for the incompetent research subject.

Federal Law

Under the guidance of the Commission, the Department of Health and Human Services (DHHS) promulgated rules that define protections for human research subjects.[7(Sec.101et seq.)] Institutions must comply with these rules when research is federally funded.[7(Sec.101(a))] Most institutions, however, also apply the policy of the federal rules to privately funded research to avoid the difficulty of administering two different sets of administrative rules for research.[2(Sec.23-2)] In recognition of the Commission's enunciation, the DHHS established the requirement of a participant's informed consent as a necessary criterion for research approval. DHHS requires that each prospective research subject, or a subject's legally authorized representative, provides a legally effective informed consent to participation in the project.[7(Sec.111(a)(4),116)] To be legally effective, the consent must meet both federal and state requirements for informed consent and, when applicable, for surrogate decision making.[7(Sec.102(d),116(e))] Federal law provides basic procedural protections and defers to more restrictive state procedure.[7(Sec.116(e))] State law provides the substantive law of informed consent and the law governing surrogate decision making.

Although federal law details the essential elements of informed consent, including those elements that must be explained to a research subject or representative,[7(Sec.116(a))] the law falls short in defining the "surrogate decision maker" and the protections that researchers should afford the incompetent patient. The law recognizes and allows the participation of a surrogate decision maker in the informed consent process but defers to state law to define the "legally authorized representative."[7(Sec.102)] Problematically, state law may or may not more fully define either the doctrine of informed consent or the surrogate decision maker.

Federal law also requires that the IRB approve and oversee human subject research through a process that reflects local conditions and values.[2(Sec.23-3)] The law requires that the board include sufficient scientific and nonscientific expertise, but also diversity in race, gender, and cultural backgrounds and sensitivity to issues such as *community attitudes*.[7(Sec.107(a)=(c))] As such, the IRB policy and procedure on informed consent or the incompetent research subject should reflect both the law and public policy of the state in which it operates.

State Law

All states, including the District of Columbia have enacted guardianship and advance directive laws. Only a handful of states have additional surrogate decision-making laws that construct a hierarchy of decision-makers when there is no legal guardian or agent under an advance directive. Given the fact that most individuals do not have a court-appointed guardian, and have not executed an advance directive, and given the fact that the vast majority of states fail specifically to address surrogate consent in medical research, most research institutions are forced to structure consent policies and procedures without the benefit of legislative guidance.

To establish institutional principles and procedures that reflect local conditions and values and to provide liability protection to the institution and to the researcher, institutions should look first to any relevant laws of the state for guidance. Specifically, the institution should look for (1) a specific prohibition of the informal appointment of a surrogate, such as a family member or close friend, (2) limitations on the consent power of the formally appointed surrogate, and (3) prescribed standards for the decision-making process. New Hampshire state law is reviewed here as a model for the type of analysis that interested parties in other states will need to conduct when establishing research policy.

Guardianship

A court-appointed guardian is a surrogate decision maker appointed by a court to protect the interests of and make decisions for a person who has been adjudicated incompetent. In most cases, a qualified and properly motivated relative, friend, or other interested person will serve as guardian. In New Hampshire, when there is no family member or interested party, a guardian can be found through the Office of Public Guardian. Similar offices exist in other states.

From the standpoint of a clinical investigator who is interested in enrolling an incompetent patient in a research study, there are two main problems with establishing a court-appointed guardian. First, although it is possible to establish temporary guardianship in a few days, it often takes much longer. For example, in New Hampshire, the guardianship process takes at least a month, often longer. Second, establishing legal guardianship is a complex and expensive process. In most cases, the party wanting to establish guardianship must hire a lawyer to direct the appointment process. In 2005, the legal fees associated with an uncomplicated guardianship appointment in New Hampshire were approximately $3,500–$4,500.

The New Hampshire court appoints a guardian to a person only after finding all of the following *beyond a reasonable doubt*: (1) the person is incapacitated and will or has come to substantial harm as a result; (2) guardianship is necessary to provide continuing care, supervision, and rehabilitation; (3) there are no available alternative resources suitable to the welfare, safety, and rehabilitation of the person; and (4) guardianship is the least restrictive form of intervention consistent with preserving the civil liberties of the person.[8[Sec.9III(1992)]] The court determines incapacity through a measure of a person's functional limitations.[8[Sec.2XI(1992)]] Finally, because courts seek the least restrictive form of intervention, the guardianship imposes only the limitations necessary to provide needed care and rehabilitative services.[8[Sec.2XIV(1992)]]

The purpose and limited scope of the New Hampshire guardianship law suggests intent to provide due process protections when needed and guardianship only as a last resort, allowing the coexistence of the law with, for example, the practice of family consent.[9] In its purpose statement, the law clearly is intended to "provide procedural and substantive safeguards for civil liberties."[8[Sec.1(1992)]] The nature of the court's inquiry, however, suggests that guardianship is a last remedial resort.

A New Hampshire court-appointed guardian probably does not have the authority to consent to medical research participation on behalf of a ward. A purpose of the guardianship law in New Hampshire is "to encourage rehabilitative care" for incapacitated individuals.[8[Sec.1(1992)]] If authorized by the court, the New Hampshire guardian may give or withhold consent to health care on behalf of the ward.[8[Sec.25I(c) (Supp.1997)]] No guardian, however, may consent to psychosurgery, electroconvulsive therapy, sterilization, or *experimental treatment* without prior court approval [emphasis added].[8[Sec.25I(c)(Supp.1997)]] Although the guardianship law does not define "experimental treatment," a plain language and conservative interpretation of the term suggests the guardian may not consent to research participation without judicial approval.

Additionally, guardians must adhere to the terms of a valid living will or DPAHC.[8[Sec.25I(d)(Suppl.1997)]] The guardian must adhere to any express wishes of the executor, including wishes made in regard to research participation. This requirement demonstrates state deference to the express wishes of the executor of the document, the patient for whom the court appoints a guardian. The wishes of the patient, expressed when competent, appear to override even court-appointed authority.

The New Hampshire guardianship law indirectly reflects the state's policy on the informally appointed surrogate in medical research consent. The law does not prohibit the appointment of a family member or close friend. Guardianship law, however, does prohibit consent to experimental treatment without judicial approval, reflecting heightened state concern in such matters. The law is silent on the process by which the guardian decides about routine health care matters. The exception is that the guardian must defer to the express wishes of the patient as stated in a valid living will or DPAHC.

DPAHC

A DPAHC is a document executed by a competent person (principal) delegating decision-making authority to another person (agent) in the event the principal becomes incapacitated. The principal may limit durable powers in time, scope, or method of decision making.[2(p.17–22)] State statutes regulating the DPAHC vary in scope and often expressly provide immunity to the institution and physician that rely in good faith on the consent of the DPAHC agent.

The New Hampshire DPAHC statute reads as follows:

> The durable power of attorney shall be in substantially the following form:
> I, ____, hereby appoint ____ of ____ as my agent to make any and all health care decisions for me, except to the extent I state otherwise in this document or as prohibited by law.[10[Sec.15(1996)]]

Researchers encounter two difficulties in regard to the New Hampshire DPAHC. First, most people do not establish a DPAHC. A DPAHC is an advance directive, which means that it must be executed before the principal is either clinically or legally incompetent. Although the need for an advance directive has received increased attention nationwide, especially after the Florida case involving Terri Schiavo, most patients will not have executed a DPAHC before becoming incapacitated.

Second, most DPAHC agreements do not mention research. Standard DPAHC language does not include reference to medical research consent as a health care decision, and unless the principal has the foresight to include such direction, difficulties in obtaining consent may ensue. New Hampshire enacted the DPAHC law "to enable adults to retain control over their own medical care during periods of incapacity."[10[Sec.2III(1996)]] The New Hampshire DPAHC agent may make any health care decision the principal could make, with some exceptions.[10[Sec.2I(1996)]] "'Health-care decision' means consent, refusal to consent, or withdrawal of consent to any care, treatment, admission to a health-care facility, any service or procedure to maintain, diagnose, or treat an individual's physical or mental condition except as prohibited in this chapter or otherwise by law."[10[Sec.1VI(1996)]] The agent may not make decisions expressly prohibited in the DPAHC or the principal's living will.[10[Sec.2I(1996)]] In addition, the agent may not consent to a voluntary admission to a state institution, voluntary sterilization, or with some exceptions, to withholding life-sustaining treatment from a pregnant patient.[10[Sec.2V(1996)]] Experimental treatment is not mentioned as it is in the guardianship statute. Overall, despite the few carved out exceptions, the agent may exercise broad power in health care decision making.

Despite the agent's broad decision-making power, the law prescribes the manner in which the agent should make that decision.[10[Sec.J:2II]] The law requires that the agent make health care decisions in consultation with the principal's health care provider, as well as "in accordance with the agent's knowledge of the principal's wishes and religious or moral beliefs, as stated orally or otherwise by [the] principal to [the] agent."[10[Sec.J:2II]] When the principal's wishes are not known, the agent must decide in accordance with accepted medical practice and an assessment of the principal's best interest.[10[Sec.J:2II]]

The New Hampshire DPAHC law, like the guardianship law, indirectly reflects the state's policy on the informally appointed surrogate in medical research consent. The law does not prohibit the appointment of a family member or close friend, nor does the law prohibit consent to experimental treatment. Notably, the DPAHC law prescribes the process by which the agent should consent to health care matters: either by substituted judgment when the principal's wishes and beliefs are known or by a best-interest standard in conjunction with accepted medical practice when the principal's wishes are not known.

Family or Friend as Surrogate

In the absence of a formally designated surrogate, researchers may wish to seek consent for research participation from a family member. Although it has long been standard medical practice to seek consent to health care from family, there is no basis for this practice in common law. Policy arguments exist for and against the practice. Some states have clarified the allowance through "family consent laws" or "surrogate laws" that include relatives or friends in a hierarchical list of allowable health care decision makers for the incompetent patient. The statute may or may not specifically mention medical research. When a state has not enacted such a law, such as New Hampshire, institutions must decide if and when it is acceptable to allow an informally appointed decision maker to consent to a clinically incompetent person's participation in a medical research study.

The National Commission for the Protection of Human Subjects of Biomedical and Behavioral Research, in a 1983 report, proposed reasons for the legal deference to family consent to health care for the incompetent patient.

1. The family is generally most concerned about the good of the patient.
2. The family will also usually be most knowledgeable about the patient's goals, preferences, and values.
3. The family deserves recognition as an important social unit that ought to be treated, within limits, as a responsible decision maker in matters that intimately affect its members.
4. Especially in a society in which many other traditional forms of community have eroded, participation in a family is often an important dimension of personal fulfillment.
5. Because a protected sphere of privacy and autonomy is required for the flourishing of this interpersonal union, institutions and the state should be reluctant to intrude, particularly regarding matters that are personal and on which there is a wide range of opinion in society.[11(pp.127–128)]

Even if family members are somehow disqualified as decision makers, the Commission continued, it may be appropriate to consult with them in the decision-making process.[11(pp.128–129)]

James Bopp, president of the National Legal Center for the Medically Dependent and Disabled, recently listed eight reasons why family members may not always appropriately make health care decisions for incompetent relatives.[12(pp.133,141–151)]

1. The family may lack information in the decision-making process because of an inability to obtain or assimilate the information.
2. Family decisions may be influenced by emotional reactions, such as shock, denial, anger, or guilt.
3. Family members may be unable to separate their interests from the interests of the patient.
4. Family financial interests may present a conflict of interest in the decision-making process.
5. Family may inaccurately predict the patient's wishes because of lack of discussion on these topics, difficulty assessing the patient's quality of life, or an inability to predict the wishes of an older person.
6. Family decisions may fail to recognize the changing interests of patients.
7. Family health care decision making may be emotionally burdensome, more so when there is disagreement in the family on the decision.
8. Deference to family may falsely assume a familial bond when there is none.

A balancing of the arguments for and against the family as a surrogate health care decision maker presents no obvious test for the appointment of a surrogate. The familiar and beneficent family, a critical social unit essential to the personal fulfillment of many, deserves the respect and deference of the state and the medical profession. Nevertheless, even the Commission recognized the necessity of limiting such deference. In difficult and emotional times, family must seek out and assimilate technical information and disregard personal or conflicting interests in order to decide, with questionable predictive accuracy, what their incompetent relative would want. Deference to that decision may arise out of a false presumption of familial bond. In the interest of all parties concerned, a structured policy that promotes the proper selection of a surrogate, specific standards of decision making, and limitations on consent power seems appropriate to support and maximize appropriate decision making.

A Decision Maker Who Is Not Family

The person closest to the patient and most knowledgeable about the patient's wishes may not be a "family member" in the traditional sense. As the law generally lags behind societal changes, it often fails to recognize the evolution of new and different units of family.

Unmarried domestic partners or an individual with whom the patient has a long-term, committed relationship may, though not commonly, appear on the priority list of surrogate consent laws.[13,14] Some states recognize the close friend as a possible surrogate in health care decision making, although this person is usually at the bottom of the priority list.[13-19] The nonfamily member often is described as an adult who has exhibited special care and concern for the patient, is familiar with the patient's values and desires, and is reasonably available.

Surrogate Decision-Maker Hierarchies

Some states have codified their policy for acceptable, informally appointed surrogates through family consent laws or surrogate laws.[13-21] These laws establish a hierarchy of acceptable surrogate decision makers which may look something like this:

1. Spouse
2. Adult children
3. Parents
4. Adult siblings
5. Grandparents

Given the fact that most patients have not taken the initiative to execute advance directives, the establishment of formal legal rankings may be useful for anxious physicians and IRBs who are looking for legal guidance, especially when multiple family members disagree about treatment. On the downside, in some cases, the individual identified by statute may not know the patient best. In these states with surrogate decision-making laws, physicians should make sure that patients understand that if they do not execute advance directives, the state will act for them.

Recommendations

1. IRB members and research investigators should understand the legal and ethical controversies associated with choosing a surrogate decision maker when medical research involves participants who are not competent to give informed consent.

2. Institutions responsible for formulating research policy should review state law on guardianship, informed consent, surrogate decision making (if it exists), and advance directives to understand which agents are legally authorized to make health care decisions for incompetent patients. Important questions to answer include the following:

    a. *May a court-appointed guardian consent to research-related activities, or must the guardian refer such decisions to probate court?*

    Some states include "experimental treatment" in the list of activities that are beyond the authority of a guardian. Although one may argue that medical therapy should not be considered experimental simply because it is delivered as part of a research protocol, federal law and most state laws do not distinguish between "experimental" and "research" therapy. A conservative interpretation of those laws would require a guardian to obtain permission from the court to enroll an incompetent patient in a medical research study.

    b. *Is there legislation on the DPAHC? If so, does it address participation in experimental therapy or medical research?*

    Researchers should examine the DPAHC document to determine the situations in which a DPAHC agent is not authorized to consent to research participation. For example, in New Hampshire, DPAHC authority would not extend to consent for participation in medical research under two circumstances: (1) when the executor of the DPAHC has added a statement that specifically limits the agent's authority to consent to participation in medical research and (2) when research involves an activity that is prohibited by law (psychosurgery, sterilization, commitment to a state institution, or termination of treatment under certain well-defined circumstances when the principal is pregnant). In the absence of any of these situations and if not defined otherwise, the phrase "any and all health care decisions" gives the DPAHC agent legal authority to consent to participation in any type of medical research study, including research that involves the use of experimental therapy.

    c. *Is there legislation that authorizes health care providers to act on consent of a family member or friend not formally appointed by a court or DPAHC?*

    In states with surrogate decision-maker hierarchies, the argument that designated surrogates are legally authorized to consent to participation in medical research may be easier to support. However, as discussed earlier, in addition to defining who is legally authorized to make health care decisions for incompetent patients, it is important to know whether the law prohibits certain decisions made by these agents. For example, in New Hampshire an agent under a DPAHC is not authorized to consent to psychosurgery. In states with surrogate decision-maker statutes, it is likely that the law will limit the authority of informally appointed surrogates in similarly sensitive situations.

3. Research policy should recognize the authority of a family or friend to participate in health care decisions, including participation in medical research. The pros and cons of

family involvement in health care decisions were discussed earlier. Local policy should embrace the growing national acceptance of the family-centered philosophy of care by recognizing the right of a properly motivated relative or close friend to participate in the full range of health care decisions in the absence of a formal legal appointment.

4. Institutional policy regarding the use of consent from surrogate decision makers should hold research to a higher standard than general medical practice. In *The Belmont Report*, the National Commission for the Protection of Human Subjects of Biomedical and Behavioral Research argues that the ethical conduct of research requires that individuals with diminished autonomy be given added protection under the law to help protect their rights and welfare. In New Hampshire, state law places limitations on consent that reflect heightened standards for research and the primacy of self-determination. The New Hampshire guardian may not consent to experimental treatment without court approval, demonstrating the legislature's recognition of heightened standards specific to the research setting. The guardian's power of consent is further limited by a valid DPAHC, establishing the primacy of self-determination.

5. The decision to use consent from an informally appointed surrogate to enroll a clinically incompetent person in a medical research study should be based on three factors: the risk of harm, the probability of direct benefit, and the implications of delaying study participation for the time it would take to appoint a legal guardian. IRBs and research investigators need unambiguous criteria that define the circumstances under which consent from a person who is not a court-appointed guardian or agent under a DPAHC may be used to enroll a clinically incompetent patient in a medical research study. For example, the Dartmouth College IRB requires that all investigators who want to enroll incompetent patients in research answer a series of questions that evaluate the issues critical to the choice of surrogate decision makers.

    a. *Will participation in the study increase the risk of harm or discomfort compared with what would be expected if the subject were managed outside the setting of a research protocol?*

    The distinction between absolute and relative risk is critical when evaluating medical research that involves surrogate consent. The absolute risk of a given form of medical treatment is irrelevant. The important factor to evaluate is the difference in risk associated with research participation. The goal of research laws and regulations is to protect research subjects from harm. When there is no risk differential, a liberal interpretation of legal limits on surrogate decision-maker authority is appropriate. When research participation is associated with a meaningful increase in risk, maximum ethical safeguards should be required for the incompetent patient.

    b. *Will participation in the study increase the chance of a favorable outcome compared with what would be expected if the subject were managed outside the setting of a research protocol?*

    As with risk, when evaluating the potential benefits of research participation, it is important to look at relative rather than absolute outcome. In some situations, research therapy is likely to be better than what would be obtained outside the research setting. Denying patients access to beneficial treatment is harmful.

    c. *The process of appointing a legal guardian may take months. Would this type of delay compromise patient care?*

    When there is a meaningful chance of direct benefit to the research subject, over and above what could be obtained outside the setting of a research protocol, a requirement that consent be obtained from a formally appointed surrogate may limit access to potentially beneficial therapy. In this situation, IRB members must use their judgment to decide whether to allow consent from an informal surrogate. When a study is likely to have a favorable risk/benefit ratio (compared with standard therapy), and it would be detrimental to delay for the time it takes to appoint a guardian, the Dartmouth IRB accepts consent from a family member.

    d. *What benefit will future patients experience as a result of the subject's participating in this study?*

    This question is only important when research participation does not have a chance of increasing direct benefit for the participant. The Dartmouth policy is that it is never acceptable to conduct research on a clinically incompetent patient when research participation increases risk and there is no chance of direct benefit for the participant. Regardless of how strongly a surrogate believes the incompetent person would wish to participate in research for the benefit of future patients, the presence of increased risk establishes an ethical boundary to surrogate authority that should not be crossed.

There are acceptable situations where participation in research does not increase risk or offer the potential for direct benefit. Studies that involve the prospective collection of data from routine medical care frequently fall into this category. When a study does not increase risk, the Dartmouth IRB will approve the involvement of incompetent subjects based on consent from a family member.

Conclusion

It is frequently difficult to determine which surrogate decision-makers are legally authorized to consent for an incompetent patient to participate in medical research. Some states have surrogate decision-maker statutes that clearly define the role of a surrogate in general medical practice, but it may be difficult to decide how such laws apply to medical research. As most states will not have legislation on this point, institutions in these states must establish a policy that defines the "legally authorized representative." Such policy should be rooted in the principles enunciated by the Commission and in the institution's state law and state public policy.

Acknowledgment
The authors thank Michelle Winchester for extensive legal research and editorial revision. An abbreviated version of this chapter is published in *IRB: A Review of Human Subjects Research* 22(4):7–11, 2000. Used with permission.

References

1. Mary E. Schloendorff, Appellant, v. The Society of the New York Hospital, Respondent. *Schloendorff v. Society of New York Hospital.* (105 N.E. 92, 93). 1914. Court of Appeals of New York. Affirmed.

2. Furrow BR, Greaney TL, Johnson SH, Jost TS, Schwartz RL. *Health Law,* Vols. 1 and 2. St. Paul, MN: West Publishing Co. Hornbook Series; 1995.

3. 93rd Congress. National Research Act of 1974. PL93-348. 1974.

4. National Commission for the Protection of Human Subjects of Biomedical and Behavioral Research. *The Belmont Report: Ethical principles and guidelines for the protection of human subjects of research.* DHEW Publication No. (OS) 78-0013 and (OS) 78-0014.4. Washington, DC: U.S. Government Printing Office, 18 April, 1979. Access date: March 22, 2001. http://ohsr.od.nih.gov/mpa/belmont.php3

5. Wichman A. Protecting vulnerable research subjects: Practical realities of institutional review board review and approval. *J Health Care Policy* 1(1):88–104, 1998.

6. Busby-Mott S. The trend towards enlightenment: Health care decision making in Lawrance and Doe. *Conn L Rev* 25(4):1159–1225, 1993.

7. Code of Federal Regulations. Title 45A—Department of Health and Human Services; Part 46—Protection of Human Subjects. Updated 1 October, 1997. Access date: April 18, 2001. http://www4.law.cornell.edu/cfr/45p46.htm

8. New Hampshire Revised Statutes Annotated. Title XLIV. Guardians and Conservators. Chapter 464-A. Guardians and Conservators. RSA 464-A (2000), 1–25. 2001.

9. Simon MM, Blais VL. The role of family in health care decisions: NH law. *New Hampshire Bar J* 36:34–37, 1995.

10. New Hampshire Revised Statutes Annotated. Title X. Public Health. Chapter 137-J. Durable Power of Attorney for Health Care. RSA 137-J, 1–15. 2000.

11. President's Commission for the Study of Ethical Problems in Medicine and Biomedical and Behavioral Research. *Deciding to Forego Life-Sustaining Treatment: A Report on the Ethical, Medical, and Legal Issues in Treatment Decisions.* Washington, DC: Superintendent of Documents; 1983:554.

12. Bopp J Jr, Coleson RE. A critique of family members as proxy decision makers without legal limits. *Issues Law Med* 12(2):133–165, 1996.

13. Arizona Revised Statutes. Title 36. Public Health and Safety. Chapter 32. Living Wills and Health Care Directives. Article 3. Surrogate Decision Makers. A.R.S. 36-3231 (2000) (Suppl. 1997), 2000.

14. New Mexico Statutes Annotated. Chapter 24. Health and Safety. Article 7A. Uniform Health-Care Decisions. Section 24-7A-5. Decisions by surrogate. N.M. Stat. Ann. 24-7A-5 (2000). 2000.

15. Delaware Code Annotated. Title 16. Health and Safety. Part II. Regulatory Provisions Concerning Public Health. Chapter 25. Health-Care Decisions. Section 2507. Surrogates. 16 Del. C. 2507 (2000) (Suppl. 1996). 2001.

16. Florida Statutes 2000. Title XLIV Civil Rights. Chapter 765 Health Care Advance Directives. Part IV Absence of Advance Directive. Section 401 The Proxy. Fla. Stat. 765.401 (2000) (West 1997). 2000.

17. Illinois Compiled Statutes Annotated. Chapter 755. Estates. Health Care Surrogate Act. Section 40/25. Surrogate decision making. 755 ILCS 40/25 (2000) (Smith-Hurd Suppl. 1998). 2000.

18. Maine Revised Statutes. Title 18-A. Probate Code. Article V. Protection of Persons Under Disability and Their Property. Part 8. Uniform Health-Care Decisions Act. Section 5-805. Decisions by surrogate. 18-A M.R.S. 5-805 (2000). 2000.

19. Maryland Annotated Code. Health-General. Title 5. Death. Subtitle 6. Health Care Decisions Act. Section 5-605. Surrogate decision making. Md. Health-General Code Ann. 5-605 (2001). 2001.

20. Connecticut General Statutes. Title 19A. Public Health and Well-Being. Chapter 368W. Removal of Life Support Systems. Section 19a-570. Definitions. Conn. Gen. Stat. 19a-570 (1999) (West 1997). 2000.

21. Kentucky Revised Statutes Annotated. Title XXVI. Occupations and Professions. Chapter 311. Physicians, Osteopaths, and Podiatrists. Kentucky Living Will Directive Act. Section 631. Responsible Parties Authorized to Make

Research-Related Injuries

Daniel R. Vasgird

INTRODUCTION

Currently, research institutions are not mandated to provide free medical care or compensation to research participants for research-induced injuries. The Code of Federal Regulations addresses the issue of the medical liability of research institutions to their subjects.[1[Sec.116(a)(6)]] Under the regulations, research institutions are only responsible for explaining whether medical treatments are available and whether any compensation will be provided to the research subject in the event that the individual should sustain an injury as a result of his or her participation in the study. In essence, the clause does not require research institutions to provide free medical care to research subjects for research-related injuries.

From a practical standpoint, there are two points for institutional review board (IRB) members and administrators to keep in mind related to this issue. First, IRBs have the ethical responsibility to raise the bar when necessary to ensure the adequate provision of free or compensated medical care for research-related injury, and second, they have the regulatory authority to enact these provisions as they see fit.

Ongoing Debate

National commissions of bioethics have debated this issue for decades and have even gone so far as to endorse a recommendation that compensation should be provided to research subjects for injuries that include harm, disability, or death directly and proximately caused by their participation in a research study.[2,3] This has all been to no avail, however, with the past 20 years marked by increasing responsiveness to the research needs of business and industry and less focus on the concerns of the research subject.[4-6]

Recently, this concern has grown to international proportions as well. Although the question of compensation to persons injured in research in developing countries is often overshadowed by the issue of comparable standard of care, participants in the 2001 *Conference on Ethical Aspects of Research in Developing Countries* examined the issue with unusual purpose and depth. In response to the question of compensation to persons injured in international research, a guidance paper was written entitled, "Moral Standards for Research in Developing Countries: From Reasonable Availability to Fair Benefits." Here it was argued that effective intervention must be both reasonably available and offer a fair benefit. The prevention of the exploitation of participants is the key to fair benefits, and this notion was extended to the idea of compensation.

Within the fair benefits framework, the usual conditions for research exist—individual informed consent and independent review by an institutional review board or ethics committee—yet the research should be *beneficial*. Thus, "research should have social value, subjects should be treated fairly, and the research should have a favorable risk-benefit ratio." Perhaps most importantly, these benefits should be extended to research participants both during and after the research project to avoid exploitation, a suggestion that has initiated heated debates and major concern in discussions of informed consent.[7]

Vulnerability

Study subjects often do not understand the full implications of the decision to participate in research.[8] Informed consent forms are often abstract and filled with medical and scientific jargon that is confusing to many research subjects. At the same time, it is evident that a growing number of research subjects in high-risk studies are drawn from lower socioeconomic status groups.[9] Therefore, the issue of whether these individuals understand when they will not receive compensated or free medical care for injuries sustained as a result of their participation in a study is of great importance if we are to safeguard their rights.

Case in Point

To illustrate how important this topic is, let me recount an incident that happened about 10 years ago. I had just begun a decade-long tenure as chairperson of the New York City Department of Health's IRB. About the same time that I started as chair, a series of quinolone antibiotic studies were submitted for IRB review. The principal investigator (PI) was a well-known researcher who had received funding from a pharmaceutical company and wanted to use departmental treatment clinics for tuberculosis and sexually transmitted diseases to recruit subjects for his studies, something he had done a number of times in the past. When I read through the first protocol, I noted that everything seemed to be in order. However, when I reached the end of the informed consent form, I noticed a clause that essentially stated that should anything go wrong, the research subject was responsible for the costs of any required medical care in the event he or she was not insured.

This struck an immediate chord of sensibility, and thus, I looked into past studies and made some inquiries. What I found out was not reassuring. Federal regulations were minimal in this area, requiring only that the subject be told that he or she would not receive free medical care or be compensated for research-related injuries or problems.

On the other hand, Office for Human Research Protections (OHRP) (formerly the Office for Protection from Research Risks) was clear that we were entitled to be more exacting if necessary. Further inquiry within our department revealed that over 70% of individuals using our clinical services had no health insurance whatsoever, as opposed to roughly 20% of the population in general. In addition, a careful reading of the risk section of the consent document made it obvious that the side effects from the proposed drugs could be serious enough to necessitate seeking medical care. When we broached this with the PI, insisting that he provide free medical care in the event of problems, he was insistent that this was standard operating procedure for all medical research and argued that our IRB was overstepping its bounds in making these demands. After prolonged and sometimes heated discussion, the PI ultimately had the pharmaceutical company agree to pay any medical costs stemming from the research, and this was included in the consent form.

The Nuremberg Code and *The Belmont Report*

The fourth provision of the Nuremberg Code addresses the issue of compensation for research-related injuries: "The experiment should be so conducted as to avoid all unnecessary physical and mental suffering and injury."[10] Drawn from the Nuremberg Code, *The Belmont Report* explicitly supports the view that its three ethical principles should serve as the criteria by which decisions on changes in policy governing human research can be justified. These principles of respect for persons, beneficence, and justice were constructed to "provide a basis on which specific rules may be formulated, criticized, and interpreted."[11] Specifically, the principles of beneficence and justice inform us of our responsibility to address the issue of medical liability. In my opinion, they provide grounds for requiring research institutions to provide free medical coverage to human subjects.

Beneficence

The principle of beneficence calls on us to secure the well-being of human subjects by reducing the risks involved in studies. These efforts are not simply acts of kindness or charity, as the word beneficence might suggest, but rather an expression of our moral obligation. If we fail to respond to an opportunity that would reduce the involved risks without compromising the potential benefits that are likely to be generated by research, we have violated the principle of beneficence at the outset. In some situations, mandating free medical coverage for research-related injuries would limit study accrual and thereby decrease societal benefit. Such a compromise is justified in deference to the protection of individual welfare in this setting. The ethical mandate to require coverage of medical care related to research injury is particularly strong when research is conducted in a setting with a high potential for coercion resulting from the lack of access to comparable care outside the setting of a research protocol.

Justice

In its most simple terms, the lack of compensation for medical care to individuals who are injured as a result of their involvement in a research study is ethically indefensible because it is unjust. There is a matter of relativity in this issue, however, and those who are financially most vulnerable among us run the greatest risks. In its *IRB Guidebook*, the OHRP's interpretation of the *Belmont* principle of justice explicitly states that "considerations (of the principle of justice) may be appropriate to avoid the injustice that arises from social, racial, sexual, and cultural biases institutionalized in society."[12] As is often mentioned when this matter is discussed, if we had national health insurance, this would be a nonissue. However, we do not, and the present does not bode well for such an initiative in the near future. Injustice related to a lack of coverage for research-related injury can be prevented by IRBs' accepting ethical responsibility and understanding their authority in this regard.

Sample IRB Policy Statement for Researchers Regarding Research-Related Injury

The following statement (or one similar) might be adopted as a component of IRB policy.

Investigators must include a statement in the consent document explaining that medical treatment will be provided free of charge to research subjects should they sustain any injury as a consequence of their participation in the study. Any statements that waive or appear to waive the subject's rights and release the investigator from any liability should not be included in the informed consent form.

By federal regulation 45 CFR 46[1[Sec.116(a)(6)]] research institutions are only responsible for providing "an explanation as to whether any compensation and an explanation as to whether any medical treatments are available if injury occurs, and, if so, what they consist of, or where information may be obtained for research involving more than minimal risk."

This clause outlines only a minimum federal standard that must be met by research institutions. It is federal policy that individual IRBs can exceed that standard as they deem appropriate. The IRB of [name of institution] requires all research involving human subjects to provide medical treatment to subjects who are injured as a result of participation in that research, regardless of the risk involved. Consent forms lacking this requirement will be denied approval from this IRB.

Sample Wording for Informed Consent Form

Wording suggested for use in the consent document follows:

What will it cost me to participate?
There is no cost to you for participating in this study. Medical treatment will be provided free of charge should you sustain an injury as a consequence of your participation in the study.

Conclusion

As the research industry continues to proliferate and the proportion of uninsured and underinsured individuals in the United States population remains a growing problem, the only practical approach is to educate our colleagues and encourage individual institutions to realistically appraise the potential for injury, insisting that researchers make provisions for free care in circumstances that dictate as much. By necessity, it is a decentralized approach, allowing for flexibility and discretion on the one hand but, unfortunately, self-serving or uninformed disregard on the other. Certainly, this is such a fundamental and extraordinarily important ethical requirement that it should be federally mandated and not left to the inconsistent discretion of individual IRBs. However, present circumstances dictate a more singular approach. There certainly is precedent now for institutions to rectify this ethical lapse. The University of Washington in Seattle has had such a policy in place for a number of years, and in 1998 the Department of Veterans Affairs amended its medical regulations to provide free medical treatment to human subjects injured as a result of their participating in Department of Veterans Affairs clinical research projects.[13]

In conclusion, this chapter presents the view that research subjects should receive free medical treatment if their participation in the research results in adverse health effects. The benefits that result from a study often are indirect and are primarily for the good and benefit of society. Thus, society has a responsibility to subjects who suffer research-related injuries, especially those in vulnerable population subgroups, who face an additional—and heavier—burden of research risk because they lack adequate health insurance. It is unlikely that these truly vulnerable groups would have the skills to negotiate the legal pathways to obtain reimbursement for medical care for research-related injuries. Although the debate over universal health care—that is, health care as a right versus health care as

privilege—will continue, the question of providing free medical care for research-related injuries is an issue of present social and moral responsibility. It is the obligation and right of IRBs to seize opportunities in which they can minimize these inequities and prevent additional burdens.

References

1. Code of Federal Regulations. Title 45A—Department of Health and Human Services; Part 46—Protection of Human Subjects. Updated 1 October, 1997. Access date 18 April, 2001. http://www4.law.cornell.edu/cfr/45p46.htm

2. President's Commission for the Study of Ethical Problems in Medicine and Biomedical and Behavioral Research. *Compensating for Research Injuries,* Vols. 1 and 2. Buffalo, NY: William S. Hein & Co.; 1982.

3. McCarthy CR. Challenges to IRBs in the coming decades. In: Vanderpool HY (ed.). *The Ethics of Research Involving Human Subjects: Facing the 21st Century.* Frederick, MD: University Publishing Group; 1996:140–141.

4. Havighurst C. Compensating persons injured in human experimentation. *Science* 169:154–155, 1970.

5. Vasgird DR. Protecting the uninsured human research subject. *J Public Health Manage Pract* 6(6):37–47, 2000.

6. Anna GJ. *The Rights of Patients: The Basic ACLU Guide to Patient Rights,* 2nd ed. Carbondale, IL: Southern Illinois University Press; 1989:154.

7. The Hastings Center Report. "Moral Standards for Research in Developing Countries." Volume 34(3):17–27, 2004.

8. Pullman D. General provisional proxy consent to research: Redefining the role of the local research ethics board. *IRB: A Review of Human Subjects Research* 21(3):1–9, 1999.

9. Darity WA. Ethics in human experimentation in health care delivery. In: National Commission for the Protection of Human Subjects of Biomedical and Behavioral Research. *Ethical Guidelines for the Delivery of Health Services.* Washington, DC: Government Printing Office; 1978.

10. The Nuremberg Code. Chapter 12: Permissible medical experiments. *Trials of War Criminals Before the Nuremberg Military Tribunals Under Control Council Law No. 10, Vol. 2.* Washington, DC: U.S. Government Printing Office; 1949: 181–182. Access date 20 August, 2001. http://www.ushmm.org/research/doctors/Nuremberg_Code.htm

11. National Commission for the Protection of Human Subjects of Biomedical and Behavioral Research. *The Belmont Report: Ethical Principles and Guidelines for the Protection of Human Subjects of Research,* 18 April, 1979. Access date 22 March, 2001. http://ohsr.od.nih.gov/mpa/belmont.php3

12. Penslar RL, Porter JP, Office for Human Research Protections. *Institutional Review Board Guidebook,* 2nd ed. 6 February, 2001. Access date 29 March, 2001. http://ohrp.osophs.dhhs.gov/irb/irb_guidebook.htm

13. Department of Veterans Affairs. Treatment of research-related injuries to human subjects (38 CFR Part 17). *Fed Regist* 63(44):11123–11124, 1998. www.access.gpo.gov/nara/cfr/cfrhtml_00/Title_38/38cfr17_main_00.html

Informing Subjects About Research Results

Thomas G. Keens

INTRODUCTION

This explains the decisions that institutional review boards (IRBs) face regarding informing subjects of study results. It is best to start with case discussions.

Case 1

Investigators wish to determine whether a specific genetic mutation is associated with an increased risk for heart disease. To do this, they will sample blood from a large number of normal individuals. They will then wait to see who develops heart disease and correlate the information with the genetic finding. It is not now known whether this gene is related to heart disease, although the investigators have some reason to believe that this might be true.

Should the subjects in the study be told whether or not they have the gene mutation? On one hand, informing subjects that they have the mutation might motivate them to do things to decrease their risk of heart disease, such as stop cigarette smoking, eat less fat, and exercise more. However, informing subjects that they do not have the genetic mutation may lull some into complacency in the belief that they will not get heart disease. On the other hand, it is not known whether the genetic mutation is truly associated with a higher risk of heart disease. Therefore, the implications of having the genetic mutation are not known, but knowledge that one has the mutation might cause undue anxiety or distress in subjects who would then believe they are destined to die of heart disease.

Should the research subjects be told whether or not they have the genetic mutation? Do the subjects have a right to know? Do the investigators have an obligation to tell the subjects? Do the investigators have a right to withhold this information?

Case 2

Urinary tract infections in newborn infants are a known cause of neonatal jaundice. Investigators wish to determine how often undetected urinary tract infections are present in otherwise asymptomatic infants who are seen in the emergency department for persistent neonatal jaundice in the first week of life. They will perform urinalyses and urine cultures on all such infants seen in the emergency

department. This testing is not the clinical standard of care in this setting. The urine culture will accurately determine whether an infant has a urinary tract infection. Current medical practice would recommend that such urinary tract infections should be treated with antibiotics.

Should the investigators be required to inform the parents of the research subject, or their doctor, if the subject has a urinary tract infection? Informing them will give subjects the opportunity to receive treatment. Do the parents of the subjects have a right to know? Do the investigators have a right to withhold this information?

Case 3

Infants born to mothers who used cocaine during pregnancy have an increased risk of dying of sudden infant death syndrome (SIDS). Some researchers believe that SIDS may be related to abnormal breathing patterns or pauses in breathing during sleep, but this is not proven. The investigators wish to record breathing patterns in infants born to mothers who used cocaine during pregnancy to see if they are abnormal. These investigators do not believe that clinical care should be changed based on breathing pattern results. Other experts, however, would put babies with abnormal breathing patterns on electronic monitors or alarm systems when they sleep.

The investigators inform the IRB that they will not disclose the results of these recordings to the families. Should the families be told the results of these research tests? If the parents are told the results of the research study, some may monitor their infants. Some may needlessly worry about information that the researchers do not believe has any predictive value. If these recordings are ultimately shown to relate to the risk for SIDS, not being told the information may deprive families of the opportunity to do something to prevent SIDS. Should the families be told the research results? Do the parents have a right to be told? Do the investigators have an obligation to tell the parents? Do the investigators have a right to withhold the results?

Clinical Care Versus Research

In clinical care, physicians and health care professionals have a primary obligation to place the interests of their patient foremost. All diagnostic tests and therapeutic procedures are performed with the best interests of the patient in mind. Although medicine is not an exact science with predictable laws like physics, patients believe to some degree that they can rely on medical knowledge to guide their medical care. For most medical conditions, diagnostic tests are performed because the results will have an impact on the patient's situation. The information derived from these tests may allow a physician to select the most appropriate therapy, to guide treatment, or to give a prognosis. Because diagnostic tests in medicine are being performed to benefit the patient, physicians generally have an obligation to inform patients about the results of these tests.

Research, by its very nature, deals with the unknown. There is less certainty. Research information is more speculative than information derived from medical tests performed for clinical care. A primary goal of research is always to benefit society in general. Although some studies have the potential to directly benefit current subjects, in many situations, altruism is the main reason to participate in research. Thus, tests and procedures may be performed primarily to benefit the research study, and not because the results will have an impact on the patient's disease. The information derived from these tests will not allow a physician to select the most appropriate therapy, to guide treatment, or to give a prognosis. When diagnostic tests in research are not being performed to benefit the subject, it is reasonable to suggest that researchers do not have an obligation to inform subjects about the results of these tests. A more difficult issue is the ethics of refusing to give research results to subjects who understand the uncertainty involved.

Federal Regulations

Federal regulations on protecting human subjects are silent on the issue of whether or not subjects should be given research results.[1] International codes on the ethical conduct of human research similarly do not comment on whether research subjects should be told research results.[2–4] These codes do indicate information that subjects should be given before consenting to participation in a research study. In some cases, the regulations require that the investigators explicitly tell potential subjects whether or not they will be given the research results and, if so, how and by whom.[1] The regulations, however, do not say that research subjects are always entitled to receive such results. They do not say that investigators are always obligated to communicate such results nor that they are entitled to withhold such results.

The one situation in which federal regulations require that subjects be informed about research results is when the new findings developed in the course of the study may change the balance of risks versus benefits to the subject.[1[Sec.116(b)(5)]] In this case, the following information shall be provided to research subjects:

> Significant new findings developed during the course of the research which may relate to the subject's willingness to continue participation will be provided to the subject.

Thus, investigators have an obligation to inform subjects about results from the study that may change their decision to participate. This is a different issue than whether or not to inform a research subject about test results performed on him or her as part of research. Therefore, regulations on protecting human research subjects do not guide the IRB in deciding which research information, if any, should be communicated to subjects.

Other Legal Requirements in Specific Cases

There are situations where state law requires the reporting of information whether it is collected for research or nonresearch purposes. There are limits to confidentiality. For example, if a research study determines that child abuse has occurred or that a subject may be a danger to himself or others or that reportable communicable diseases are present, the investigator has a legal obligation to report such findings to appropriate authorities. It is important to note that in situations where the law requires the reporting of test results or evaluations, the information carries the same degree of certainty as information obtained as part of medical care. Disclosure of this type of information will benefit the subject and/or others. Therefore, disclosing this type of information is analogous to informing patients about their own medical test results.

Ethical Principles

The Belmont Report is the classic reference for the three basic principles underlying the ethical conduct of human research and the protection of human research subjects.[5] Of these principles, respect for persons and beneficence address the issue of informing subjects about research results. At first glance, these principles appear to present competing obligations.

Respect for Persons
The principle of respect for persons acknowledges the freedom and dignity of every person. A person should be able to choose what will and will not happen to him or her. Respect for persons motivates ethical research to require that subjects understand the full implications of their decision to participate in research. There are two ways one could apply the principle of respect for persons to the question of informing subjects of research results. One might argue that respect for persons requires that researchers give each subject the option of being informed of research results, with a full explanation of the potential implications of this decision. From this perspective, researchers would be ethically obligated to report research results to any subject who wants them.

The alternative view interprets the principle of respect for persons to mean that informed consent requires the potential subjects to understand if they will or will not be informed of research results. There is, however, no ethical justification for requiring result disclosure per se. Subjects are not required to participate in research. It is perfectly ethical to allow people to exercise their right as autonomous agents to decline to participate in a research study because they do not agree with the plan to limit access to research results.

Beneficence

Beneficence recognizes the obligation to maximize potential benefits and minimize potential risks. One should not injure a person despite the possibility of benefit to others, such as to society. Research-related risks to subjects must be reasonable in light of expected benefits to the subject or to society. Risks to subjects should be minimized. This principle argues that investigators should do what is best for the subject. Beneficence dictates that an investigator is obligated to provide a subject with research information if that information will maximize benefits or minimize risks to the subject. Beneficence also argues that the investigator should not inform the subject about research results if that information would cause harm. If we apply this argument to the three case studies at the beginning of this chapter, the outcome is not definitive. One can support an argument that it is ethical to not inform subjects of research results in cases where there is uncertainty about the importance of these results to clinical issues that would affect the welfare of the subject. In case 1, the research results are not known to benefit individuals, and they may be harmful; thus, the investigator should not inform the subject. In case 2, informing the subject would clearly maximize benefits and minimize harm, and thus, the investigator would be obligated to inform the subject. In case 3, the interpretation of these research results varies according to different experts. Therefore, the investigator may be obligated to inform or not inform subjects, depending on the investigator's considered opinion. The take-home message from this analysis is that the critical issue in evaluating the ethics of a study that would withhold information about research results from subjects is the level of confidence in the accuracy of the information at the time that the study is being conducted.

Research Information: Knowledge or Speculation

Information derived from subjects through research may constitute knowledge or potentially relevant information, or it may constitute speculative data of little relevance to the individual subject. In case 1, the information derived about each subject is speculative at best. It is not known whether this information truly predicts any clinical outcome. Furthermore, there may be harm in providing this information to subjects if they are then misled to believe that they are at risk. Therefore, as a generalization, for speculative information, not proven to have clinical relevance to the subject, the investigator is not obligated to inform the research subject. Because providing subjects with this information may cause harm, one can make a strong argument that the investigator has an ethical obligation to withhold such information from the research subject.

In case 2, the information has direct clinical implications for the subject. The information is not speculative but has specific and agreed-on clinical implications. Therefore, it is likely to be in the best interest of research subjects to have research results disclosed to the parents of the subjects or their physicians. In general, the investigator is obligated to inform the subject of research results when there is little or no question that access to the information could benefit the subject.

Case 3 provides an example with more ambiguity. Some experts believe that the research information has clinically relevant predictive value and that treatment may be implemented based on this information. Other experts believe this information has no clinical relevance and that treatment should not be based on this information. This study was actually performed by investigators at two institutions, and therefore the study was reviewed by two IRBs. Both IRBs approved the study. At institution A, the IRB agreed with the investigators' assessment that the research information had no clinical utility and that it might worry some parents. Therefore, the study was approved at institution A, provided parents were not given the results of the research study, and the parents were informed that they would not receive the research results. At institution B, the IRB sided with experts who believed the research results might have potential predictive value and/or clinical relevance. Therefore, the study was approved at institution B, provided that parents were given the results of the research study, and the parents were informed that they would receive these results. Both IRB decisions were correct. Both IRBs acted on their views of the strength of the research information and its relevance to the subjects' clinical care.

The bottom line is that subjects should always understand whether they or their physicians will or will not be informed of research results. Sometimes it may be appropriate to offer subjects a choice about whether they wish to have the information disclosed after they have been informed about the nature of the information. An example of this would be a population study on the incidence of the Huntington's disease gene. Huntington's disease is an incurable, degenerative neurologic disorder that is inherited and ultimately fatal. If a subject has the gene, he or she will develop Huntington's disease in middle age. Some subjects want to know this information in young adult life, when they are still asymptomatic. Other subjects do not want to know such information. Although the information is certain (correlates absolutely with the development of Huntington's disease), there is nothing subjects can do to prevent or modify the fact that they will develop this fatal disease if they have the gene. In such a study, the IRB could permit the subjects to decide whether or not they want to have the information disclosed after informing them of the implications.

Conclusion

As part of their review of human research protocols, IRBs must decide whether or not research information should be given to subjects. To help in this determination, the IRB should consider the following:

1. A complete understanding of the extent to which research results will be disclosed to the subjects and/or their physicians is an absolute requirement of ethical research.

2. When considering the ethics of withholding research results from study subjects, an important consideration is the level of certainty that this information will impact the diagnosis, management, or prognosis of the subject.

3. Disclosing research results to subjects may harm research subjects. Risks may be the dominant factor when the accuracy of research results is in question.

4. In some situations, it is appropriate for the research plan to allow the subjects to choose whether research results will be given to them or their physician.

5. When research results are disclosed to subjects, the process should always be structured in a way that respects privacy, offers appropriate support when news is bad, and involves persons knowledgeable about all of the implications of the information with respect to the subject's disease or disorder.

References

1. Code of Federal Regulations. Title 45A—Department of Health and Human Services; Part 46—Protection of Human Subjects. Updated 1 October, 1997. Access date 18 April, 2001. http://www4.law.cornell.edu/cfr/45p46.htm

2. U.S. Supreme Court. Order denying writ of habeas corpus, October 20, 1947. *Trials of War Criminals Before the Nuremberg Military Tribunals Under Control Council Law, Volume 2, Chapter 10*. 1949: 888.

3. World Medical Association. *Declaration of Helsinki: Ethical Principles for Medical Research Involving Human Subjects*. First adopted in Helsinki, Finland, in 1964. Updated 10 July, 2000. Access date 20 March, 2001. http://www.wma.net/e/policy/17-c_e.html

4. Council for International Organizations of Medical Sciences, World Health Organization. International ethical guidelines for biomedical research involving human subjects. In: Vanderpool HY (ed.). *The Ethics of Research Involving Human Subjects: Facing the 21st Century*. Frederick, MD: University Publishing Group; 1996:501–510.

5. National Commission for the Protection of Human Subjects of Biomedical and Behavioral Research. *The Belmont Report: Ethical Principles and Guidelines for the Protection of Human Subjects of Research*, 18 April, 1979. Access date 22 March, 2001. http://ohsr.od.nih.gov/mpa/belmont.php3

Explaining the Cost of Research Participation

Kevin M. Hunt

INTRODUCTION

Just after my first institutional review board (IRB) meeting, I was attempting to describe to a colleague what had happened there. I related the efforts required for reading copious amounts of esoteric research and the nature of the debates at the meeting. I questioned how my financial focus intersected with this process. My colleague's response to my doubts was to declare, "This is where the rubber meets the blue sky."

As the former Director of Patient Financial Services at a prestigious academic medical center, I spent more than 5 years participating with the Committee for the Protection of Human Subjects. I have found the work on the IRB to be both rewarding and meaningful. In contrast to the doubts that characterized my earlier participation with the IRB, I am now convinced that the complete and accurate disclosure of research-related costs is critical to the essential protections that must be offered to all human subjects. I further believe that this same level of disclosure of research-related costs is critical to the compliance protections that need to be in place for the medical organizations where the research is taking place. Finally, the complete disclosure of research-related costs will help to minimize any possible potential conflict of interest issues that could adversely impact the research participant.

There has been a dramatic evolution in the collective thinking of IRB members regarding the numerous issues related to explaining research-related costs. The progression in member's thinking has gone from considering the issues of research-related costs as little more than an administrative burden, demanding slight attention, to such issues being an essential component of every deliberation on every protocol submitted to the IRB. The purpose of this chapter is to review and examine the IRB's responsibility to extend protections regarding research-related costs to human subjects. I also discuss the role that the IRB must play in protecting the institution's exposure as it pertains to research-related costs.

Disclosure of Research-Related Costs to Human Subjects

The cost associated with research participation directly affects every human subject enrolling in a research study.

Research-related costs are all potential out-of-pocket expenses to participants resulting from their participation in a research protocol. These costs typically include coinsurance and deductible payments and potentially the costs of noncovered services as defined by the participant's insurance carrier. Other first-dollar expenses may be associated with their participation in a protocol, such as travel or payment for explicit research services, drugs, or supplies. For participants who are uninsured, all costs will be first-dollar expenses for all care being rendered during the course of a study.

Most studies provide varying degrees of financial coverage from the industrial sponsor for those drugs or procedures being studied within the research design. However, studies that do not clearly distinguish services that are medically necessary from those services being provided to advance research objectives can result in costs being shifted to the research participants. Payment for these services may be denied by the insurance carrier and then be billed to the participant.

Sometimes participants may incur substantial research-related costs. For example, a Phase I cancer drug trial was proposed to our IRB that required both inpatient hospitalization and extensive outpatient follow-up, testing, and monitoring. The study was well received by the scientific community, but it had no corporate or industrial sponsor. The protocol consent documents did not address the research-related costs because the principal investigator's intended to find a sponsor. What should an IRB do in such a case? Given the scientific merits of the investigation, and that adequate safety monitoring was available to the human subjects, should the IRB approve the study? Should the IRB table the protocol until a sponsor is found? Might the IRB approve the study because its first mission to protect human subjects had been met, and let the individual research participant make the final determination as to his or her enrollment in the study? There may be more than one right answer to these questions, but this protocol, as presented, placed the research participant at significant financial risk. The research-related costs in this study were estimated to be in the range of $10,000 to $20,000. The financial effects on the participants were simply too great. The total expenses, in my opinion, clearly crossed a threshold of unreasonableness. What, however, should a reasonable cost threshold be? IRBs easily recognize when research stipends are too high and constitute a coercive inducement. However, IRBs have not developed similar vigilance regarding reasonableness standards as they apply to transferring research-related costs to participants. Perhaps we want to believe that if the research participant has insurance, then all research-related expenses are covered. I would argue that this point of view is no longer sufficient if we want to provide reasonable protections to human subjects and to the research institution. The devil is in the details. Although it is difficult to know to what extent insurance plans will provide coverage, we need to do a better job than we are doing today.

Informed Consent Language

My opinion is that research participants should be routinely informed that their participation in a clinical trial may result in the refusal of their insurance company to pay any costs of their medical care, unless we explicitly know otherwise. Ironically, Medicare has the most comprehensive coverage policy for beneficiaries who participate in research, whereas many commercial carrier insurance policies typically extricate the plan from providing any coverage for any investigational, experimental, or research-related services. However, a U.S. General Accounting Office (GAO) report to Congress indicated, "Insurers may unknowingly pay for trial-related care for patients who enroll without the insurer's explicit approval."[1] Having insurance plans unwittingly pay for research-related costs is definitely not the correct approach for providing protections to human subjects. At my institution a few years ago, the informed consent form language from the "financial consideration" section was very clear. Then, the consent document stated, "All costs associated with this study will be billed to you or your insurance carrier. Your insurance company may not pay the costs for medical treatment as a result of your enrollment in a research study."

It is remarkable that anybody enrolled in a research protocol when statements such as this were included. Clearly, human subjects are willing to risk a great deal if they believe their health or life may hang in the balance. Participants may even believe that the services being provided to them in a research protocol are superior to standard care. Clearly that is not the case, and this is where a participant's altruism, health care needs, and hopes make him or her part of a very vulnerable population. IRBs often approve studies where research participants must be willing to incur research-related costs in order to receive a placebo.

IRB members must question whether human subjects in research protocols are being adequately protected if the protocols include exposures to unreasonable research-related costs. Each IRB needs to articulate its own standards for financial reasonableness in research-related costs in order to evaluate when this line has been crossed. Evidence that IRBs are moving in this positive direction can be found in the wording of a current "financial considerations" section of the informed consent when it paraphrases the following statement.

You will not be charged, nor will your insurance carrier be charged, for any test or visit that is completed solely for the purpose of this study. The sponsor of the study will pay for all costs associated with the research component of this study. The tests that you will not be charged for include. . . . The parts of your care that would normally be done as standard treatment, such as . . . will be billed to your insurance company.

This type of explicit disclosure may place a greater burden on the sponsor, the principal investigator, or perhaps even the research participant. However, the specific wording, as to who will be paying for what, is essential if the IRB is to evaluate the reasonableness of research-related costs before they are passed along to the participant.

Supporting the explicit disclosure of research-related costs to research participants is one thing, but actually getting to a detailed and explicit accounting of these costs has proven to be even more difficult. In most medical centers, if the concept of providing explicit disclosure is still not open to controversy, *it certainly is still open to noncompliance.*

When an individual either elects or considers enrollment in a research protocol that his or her physician is helping to direct, the relationship between patient and physician changes. The relationship is now not doctor and patient but is more accurately described from the ethical standpoint as researcher and participant. Researcher and participant need to discuss fully and collaboratively all financial concepts: incentives to the researcher, complex billing issues, and conflicts of interest. Although these discussions do form the basis of responsible patient advocacy, they may not be sufficient to fulfill the IRB's mandate for protecting human subjects. I would argue that explicit disclosures that are discussed must also be in writing, be easily understood, and be incorporated into the informed consent process. The principal investigator (PI) is in the best position for crafting such an explicit disclosure. The PI can distinguish services that are routinely part of the standard of care for the patient population being studied and those services and procedures that are solely conducted to advance research objectives. The PI can also reveal all financial incentives for the researcher or for the institution, as well as any potential conflicts of interest. Without this explicit and detailed input to the IRB from the PI, the IRB will be hampered in determining whether its reasonableness standard for incurring research-related costs has been exceeded.

Disclosure in the Informed Consent

Should this information be explicitly detailed in the study's informed consent document? Could the financial disclosure information be an addendum to the consent but reviewed by the IRB? Should all disclosures be reconciled against the research grant or contract? Would a group other than the IRB more appropriately handle these administrative tasks? Each of these questions must be answered in order to strengthen the IRB process and to ensure the protection of human subjects pertaining to research-related costs. Failure to meet these new and emerging standards for financial disclosure could ultimately jeopardize enrollment in future clinical trials, especially if the public believes researchers and research institutions are not forthcoming with full and complete financial disclosures.

An illustration of this is found in a recent national investigational product study that moved from the clinical trial status to an approved device implantation procedure. This type of outcome and approval is the goal of many clinical trials being reviewed by IRBs. The original protocol provided for a 5-year follow-up period in which a greater number of magnetic resonance imaging (MRI) scans would be performed than was then the standard of care. Now that the procedure has been approved, the greater number of MRI scans has become the new standard of care. Consequently, even though no new participants were being enrolled in these studies, the sponsor and the PI sought to have patients sign a new consent allowing the patient's insurance to be billed for all subsequent MRI scans. The reaction from the research participants/patients resulted in a significant number of withdrawals from the studies. Participants were angry that they were suddenly going to incur greater out-of-pocket costs. One participant agreed to sign the new consent but explicitly demanded that none of his follow-up data be forwarded to the industrial sponsor. Other participants refused to sign the new consent or to comply with the new standard of care because they could not afford the extra MRIs.

This example raises some very troubling and important disclosure issues. What financial and clinical obligations does a sponsor have to its original participants if the product or procedure is subsequently approved for commercial use or becomes the new standard of care? Do the original consent and its care provisions remain in effect if the participant refuses to sign the new consent? What provisions should there be in this process for participants who no longer have insurance and are medically indigent?

These questions should be considered by IRBs in evolving their policy positions regarding research-related costs, as well as in preparing revisions to the "financial considerations" section of the informed consent. My recommendation is that the consent document should contain language that reflects the following principles. (Reasonable people will disagree with some of these statements. Every IRB must make its own decisions.)

1. Patients should be charged only for medically necessary services or for services for which they agreed in advance to incur the direct cost.
2. The cost of services solely for advancing the objectives of the research should be borne by the research sponsor. There is a legitimate argument against this point of view. People are

not required to participate in research. As long as a person understands the implications of the decision to participate in a study, one can argue that it is ethically sound to charge participants for research costs.

3. Enrollment in a study protocol should never be exclusionary based on a person's ability to pay. Wealth should not be a defining issue in gaining access to needed care, including research.
4. It should always be clearly and simply stated, down to a visit/charge level of detail, which services are part of a patient's standard of care and which services are necessary to advance the research objectives.
5. Research participants should be reassured that sufficient research dollars are available to cover all research-related costs and that the research protocol will not be curtailed for financial reasons. These types of guarantees may place the institution where the research is being performed at some financial risk.
6. Research participants should be informed about any financial incentives being provided to the researcher or the research institution from the industrial sponsor or the grant. This includes per capita payments to researchers for subject enrollment.
7. Participants should be explicitly informed of any and all potential conflicts of interest as identified under the institution's policies.
8. Research participants should have access to financial counselors who are able to advise them, based on the explicit disclosure, about the extent of their financial exposure. Financial counseling is an essential part of the consent process in many studies and therefore should be available both before the initial decision to participate in research and during the course of the study.

Protecting the Institutions

Several years ago, I received a mandatory request from the Medicare fiscal intermediary (FI) demanding a complete listing of all Medicare beneficiaries actively enrolled in research protocols taking place at my medical center. This request raised some institutional consciousness because it required a mandated response from every PI on campus within 30 days. At that time Medicare reimbursed only items and services that were medically necessary and reasonable, specifically excluding payment for research-related costs. Section 1862(a)(1)(A)[2] of the Medicare regulations states this:

> Notwithstanding any other provision of this title, no payment may be made under Part A or Part B for any expenses incurred for items or services which are not reasonable and necessary for the diagnosis and treatment of illness or injury or to improve the functioning of a malformed body member.

Medicare interprets "reasonable and necessary" to mean "safe, effective, and not experimental," as noted in the presentation by S.T. Nicholson entitled "Medicare Reimbursement for Research-Related Activities," given to the Dartmouth Hitchcock Medical Center Hematology/Oncology section retreat on September 3, 1998.

Medicare compliance initiatives regarding research as well as investigations from the Office of the Inspector General have resulted in research-related prosecutions and settlements under the Federal False Claims Act, many of which have appeared as unfortunate headlines on a regular basis. However, my focus in this section is not to further detail these compliance risks but to begin to convey how these emerging legal and ethical realities should be influencing the IRB to take steps to protect the institution as it protects human subjects.

The IRB may not assume that the financial and administrative requirements to assure compliance with federal regulations, local medical review policies (LCD/LMRPs), third-party contracts, and appropriate state laws are automatically happening within its institution. However, the IRB must clearly understand how these responsibilities have been delegated to other administrative units within the organization. It must be sure that the division of responsibilities is clear, well-coordinated, and integrated with each operational unit. IRBs may, at times, be appropriately risk averse to taking a leadership role in advancing new administrative standards or advocating for new regulatory mandates, but IRBs must understand that avoiding or ignoring these mandates is not an option. Because the IRB is in a position to meld patient interests, public interests, clinical interests, research interests, and financial interests, it must become an essential voice in bringing about institutional change.

IRB Review

Most probably, the IRB usually does not know the capacity of its institution's health information system for carrying out its emerging and changing policies having to do with research-related costs. Medical centers are typically large, complex organizations. Some have decentralized administration. Compliance exposures can occur if management controls are not sufficient or properly monitored. The IRB can be integral in examining these types of issues by exercising its prerogative to conduct reviews of approved protocols. These reviews might include a review of claims to ascertain whether human subjects are being charged in a manner prescribed by the protocol. Other reviews might involve extended interviews with research participants regarding how clearly they were informed about research-related costs. Although the complexity of the role of the PI is increased by such audits, all functions in the continuum of patient care related to research should be monitored if the numerous and burgeoning compliance demands are to be met by our institutions.

For example an audit of approved protocols where Food and Drug Administration–approved class B investigational devices/implants were employed would have been particularly revealing of both the complexity of issues and the potential exposures created for the institution. Use of investigational implants invariably requires IRB approval. Even though the Food and Drug Administration has approved class B implants and has issued a corresponding

Investigational Device Exemption (IDE) number, local FIs maintained the prerogative to approve, or disapprove, payment for these devices. Furthermore, LCD/LMRPs issued by the Medicare FI frequently prescribe additional steps to be taken by the institution subsequent to IRB approval, if a patient claim was to be submitted for payment. It is essential that when it approves a research protocol the IRB find a means to assure that the protocol is not only safe to be pursued with human subjects, but also is coordinated with the administrative and regulatory processes that are downstream from its approval.

In August 2000, the government published the National Coverage Decision for Medicare Coverage of Clinical Trials.[3] These new regulations provide the framework that institutions must use to integrate all of their research-related activities, including the activities of the IRB. No longer will the lack of administrative rules be a haven from compliance demands. All patients enrolled in research protocols have to be tracked through the institution's health information system. Financial coverage decisions must be rendered for each Medicare patient visit and each patient service provided during the course of a clinical trial. Billing modifiers must be attached to all routine medically necessary services provided during the course of a clinical trial. Although IRBs have been typically removed from these bureaucratic burdens, research participants will now be entitled to a new level of information. From increased levels of information, new advocacy rights will also emerge requiring an improved informed consent process.

Conclusion

In this chapter, I have attempted to make a case to expand the IRB's patient advocacy role in closely looking at research-related costs routinely passed along to participants. The same level of diligence that an IRB applies to assuring the safety monitoring of a clinical trial must be applied to all potential financial impacts. Overlooking or not thoroughly examining research-related costs would be to short circuit a very critical step of the continuum of patient care. The examination of research-related costs is not entirely new territory for IRBs, but there are newly added regulatory and compliance reasons to elevate the need for explicit and detailed financial disclosures. Furthermore, improved disclosures are not only the best steps to take for extending protections to human subjects, but the same practices required to craft more complete disclosures should also extend added protections to research institutions. New administrative or policy burdens may be placed on the IRB when fulfilling these mandates, but it is not an option to ignore the numerous issues associated with research-related costs.

To the average person, health care billing is virtually unintelligible. Adding a dash of research-related costs to routine health care claims is to take an already confusing situation and make it worse. I therefore recommended the IRB have a knowledgeable member from the patient financial services department join the committee. This will provide a means for extending important patient/participant advocacy discussions of research-related costs. Most organizations have a very long way to go to improve and to make understandable the cost, reimbursement, and billing of research-related services.

References

1. General Accounting Office. NIH clinical trials: Various factors affect patient participation (report No. GAO/HEHS-99-182), September 1999. Access date 21 August, 2001. http:frwebgate.access.gpo.gov/cgi-bin/useftp.cgi?IPaddress5162.140.64.21&filename5he99182.pdf&directory5/diskb/wais/data/gao

2. United States Code. Social Security Act. Title XVIII—Health Insurance for Aged and Disabled; Part D—Miscellaneous Provisions; Sec. 1862(a)(1)(A) Exclusions from coverage and Medicare as secondary payer. Updated 1 January, 1999. Access date 22 August, 2001. http://www.ssa.gov/OP_Home ssact/title18/1862.htm

3. Health Care Financing Administration. Medicare coverage policy—Clinical trials. Final national coverage decision, 19 September, 2000. Access date 22 August, 2001. http://www.hcfa.gov/coverage/8d2.htm

Improving Informed Consent

Jeffrey A. Cooper and Pamela Turner

INTRODUCTION
The quality of informed consent can be improved by following the four basic steps that would be used to improve the quality of any process:

1. Establish a baseline measurement for the quality of informed consent and determine a hypothesis by which informed consent can be improved.
2. Implement an intervention designed to improve informed consent.
3. Monitor the effectiveness of that intervention by continuously measuring the quality of informed consent and evaluating for any changes from the baseline.
4. Act on the results of measurements and standardize the plan if successful. Continue the cycle for further improvement. This is commonly referred to as the Plan-Do-Check-Act cycle (Figure 6.11.1).[1]

Elements of Informed Consent Quality

In evaluating the quality of informed consent, three areas should be considered: structure, process, and outcome. These three items have a serial relationship, where process depends on structure and outcome depends on process (Figure 6.11.2).[2]

Structure
Structure refers to the tangible elements required to have a good informed consent. Such tangible elements would include recruitment materials, consent documents, addenda to consents, and any other written or visual information used to convey information and understanding to subjects about the research. The regulations define a specific structure for informed consent documentation.[3(Sec.117),4(Sec.27)] The regulatory mandated structure should be considered a minimum standard, and additional structural features may be required for a high-quality informed consent. The relationship of the informed consent documentation and the quality of the informed consent process is controversial.

Process
Process refers to the actions necessary to obtain a high-quality informed consent. These actions include recruitment, the presentation of the study, and the provision of additional information about the research. In evaluating these actions, one needs to consider the five questions of "who," "what," "where," "when," and "how" applied to a quality informed consent. Who should provide information to the subject? What information should be presented? Where should the information be given? In what time sequence should the research staff present the information? How should the information be presented? The answers to these questions are much debated.

Outcome
Outcome refers to the actual results of a high-quality informed consent. It is the answer to the question: "How do

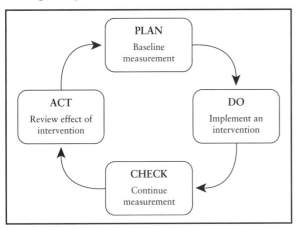

Figure 6.11.1 Four Basic Steps to Improve the Quality of Any Process
Source: Data from Graham N.D.

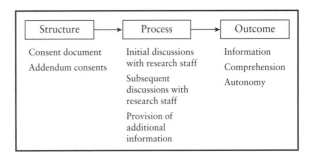

Figure 6.11.2 Serial Relationship of the Basic Elements of the Informed Consent Process
Source: Data from Donabedian A.

you know a subject had a good informed consent?" This question can be evaluated several different ways. For example, did the subject gain adequate knowledge and comprehension of the research because of the informed consent process? Was the subject satisfied that all questions were answered during the informed consent process? Did the subject's experiences in the research match the information provided during the informed consent process?

In the final analysis, the outcome of the informed consent is more important than the structure or process of informed consent.[5] However, the outcome of informed consent is difficult to define and measure. For example, it is easier to determine whether the risks of a research project are listed in the consent documentation or conveyed orally to a prospective subject than it is to determine whether the subject understood the risks and used the information to make a knowledgeable decision about participation in the research. The regulations focus on the structure of informed consent (the requirements of consent documentation) and the process for approval of the structure (institutional review board [IRB] review of the protocol and consent document), but have no requirements for the outcome of informed consent. If we wish to improve informed consent, then we will have to define the desired outcomes of informed consent and learn how to reliably measure the presence or absence of these desired outcomes. We can use that metric to determine the structure and process that result in the desired outcomes and assess the quality of the necessary structure or process as a proxy for the quality of the outcome.

We know very little about the structure and process that lead to the desired outcome of informed consent. Interventions that manipulate the structure or process without measuring outcome should be avoided.

The Belmont Report

The Belmont Report clearly articulates the desired outcome of informed consent: "Respect for persons requires that subjects, to the degree that they are capable, be given the opportunity to choose what shall or shall not happen to them."[6] Subjects should be provided information, understand the information, and based on their comprehension of the information, make a voluntary decision to participate in research.[7–9]

The consent process includes communication of information to the subject, which the subject should take away in the form of knowledge. The ideal state might be that all subjects know everything in the consent document; however, this is clearly an unrealistic expectation. Few investigators or IRB members can recite all knowledge contained in any arbitrary consent document. Knowledge may also be time limited. Subjects may know at the time of a decision the specific information provided to them, but after the decision has been made, they may readily forget that information. As Levine[7] has pointed out, when we make decisions about which car to buy or college to attend, we may do a great deal of in-depth research and gain

a large amount of knowledge that allows us to make an informed decision. However, after the decision is made, we may forget the specific knowledge that we used to make such a decision. On the other hand, there are some items of knowledge that subjects should know throughout a research study. For example, we expect subjects to know that they are participating in research, that they made a choice to participate and that they may withdraw from the research at any time without penalty. Therefore, we need to be circumspect about what kind of knowledge subjects should be expected to recollect after agreeing to participate in a research study.

Comprehension of Consent Process

As part of the consent process, subjects should comprehend important elements of the information provided. Comprehension is more than just knowledge. Memorization of knowledge does not equate with comprehension. Comprehension requires an ability to interpret the knowledge imparted in the consent process and it requires subjects to be able to perceive meaning and ascribe significance to the knowledge that they have gained.[7]

Another desired outcome of the consent process is the autonomy of the subject in making a free choice regarding participation in a research study. This requires a subject to exercise his or her free will. Subjects must choose freely for themselves with no restraint or coercion.

The autonomy of the subject's informed consent can also be evaluated in terms of the subject's satisfaction with specific elements of the process. The evaluation of satisfaction examines the outcomes of the research experience relative to the subject's expectations, as well as the information and understanding by the subject during the consent process. Satisfaction with the consent process does not mean that the subject's expectations of the research were fulfilled, such as expecting a cure of one's cancer. Instead, satisfaction with the consent process means that the subject believes that the consent process provided adequate explanation and preparation for the eventual research experience. An important limitation of the use of satisfaction measurements is the difficulty of assessing satisfaction with rare events. For example, there may be a rare, but serious, adverse event in a research study, and the research staff may poorly communicate the possibility of that event to subjects. However, measurement of satisfaction may not detect that limitation of the informed consent process, if none of the subjects in that research study experienced the rare event.

To improve the quality of informed consent, the IRB should focus on strategies that improve the outcome of informed consent and manipulate the structure and process to improve the outcome. An IRB must assess and improve the structure and process of informed consent mandated by the regulations but should not make the assumption that meeting the regulatory standards guarantees the desired outcome of informed consent.

Measurement of Consent Quality

The quality of the structure of informed consent is generally measured through audits and inspections. The IRB can audit the informed consent documents of subjects who have agreed to participate in research and measure how often the consent has the appropriate signatures, how often the approved consent was used, and how often the date of the consent precedes the date of research procedures. The IRB can also re-review a sample of approved consent documents and measure how often the IRB approves a consent document with a missing element, overly technical language, absence of relevant risks, exculpatory language, or other deficiencies. Similar data can be collected during the process of continuation review. The IRB can also assess the structural quality of the consent document by measuring the reading level using several commercially available tools.

The measurement of process quality can be performed through audits, monitoring, interviews, or surveys. The IRB can audit protocols to determine how often additional information discovered during the course of research that might have influenced subjects' willingness to continue participation was presented to subjects. The IRB can use a consent monitor to determine that all elements of informed consent were provided to prospective subjects, that prospective subjects were given the opportunity to ask questions, the prospective subjects' questions were answered correctly and appropriately, and that consenting subjects made an autonomous decision. The IRB can also conduct a postconsent survey or interview with subjects. The survey or interview can be used to measure the amount of time allocated to the informed consent process. It can also determine whether the subject had any unanswered questions about the research and if specific elements of consent were discussed with the subject.

The quality of the outcome of informed consent can be measured with retrospective surveys and interviews of subjects. The surveys can focus on knowledge, understanding, autonomy, and satisfaction. The literature contains validated surveys that IRBs can use to measure the outcome of informed consent.[5,10] IRBs should have a clear understanding of survey development before developing their own tools.[11,12]

Throughout the course of a research study, one can evaluate the subject's knowledge of his or her rights as a research subject. Does the subject know that he or she took part in a research study? Does the subject know that he or she gave voluntary consent to take part in a research study? Does the subject know that he or she has the right to withdraw from the research at any time without penalty or loss of benefits?

Other issues to evaluate after informed consent include the subject's knowledge of the research protocol itself. Does the subject understand the research purpose of the procedures being performed? Does the subject know the duration of his or her participation? Does the subject know that some procedures are being performed solely for research? Does the subject know that taking part in the research entails risk or potential benefits? Does the subject know that detailed information about the research is contained in the informed consent document? Again, subjects are unlikely to remember specific details about the research. Therefore, the best knowledge issues to evaluate are likely those that are quite general.

Several elements of subject comprehension may be useful to evaluate immediately after informed consent or at any time during or after the subject's participation in research. Does the subject understand the concept of research? Does the subject understand his or her rights as a research subject? Does the subject understand the elements of consent? The measurement of understanding independent of knowledge is difficult and likely involves the assistance of a knowledgeable educator.

Various elements of the subject's autonomy might be useful to evaluate either immediately after informed consent or at any time during or after participation in the research. Did the subject agree to take part in the research? Who, according to the subject, made the decision to take part in the research? Did the subject make the decision for himself or herself? Because subjects may express their autonomy through delegation, the IRB should also ask if the subject freely delegated the decision to take part in research to a third party.

The information, knowledge, and autonomy of subjects can be evaluated in part through questions directed at their satisfaction with the consent process. Was the subject satisfied with the information that was provided during the informed consent process about what would happen during the research? Was the subject satisfied with the information provided about the risks or potential benefits of the research? Was the subject satisfied with the information provided about the alternative to participation in the research? The IRB can ask subjects how well their experiences in the research met their expectations and if there were any surprises during the research.

Benchmarking

After the IRB has developed baseline measurements, it can use benchmarking to generate hypotheses about how the outcome of informed consent could be improved and to implement interventions in the structure or process of consent based on those hypotheses.[1,13] In benchmarking, the IRB measures the outcome of informed consent against other institutions and determines a structure or process associated with better outcomes. The interventions can be stratified according to those related to structure, process, and outcome. The five strategies for implementing interventions, in order from greatest to least effectiveness, include peer-based feedback, rewards and punishments, involving people in the change process, administrative rules, and education.[14,15] Generally, providing IRB members or research staff with a scorecard that allows them to compare their quality outcomes relative to their peers' is most effective in changing behavior. Administrative rules and education, despite their popularity among IRBs, are the two least effective methods for changing behavior.

Structural Interventions

Structural interventions change the tangible aspects of informed consent. Examples of structural interventions include the development of a consent template, standardized consent language, or a glossary of lay definitions; increasing or decreasing the amount of information in the consent document; and lowering the reading level of the consent document. With each of these interventions, the IRB can assess the impact on outcome by measuring subject knowledge, comprehension, autonomy, and satisfaction. The IRB can provide feedback to committee members on deficiencies observed in audits of approved consent documents. The IRB can also develop other promising structural interventions by measuring outcomes across a variety of research studies.

Process interventions include requiring that qualified personnel conduct the informed consent process, that subjects are given a minimum amount of time to make a decision regarding participation, that information is repeated to subjects, or that subjects discuss the research with their primary care physician. The IRB can involve investigators and research staff to develop strategies to improve informed consent and can also develop other promising process interventions by measuring outcomes across a variety of research studies. For example, IRBs can evaluate the influence of repetition of information given by research coordinators and principal investigators to subjects on the retention of knowledge or comprehension.

When the IRB implements an intervention, it must re-evaluate the outcome of informed consent and look for changes from the baseline measurement. Statistical process control charts represent a statistically valid technique for determining changes in a baseline[16,17] and are beyond the scope of this chapter. Many institutions have quality-improvement departments that can provide support for statistical process control charts, and the reader should refer to the references for further assistance.

When evaluating the effect of structure and process on outcome, many structures or processes will vary without a clear or known effect on outcome. This is referred to as unexplained variation[18] and is common among IRBs. For example, IRBs have different requirements for boilerplate language and the format of consent documents. Researchers have different methods of obtaining informed consent, none of which have been demonstrated to have advantageous effects on outcome. Unexplained variation has several negative side effects and can cause researchers and sponsors to lose respect for the authority of the IRB when a structure or process acceptable to one IRB is not acceptable to another. Unexplained variation also minimizes the likelihood that IRBs or researchers will adhere to effective procedures. When the IRB detects variability in its structure or process, the IRB should determine whether the variability is explainable in terms of outcome or represents unexplained variation. In the case of unexplained variation, the IRB should measure the outcome and choose the structure and process that leads to the best outcome. If two or more structures or processes lead to equivalent outcomes, the IRB should choose one to maximize compliance and therefore maximize outcome.

The Environment of Quality

When improving any function, several recurring themes emerge as key elements to success.[19] The IRB and the institution must be committed to quality improvement. Frontline research personnel must be involved in the change process and have ownership of the process. Measurements should be kept simple and reliable to maximize the validity of the measurement and to maximize the likelihood that the measurement will be performed consistently. In general, 80% of the improvement can be achieved with 20% of all possible changes that can be made.

Conclusion

In summary, the quality of informed consent can be measured by considering the structure, process, and outcome of informed consent. IRBs tend to focus on structure and process because that is the focus of the federal regulations. However, to improve the informed consent structure and process, we must develop measurements of the outcome of informed consent as defined in *The Belmont Report*.[6] From those outcome measurements, we can implement interventions that will allow us to discover the ideal structure and process of informed consent.

References

1. Graham ND (ed.). *Quality in Health Care: Theory, Application, and Evolution.* Gaithersburg, MD: Aspen Publications; 1995.

2. Donabedian A. The role of outcomes in quality assessment and assurance. *QRB Qual Rev Bull* 18(11):356–360, 1992.

3. Code of Federal Regulations. Title 45A—Department of Health and Human Services; Part 46—Protection of Human Subjects. Updated 1 October, 1997. Access date 18 April, 2001. http://www4.law.cornell.edu/cfr/45p46.htm

4. Code of Federal Regulations. Title 21, Chapter 1—Food and Drug Administration, DHHS; Part 50—Protection of Human Subjects. Updated 1 April, 1999. Access date 18 April, 2001. http://www4.law.cornell.edu/cfr/21p50.htm

5. Joffe S, Cook EF, Cleary PD, Clark JW, Weeks JC. Quality of informed consent: A new measure of understanding among research subjects. *J Natl Cancer Inst* 93(2):139–147, 2001.

6. National Commission for the Protection of Human Subjects of Biomedical and Behavioral Research. *The Belmont Report: Ethical Principles and Guidelines for the Protection of Human Subjects of Research,* 18 April, 1979. Access date 22 March, 2001. http://ohsr.od.nih.gov/mpa/belmont.php3

7. Levine RJ. *Ethics and Regulation of Clinical Research,* 2nd ed. Baltimore, MD: Urban and Schwarzenberg; 1986.

8. Beauchamp TL, Childress JF. *Principles of Biomedical Ethics,* 4th ed. New York: Oxford University Press; 1994.

9. Meisel A, Roth LH, Lidz CW. Toward a model of the legal doctrine of informed consent. *Am J Psychiatry* 134(3):285–289, 1977.

10. Miller CK, O'Donnell DC, Searight HR, Barbarash RA. The Deaconess Informed Consent Comprehension Test: An assessment tool for clinical research subjects. *Pharmacotherapy* 16(5):872–878, 1996.

11. Alreck PL, Settle RB. *The Survey Research Handbook: Guidelines and Strategies for Conducting a Survey,* 2nd ed. Chicago: Richard D. Irwin; 1995.

12. Sudman S, Bradburn NM. *Asking Questions.* San Francisco, CA: Jossey-Bass Publishers; 1982.

13. Lenz S, Myers S, Nordlund S, Sullivan D, Vasista V. Benchmarking: Finding ways to improve. *J Comm J Qual Improv* 20(5):250–259, 1994.

14. Greco PJ, Eisenberg JM. Changing physicians' practices. *N Engl J Med* 329(17):1271–1273, 1993.

15. Oxman AD, Thomson MA, Davis DA, Haynes RB. No magic bullet: A systematic review of 102 trials of interventions to improve professional practice. *Can Med Assoc J* 153(10):1423–1431, 1995.

16. Wheeler DJ, Chambers DS. *Understanding Statistical Process Control,* 2nd ed. Knoxville, TN: SPC Press; 1992.

17. Plesk PE. Tutorial: Introduction to control charts. *Qual Manage Health Care* 1(1):65–74, 1992.

18. Berwick DM. Controlling variation in health care: A consultation from Walter Shewhart. *Med Care* 29(12):1212–1225, 1991.

19. Carman JM, Shortell SM, Foster RW, Hughes EF, Boerstler H, O'Brien JL, O'Conner EJ. Keys for successful implementation of total quality management in hospitals. *Health Care Manage Rev* 21(1):48–60, 1996.

Informed Consent Evaluation Feedback Tool

Elizabeth A. Bankert and Robert J. Amdur

"Most codes dealing with human experimentation start out with the bland assumption that consent is ours for the asking. This is a myth. The reality is that informed consent is often exceedingly difficult to obtain in any complete sense. . . . Nevertheless, it remains a goal toward which one must strive for sociological, ethical, and legal reasons." –Henry Beecher, MD, 1966

INTRODUCTION

In 1998, we started an interview process to determine how well participants understand what they are supposed to understand about research. Our goal was to find a simple and user-friendly way to evaluate the quality of informed consent of people who had recently decided to participate in a research project. Our motivation for doing this was more operational than academic. Our institutional review board (IRB) was spending considerable time and energy evaluating and revising the consent document as part of the process of initial protocol review. The experience of many of the clinician–investigators at our medical center suggested that we were overestimating the importance of the consent document in the consent process. Research participants often told us that they obtained important information about the study from sources other than the consent document. Detailed interview studies at other institutions suggested that, in spite of detailed consent documents, many research participants do not understand the essential elements of informed consent to the degree that we would like.

To get the information that we needed to direct our process of IRB review, as well as to find ways to improve the quality of informed consent in research participants, we focused our attention on developing a survey tool that would evaluate comprehension of research issues. Our efforts evolved through several stages. We worked with educational psychologists and piloted several different evaluation tools. We started with a very detailed and complex survey that covered many aspects of informed consent in detail. This proved to be both difficult to administer and poorly accepted by research subjects. As the program evolved, the survey instrument became progressively simpler and shorter.

The first phase of the project included the use of an informed consent evaluation form with approximately 75 research participants. We asked individuals who had recently enrolled in a research project to respond to a one-page survey that tested comprehension of the eight basic elements of informed consent as described in the federal regulations. These initial surveys convinced us that many of the people who participate in biomedical research do not understand the essential elements of informed consent. The structure of our interview system did not involve research methods, and thus, it would not be appropriate to present quantitative results here.

The reason to mention this qualitative experience is that it was a turning point in the direction of our project. In our minds, the more important question is how to improve the consent process so that subjects do not enroll until they are well informed. To this end, we directed our attention to developing a program that could be used by members of the research team as a routine part of the consent process to evaluate and improve the quality of informed consent before participant enrollment. We have enough experience with a particular survey instrument to be optimistic.

Informed Consent Evaluation Feedback Tool

We have been using a survey instrument that we call the Informed Consent Evaluation Feedback Tool (ICE FT)(see

Figure 6.12.1 at the end of the chapter). We pronounce this acronym "ice foot." The primary goal of the ICE FT is to focus the attention of potential research participants on the basic elements of informed consent as described in the federal regulations. The ICE FT is a simple list of questions the researcher uses to obtain information during the consent process about the level of comprehension of the potential research participant. The main purpose of the ICE FT is to guide the dialogue between the researcher and potential participant. It is not a test to be taken and then graded by the researcher. There are two basic ways to use the ICE FT to evaluate and improve the quality of informed consent.

Use the ICE FT to Guide the Initial Discussion During the Consent Process

The ICE FT is given to the potential participant before discussing the details of the research study with a statement such as, "We are about to discuss a research project. There are good reasons to participate in this research study, but the study is not right for everyone. It is not the kind of situation where we can just tell you what you should do. It is important that you make the final decision about taking part in this study, and that means you need to understand what the study is all about. We know this is new information for you, and people often need to ask questions and hear things explained more than once before they feel like they understand what they want to know. I am going to go over a list of questions with you. This list of questions will help us discuss the study. Please take a look at the questions before we get started."

The researcher then uses the ICE FT tool throughout the consent process as a prompt to encourage an interactive dialogue. The intent is to create an atmosphere where the potential participant is comfortable asking questions and interacting verbally about the study. The subject's questions and responses are used to determine the general level of comprehension of specific issues. There is no grading system. The researcher should think in terms of a pass/fail model for evaluating comprehension in this setting.

The session begins with the researcher's asking the participant to explain the purpose of the study. In most cases, the researcher and potential subject will need to discuss possible answers before the potential participant will be able to demonstrate that he or she understands the study well enough to go on to the next question.

Use the ICE FT After the Initial Study Discussion

Without mentioning or showing the potential subject the ICE FT, the researcher explains the study, including the essential elements of informed consent. Questions are answered, and comments are discussed. After the researcher is satisfied that the potential subject is adequately informed, the researcher explains the ICE FT. At this point, the basic format for the discussion is as described in the previous example. The researcher asks the potential participant to answer each of the ICE FT questions either verbally or in writing (researcher preference). It may be desirable for the potential participant to take the ICE FT home to think about the questions and discuss them with family members. Before enrolling a person in the study, the researcher reviews the potential subject's answers to the ICE FT. This review is an interactive dialogue that further educates the potential participant and allows the researcher to determine whether the person is informed to the point that it is ethically acceptable to allow enrollment in the study.

The primary purpose of the ICE FT is to evaluate and improve the level of comprehension of potential research subjects in real time. We do not recommend asking research subjects to sign the ICE FT, as this gives people the impression that its purpose is to help defend the researcher or organization from legal liability. The consent document already suffers from this problem, and it will compromise the effectiveness of the ICE FT to have it viewed as anything other than a tool to promote subject education and to increase dialogue between researcher and subject.

Our Experience with the ICE FT

The ICE FT has been used by protocol nurses in the oncology, cardiology, and psychiatric departments at the Dartmouth Hitchcock Medical Center in Lebanon, New Hampshire. We appreciate and acknowledge the time and effort these research teams have contributed to all phases of the ICE FT project. To date, the feedback we have received has been extremely positive. The research nurses say that it facilitates the informed consent discussion from their standpoint in terms of saving time as well as identifying people who are not good candidates for the study under consideration.

As previously mentioned, the ICE FT project has never been pursued as a research effort, and thus, we have no control group for comparison or outcome measurements. The potential participants seem to like it based on the positive comments that have been written at the bottom of the ICE FT form: "I would not have known what to ask if it was not for the list of questions" and "If you have to answer questions, it forces you to read what you are signing." This kind of feedback is enough for us to continue working with the ICE FT at Dartmouth. We are in the process of educating all of the research groups at our institution about the need to evaluate the quality of informed consent during the initial consent process. We present the ICE FT as a way to help researchers accomplish this goal.

Conclusion

Major improvements in the protection of research subjects will require the evaluation of the endpoints of ethical behavior. As informed consent is one of the most important requirements for ethical research, it is important to develop tools that allow both researchers and the IRB to evaluate the quality of the informed consent process prior to starting research procedures. The Informed Consent Evaluation Feedback Tool described in this chapter is a simple set of questions that helps direct and evaluate the informed consent process. Our initial experience with it suggests that it is useful for both research investigators and research subjects.

The Informed Consent Evaluation Feedback Tool (ICE FT)*

IRB # _____ Title of the study _____

1. The purpose of this study is to:

2. Possible benefits of the research include:

3. Possible risks of the research include:

4. There are no other options for my health care:
    ❏ True   ❏ False

5. The costs of the research will be paid for by the sponsor:
    ❏ True   ❏ False

6. Alternatives to participating in this research include:

7. If I do decide to participate in this study, I can change my mind and withdraw from the study at any time:
    ❏ True   ❏ False

8. Participation in this research is voluntary.
    ❏ True   ❏ False

9. Researchers directing this study and individuals from the government who are responsible for being sure that research is done correctly have the right to review my records from this study.
    ❏ True   ❏ False

10. I have these questions for the research team:

Figure 6.12.1 Informed Consent Evaluation Feedback Tool
*This template includes a sampling of basic questions only, it should be modified to be appropriate for the specific study, e.g., randomization, placebo.

Source: ©Dartmouth College. Used with permission.

PART 7

Continuing Review

Revisions to an Approved Study

Sherry Bye and Ann O'Hara

INTRODUCTION

Revisions range from a request to correct a simple typographical error in the consent form to a significant change in the study design. Each change must be reviewed and approved by the institutional review board (IRB) prior to initiation. Researchers must be informed that all revisions need to be approved by the IRB before implementation. This chapter addressed the IRB requirement to review revisions to an approved study. Amendments, modifications, revisions, addenda, updates, administrative changes, additions, and other labels are identified with study changes. Throughout this chapter, the term *revision* will be used to refer to all of these changes.

Federal Regulations

Why do study revisions need to be approved by the IRB? Food and Drug Administration guidelines[1][Sec.108(a)(3)] state that the IRB shall follow written procedures "for ensuring prompt reporting to the IRB of changes in research activity; and for ensuring that changes in approved research, during the period for which IRB approval has already been given, may not be initiated without IRB review and approval except where necessary to eliminate apparent immediate hazards to the human subjects." The Department of Health and Human Services regulation has similar wording.[2][Sec.102(b)(4)(iii)] In addition, the Food and Drug Administration information sheet for IRBs and clinical investigators, "Continuing Review After Study Approval," item 4, "Process for Reviewing Changes in Ongoing Research During the Approval Period," provides further guidance.[3] To comply with these regulations, the IRB operating manual should include a written procedure for submitting, reviewing, and approving revisions in an approved study. The IRB approval letter should include a statement that IRB approval is required before implementing a revision in a study. A sample statement for inclusion in an approval letter is as follows: "Procedural changes or amendments must be reported to the IRB, and no changes may be made without IRB approval except to eliminate apparent immediate hazards to the subject."

Types of Revisions

For triage at the IRB office, revision requests can be divided into two types: minor revisions (involves no more than minimal risk) and substantive revisions (more than minor changes and/or changes increase risks to subjects).

Minor Revisions

Minor revisions involve procedures that are no more than minimal risk, or risks to subjects are not increased, and/or the revision is not a significant alteration of the study design. Minimal risk[2][Sec.102(I)] means that the probability and magnitude of harm or discomfort anticipated in the research are not greater than those ordinarily encountered in daily life or during the performance of routine physical or psychologic examinations or tests. The IRB office can use the expedited review procedure to review and approve.[2][Sec.110(b)(2)] To allow for an efficient review of minor changes, many IRBs designate an experienced office staff member as an IRB member. This individual may then approve a minor revision to an approved study as the designee for the chairperson. Examples may include changes in telephone numbers, the addition or deletion of associates or staff, the reduction in the number of research participants, or the deletion of questions in a survey.

Substantive Revisions

Any revision to a study that involves increased risk to subjects or significantly affects the nature of the study must be reviewed by the full IRB. Examples may include the revisions to the recruitment plan, adding, revising eligibility criteria, adding a research site, changing the principal investigator, or changing the consent form to include a newly identified side effect or adverse event related to the study drug.

Submission of Revision Requests

The request for a revision to an approved study is usually submitted using a form provided by the IRB office. The Dartmouth Revision Request Form may be found at www.dartmouth.edu/~cphs/tosubmit/forms. The revision request form should identify the principal investigator, the title of the study, and the internal IRB number for tracking purposes. It must also include a description of and justification for the requested revision(s) and information about any change in the level of risk to the study participants. Many IRB offices are beginning to handle revision requests in electronic format; however, in any format, requests must be justified and must be clearly described. The ultimate result of an IRB-approved revision request is revised documents with the revision incorporated into the study documents. This requires the researcher and the IRB office to have the most current version of both the study protocol and the consent form.

Review Procedures

When a request for revision arrives in the IRB office, the IRB staff should review the material to determine the level of review required. To determine the appropriate level of review, the IRB staff and the IRB chair must be familiar with the federal guidelines related to the review of revisions. All changes to a protocol, regardless of how minor, must be approved according to either the expedited or full-board process as specified in the regulations. The IRB administrator and/or IRB chair or a designated IRB member must make this determination.

Expedited Review and Approval

Federal guidelines[1][Sec.110(b)],[2][Sec.110(b)] state, "An IRB may use the expedited review procedure to review . . . (2) minor changes in previously approved research during the period (of one year or less) for which approval is authorized."

Because the expedited review procedure described previously here allows the IRB chair and/or an experienced member of the IRB to review the revision and determine approval, some revisions that qualify for expedited review may be approved by an IRB staff member, if this person is a voting member of the IRB and is designated by the chair to perform this function.[2][Sec.110(b)(2)] A revision cannot be disapproved by expedited review; however, the chair or IRB member can recommend that the revision be reviewed by the full IRB.

Full-Board Approval

When the revision is substantive, that is, it increases risks to participants beyond minimal risk, or is a significant change in the study design, the revision must be reviewed by the full IRB. This review should follow the IRB's procedure for full-board review for a research study; for example, it should appear on the agenda. The researcher should provide written documentation of the reason for the revision, how it will change the study, how it will affect the risks to the study participant, and what safeguards will be implemented to protect the study participant from the additional risks. This document should include information about how the revision will affect currently enrolled study participants. If appropriate, the researcher should provide references to support the revision. If the revision involves a change in the consent form, a revised consent form should be submitted with the revision to the full IRB. The IRB should determine whether the revision affects previously enrolled study participants and whether it might affect their willingness to continue in the study. In this case, study participants should be contacted and presented with a revised consent form.

After the IRB review, members will vote on the revision. The discussion of controverted issues and the vote should be included in the IRB minutes. If additional revisions are required, the researcher should be notified in writing whether the IRB expects the researcher to resubmit them in writing and whether the researcher must appear at an IRB meeting. When the revision has been approved by the IRB, an IRB revision approval document should be sent to the researcher indicating that the revision has been reviewed and approved by the full board. A copy of this document should be placed in the study file.

Documentation

All members of the IRB must be informed of revisions to study protocols approved by the expedited review procedures.[2][Sec.110(c)] Expedited revisions should be included in the IRB agenda and minutes. An IRB revision approval document should be sent to the researcher indicating approval by the IRB. At Dartmouth College, approval letters are issued for revisions that are reviewed by the full committee. For revisions reviewed via the expedited procedure, the revision form is signed indicating approval. We found that this process saves significant office paperwork. Copies of the revision approval in either format are sent to the principal investigator and to any designated contact people, that is, study coordinators. The original copy of the revision form and all accompanying documents are kept in the study file. If a new consent form is approved as part of the revision, it will be stamped with an IRB approval stamp indicating the approval date. This IRB-stamped, approved consent form can be machine copied, which assures that the most recently approved consent form is used for enrolling subjects. At many institutions, including Dartmouth College, researchers are required to use the stamped, approved consent form when enrolling subjects. For all revisions, it is important to remember that the revision approval is effective only until the expiration date of the most recent continuation review. As already mentioned, the advent of electronic systems will change the need for multiple paper copies and hand date-stamping of consent forms. A welcome innovation would be electronic archiving of study documents in order for researchers and IRBs to have easy access to the most current IRB-approved versions.

Continued Enrollment During IRB Review of Protocol Revision

When the researcher has a currently approved study, enrollment may continue under the study as approved by the IRB. The revisions cannot be made in the protocol or the consent form, however, until the IRB approves them. An exception would be if there were immediate hazards to the subject. In this case, the change must be made without waiting for IRB approval. A common area of misunderstanding is the situation in which a researcher wants to enroll a subject who does not meet all of the inclusion criteria stated in the IRB-approved protocol or study description. Some researchers think that it is acceptable to waive certain inclusion criteria based only on approval of the study sponsor. From the regulatory standpoint, the act of waiving an inclusion criterion without prior IRB approval is no different than ignoring IRB-approved conditions. Revising inclusion criteria, or any other aspect of the protocol, even for a single subject, requires prospective IRB approval.

Conclusion

It is important for IRBs and researchers to understand that federal regulations require IRB approval before implementing a revision to an approved research study. Eliciting appropriate information related to the revision will assist in determining the review designation for the IRB. An efficient and effective way to handle revisions is important in the IRB office as the number of revisions is significant and researchers want to implement revisions in a timely manner. At the same time, it is important to review carefully all revisions to ensure the safety of research subjects.

References

1. Code of Federal Regulations. Title 21, Chapter 1—Food and Drug Administration, DHHS; Part 56—Institutional Review Boards. Updated 1 April, 1999. Access date 27 March, 2001. http://www4.law.cornell.edu/cfr/21p56.htm

2. Code of Federal Regulations. Title 45A—Department of Health and Human Services; Part 46—Protection of Human Subjects. 1 October, 1997. Access date 18 April, 2001. http://www4.law.cornell.edu/cfr/45p46.htm

3. Food and Drug Administration. Information Sheets: Guidance for Institutional Review Boards and Clinical Investigators. Updated September, 1998. Access date 9 April, 2001. http://www.fda.gov/oc/oha/IRB/toc.html

Protocol Renewal

Karen M. Hansen

INTRODUCTION

An institutional review board's (IRB) review and approval of a new study is intended to ensure that, where appropriate, ethical principles and safeguards for research participants are considered and applied. These initial steps are only the first in a series of shared, ongoing monitoring activities extending throughout the life of a study.

The research investigator's and/or participant's experience(s) inevitably reshapes and changes the course of a study. Feedback from participants, adverse event reports, drug toxicities, or preliminary findings may alter the study's design and/or methods. Each new study requires ongoing monitoring by the investigator and the IRB. Renewal of protocols through the IRB occurs at intervals specified by the IRB and no less than annually. It is an inherently sound, ethical process that is also federally mandated. The Office for Human Research Protections (OHRP) has released guidance entitled "What Constitutes Substantive and Meaningful Continuing Review?" It is found at http://www.hhs.gov/ohrp/humansubjects/guidance/contrev2002.htm#what%20constitutes%20substantive%20and%20meaningful.

What Is Protocol Renewal?

Protocol renewal is a form of continuation review. At IRB-defined time intervals, the investigator reports the study's progress and findings to date. It is a monitoring mechanism that assures that continuing safeguards are in place to protect the rights and welfare of study participants. It is often not possible to predict the complex interactions and evolution of a study solely at the development stage. Periodic review of findings allows the IRB and investigator to determine whether the benefits and risks of the research have changed as the study has progressed. Simply put, it is an opportunity to revisit and reapply the ethical principles and norms[1(p.326)] outlined in *The Belmont Report*[2] and federal regulations for the protection of human subjects. As noted by Levine,[1(p.342)] each IRB is an agent of its own institution. Therefore, IRBs should specify their own requirements while factoring in the regulatory or policy requirements and other issues necessary to safeguard the rights and welfare of human subjects.

Federal Regulations and International Guidelines

Office for Human Research Protection

The United States Department of Health and Human Services OHRP (formerly known as the Office for Protection from Research Risks) offers guidance[3] about their continuing review expectations. Federal regulations outline initial IRB review criteria that include determinations regarding risks, potential benefits, informed consent, and safeguards for human subjects. The OHRP has stated that the same review criteria are required during continuing review as well. The OHRP specifies the following review parameters:

In conducting continuing review, the IRB should review, at a minimum, the protocol and any amendments as well as a status report on the progress of the research, including (a) the number of subjects accrued; (b) a description of any: adverse events or unanticipated problems involving risks to subjects or others, withdrawal of subjects from the research, or complaints about the research; (c) a summary of any recent literature, findings, or other relevant information, especially information about risks associated with the research; and (d) a copy of the current informed consent document. Primary reviewer systems may be employed, so long as the full IRB receives the above information. Primary reviewers should also receive a copy of the complete protocol including any modifications previously approved by the IRB.[3]

Food and Drug Administration

The Food and Drug Administration (FDA) provides the following guidance:

Routine continuing review should include IRB review of a written progress report(s) from the clinical investigator. Progress reports include information such as the number of subjects entering the research study and a summary description of subject experiences (benefits, adverse reactions); numbers of withdrawals from the research; reasons for withdrawals; the research results obtained thus far; a current risk–benefit assessment based on study results; and any new information since the IRB's last review. Special attention should be paid to determining whether new information or unanticipated risks were discovered during the research. Any significant new findings that may relate to the subjects' willingness to continue participation should be provided to the subjects in accordance with 21 CFR 50.25(b)(5). The IRB should obtain a copy of the consent document currently in use and determine whether the information contained in it is still accurate and complete, including whether new information that may have been obtained during the course of the study needs to be added."[4]

Frequency of Protocol Renewal

The OHRP, FDA, and International Conference on Harmonisation (ICH) Guidance for Industry, E6 Good Clinical Practice (GCP): Consolidation Guidance reiterate the expectation that IRB review occur at least once every 365 days, or more frequently, if specified by the IRB. ICH guidelines are discussed in detail in Chapter 8-3.

Both OHRP and FDA regulations describe timing for continuation review. Specifically, human-subject studies funded by the National Institutes of Health or regulated by the FDA must undergo continuation review after approval by the IRB in compliance with regulations[5[Sec.109(e)],6[Sec.109(f)]] that state the following: "An IRB shall conduct continuing review of research covered by this policy at intervals appropriate to the degree of risk, but not less than once per year."

Furthermore, the ICH E6 GCP Guidance[7(Sec.4.10.1)] states, "The investigator shall submit written summaries of the trial status to the IRB/IEC annually, or more frequently, if requested by the IRB."

Administering Protocol Renewal

Timing of IRB Review

Send timely renewal notices to the investigator. Some IRBs meet weekly, whereas others may meet quarterly. Thus, the timing of the continuation reviews may cycle differently at each organization/institution. It is up to your institutional infrastructure and operations to assure that protocol renewal review occurs annually. The IRB's administrative office must have an operating system in place for tracking time frames of protocol approvals and ensuring that renewal notices are sent out to investigators on time.

Deadlines for Renewal

Advance notices may be sent to investigators 2 and 3 months before the expected IRB review date for the protocol renewal. It is important to anticipate your investigators' real-time response rates and office staff needed to track renewal notices and their receipt for IRB review.

Specify the documents to be submitted for protocol renewal review. Request the research study documents (i.e., current protocol, consent form, questionnaire, or survey instrument) and, if applicable, completed protocol renewal form. Protocol renewal forms are an efficient way for the investigator and IRB to evaluate data from the study and make determinations about the study's continued approval through the IRB.

State the consequences of failing to comply with protocol renewal requirements. The renewal notice letter can help inform and educate the investigator about the importance of complying with the protocol renewal request. Failure to provide a continuation review report could lead to study suspension, a loss of funding and/or publication possibilities, or reporting of noncompliance to sponsors or funding agencies.

Issues to Evaluate at Protocol Renewal

It is useful for the IRB to have an institution-specific form to facilitate the protocol renewal process. Some of the topics or questions to include on the institution-specific form are described here.

Accrual

1. Has accrual progressed as planned? If not, will this impact the ability of the researcher to complete the study?
2. If the study objectives cannot be met and the study involves more than minimal-risk interventions, is it reasonable to continue accrual?
3. If the study is a multisite trial, has the investigator provided you with trial-wide accrual data in addition to local accrual data?

Revisions

1. Are new revisions being submitted at the time of continuation review/protocol renewal?
2. Will each committee member get a full copy of the revised protocol, or is the revision a minor change in previously approved research?

Unanticipated Toxicity

1. How many serious and unexpected toxicities have occurred since the trial's initiation?
2. If the toxicities (in type or number) are linked to the study intervention, are new toxicity risks described in the consent form?
3. Will the information about unanticipated toxicity(s) impact the risk/benefit ratio and continued study approval?

Subject Complaints

1. Were there concerns about approach or contact for the study?
2. Have subjects withdrawn because of disappointing interactions with the study team?
3. Is there a need to modify procedures or re-educate staff because of these concerns?
4. Do study team members know whom to contact with questions about the rights of research participants?

New Information or Findings Relating to Risk/Benefit Assessment

1. Are safety and risk factors for participants adequately described in the consent form based on findings to date? If not, is the informed consent process or document still acceptable or does it require revision?

2. Has any new institutional policy or regulation been instituted since the last IRB review? If so, does this influence the future conduct of the study?

Interval of Renewal
Should renewal review be done annually or more frequently? The risk to subjects determines the renewal interval.

Other Continuation Review Considerations

Each institution's infrastructure, history, policy development, and state law may impact the process of protocol renewal and the information requested. For example, comprehensive cancer center grants require clinical trial review by a scientific review committee as well as a protocol data and monitoring committee separate from the IRB. Collectively, these committees conduct continuation review in addition to the IRB. A dual system of protection is in place.

Coordinating centers for multisite trials also provide IRBs with reports from data safety monitoring boards and/or statistical centers at the time of continuation review. These reports enable the IRB review process and provide trial-wide data findings that may impact the risk/benefits assessment at the local IRB level. For this reason, IRBs request both local and trial-wide data on continuation review report forms.

A private hospital may not be involved in multisite trials or rely on a separate protocol monitoring committee within the institution. In this situation, careful reassessment at continuation review hinges primarily on the investigator and the IRB.

Full-Board or Expedited Review?

Initial Full-Board Review
Studies that initially went through a convened meeting of the IRB will continue with full-board review at the time of protocol renewal. However, *expedited review may be used for continuation review of studies that initially underwent full review in the following circumstances:*[8]

1. (a) Research is permanently closed to the enrollment of new subjects; all subjects have completed all research-related interventions; and research remains active only for long-term follow-up of subjects; or (b) no subjects have been enrolled and no additional risks have been identified; or (c) the remaining research activities are limited to data analysis.

2. Protocol renewals may also undergo expedited continuation review in specific circumstances. The following categories of research qualify for expedited review unless the IRB, sponsor, or other study-related party requires full review: continuing review of research not conducted under an investigational new drug application or investigational device exemption where categories 2 through 8 of the expedited review categories[8] do not apply; however, the IRB has determined and documented at a convened meeting that the research involves no greater than minimal risk and no additional risks have been identified.

Initial Expedited Review
Research activities that initially qualified as minimal risk and underwent initial expedited review and approval can continue as expedited review activities at protocol renewal unless changes in procedures or intervention cause the activity to be more than minimal risk. A more detailed discussion of expedited review categories is the subject of Chapter 4-2.

Conclusion

Ongoing protocol review is an important—some would say the most important—aspect of the IRB's role in protecting the rights and welfare of research participants. Guidelines for protocol renewal by IRBs are presented in this chapter with an emphasis on the administration of the renewal process. By establishing standard operating procedures that focus attention on evaluating study progress in view of the major ethical standards, the IRB will comply with federal regulations and fulfill its institutional commitments. The documentation of the continuation review process is a complex task that requires attention to the details of several different sections of the federal regulations that apply to the IRB review process.

References
1. Levine RJ. *Ethics and Regulation of Clinical Research*, 2nd ed. Baltimore, MD: Urban and Schwarzenberg; 1986.
2. National Commission for the Protection of Human Subjects of Biomedical and Behavioral Research. *The Belmont Report: Ethical Principles and Guidelines for the Protection of Human Subjects of Research*, 18 April, 1979. Access date 24 January, 2005. http://www.hhs.gov/ohrp/humansubjects/guidance/belmont.htm
3. Office for Human Research Protections. Guidance on Continuing Review. Dated July 11, 2002. Access date 24 January, 2005. http://www.hhs.gov/ohrp/humansubjects/ guidance/contrev2002.
4. Food and Drug Administration. Information Sheets: Guidance for Institutional Review Boards and Clinical Investigators, September 1998. Access date 24 January, 2005. http://www.fda.gov/oc/ohrt/irbs/default.htm
5. Code of Federal Regulations. Title 45A—Department of Health and Human Services; Part 46—Protection of Human Subjects. Revised 13 November, 2001. Access date 24 January, 2005. http://www.hhs.gov/ohrp/ humansubjects/guidance/45cfr46.htm
6. Code of Federal Regulations. Title 21, Chapter 1—Food and Drug Administration, DHHS; Part 56—Institutional Review Boards. Updated 1 April, 2004. Access date 24 January, 2005. http://www.fda.gov/oc/ohrt/irbs/appendixc.html
7. Food and Drug Administration. International Conference on Harmonisation: Guidance for Industry, E6 Good Clinical Practice (GCP): Consolidation Guidance. http://www.fda.gov/cder/guidance/959fnl.pdf
8. Department of Health and Human Services. Protection of human subjects: Categories of research that may be reviewed by the Institutional Review Board (IRB) through an expedited review procedure. *Fed Regist* 63(216):60364–60367, 1998. http://www.hhs.gov/ohrp/humansubjects/guidance/ expedited98.htm

Institutional Review Board Review of Adverse Events

Christopher J. Kratochvil, Ernest D. Prentice, Kevin J. Epperson, and Bruce G. Gordon

INTRODUCTION

The Department of Health and Human Services (DHHS) regulations for the protection of human subjects[1][Sec.109(e)] and the corollary Food and Drug Administration (FDA) regulations[2][Sec.109(f)] require the institutional review board (IRB) to conduct "continuing review of research . . . at intervals appropriate to the degree of risk but not less than once per year." The IRB is also required[1][Sec.111(a)(6)],2[Sec.111(a)(6)] to ensure that "when appropriate, the research plan makes adequate provision for monitoring the data collected to ensure the safety of subjects." Depending on the size and nature of the research, monitoring may be performed by the investigator, a data and safety monitoring board (DSMB), or even the IRB itself.

The purpose of continuing to review and monitor ongoing studies is to ensure that the research remains justified and that the rights and welfare of the participants continue to be fully protected. Accordingly, it is of paramount importance that the IRB is assured as the study progresses that the risks are minimized, the benefits are maximized, and the risk/benefit relationship of the research continues to be acceptable. Indeed, these are the cardinal responsibilities of the IRB.

From a practical standpoint, change in the risk/benefit relationship of ongoing research, particularly in the early stages, is most affected by the occurrence of adverse events (AEs) that impact subject morbidity and mortality. Thus, it is important for the IRB to be able to perform a valid review of AEs and determine their impact on continuation of the research, whether the informed consent form requires revision, and whether subjects already enrolled in the research should be reconsented. Although IRBs recognize and acknowledge this responsibility, many are not equipped to deal effectively with the avalanche of external AE reports (AERs) that are generated during the course of multicenter trials, particularly those involving investigational drugs. These AERs are sent routinely by study sponsors to all IRBs of record, via local investigators.

It is important to note that when the federal regulations were framed in the late 1970s, large multicenter trials were not the norm. This chapter addresses the DHHS and FDA regulations that apply to AE reporting and the IRB review of AEs. Inconsistencies and problems in interpreting the federal regulations are discussed, and practical suggestions are offered on how IRBs could effectively and efficiently review AERs.

Federal Regulations

An institution is required by the DHHS[1][Sec.103(b)(5)] and the FDA[2][Sec.108(b)(1)] to establish written procedures for ensuring "prompt reporting" to the IRB and appropriate institutional officials about "any unanticipated problems involving risks to subjects or others. . . ." This reporting requirement is unclear, however. The meaning of *prompt* is not defined, and there is also no minimum risk threshold for reporting a problem. Also, the term *any* implies that all unanticipated problems involving risk must be reported to the IRB regardless of the level of risk and irrespective of any causal relationship between the problem and the research.

Thus, using a literal but clearly impractical interpretation of the federal regulations, even a minor unanticipated AE should be reported regardless of its relationship to the research. Few IRBs, however, require either minor or unrelated AEs to be reported. Although this position may not be totally consistent with the written requirements of the regulations, it is a feasible and practical approach, with little danger that the rights and welfare of research subjects would be compromised. For example, if a subject suffered an unanticipated, transient, minor headache in a drug study, the investigator should certainly evaluate this AE, but it is not necessary from a subject safety standpoint to report the event to the IRB.

The aforementioned sections of the DHHS and FDA regulations do not use the term *adverse event*. Instead, the broader phrase *problems involving risk* is used. Clearly, any unanticipated problem involving "risk" that ultimately results in harm to the subject and is related to a research intervention encompasses a reportable AE. For example, an unexpected cardiac arrest in an exercise study or a corneal ulcer in a glaucoma study is obviously reportable to the IRB. The term *problems involving risk*, however, could also be construed to mean a problem involving risk to the subject that does not actually result in any harm. Indeed, the word *risk* literally means only the *possibility* of harm occurring, as opposed to the actual occurrence of harm. For example, the loss of a subject's research records that contain identifiable private information would be a reportable event. There is a risk of a breach of confidentiality, which may or may not occur. Thus, IRBs should be aware of the fact that, technically, under the federal regulations, an unanticipated risk to which a subject is exposed is a reportable event, and actual harm is not required.

Risk to "Others"

The regulations also require that unanticipated problems involving risk to "others" must be promptly reported. For example, if a research technician is inadvertently exposed to a low level of radiation during a study, this would be a reportable event. The term *others* could also be interpreted to mean other subjects enrolled in the same clinical trial or receiving the same drug or device at another study site. The implementation of this interpretation by pharmaceutical companies and device manufacturers, however, has been problematic. Without objection or clarification by federal regulators, a massive number of AERs are being sent to IRBs across the nation, even though it is generally acknowledged that IRBs cannot effectively review many of these AERs, particularly in the context of a multicenter clinical trial. Individual AERs often do not contain sufficient information about the AE to allow the IRB to make an informed assessment of its significance. An AER without a denominator and unblinding of its study arm assignment handicaps the IRB and can lead to errors in judgment that can either affect subject safety or unnecessarily impede the progress of the research.

On the other hand, even in the absence of clinically meaningful data, certainly an unanticipated, serious AE that "may" be related to the drug or device that occurs at an external site cannot be ignored by the IRB. This is obviously for subject safety as well as legal reasons. It is entirely possible that prompt review of an AER by the IRB could prevent other subjects from suffering the same AE and make the investigator more aware of the need for surveillance for a particular problem. If changes to the consent form result, it may help current subjects appropriately reevaluate their participation and new subjects make a more informed decision regarding entering a study. Disclosure in the consent document of a previously unidentified risk will also help protect the investigators and their institution against liability for breach of fiduciary duty, that is, failure to disclose all known risks. Thus, whenever the IRB receives a safety report or other information about an AE that occurred in a multicenter trial, the board is obligated under the current interpretation of the regulations to perform the best review possible even when the data are not yet complete or statistically valid. This is a difficult situation plaguing every IRB that reviews AERs from multicenter trials. The problem is obviously very significant at large institutions, which commonly receive thousands of AERs annually. It is reasonable to speculate that some pharmaceutical companies are asking IRBs to review AERs for primarily liability reasons as opposed to any real expectation that the IRB can actually perform a consistently valid review of the AE.[3]

AE Reporting by the Institution to Federal Agencies

AE reporting requirements extend beyond the IRB and institutional officials. DHHS regulations[1][Sec.103(b)(5)] and FDA regulations[2][Sec.108(b)(1)] also require the institution to have a procedure in place for prompt reporting of any unanticipated problems involving risk to the subject or others to the appropriate "department or agency head." In the case of research that is subject to DHHS regulations, the AE must be reported to the Office for Human Research Protections (OHRP), which acts on behalf of the Secretary of DHHS. AEs must also be reported to federally funded cooperative research groups in accordance with their requirements. For example, the National Cancer Institute's Cancer Therapy Evaluation Program has comprehensive guidelines on AE reporting, specific to their Institute.[4] When AEs occur in research regulated by the FDA, then the event must be reported to the FDA. This reporting is normally accomplished through established reporting channels from the investigator, to the sponsor, to the FDA, in accordance with the requirements of all applicable FDA regulations. If, however, the investigator holds the investigational new drug (IND) application or investigational device exemption (IDE), he or she should report the AE directly to the FDA or to the FDA through the investigator's IRB.

As mentioned previously, federal regulations for the protection of human subjects do not base reporting requirements on a risk threshold. Theoretically, this should result in a tremendous number of AERs being sent to the FDA and OHRP. However, with the exception of any sponsor requirements to the contrary, institutions in general do not routinely submit AERs or reports of unexpected problems involving risk to federal authorities unless the event is serious and related to the research. As a matter of fact, very few IRBs ever report problems involving risk where there is no concomitant harm to the subjects. Clearly, neither the OHRP nor the FDA has the resources to review all AEs or problems that occur during the conduct of research. It is equally clear that comprehensive review of AEs at the federal compliance oversight level is neither warranted nor cost effective. Thus, it is not surprising that OHRP and the FDA have never enforced the "letter of the law."

AE Reporting by the Sponsor

As previously pointed out by Gordon and Prentice,[5] sponsors of FDA-regulated research involving drugs or biologics are required[8][Sec.32(c)] to notify the FDA and all participating investigators in a written IND safety report of any AEs associated with the use of the investigational drug/biologic that are both serious, related and unexpected.

Although this regulation does not require the sponsor to notify IRBs at participating study sites, it is nevertheless routine to do so. Sponsors instruct investigators to provide a copy of the safety report to the IRB or send a copy of the report directly to the IRB. Although this involvement of the IRB may be perceived by sponsors as helping to manage their liability, it is unrealistic to expect IRBs to act as "quasi-DSMBs." This is particularly true with the burgeoning numbers of AEs being submitted as multicenter clinical trials have become the norm and more trials are being conducted. Neither the FDA nor the OHRP have issued clear official guidance on this issue, but "advice" by Michael Carome, OHRP, offers some practical guidance, "With respect to reports of adverse events involving subjects who are not participating in research at your institution (hereafter referred to as external adverse events), unless these external adverse events represent unanticipated problems involving risks to subjects participating in research (or to others) at your institution, such events do not need to be reported to, or reviewed by, your IRB under HHS regulations at 45CFR46.103(b)(5)."[7]

In contrast to the FDA regulations for the protection of human subjects,[2][Sec.108(b)(1)] the FDA IND regulations[6][Sec.32(c)] include a risk-reporting threshold. That is, the AE must be serious and unexpected and must be associated with the use of the drug/biologic, all as defined in 21 CFR 312.[6][Sec.32(a)] It is interesting to note that the FDA requirements for AE reporting in device studies are similar to 21 CFR 56[2][Sec.108(b)(1)] but differ from 21 CFR 312[6][Sec.32(c)] in terms of reporting criteria. The FDA IDE regulations[8][Sec.150(b)(1)] require the sponsor to report any unanticipated adverse device effects (i.e., an AE that occurs in a device study which was not previously identified as a potential risk), to all reviewing IRBs and participating investigators, regardless of severity. This more comprehensive AE reporting requirement is undoubtedly because many medical devices are implanted and, thus, the risk may persist over time.

Although there is no reference to causality in the IDE regulations, any unanticipated AE that could possibly be related to the device should be considered a reportable adverse device effect.

IRB Policies and Procedures for Review of AEs

Every IRB should have written policies and procedures concerning review of AERs. Given the impracticalities and inconsistencies in the applicable DHHS and FDA regulations as well as a distinct lack of written guidance from OHRP and FDA, many IRBs are struggling to deal with an overwhelming number of AERs. It is, therefore, not surprising that there is little consistency in the way IRBs review AERs. This section provides general guidance to facilitate efficient and effective IRB review of AEs. This guidance is based on the experiences of the authors who have implemented these guidelines as a part of the University of Nebraska Medical Center (UNMC) IRB's policies and procedures for review of AERs.[3,5]

Two separate and specific review forms for AEs are used: one for AEs that occur at institutions served by the IRB and another for those that occur at external unaffiliated study sites (Table 7.3.1). These IRB AER forms are referred to as "internal" and "external" and are designed so that the investigator provides the IRB with a reasonably detailed analysis of the AE. Clearly, the investigator, as opposed to the IRB, is usually in a better position to assess the significance of the AE in terms of whether the protocol requires modification to minimize risk, whether the consent form should be revised, or if subjects should be reconsented. Thus, an IRB should use the expertise of its investigators as an integral part of the review, particularly in cases in which there is little available information concerning the AE.

Important AE Terminology

- Unanticipated: the specificity or severity of the AE is not consistent with the current investigator's brochure or with other current risk information (based on 21 CFR 312.32(a)).

- Related or possibly related: there is a reasonable possibility the AE may have been caused by the drug or intervention or it is possible that the AE may have been caused by the drug or intervention, but there is insufficient information to determine the likelihood of this possibility (based on 21 CFR 312.32(a)).

- Serious: (1) results in death or (2) is life threatening or (3) requires inpatient hospitalization or prolongation of existing hospitalization or (4) results in serious, persistent, or significant disability or incapacity or (5) results in a congenital

Table 7.3.1 Essential Features of an IRB Adverse Event Report in Drug Studies

- Describe the adverse event in sufficient detail as to allow an informed review of the occurrence (description, causality, prognosis)
- Explain why the *external* adverse event is unexpected **and** related **and** serious (if does not meet all 3 criteria, no report necessary)
- Explain why the *internal* adverse event is unexpected **and** related (if does not meet both criteria, no report necessary)
- Describe changes to the protocol to minimize further risk, or the rationale if no changes are required
- Describe changes to the consent or the rationale if no changes are required
- Describe the plan to reconsent current participants or the rationale if no reconsent is required
- Risk/Benefit Analysis Update: Explain why the overall risk/benefit relationship of the research is still acceptable in light of the information concerning this adverse event report

anomaly or birth defect or (6) causes cancer or (7) is an overdose or (8) is any medical event which requires treatment to prevent one of the medical outcomes listed previously (based on 21 CFR 312.32(a)).

Internal Events

Investigators at UNMC submit an internal AER form for "internal" AEs or problems involving risks that are unanticipated and related or possibly related to the drug, biologic, or other research intervention. The internal event reviews require a particularly careful and thoughtful assessment, as the local IRB reviewing the event may be the only oversight other than the investigator. This is in stark contrast to a multicenter trial sponsored by a pharmaceutical company, which may have several layers of review: the FDA, the sponsor, and potentially dozens of IRBs. Thus, the risk-reporting threshold for AEs that occur at UNMC is set at a level equivalent to "more than minor," defined as an AE that requires a treatment or other intervention by a health care professional, as a reasonable standard. Other IRBs may adopt a more stringent standard in consideration of the federal regulations.[1][Sec.103(b)(5)],[2][Sec.108(b)(1)] AEs that are expected and, therefore, described in the protocol as well as the consent document should normally not be reviewed by the IRB unless an expected AE occurs more frequently than anticipated or is more serious than expected. One exception to this rule is in the case of a death. Many IRBs, including the UNMC IRB, review all deaths that occur on protocol, regardless of whether the death was related to the research.

External Events

Investigators submit an AER form for external AEs to report problems involving risk that occur at unaffiliated research sites. Our IRB does not routinely review external AEs that occur in studies of drugs or biologics unless the event is serious, related (or possibly related), and unanticipated. The difference in the risk-reporting threshold for internal versus external AEs in such studies is based on the fact that an IRB should have greater responsibility for the review of internal AEs than external AEs. Indeed, IRBs should not be required to review routinely individual external AEs except under unusual circumstances in which the sponsor has determined that immediate IRB review is necessary to reassess risk or disclose new risks to subjects.

Finally, it should be reiterated that the AE reporting requirements for device studies are different from the requirements for studies that involve investigational drugs or biologics. FDA regulations[8][Sec.150(b)(1)] require the sponsor to report any unanticipated adverse device effects that occur during device studies to all reviewing IRBs. Thus, the IRB cannot review only serious, unanticipated adverse device effects.

The Role of the Data and Safety Monitoring Board

The DHHS and FDA regulations that require the reporting and IRB review of AEs are complex, inconsistent, and out of touch with the realities of modern-day clinical research. Perhaps this is in part because the regulations for the protection of human subjects were issued in 1980 and have never been revised to accommodate the nature of large, multicenter, clinical trials. Even if local IRBs received complete information about every AE in a timely fashion and the board possessed the required expertise, it is both unrealistic and inefficient to expect each IRB to perform this time-consuming task. Although IRBs should perform a thorough review of all unanticipated AEs that are more than minor in terms of health-related significance and occur at the institution(s) under their jurisdiction, this responsibility should not be extended to AEs that occur at other institutions.

The responsibility for safety monitoring in a multicenter clinical trial should rest with a data and safely monitoring board (DSMB). As Bankert and Amdur pointed out, "The IRB is not a data and safety monitoring committee."[9] To attempt to put an IRB in this role is inappropriate.

A DSMB is composed of an *independent* group of experts that reviews the ongoing conduct of a clinical trial in order to identify any safety problems rapidly, ensure the quality and integrity of the data, and determine when trial objectives have been met. DSMBs are generally set up by the sponsor, report to the sponsor, and follow operational rules that are study specific. Although all clinical trials need monitoring, not all trials need DSMBs, which are more common in Phase III studies. When used for a trial, DSMBs should be required to provide IRBs with safety information in a digestible format, at appropriate intervals that will allow IRBs, together with their investigators, to perform a more reliable assessment of the significance of AE data in terms of the protection of human subjects. The DSMBs generally have access to all of the available data, including the treatment arm when appropriate in blinded studies, which helps them make an informed decision, as opposed to local IRBs who are forced to make decisions based on limited and often anecdotal information. The National Institutes of Health have taken a step in this direction by requiring that a DSMB be in place for multicenter clinical trials and that DSMB reports be given to the IRBs with ongoing oversight responsibilities.[10] It should, however, be emphasized that although the DSMB and the sponsor clearly have the authority to amend or halt a study, the reviewing IRB that approved the protocol bears the ultimate responsibility for ensuring that the rights and welfare of subjects at their institution are fully protected. Thus, IRBs need to communicate with investigators, DSMBs, other IRBs, and federal regulators as the need arises.

Conclusion

Clearly, there are significant regulatory inconsistencies related to the reporting and IRB review of AEs in studies regulated by the FDA and DHHS. These inconsistencies are confusing for investigators and troubling to IRBs. Additionally, the requirements for reporting AEs as the regulations are currently written are so burdensome—

particularly in the current era of large multisite trials—that they have become extremely impractical. Therefore, both harmonization and modification of regulatory requirements are needed. In the meantime, IRBs should use a rational approach to the review of AEs that is based on a reasonable interpretation and application of the federal regulations.

References

1. Code of Federal Regulations. Title 45A—Department of Health and Human Services; Part 46—Protection of Human Subjects. Updated 1 October, 1997.

2. Code of Federal Regulations. Title 21, Chapter 1—Food and Drug Administration, DHHS; Part 56—Institutional Review Boards. Updated 1 April, 1999.

3. Prentice ED, Gordon B. IRB review of adverse events in investigational drug studies. *IRB: A Review of Human Subjects Research* 19(6):1–4, 1997.

4. National Cancer Institute Cancer Therapy Evaluation Program. National Cancer Institute guidelines: Expedited adverse event reporting requirements for National Cancer Institute investigational agents, 2001. Access date 22 December, 2004. http://ctep.cancer.gov/forms/NCI_AEReporting_Gdln_final.pdf

5. Gordon B, Prentice E. Selective review of external adverse events: One IRB's response to the avalanche of IND safety reports. *IRB: A Review of Human Subjects Research* 21(3):10–11, 1999.

6. Code of Federal Regulations. Title 21, Chapter 1—Food and Drug Administration, DHHS; Part 312—Investigational New Drug Application. Updated 1 April, 1999.

7. Personal communication, Michael Carome, OHRP, 7 July, 2003.

8. Code of Federal Regulations. Title 21, Chapter 1—Food and Drug Administration, DHHS; Subchapter H—Medical Devices; Parts 800 through 898. Updated 1 April, 1999.

9. Bankert E, Amdur RJ. The IRB is not a data and safety monitoring committee. *IRB: A Review of Human Subjects Research* 22(6):9–10, 2000.

10. National Institutes of Health. NIH Policy for Data and Safety Monitoring, 10 June, 1998. Access date 21 December, 2004. http://grants2.nih.gov/grants/guide/notice-files/not98-084.html

Data and Safety Monitoring

J. Allen McCutchan

INTRODUCTION

Institutional review boards (IRBs) are tasked with the "continuing review" of research (i.e., monitoring studies after their initial approval) but face a multitude of problems in trying to do so. This chapter attempts to clarify the responsibility of investigators, sponsors, and IRBs for monitoring the conduct of studies after their initial approval. It advocates a central role for data and safety monitoring boards (DSMBs) in the monitoring of complex or potentially risky studies.

Data and Safety Monitoring Boards

A DSMB is a multidisciplinary group that is usually composed of three to six experts in at least two areas: (1) medical issues (the disease, drug, device, procedure, or outcome measures) and (2) method issues (clinical trials design, data management, and statistical analysis). For some studies, expertise in research and biomedical ethics is also required. DSMBs can monitor the timeliness of accrual, the quality of data collection and management, and the accumulating outcomes to assure the safety of participants and the scientific integrity of the study.

The terms *DSMB* and *independent DSMB* are used interchangeably because a criterion for serving on a DSMB is a lack of ties, affiliations, or interests that might create bias when evaluating data or making recommendations. The independence of the DSMB requires that its members have no professional or financial interest in the outcome of the studies it monitors. On the other hand, the sponsors or investigators convene and support the DSMB, selecting and compensating its members for their services. Moreover, the data that the DSMB reviews are usually processed and presented by data managers who are employees or contractors of the sponsors or investigators. Thus, the DSMB depends on the professional integrity of the data managers for the accuracy of data it reviews.

When Is a DSMB Needed?

IRBs are currently without meaningful guidance on when to require a DSMB as opposed to other models of data oversight. A definitive evaluation of this issue is beyond the scope of this chapter. In general, the factors that suggest that a DSMB is the most appropriate way to monitor data include these:

1. *A large study population.* Many persons may be harmed before problems are recognized.
2. *Multiple study sites.* When no investigator treats more than a fraction of the participants, it is difficult to recognize a pattern of increased or unusual problems.

3. *Highly toxic therapies or dangerous procedures.* This is a critical determinant of how frequently and intensely participants should be monitored for adverse effects.
4. *High expected rates of morbidity or mortality in the study population.* Problems related to the natural history of disease or aging may obscure adverse events caused by the intervention.
5. *High chance of early termination.* There is a reasonable likelihood that the study may be terminated early for reasons of safety, futility, or efficacy.

What Does a DSMB Do?

DSMBs usually review data at predetermined intervals during the study, sometimes operating under protocol-specified rules for considering whether or not the study should continue. The DSMB may specify the type and form of data presented, examine the blinded data by group (without being told which group is which), and/or completely unblind the study. Their decisions are rendered as suggestions to the sponsors or investigators and are subject to review and negotiation before their implementation.

Meetings of a DSMB are often divided into an open session attended by the investigators and sponsors and a closed session limited to the members of the DSMB. During the open period, issues of data quality may be discussed. In addition, the rates of accrual of participants, outcomes (such as deaths, relapses, or responses), and adverse events may be reviewed for the study as a whole. In a closed session, the DSMB may see the rates of these events in each study arm and discuss the issues of modifying or stopping the study.

DSMBs may conclude that the study should be stopped for one of several reasons.

1. Efficacy—With high certainty, the study question has been answered (e.g., one group is doing better than the others, or no group is likely to do better than any other).

2. Futility—The study question will not be answered when the study is completed, for example, because too many of the patients have been lost to follow-up or stopped the intervention.

3. Safety—Risks to patients are too high.

Most investigators and sponsors immediately accept and implement the conclusions of the DSMB, but occasional disagreements require negotiation. The IRB should insist that it be notified immediately of the DSMB's recommendations to modify or stop a study.

DSMBs and the IRB

DSMBs can monitor the safety of study participants more rigorously and more easily than IRBs and should routinely communicate their findings and recommendations to all of the IRBs involved in multisite studies. The frequency and content of the reports will vary depending on the safety issues and specific monitoring plan proposed for each study. IRB members and administrators have persuasively advocated this approach in several recent articles.[1,2] Moreover, the National Institutes of Health (NIH) has adopted this policy.[3]

DSMBs can assist IRBs in their oversight of studies because DSMBs have greater access to the accumulating data than IRBs and can unblind the treatment assignments of either individuals or groups of participants. Because unblinding can be independent of the investigators or sponsors of the study, safety issues may be addressed without compromising the objectivity of the investigators. Knowing the group assignment of individuals in blinded treatment studies is often invaluable for assessing an individual adverse event. DSMBs can make informed decisions that the IRB could not attempt. For example, review of unblinded data by a DSMB can detect excess morbidity or mortality in one arm of a large trial that is not apparent to the IRB or investigators. As discussed earlier, DSMBs may also terminate a study earlier than scheduled because the study has already reached a clear outcome or is very unlikely to do so even if completed. This unique insight of the DSMB contributes to safety because it minimizes the exposure of patients to more risky or less effective therapies.

DSMBs have become standard in the monitoring of most NIH-sponsored and many industry-sponsored Phase III clinical trials over the past decade. Large, multisite clinical trials groups such as the AIDS Clinical Trials Group of the National Institute of Allergy and Infectious Diseases routinely review their interventional studies.[4] Guidelines for monitoring of Phases I, II, and III studies are available on the Web.[5,6] Despite this widespread appreciation of their usefulness by the NIH, their DSMBs do not routinely communicate with local IRBs, and many IRBs are unaware of their existence.

How Can DSMBs Be Integrated into IRB Procedures?

The time to deal with the DSMB issue is at the time of initial protocol review. This is the subject of other chapters in this book. Initially, IRB members and administrators may be unfamiliar with the functions of DSMBs and their advantages for investigators and the IRB. Data-monitoring plans, including consideration of the need for a DSMB, should be a routine part of evaluating the data management and statistical section of protocols. This may require that the IRB sponsor training, for both investigators and IRB members, addressing the need for DSMBs, and that reminders be added to the instructions for protocol submission and review.

Negotiations with the sponsors of studies to establish a DSMB, ask for reports on their reviews, or request unblinded reviews of serious adverse events (SAEs) are usually conducted via the principal investigator (PI) of the study at the IRB's institution. The PI may not be able to convey the rationale for the IRB's request to the sponsor without help. IRBs should provide explicit reasons for requesting establishment of or action by a DSMB in writing to the PI. These requests may explain (1) the features of the study that require establishment of a DSMB, (2) the specific reports required from the DSMB, (3) the reason that SAEs need to be evaluated by the DSMB, or (4) additional information required by the IRB, such as "stopping rules" for the study.

For example, the letter to an investigator might contain remarks like the following:

The plan and resources for data collection and monitoring were not adequately outlined in your submission. Please indicate the personnel, site, computer resources, and monitoring procedures you will employ as required in the data and monitoring section of the outline for submission of protocols to the IRB. Your submission indicates that (DRUG X) has been associated with (SEVERE TOXICITY) in a substantial proportion of patients in prior studies and that you intend to treat patients at a more advanced stage of disease than in prior studies. For these reasons, the board suggests that you convene a DSMB to review the safety of the study. Specifically, after treating the first 50 patients and after each group of 50 patients thereafter, the DSMB should assess and compare the accumulating rates of (SEVERE TOXICITY) in the two arms of your study and communicate to the IRB that continuation is appropriate. Also indicate and justify in the protocol what rate of toxicity in the DRUG X arm would trigger the DSMB to stop enrollment and reevaluate the safety of the study.

Approval or continuation of the protocol should depend on an adequate response to the IRB's requests for better definition of the monitoring plan. Investigators at cautious institutions may be unable to participate in the study if the sponsor or DSMB is unwilling to respond to such requests. Because individual IRBs require that DSMBs be convened and communicate regularly with IRBs, they may be perceived initially as "difficult" by study sponsors or local investigators. This may appear to place local investigators in an awkward position, especially if they have no control over the content of the study protocol. However, the protections afforded to the research subjects, the investigators, and the institution greatly outweigh this disadvantage. Moreover, as multiple IRBs make similar requests, investigators and sponsors will understand that, for many studies, regular monitoring by a DSMB is the standard of practice.

Conclusion

Data and safety monitoring is one of the most complex and important aspects of the process of protecting human research subjects. The role of the IRB in the data safety monitoring process is discussed in detail in several other chapters in this book. This chapter has focused on the most rigorous approach to ongoing data monitoring, the data and safety monitoring board. For IRBs to function optimally from the standpoint of protecting research participants in compliance with federal regulations, it is important for the IRB to understand when it is appropriate to require a DSMB as part of the initial research plan and how the IRB and DSMB should interact during the life of the study.

References

1. Gordon VM, Sugarman J, Kass N. Toward a more comprehensive approach to protecting human subjects: The interface of data safety monitoring boards and institutional review boards in randomized clinical trials. *IRB: A Review of Human Subjects Research* 20(1):1–5, 1998.

2. Bankert E, Amdur RJ. The IRB is not a data and safety monitoring committee. *IRB: A Review of Human Subjects Research* 22(6):9–10, 2000.

3. National Institutes of Health. Guidance on reporting adverse events to institutional review boards for NIH-supported multicenter clinical trials (from NIH Guide for June 11, 1999). Access date 29 March, 2001. http://grants.nih.gov/grants/guide/notice-files/not99-107.html

4. Ellenberg SS, Myers MW, Blackwelder WC, Hoth DF. The use of external monitoring committees in clinical trials of the National Institute of Allergy and Infectious Diseases. *Stat Med* 12(5–6):461–467, 1993.

5. National Institutes of Health. NIH policy for data and safety monitoring, 10 June, 1998. Access date 29 March, 2001. http://www.grants.nih/gov/grants/guide/notice-files/not98-084.html

6. National Institutes of Health. Further guidance on a data and safety monitoring board for Phase I and Phase II trials, 5 June, 2000. Access date 29 March, 2001. http://grants.nih.gov/grants/guide/notice-files/NOT-OD-00-038.html

Noncompliance, Complaints, Deviations, and Eligibility Exceptions

Lucille Pearson and Tracy Ostler

INTRODUCTION

The principal investigator is responsible for ensuring that research is carried out according to the institutional review board (IRB)-approved study design and consent process. During the course of the study, however, not everything will go according to plan. The purpose of this chapter is to explain how the IRB should address a report of noncompliance, a complaint, a report of a deviation, or an eligibility exception notice. These reports may come to the IRB from a range of sources. A participant or family member may complain. A whistle-blower may call the IRB. A member of the research team may contact the IRB, or noncompliance may be suspected as a result of an internal IRB audit. This chapter does not address the issue of the origin of the report but addresses a procedure for responding to these reports once they are received by the IRB.

Federal Regulations

Title 45 CFR 46.103 (b)(5)

Written procedures for ensuring prompt reporting to the IRB, appropriate institutional officials, and the Department or Agency head of (i) any unanticipated problems involving risks to subjects or others, as well as any serious or continuing noncompliance with this policy or the requirements or determinations of the IRB, and (ii) any suspension or termination of IRB approval.

Title 45 CFR 46.113 (analogous to Food and Drug Administration [FDA] regulation 21 CFR 56.113)

Suspension or termination of IRB approval of research. An IRB shall have the authority to suspend or terminate approval of research that is not being conducted in accordance with the IRB's requirements or that has been associated with unexpected serious harm to subjects. Any suspension or termination of approval shall include a statement of the reasons for the IRB's action, and shall be reported promptly to the investigator, appropriate institutional officials, and the Department or Agency head.

IRB Written Policy

How does the IRB address the regulations and review the myriad of reports in a timely manner? The first step is to develop clear procedures to describe institutional policy. Ensure that the policy becomes a written part of your internal IRB guidance. To create the policy, individuals with knowledge of federal regulations and institutional requirements should meet to compile the procedures as appropriate for your institution. The IRB is part of the institution, and thus, internal IRB policies should agree with those of the greater institution. For example, ensure that there is consideration of the Scientific Misconduct Policy or Conflict of Interest Policy if applicable. The importance of establishing a written policy is that adherence to it will ensure consistency. This policy should outline in advance how each report will be handled, thus eliminating any confusion when an actual report arrives at the IRB office.

Distribute the Policy

After the policy is written, it is extremely important that the information be distributed to the research community. This can be accomplished in several ways. The information can be added to a website, added to a researchers' reference guide, or referred to in the IRB approval letter. The IRB should provide contact information so that individuals have a clear understanding of how to make these reports.

IRB Office Receipt of the Reporting Form

All reports are important to review; however, each instance need not be subjected to the same level of scrutiny. Some reports will clearly be more serious than others. For example, forming a subcommittee and conducting an extensive audit would not be appropriate for the isolated use of an outdated consent form. It is appropriate to investigate and respond to the complaint or report of noncompliance relative to its level of seriousness.

Content of the Reporting Form

Because of the need to triage the reports, the information received from the researcher or subject should contain important information such as the date of the event, a thorough description of the event, and whether the sponsor has been notified. There are other important points as well: Have the rights or welfare of the participants been affected, and have risks to subjects been increased? The Dartmouth Reporting Form can be found at: www.dartmouth.edu/~cphs/tosubmit/forms.

Review Process

When Suspension Is Not Necessary

If the situation does not merit suspension of the research study, a summary of the report is completed, and an internal review form is attached. The letter *a* is circled, dated, and initialed by the IRB administrator, the IRB chair, or a designee. The form is filed in the study folder, and the primary reviewer reviews all reports at the time of renewal. A sample statement follows:

> **a.** Suspension not merited: If the IRB director and IRB chair agree that suspension is not merited, the issue will be resolved among any combination of the following individuals: IRB director, IRB chair, PI, PI's department chair. All communication will be documented.

When Suspension Is Necessary

If the report does merit suspension of the research study, further steps are required. The letter *b* is circled on the internal review form, dated, and initialed by the IRB administrator, the IRB chair, or a designee. These steps are followed:

> **b.** Notice of suspension effective immediately will be sent to the PI, co-PIs, department chair, grants and contracts department, IRB institutional official, and IRB chair. The notification includes the requirement to halt further participant enrollment.
>
> Within 2 days, a meeting should be called and attended by any combination of the following individuals: IRB director, IRB chair, PI, PI's department chair. The attendees should discuss the nature of the situation and determine whether a designation of serious or continuing noncompliance is warranted. At this meeting, it should also be determined whether any other studies being conducted by the PI should be suspended.
>
> To make the determination of serious or continuing noncompliance, an audit of study records may be needed. The PI will be required to produce, at a minimum, (1) all signed consent forms and (2) all data related to the study project.

The results of the review of study records and discussions with the PI will determine whether the situation is of a nonserious and noncontinuing nature.

> **i.** Nonserious and noncontinuing problem: If the problem appears to be isolated or is a misunderstanding of a nonserious and noncontinuing nature, the incident will remain internal. A letter from the IRB office to the PI describing a summary of the audit will be written. A response from the PI describing corrective actions is also required. This will be considered the final step if the incident is considered nonserious and continuing noncompliance was not found. Suspension of patient enrollment will be lifted.

If a designation of "nonserious and noncontinuing" is applicable, a summary of the proceedings must be added to the noncompliance/complaint form. The letter *i* must be circled, dated, and initialed by the IRB administrator and IRB chair (or designee). The IRB office should feel confident in requiring any further overview of the research.

> **ii.** Serious or continuing: If the audit indicates noncompliance that is serious or continuing, the Office for Human Research Protections (OHRP) will be notified within 48 hours, regardless of the funding source. If applicable, the FDA will be notified. This will be a phone call to OHRP (or FDA) to inform the office of the incident of serious, continuing noncompliance. A letter will follow the phone call within 48 hours. The letter will briefly describe the incident, the preliminary steps taken, and an indication of the time frame for full audit and full report to follow, including corrective actions for this specific incident as well as for the research program in general at [name of institution] to ensure that similar incidents will not occur again.
>   **a.** An audit will be performed of all research conducted by the PI.
>   **b.** Communication with PI, OHRP, FDA will occur.
>   **c.** Notice to the internal committee for misconduct in science will be given.
>   **d.** Suspension of patient enrollment will be lifted once the audit process and communication process are completed to the satisfaction of the IRB.

If a designation of serious or continuing noncompliance is found to be applicable, the steps previously described must be initiated. The letters *ii* should be circled, dated, and initialed by the IRB administrator and the IRB chair or her or his designee.

Research Audit

If the IRB determines that an audit is necessary, what mechanism will the IRB use to conduct the audit? This may depend on the size of your organization. In a large institution with the responsibility of monitoring thousands of protocols, a single individual cannot accomplish this task. In a small community hospital setting, it is not unusual for the IRB administrator to be given the task of auditing the researcher and the study and reporting the findings to the IRB. Some organizations have a regulatory compliance officer whose job is to investigate issues of noncompliance. In a large institution, the IRB may appoint an audit subcommittee consisting of IRB members and nonmembers, if appropriate, to ensure fairness and expertise. An audit report may include any or all of the following:

1. Review protocol(s) in question.
2. Review FDA audit report of the investigator/study, if appropriate.

3. Review any relevant documentation, including consent documents, case report forms, subjects' investigational, and/or medical files, as they relate to the investigator's execution of his or her study involving human subjects.

4. Interview subject(s) involved in the study, if appropriate.

5. Interview appropriate study or hospital personnel, if necessary.

6. Prepare either a written or oral report of the subcommittee's findings that is presented to the full IRB at its next convened meeting.

7. Recommend actions to the full IRB, if appropriate, based on its findings.

The IRB then makes the final determination of the appropriate action(s) to be taken in the case based on its own knowledge of the facts and the additional facts gathered by the subcommittee during the course of its audit and investigation.

Reporting Audit Results

After the final determination is made by the IRB, the investigator is informed in writing. If the determination includes suspension of an investigator because the research was not conducted in accordance with the IRB's requirements or has been associated with unexpected serious harm to subjects, the IRB, under federal regulations,[1][Sec.113] has the responsibility to report that suspension promptly to the OHRP. If the study in question involves an investigational drug, biologic, or device, regulations[2][Sec.113] also require a report to the FDA.

When reporting the suspension to either the OHRP or FDA, you must include your reasons for the IRB's action. You also have the regulatory responsibility to report the IRB actions to the appropriate institutional officials. In an academic medical setting, this would include the institutional official for human subjects, the chancellor or president of the institution, the dean of the medical school, and the investigator's department chair. In a community hospital setting, it could include the chief executive officer, the president of the hospital, the hospital's medical director, and, in some institutions, the hospital's board of directors.

Continuing Review

At the time of study renewal, all reports should be provided to the primary reviewer and in summary format to the IRB members. Although at the time of initial review each report is treated as a single event, the existence of multiple reports can be important. For example, as described previously here, if a researcher submits frequent requests for exceptions to eligibility criteria, it may be cause for a discussion (e.g., perhaps the eligibility requirements should be expanded or changed). A part of the ongoing review of a project is to evaluate the number of reports and the level of seriousness of the report and respond accordingly. It may be time for a proactive visit if numerous reports are filed. This is time for respectful interaction with the research team—we want to encourage reporting but at the same time the research team needs to be aware that the study needs to adhere to approved processes.

Eligibility Exceptions

A special note related to this topic: Noncompliance, complaints, and deviations are reported to the IRB after the event occurs. Eligibility exceptions are a special category in that many IRBs now require preapproval of subjects who do not meet the eligibility criteria. Historically, IRBs were not notified of eligibility exceptions. It was primarily a discussion between the researcher and the sponsor of the study. This practice has undergone increased scrutiny based on the tragic death of Jesse Gelsinger. If a researcher wishes to enroll an individual who does not meet the eligibility criteria, an eligibility exception request is completed which includes the protocol title, investigator's name, the reason for eligibility deviation request, and, if applicable, whether the eligibility exception has been approved by the sponsor. The only exception to this policy is when the eligibility exception is necessary to eliminate apparent immediate hazards to the subject. Electronic communication allows for a relatively timely review of the eligibility exemption request by the IRB chair or appropriate medical designee. Notice of IRB concurrence is returned to the investigator via e-mail as well.

Issues remain with eligibility exemptions related to the restrictions of the inclusion criteria. If the inclusion criteria are based on sound medical information, is it indeed appropriate to enroll a patient not meeting these requirements? Is it safe for the subject? How is the data analysis affected? These are questions that must be at the forefront of discussions between the IRB and researcher when the request is submitted, especially if several eligibility requests are submitted for the same study.

If an eligibility deviation has occurred without prior IRB approval, the deviation must be reported to the IRB as noncompliance. The IRB cannot retrospectively approve the eligibility exception request and, therefore, must review the exception as a protocol deviation, following the same steps outlined in this chapter.

Conclusion

Reports of noncompliance, complaints, deviations, and eligibility exceptions arrive into the IRB office at a steady rate. With a written policy in place, the steps to take once a report is received will enable the review to occur with a consistent approach. Treat each report in a prompt, professional, and fair manner. Doing so will promote an environment where subjects feel comfortable voicing their concerns and researchers feel comfortable bringing problems to the IRB.

References

1. Code of Federal Regulations. Title 45A—Department of Health and Human Services; Part 46—Protection of Human Subjects. Updated 1 October, 1997. Access date 18 April, 2001. http://www4.law.cornell.edu/cfr/45p46.htm

2. Code of Federal Regulations. Title 21, Chapter 1—Food and Drug Administration, DHHS; Part 56—Institutional Review Boards. Updated 1 April, 1999. Access date 27 March, 2001. http://www4.law.cornell.edu/cfr/21p56.htm

Institutional Review Board Closure of Study Files

Sandra P. Kaltman and John M. Isidor

INTRODUCTION

What guidance do the regulatory agencies provide regarding when an institutional review board (IRB) may close a study file and consider its oversight responsibilities completed? The answer is not entirely clear.

Applicable Food and Drug Administration and Office for Human Research Protection Regulations and Guidance

The Food and Drug Administration (FDA) regulations are silent regarding an IRB's responsibility to close study files. The Investigational Device Exemption regulations require an investigator to submit a final report to the IRB within 3 months after termination or completion of a study or of the investigator's part of a study.[1] These regulations do not define what constitutes study closure. Unlike the Investigational Device Exemption regulations, the FDA Investigational New Drug Application regulations do not require investigators to submit final reports to IRBs.[2]

The 1998 FDA Information Sheets mention that clinical investigators are required to report to the IRB when a study has been completed, citing 21 CFR 56.108(a)(3). That regulation requires prompt reporting to the IRB of changes in a research activity. The FDA notes that a final report/notice to the IRB allows it to close its files and also provides information that may be used by the IRB in the evaluation and approval of other studies.[3]

Office for Human Research Protections (OHRP) regulations do not directly address when an IRB may or should close a study file. However, in their Guidance on Continuing Review, OHRP lists conditions under which IRB files should remain open.[4] Expedited review category 8 provides for expedited continuing review where the research is permanently closed to the enrollment of subjects, where all subjects have completed all research-related interventions, and where the research remains active only for long-term follow-up of subjects, *or* where no subjects have been enrolled and no additional risks have been identified, *or* where the remaining research activities are limited to data analysis.[*] After considering this guidance on when continuing review can be done by expedited review, one can infer that an IRB should keep its files open until those conditions no longer exist.

Category 8 includes data analysis as requiring continuing review because as long as identifiable data are being analyzed, continuing IRB oversight is necessary to ensure that the appropriate confidentiality is being maintained. After the data analysis is complete, and the data will not be used for additional research purposes, the study can be closed. Continuing review is required because of confidentiality concerns for identifiable data, therefore may also be closed if the data are de-identified.

If, after the study is closed, identifiable data are to be retained which may be used for additional research studies beyond the original intent, then the data set is considered a data repository and should be under the oversight of the IRB and receive continuing review. The OHRP has guidance on IRB oversight over data repositories.[5,6]

Informal Survey of IRB Practices Regarding Study Closure

An informal survey revealed no uniformity in IRB practices. Some IRBs have a formal standard operating procedure (SOP); others do not. Most IRBs perform study closure as an administrative procedure, but at least one requires board authorization. Some IRBs have the investigator fill out a final review form; others require only a simple e-mail notification to the IRB. Some IRBs send a closure letter or other type of notification to the investigator; others do not. Some IRBs provide formal notification to IRB members regarding closure; others do not. The most significant difference in

---

[*]An example of a study that would fit under category 8 for expedited continuing review is an oncology study in which all research activities have concluded with the exception of the collection of survival data on all enrolled subjects.

practice among IRBs is the identification of the point after which the IRB no longer has oversight responsibility for a study. Some IRBs end their oversight when all study-related subject activities are concluded. Others require notification from the investigator that all analyses by the investigator of identifiable subject data have concluded.

A number of institutions include items within their renewal/termination form to assist in the identification of whether or not IRB review should continue. After considering regulatory requirements and guidance, below is a section from the continuing review form used at Dartmouth (www.dartmouth.edu/~cphs/tosubmit/forms/), which was developed to assist in the determination of study closure:

____ Enrollment is closed. Data collection is complete. Attach any summary reports or closure notifications, and consent form if there was any enrollment in the last year. Complete items #5 through #9. Check as applicable and respond as appropriate to the following:

____ Data is deidentified per HIPAA (see list). There is no identifiable protected health information being maintained or analyzed. Describe below and IRB review of this study will be terminated.

____ Data is being maintained and such that identifiers are separated from protected health information via the use of a coding system AND there is no additional research beyond the original intent planned for this data. Describe below and IRB review of the study may be terminated.

____ Data is being maintained and/or analyzed such that identifiers are not separated from protected health information and/or there is a plan for continued or future research other than the original intent using the data obtained from this project. Describe below and IRB will continue review of the study/data per expedited category 8(c).

Describe the current status of data maintenance as checked above:

Note: Once terminated from IRB review, it is the continued responsibility of the research team to maintain the confidentiality of the data. Please contact the IRB Office if stored data is accessed for research purposes other than the original intent.

Recommendations

It would be helpful to develop best practices in accordance with federal regulations and guidance so that IRBs can maintain a consistent process to handle study closures.

IRBs may consider the following items:

1. Develop a formal or administrative policy and procedure regarding what constitutes study closure by the IRB.

2. Describe in such a policy:
   a. The type of guidance that is provided to the investigator regarding what constitutes study closure.
   b. The type of notification that is required from the investigator, including consideration of whether the investigator should formally attest to the fact that all research-related activities are concluded.
   c. Whether it is a formal board action or an administrative procedure to close a study.
   d. Circumstances that could require a study to be reopened.**
   e. Procedures that will be used if an IRB study file needs to be reopened.
   f. Considerations that arise when a study is closed because of investigator noncompliance.
   g. The type of notification that will be provided to the investigator regarding IRB closure of its study file.
   h. Whether it is necessary to inform members of the IRB regarding IRB closure of a study file.

Conclusion

Until IRBs develop best practices there will continue to be widespread inconsistencies in the formula for study closure. Under these circumstances, it is prudent for each IRB to develop clearly defined internal policies and procedures based on federal regulations and guidance and to follow them consistently. This chapter has provided suggestions for a best practice process for study closure, further discussions are needed.

References

1. Code of Federal Regulations. Title 21—Food and Drug Administration, DHHS; Part 812—Investigational Device Exemptions, Section 150(a)(6).

2. Code of Federal Regulations. Title 21, Chapter 1—Food and Drug Administration, DHHS; Part 312—Investigational New Drug Application. Updated 1 April, 1999.

3. 1998 FDA Information Sheets, Response to Question 19; http://www.fda.gov/oc/ohrt/irbs/faqs.html. Updated 17 April, 2001.

4. Office for Human Research Protections. Department of Health and Human Services. Guidance on Continuing Review. http://www.hhs.gov/ohrp/humansubjects/guidance/contrev2002.htm. Updated 11 July, 2002.

5. Office for Protection from Research Risks. Issues to Consider in the Research Use of Stored Data or Tissues. November 7, 1997. http://www.dhhs.gov/ohrp/humansubjects/guidance/reposit.htm. Updated 7 November, 1997.

6. Office for Human Research Protections. Department of Health and Human Services. Guidance on Research Involving Coded Private Information or Biological Specimens. http://www.dhhs.gov/ohrp/humansubjects/guidance/cdebiol.pdf. Updated 10 August, 2004.

**Such a circumstance would exist if the sponsor and/or investigator seek to collect additional identifiable information from subjects.

PART 8

Administrative and Regulatory Issues

Health Insurance Portability and Accountability Act and Research

Lawrence H. Muhlbaier

INTRODUCTION

The Health Insurance Portability and Accountability Act (HIPAA), originally known as the Kassebaum-Kennedy Act of 1996, had two main goals: to make health insurance *portable* and to increase accountability in Medicare billing. Health insurance portability enables employees who change jobs to obtain health insurance at a new job without being penalized for pre-existing conditions. Accountability efforts sought to address fraud and waste in Medicare billing.

Another section of HIPAA, concerning *administrative simplification*, mandated standards for the secure storage and transmission of health care information in electronic form. In support of these mandated standards, the Department of Health and Human Services (DHHS) wrote two new regulations: the Standards for Privacy of Individually Identifiable Health Information (the Privacy Rule) and the Security Standards for the Protection of Electronic Protected Health Information (the Security Rule). These rules, which were both specific (to be a covered entity [CE], a health care provider, payor, or clearinghouse must conduct certain types of electronic billing) and broad (all individually identifiable health information, regardless of how communicated), yielded regulation 45 CFR 160–164. Although many think that 45 CFR 160–164 is too stringent, large amounts of health information are still unprotected (e.g., health information held by many researchers, research sponsors, tumor registries, cash-only health care providers). The Privacy and Security Rules have the same intent as protections of confidentiality provided under the Common Rule, but they are much more specific. The Privacy Rule became effective in April 2003 and the Security Rule in April 2005. Although the Privacy Rule has received more attention, both regulations have led to significant changes in the environment of health care research.

According to a strict reading of the HIPAA Privacy Rule and Security Rule (45 CFR Parts 160–164), there is very little that an institutional review board (IRB) or privacy board must do to be in compliance. The primary requirements are to address waivers or alterations of authorization and review combined consent and authorization forms, particularly for central or independent IRBs. For institution-based IRBs, however, it is a much different story—anything at the institution that relates to both HIPAA and research is assigned to the IRB. This situation is complicated by the DHHS guidelines on HIPAA and research, which seem to restructure things we thought we knew about the Common Rule. This chapter addresses the broader needs.

In this chapter, we cover the elements of an authorization in the context of the Common Rule. That is followed by a discussion of other areas that do not require individual authorization and other areas of HIPAA that affect research. Relative to the Common Rule, HIPAA is a young piece of legislation, and thus, we might see some changes over the next few years. We conclude with a list of areas in which we might see change in the future.

Definition of Protected Health Information

Protected health information (PHI) is, simply, individually identifiable health information held by a CE. By now, entities should know whether or not they are CEs. However, look at the details: Mentioned are past, present, and future information about health, health care, and payment for health care, but there is not a word about *patients*. The Privacy Rule uses the term *individual*, which means that the rule applies to information about nonpatients as well. Similarly, *identifiable* has taken on a much broader scope than it does under the Common Rule, largely because of the power and availability of computers and nonmedical databases that could be linked to the PHI. For more about identifiability, see the section "De-identified Data" later here.

Authorization

Authorization is written permission from an individual allowing a CE to use or disclose specified PHI for a particular purpose. The technical requirements for authorizations have been well documented.[1,2] Many of the requirements are similar to or are a restatement of requirements under the Common Rule.

Several areas, discussed later here, have received significant discussion and may be misinterpreted by investigators.

To Whom the PHI Will Be Disclosed
The *reasonableness* standard is applied throughout the Privacy Rule. How specific is *reasonable*? Certainly the sponsor of the research must be listed. However, what about the other organizations that contract with them—clinical research organizations (CROs), monitors, and central laboratories (except Clinical Laboratory Improvements Amendments of 1988 labs, as they are specifically exempt because they have their own privacy regulations). It is not uncommon for studies to change monitoring organizations. If CROs change, then a study is in serious trouble, but does that change what is reasonable to tell the subject? Each IRB will have to decide the level of specificity they require. The sponsor, the CRO, and their contractors may be considered a reasonable statement. In addition, listing Office for Human Research Protections (OHRP), National Institutes of Health (NIH), or the Food and Drug Administration (FDA), as appropriate, could be included as disclosure in the standard language of an authorization. Although they can all review the records without authorization, listing these groups will preclude the need for disclosure tracking and serve to more fully inform the subjects.

Redisclosures Not Protected
This statement is required, even if the PHI is not expected to leave the institution. If the possible disclosure to OHRP is listed, then this statement makes more sense to the subject.

Combined Versus Separate Authorizations
The Privacy Rule allows an authorization for research to be combined with another authorization and/or with a consent for research. The choice of combined versus separate is an institutional decision and not something with which a research sponsor should be involved. An informal survey of academic medical centers showed that approximately 50% chose to keep the authorization and consent separate, and about 50% combined them. The argument for separation is that it makes both documents simpler and the authorizations do not require review by the IRB. The argument for combining is that there is significant overlap in content, and thus, combining reduces potential inconsistencies and avoids the situation of having one signed but not the other.

Tissue Repositories and Combined Authorizations
Guidance from the NIH states that separate authorizations are required if the research-related treatment is dependent on one authorization and not on the other.[3] This means that the approach used under the Common Rule to provide an initial line to store tissue for future unspecified research cannot be used under the Privacy Rule—one authorization must be provided for the well-defined study and another for the future research activities.

Designated Record Set
The part of medical records that must be disclosed to the individual is called a *designated record set* (DSR). An authorization can state that certain parts of the DSR may not be available to the individual. In such a case, it must also state when that information becomes available to the individual. In general terms, a DSR is the subset of medical information used to make decisions about or to inform the care of the individual. Research information that is specifically for the research (e.g., special lab tests for a study) is not typically part of the DSR, as it is often not available to the caregivers. The CE needs to disclose only one copy of the DSR to the individual, and clinical research information is a copy of information in the DSR. Generally, the only piece of study information that is part of the DSR is the randomized treatment in a blinded study, as that describes care that the individual received.

A secondary effect of this part of the Privacy Rule is that the actual treatment received must be returned to the CE for inclusion in the medical record. In the past, many research sponsors resisted returning the treatment received in a blinded study to the investigator (CE); they are now obligated to send it to the CE. Because most research sponsors are not subject to the Privacy Rule directly, it would be wise to state in the site contract that the sponsor is obligated to return the code to the CE.

Waiver of or Alteration to Authorization

The criterion for waiver or alteration of authorization is essentially a subset of that for the waiver of consent under the Common Rule. It refers to minimal risk to the privacy rather than minimal risk of all aspects of the study. The HIPAA waiver policy has some more explicit statements about the protections of the PHI, but they follow the Common Rule's intent to minimize risk.

Research that would have a waiver of documentation of consent under the Common Rule can be addressed under HIPAA as an alteration to the authorization. For example, if the only link of a subject to the study is their signature on a consent form, then it can be considered impracticable to the study's completion to obtain a signed authorization as such a requirement might prevent study completion.

Notice of Review Preparatory to Research

The notice of review preparatory to research (RPR) is a new construct under the Privacy Rule. RPR includes activities such as counting the number of patients who might have met study criteria in the past to help size a study or using PHI to describe a population for a grant proposal. In addition, RPR can be used to identify individuals who might be potential research subjects. The use or disclosure of PHI under the notice of RPR has several requirements:

- The use or disclosure is sought solely to review PHI as necessary to prepare the research protocol or other similar preparatory purposes.
- No PHI will be removed from the CE during the review.
- The PHI that the researcher seeks to use or access is necessary for the research purposes.

The PHI may be a disclosure even if the PHI cannot leave the CE. For instance, if the person doing the RPR is a physician with admitting privileges to a hospital and is using the hospital's records to do the RPR, the hospital (CE) is disclosing the PHI to the physician researchers (if the physician is not part of the workforce of the hospital). The disclosure is subject to the disclosure accounting provisions of HIPAA even if the disclosure would not be accounted for if that same physician were treating the patient.

The notice of RPR is a notice to the CE; approval is not required. According to the Privacy Rule, even verbal notice is acceptable, but it has to have the required statements listed previously here. However, the DHHS can audit the CE for compliance. These two statements, taken together, mean that the notice of RPR should be documented, and someone needs to verify that the required elements are included. Having a form to submit to the CE (likely represented by the institution-based IRB or the compliance office) makes it easier for both the investigator and the reviewer. At many institutions, the workforce members are aware of their responsibilities under HIPAA and are asking researchers to show they have the right to the material; thus, providing a *receipt* of the notice might be helpful. Larger research institutions should consider automating the process with, for example, a web-based form and e-mail receipt.

Similarly, as the notice of RPR is subject to the minimum necessary requirement of the Privacy Rule, having the researcher specify the data needed for the review would support the CE in an audit.

Prescreening

The activity of identifying subjects for research can be addressed in a number of ways under the Privacy Rule. However, in the context of the Common Rule, subject identification is a bit more complex. The DHHS has issued guidance stating that prescreening activities meet the Common Rule definition of human subjects research,[2] and thus, the activity must have a waiver of consent if it does not meet the exemption criteria.

In accordance with the Privacy Rule, the identification of potential subjects is accomplished with either a notice of RPR or a waiver of authorization. The waiver of authorization is easy to apply for when you are also applying for a waiver of consent. If the researcher also needs to obtain a waiver of consent, then, as the notice of RPR involves different requirements and constraints, it does not seem to gain much over a waiver of authorization.

If the prescreening activity does not involve recording any "individual private information," then it would likely be eligible for exemption under the Common Rule, and a notice of RPR is a very direct and easy way to address prescreening.

The act of contacting the individual to seek their authorization is a part of the CE's operations. Thus, if the research is not subject to the Common Rule, the researcher can identify the potential subjects with the notice of RPR and the CE can contact them to seek authorization.

Decedent Research

Much like the RPR, decedent research can be done with a notice to the CE meeting these requirements:

- Representation that the use or disclosure sought is solely for research on the PHI of decedents.
- Documentation, at the request of the CE, of the death of such individuals.
- Representation that the PHI for which use or disclosure is sought is necessary for the research purposes.

In addition, depending on the context, the CE may request that the researcher provide evidence that the individual is, in fact, dead.

Like the RPR, decedent research is also subject to the minimum necessary requirement of HIPAA, and thus, asking the researcher to specify the information needed will remind them that they can work only with information pertinent to their question. Decedent research is also subject to the disclosure-accounting provisions of the Privacy Rule (in this case, to the next of kin or the legally authorized representative).

De-identified Data

De-identified data are not subject to the Privacy Rule. The process of de-identification is part of the operations of the CE. In addition, de-identified data are not subject to either the minimum necessary criteria or to stricter state law.

Data can be de-identified in either of two ways:

1. Eighteen specific identifiers relating to the individual, the individual's household members, relatives, or employer must be removed, and the CE can have no actual knowledge that the information can be used alone or in combination with other information to identify the individual.

2. A person with appropriate knowledge of and experience in *disclosure analysis* determines that the risk of reidentification is very small and documents the methods and results of the analysis leading to that determination.

The de-identified data can have a re-identification code, but that code cannot be derived from any information about the individual. (This criterion for the reidentification code precludes the use of encrypted codes for reidentification.) The presence of a reidentification code may mean that the data are not *anonymized* in the sense of the Common Rule [.101(b)(4)].

Because the list of prohibited identifiers includes dates (any part other than year) and ZIP code beyond the third digit, de-identification has not gotten much traction in the research community. As more data become subject to the NIH grant and contract requirements to share the data derived from the study, more people will provide their data to the research community in de-identified format by precomputing all of the durations of potential interest.

Researchers can do the de-identification of PHI for their own research purposes (this is analogous to the process that might be used for declaring exemption under .101(b)(4) of the Common Rule). A person (including a researcher) who is not part of the workforce can still perform the de-identification process as a business associate of the CE.

Limited Data Set with Data Use Agreement

Researchers and others often talk about a limited data set (LDS) in terms of the identifiers that are allowed or not allowed. Another limit, arguably more important, is the data use agreement (DUA) in which the data recipient promises not to attempt to reidentify or contact the individuals. Many of the case report forms sent to research sponsors have the identifiers limited but do not have the DUA.

The LDS/DUA allows more identifiers than a de-identified data set. In particular, it allows any and all dates and additional geocoding (ZIP codes or ZIP+4 codes are allowed, but the specific street address is not allowed). This is typically all that a researcher would want. Like the de-identified data and information obtained under an authorization, the LDS/DUA does not require disclosure tracking.

Unlike the de-identified data set, the LDS/DUA is still considered PHI and is subject to the minimum necessary requirements of the Privacy Rule. To the IRB, the practical import of this difference is that the researcher should specify the information he will be using under the LDS/DUA. As a practical matter, this means that an LDS/DUA should broadly cover the domains of interest to the researcher (e.g., *laboratory values* instead of *LDL cholesterol*) and not include irrelevant domains (charge data with no cost-related question).

There are also LDS/DUAs received from non-CEs (particularly, some NIH public use files). Under recent guidance from OHRP,[4] any LDS/DUA can be declared *not human subjects* and not further subject to Common Rule oversight.

FDA Guidance

The FDA has been silent about HIPAA and research; their lone guidance was to clarify that stand-alone authorizations need not be reviewed by an IRB. The FDA has also not commented on the recruitment of research subjects.

International Conference on Harmonisation Implications

International Conference on Harmonisation (ICH) guidelines state that the IRB should review everything that is given to subjects and which is related to research. If the institution applies nonconflicting ICH guidance to all of its research, then the authorizations would need to be reviewed.

Centers for Disease Control Guidance

Most Centers for Disease Control activities are in the areas of public health, which are all allowed under the Privacy Rule [164.512(b)]. CDC guidance on the Privacy Rule includes a few statements related to research. Of interest to most of us who have lived with the OHRP interpretation of the Common Rule for many years is that the CDC defines practice (or nonresearch) if a project activity is primary practice (and, implied, secondary research), and most OHRP guidance defines a project as research if *any* portion is research.[5]

Workforce and Use Versus Disclosure

A person is considered a member of the workforce of a CE if the person's activities are under the direct control of the CE. Thus, regular employees, students, and onsite contractors would be considered part of the workforce, whereas physicians who just have admitting privileges to a hospital are not part of the workforce of that hospital. An activity performed under a waiver of authorization, notice of review preparatory to research, or notice of decedent research is considered *use* if done by a member of the workforce. A person (researcher) who is not part of the workforce can perform those same activities, but the activity is then a disclosure and subject to the disclosure accounting provisions.

Business Associate Contracts and Research

Business associate contracts (BACs) are for activities related to treatment, payment, or operations. The only research activities for which a BAC might be pertinent are obtaining authorizations and creating a limited or de-identified data set. A BAC is not indicated for a researcher to work under a waiver of authorization or other 164.512 activities in HIPAA (uses and disclosures for which an authorization or opportunity to agree or object is not required).

HIPAA Security Rule and Research

The HIPAA Security Rule, under 45 CFR 160–164, applies to systems within a CE that contain PHI. An LDS/DUA is still considered PHI and is subject to the Security Rule; similarly, the other research activities done without individual authorization are subject to the Security Rule to the extent they are done within a CE. It is arguable that PHI obtained with an individual authorization is subject to the Security Rule while still in the possession of a CE. The Security Rule under HIPAA is much more specific about what must be done than the general statements of security seen under the Common Rule. Researchers and IRBs at CEs need to be aware of this requirement, as it may call for a major change in some research operations.

Future Changes to the Privacy Rule

The Privacy Rule can be changed by DHHS once a year. At present, the Secretary's Advisory Committee on Human Research Protections is considering several recommendations, listed here, to send to the Secretary of DHHS as potential changes to the Privacy Rule.

- Remove the disclosure accounting requirement for research.
- "Safe harbor" de-identification should remove ZIP code, geographic subdivisions, and dates from the list of prohibited identifiers.
- Subject recruitment simplification in the RPR: Remove the requirement to have PHI stay at the CE.
- Future use: Have an informed consent conform to the Common Rule satisfy the authorization requirements rather than requiring a separate authorization.
- Exempt research: Research determined to be exempt under the Common Rule should be made exempt under the Privacy Rule.
- The transition provisions of the Privacy Rule should exempt research previously determined to be exempt under the Common Rule.

- Public health definition: Broaden the definition to allow disclosures *enabled* by state law rather than just those *required* by state law.

Conclusion

The HIPAA has little official impact on an IRB, but many of the HIPAA requirements of the CE related to research are assigned to institution-based IRBs. This chapter attempted to highlight the areas of concern for research and research oversight, as well as offer some practical suggestions to meet these concerns. Disclosure accounting might be the biggest long-term effort, particularly for CEs in which the researcher is not part of the workforce. Other areas add to the administrative workload of the IRB and researchers but will not cause wholesale changes to the research process.

References

1. Protecting Personal Health Information in Research: Understanding the HIPAA Privacy Rule. http://privacyrule-andresearch.nih.gov/pr_02.asp, Sponsor: NIH, Accessed: 17 June, 2005.
2. Clinical Research and the HIPAA Privacy Rule. http://privacyruleandresearch.nih.gov/clin_research.asp, Sponsor: NIH, Accessed: 17 June, 2005.
3. Research Repositories, Databases, and the HIPAA Privacy Rule. http://privacyruleandresearch.nih.gov/research_repositories.asp, Sponsor: NIH, Accessed: 17 June, 2005.
4. Guidance on Research Involving Coded Private Information or Biological Specimens/ http://www.hhs.gov/ohrp/humansubjects/guidance/cdebiol.pdf, Sponsor: OHRP, Accessed: 16 June, 2005.
5. Guidance from CDC and the U.S. Department of Health and Human Services. *MMWR* 52:1–12, 2003.

Office for Human Research Protections Federalwide Assurance

Jeffrey M. Cohen

INTRODUCTION

An assurance is a type of contract that an institution or project director has with a federal agency that establishes standards for research conduct. In the past, there were many different kinds of assurances related to institutional review board (IRB) overview of research (e.g., single project assurance and multiple project assurance). In an effort to simplify the assurance system related to research, the Department of Health and Human Services (DHHS) revised the assurance program so that there is only one kind of assurance document. The purpose of this chapter is to explain the current assurance program.

Regulatory Requirements

Each institution engaged in research that is covered by this policy and that is conducted or supported by a Federal Department or Agency shall provide written assurance satisfactory to the Department or Agency head that it will comply with the requirements set forth in this policy. In lieu of requiring submission of an assurance, individual Department or Agency heads shall accept the existence of a current assurance, appropriate for the research in question, on file with the Office for Protection from Research Risks, National Institutes of Health, DHHS, and approved for Federalwide use by that office. . . . [1[Sec.103(a)]]

Departments and agencies will conduct or support research covered by this policy only if the institution has an assurance approved as provided in this section and only if the institution has certified to the Department or Agency head that the research has been reviewed and approved by an IRB provided for in the assurance, and will be subject to continuing review by the IRB. [1[Sec.103(b)]]

As these quotations from 45 CFR 46 indicate, in order for institutions to receive federal funding for research involving human subjects, the institutions must have an approved assurance of compliance on file with the Office for Human Research Protections (OHRP) (previously known as the Office for Protection from Research Risks).

What Is an Assurance of Compliance?

Basically, an assurance is written documentation of an institution's commitment to comply with the federal regulations governing human subjects research. In December 2000, the OHRP established a new format for the assurance of compliance entitled the "federalwide assurance of protection for human subjects" (FWA). The FWA replaced the previous format, which involved considerable paperwork and was labor intensive, with a simplified document in which the institution stipulates that it will comply with appropriate ethical standards and procedural standards rather than spelling them out in a written document. Another change from the previous assurance is that international institutions have more flexibility in substituting international ethical codes and standards for U.S. codes and standards.

As the title indicates, the FWA covers all federally supported or conducted research involving human subjects. However, some federal agencies or departments other than the DHHS may have additional requirements or may require additional documentation along with the FWA. Institutions conducting human subjects research supported by another federal agency or department should contact the sponsor for details on its assurance policies.

Who Must Submit an FWA?

Each legally separate entity needs its own FWA. An institution's FWA can only cover components of that institution that are legally part of its corporate structure. Institutions that are affiliated solely through professional or collaborative arrangements must provide a separate FWA.

Questions often arise concerning performance sites and collaborating institutions. The regulations require that each institution that is "engaged" in covered research must have an FWA. Therefore, the question is whether the performance site is engaged in the research. OHRP has guidance on when institutions are engaged in research on its website.[4] In general, institutions become "engaged" in human subject research whenever their employees or agents (1) intervene or interact with living individuals for federally supported research purposes or (2) obtain individually identifiable private information for federally supported research purposes.

Awardee institutions are automatically considered to be engaged in human subject research, even if all activities involving human subjects are carried out by a subcontractor or collaborator.

What Is Included in an FWA?

Statement of Ethical Principles Governing the Institution

For most domestic institutions, this will be *The Ethical Principles and Guidelines for the Protection of Human Subjects* (*The Belmont Report*) prepared by the National Commission for the Protection of Human Subjects of Biomedical and Behavioral Research in 1979. International institutions may choose to apply "Recommendations Guiding Medical Doctors in Biomedical Research Involving Human Subjects" (*The Declaration of Helsinki*), prepared by the World Medical Assembly, which was revised in October 2000. Institutions do have the option of applying other appropriate ethical standards recognized by federal departments and agencies that have adopted the Federal Policy for the Protection of Human Subjects. If they do so, they must submit that statement along with their assurance.

An Assurance of Compliance with the Terms of the Assurance

In the FWA, the institution commits to complying with the Terms of Assurance, a separate document on the OHRP website.

The Terms of the Assurance include a commitment to do the following:

1. Comply with the appropriate federal regulations for federally supported research.

   a. Domestic institutions must apply the Federal Policy for the Protection of Human Subjects (the Common Rule) and, for DHHS-supported research, 45 CFR 46 and its Subparts A, B, C and D.[1]

   b. International institutions can also apply international standards such as the Canadian Tri-Council Policy, Council for International Organizations of Medical Sciences International Ethical Guidelines, International Conference on Harmonisation,[2][Sec.E6(1–4)] the guidelines from the Indian Council of Medical Research,[3] or another equivalent international standard.

2. Have written IRB procedures.

3. Provide IRB review of nonexempt research covered by the FWA.

4. Obtain and document informed consent unless otherwise waived in accordance with the regulations.

5. Ensure that all collaborating institutions in federally supported research operate under an approved FWA.

6. Have a formal written agreement of compliance from all nonaffiliated investigators.

7. Provide IRBs operated by the institution with sufficient resources.

In the Terms of Assurance, the OHRP strongly recommends the appropriate training of the institutional signatory official, the IRB chair, and the human protections administrator, and investigators.

Research Not Funded by a Federal Agency

Although the terms of the FWA must be met for all federally sponsored research, institutions have the option of applying the federal regulations to all of its human subjects research regardless of the source of support. Although there are multiple reasons for an institution to extend its federal assurance to privately funded research, it is important to understand that this is purely an elective move. Institutions actually have two options in this regard. If they choose to apply federal regulations to research not funded by a federal agency, they can choose to apply either 45 CFR 46 and all its subparts (A, B, C, D) or the Common Rule (which does not include the subparts).

Designation of IRBs

In the FWA, the institution must designate one or more IRBs for review of the research under the assurance. All IRBs designated in an FWA must be registered with the DHHS. To register an IRB, an institution simply completes the form available on the OHRP website and submits it to OHRP. The registration process does not involve formal commitments or evaluation; the information about the IRB is simply entered into the IRB registration database.

The IRB(s) designated in the FWA need not be local IRBs. An institution may rely on another IRB, either from another institution or an independent IRB, as long as the other IRB agrees to comply with the terms of the assurance and the guidelines for satisfactory knowledge of the local research context are met (see the OHRP website for this guidance[4]). Such reliance must be documented in writing and available for review by OHRP on request. OHRP's sample IRB authorization agreement may be used for this purpose, or institutions may develop their own agreement.

Designation of a Human Protections Administrator

The human protections administrator is an employee or agent of the FWA institution who exercises day-to-day operational responsibility for the institution's program for protecting human subjects. This individual's title and position within the institutional structure will vary from institution to institution. What is important is the individual's comprehensive knowledge of all aspects of the institution's systematic protections for human subjects. Every domestic FWA institution should have a human protections administrator, even if the institution relies totally on IRBs from other organizations.

Signature of the Institutional Signatory Official

The FWA signatory must be a high institutional official who has the legal authority to represent the institution named in the FWA, as well as all the institutional components listed in the FWA. Entities that the signatory official is not legally authorized to represent may not be covered under the FWA.

Conclusion

The FWA formalizes an institution's commitment to protect human subjects. The OHRP holds institutions responsible for all research involving human subjects covered under their assurance. The FWA makes these responsibilities clear and serves as the OHRP's primary mechanism for compliance oversight. When problems arise at an institution, the OHRP determines whether the institution is complying with the commitments it made in the FWA. If it is not, the OHRP may restrict or suspend an institution's FWA, thus limiting or prohibiting human subjects research at the institution. Therefore, it is essential that institutions ensure that everyone involved in human subjects research is knowledgeable about and understands the commitments made in the FWA.

Additional information and guidance on the FWA may be found on the OHRP website.[4]

References

1. Code of Federal Regulations. Title 45A—Department of Health and Human Services; Part 46—Protection of Human Subjects. Revised November 13, 2001. Access date 21 February, 2005. http://www.dhhs.gov/ohrp/humansubjects/guidance/45cfr46.htm

2. International Conference on Harmonisation. E6 Good Clinical Practice. ICH harmonised tripartite guidelines: Guideline for a good clinical practice, 1 May, 1996. Access date 21 February, 2005. http://www.ich.org/MediaServer.jser?@_ID=482&@_MODE=GLB

3. Indian Council of Medical Research, New Delhi, Chairperson MN Venkatachaliah. Ethical Guidelines for Biomedical Research on Human Subjects, 6 September, 2000. Access date 21 February, 2005. http://www.icmr.nic.in/ethical.pdf

4. Office for Human Research Protections. Access date 21 February, 2005. http://www.dhhs.gov/ohrp/

International Conference on Harmonisation

David G. Forster and Gary L. Chadwick

INTRODUCTION

The International Conference on Harmonisation of Technical Requirements for the Registration of Pharmaceuticals for Human Use, commonly referred to as the International Conference on Harmonisation (ICH) is designed to streamline the process for developing and marketing new drugs internationally.[1] The ICH is composed of representatives from the pharmaceutical industry and the regulatory bodies of the United States, Japan, and the European Union. In addition, observers to the process include Canada, the European Free Trade Area, and the World Health Organization.

The ICH has established several international standards of good clinical practice (GCP) for the development of pharmaceutical products. The guideline that primarily affects institutional review boards (IRBs) is E6, "ICH harmonized tripartite guideline: Guideline for good clinical practice."[2] The E6 guideline has eight parts: (1) glossary, (2) principles, (3) IRBs, (4) investigator, (5) sponsor, (6) protocol and amendments, (7) investigator's brochure, and (8) essential documents. The drafting of E6, like other guidelines, took years and several rewrites. The initial foundation for drafting the E6 guidelines was the Food and Drug Administration (FDA) regulations for the protection of human subjects.[3,4]

Legal Status and Compliance

After the guidelines were finalized, several countries adopted them as law. In the United States, however, the FDA adopted the ICH only as guidance.[5] Therefore, the ICH guidelines are not regulation and do not have the force of law in the United States. In the *Federal Register* notice, the FDA stated that the ICH guideline "does not create or confer any rights for or on any person and does not operate to bind the FDA or the public. An alternative approach may be used if such approach satisfies the requirements of the applicable statutes, regulations, or both." Therefore, compliance is voluntary, but as with any published FDA guideline, compliance is considered part of GCP.

An advantage for drug manufacturers and sponsors is that the FDA and equivalent government agencies in other countries will consider studies conducted in accordance with the ICH guidelines as meeting the regulatory requirements of the drug approval processes for all of these countries. Therefore, sponsors often want to use IRBs that meet the ICH requirements. One of the requirements of the ICH guidelines is that "the sponsor obtain from the investigator/institution . . . [a] statement obtained from the IRB/IEC that it is organized and operates according to GCP and the applicable laws and regulations."[2(Sec.5.11)]

Based on this requirement, several sponsors have issued letters to IRBs asking them to state that they comply with ICH.

Some have suggested that in response to this question IRBs can answer that inasmuch as the ICH guidelines mirror the FDA regulations, then the IRB complies with ICH. There are, however, certain requirements of ICH that are not included in FDA or DHHS regulations. A sponsor could be adversely affected if a drug agency, in a country that has adopted ICH as law, refuses to accept data in an application because the IRB that oversaw the research was not fully in compliance with the ICH requirements.

Each IRB needs to review the ICH guidelines and either adopt them, not adopt them, or adopt those parts that require minimal changes and provide an increase in human subject protection.

Differences Between ICH Guidelines and U.S. Regulations

As stated previously, the ICH E6 guidelines generally agree with the FDA regulations for IRBs and informed consent. However, in a few areas, the ICH guidelines have requirements that go beyond either FDA, DHHS, or Common Rule requirements. It is important to know what these differences are because full compliance with ICH requires some changes in IRB operations. If the written procedures include—as they should—how the IRB complies with the various requirements of the ICH guidelines, they must be followed by the IRB. The FDA only inspects IRBs to the standards of the FDA regulations, not ICH; however, the FDA can cite an IRB for not following its own written procedures. References later here are either to the ICH E6 guidelines[2] or to the FDA regulations.[3,4]

Definition of Vulnerable Subjects

ICH provides the following definition of vulnerable subjects.[2(Sec.1.61)]

Vulnerable Subjects: Individuals whose willingness to volunteer in a clinical trial may be unduly influenced by the expectation, whether justified or not, of benefits associated with participation; or of a retaliatory response from senior members of a hierarchy in case of refusal to participate. Examples are members of a group with a hierarchical structure, such as medical, pharmacy, dental, and nursing students, subordinate hospital and laboratory personnel, employees of the pharmaceutical industry, members of the armed forces, and persons kept in detention. Other vulnerable subjects include patients with incurable diseases, and persons in nursing homes, unemployed or impoverished persons, patients in emergency situations, ethnic minority groups, homeless persons, nomads, refugees, minors, and those incapable of giving consent.

The FDA describes vulnerable subjects as individuals "such as children, prisoners, pregnant women, handicapped, or mentally disabled persons, or economically or educationally disadvantaged persons."[4(Sec.111(b))]

Neither the FDA nor the ICH definition provides a complete list of vulnerable subjects, and the examples of vulnerable subjects provided in each are somewhat different. Because both definitions rely on the ethical principle of respect for persons, IRBs and investigators must consider whether the potential subject's ability to exercise free choice (autonomy) is limited in some way. Special FDA and DHHS regulations exist for children. DHHS also has additional regulations for prisoners, pregnant women, and fetuses. IRBs must decide what types of special protections are required for these and other vulnerable populations, as well as whether to extend protections to those not specifically named in the regulations or the ICH guidelines.

Confidentiality of Medical Records

ICH has broader requirements than the FDA or DHHS concerning notice to subjects about potential access to identifiable research records by third parties. The informed consent should include that "the monitor(s), the auditor(s), the IRB/IEC, and the regulatory authority(ies) will be granted direct access to the subject's original medical records for verification of clinical trial procedures and/or data, without violating the confidentiality of the subject, to the extent permitted by the applicable laws and regulations and that, by signing a written informed consent form, the subject or the subject's legally acceptable representative is authorizing such access."[2(Sec.4.8.10(n))] ICH further states that "the sponsor should verify that each subject has consented, in writing, to direct access to his/her

original medical records for trial-related monitoring, audit, IRB/IEC review, and regulatory inspection."[2(Sec.5.15.2)]

FDA regulations only state that "in seeking informed consent, the following information shall be provided to each subject: (5) A statement describing the extent, if any, to which confidentiality of records identifying the subject will be maintained and that notes the possibility that the Food and Drug Administration may inspect the records."[3(Sec.25(a)(5))]

Thus, ICH allows much broader access to research records and to otherwise confidential medical records. Some IRBs have received complaints from subjects about the extent of this access. Most consent forms approved by IRBs now permit access to research records by sponsors. Access of foreign regulatory agencies to research records is generally not troubling. However, access for these entities to subjects' medical records is problematic for both IRBs and subjects. For the sake of compliance, it is easy to change the wording in a consent form from "research records" to "research and medical records," but philosophically, it is quite different.

For research conducted at covered entities, the Health Insurance Portability and Accountability Act Privacy Rule also requires that subjects be informed of parties to whom their protected health information may be disclosed (please see the chapter on Health Insurance Portability and Accountability Act for further details about the specific requirements of the Privacy Rule).

Signature by Person Conducting the Consent Discussion

The ICH guidelines[2(Sec.4.8.8)] state, "Prior to a subject's participation in the trial, the written informed consent form should be signed and personally dated by the subject or by the subject's legally acceptable representative, and by the person who conducted the informed consent discussion." The FDA regulations only require the signature of the subject and the date the subject signed the consent form.[3(Sec.27(a))]

Many IRBs already require the signature of the person obtaining consent on consent forms, especially for greater-than-minimal-risk research. This means that many IRBs already meet this ICH requirement. If not, it is easy to include a signature line labeled "Person Conducting Informed Consent Discussion." This line should not be labeled "Investigator's Signature" if the investigator is not always the person who obtains consent.

Subject Receipt of a Signed and Dated Copy of the Consent Form

The ICH guidelines[2(Sec.4.8.11)] require that the subject or the legally authorized representative receive a copy of the signed and dated written informed consent form.

FDA regulations allow subjects to receive either a signed or unsigned copy.[6(p.11)] To be in compliance with ICH guidelines, the IRB should include notice in the consent form that the subject will receive a signed and dated copy of the consent form. Persons obtaining consent must then ensure that this procedure is followed.

Assent of Children and Mentally Incapacitated Adults

The ICH guidelines[2][Sec.4.8.12] require that:

> When a clinical trial (therapeutic or nontherapeutic) includes subjects who can only be enrolled in the trial with the consent of the subject's legally acceptable representative (e.g., minors, or patients with severe dementia), the subject should be informed about the trial to the extent compatible with the subject's understanding and, if capable, the subject should sign and personally date the written informed consent.

The FDA regulations and the DHHS regulations on the inclusion of children in research[7][Subpart D] require the assent of children for clinical research.

Neither FDA nor DHHS regulations, however, specifically require that incapacitated adults assent to research participation. Many IRBs have considered this mechanism to be an additional protection, which they have required for this vulnerable population. To meet the ICH requirement, the IRB would have to institute a policy for formally considering assent whenever a protocol allows decisionally impaired adult subjects to be enrolled. This policy can easily be modeled on DHHS regulations for children,[7][Subpart D] with similar considerations and conditions.

Impartial Witness for Illiterate Subjects

The ICH guidelines[2][Sec.4.8.9] state this:

> If a subject is unable to read or if a legally acceptable representative is unable to read, an impartial witness should be present during the entire informed consent discussion. After the written informed consent form, and any other written information to be provided to subjects, is read and explained to the subject or the subject's legally acceptable representative, and after the subject or the subject's legally acceptable representative has orally consented to the subject's participation in the trial and, if capable of doing so, has signed and personally dated the informed consent form, the witness should sign and personally date the consent form. By signing the consent form, the witness attests that the information in the consent form and any other written information was accurately explained to, and apparently understood by, the subject or the subject's legally acceptable representative, and that informed consent was freely given by the subject or the subject's legally acceptable representative.

The FDA regulations permit illiterate subjects to "make their mark" on a regular consent form. FDA also allows the use of a short-form consent document with a written summary for oral presentation, but then a witness is required.[3][Sec.27(b)(2)] The ICH guideline goes beyond the FDA regulations in requiring an impartial witness and specifying to what the witness should attest.

Most IRBs define impartial as not being connected with the study team. This allows relatives, employees of the institution who are not engaged in the conduct of the research, and similar persons to fill this role. Whatever the definition, it should be included in the IRB written procedures, and investigators must know who qualifies as impartial.

After who can function as an impartial witness has been defined, the IRB must figure out how to provide for documentation of the signature. One approach that

some IRBs have taken is to provide investigators with an IRB-approved addendum that can be used with any consent form. This approach creates some logistical problems in supplying the form or having it readily available and known to the investigator. A second approach is to have an impartial witness signature block at the end of every consent form intended to comply with ICH, with clear instructions regarding the use of the signature block. A disadvantage to this approach is that an array of signature blocks may be confusing. Other IRBs have advised having the witness sign on a signature line drawn onto the consent form, but this creates a problem by allowing a change to the consent form without prior IRB approval. Investigators might get the mistaken impression that ad hoc changes to the consent form are acceptable. Also, ensuring that the wording of the attestation is correctly inserted can be a problem with this method.

This is a good place to point out that both FDA and DHHS regulations require that no change be made to the study without prior IRB approval.[4][Sec.108(a)(4)] The ICH guidelines, in contrast, allow the investigator to make some minor changes to the protocol without prior IRB approval. As stated in the ICH guidelines,[2][Sec.4.5.2]

> The investigator should not implement any deviation from, or changes of, the protocol without agreement by the sponsor and prior review and documented approval/favorable opinion from the IRB/IEC of an amendment, except where necessary to eliminate an immediate hazard(s) to trial subjects, or when the change(s) involves only logistical or administrative aspects of the trial (e.g., change of monitor[s], change of telephone number[s]).

IRBs in the United States must continue to meet FDA and DHHS requirements in this situation because they are more stringent.

Elements of Consent

A few of the ICH guideline requirements for elements of informed consent go beyond the FDA requirements and must be included by the IRB for studies that are intended to meet ICH requirements.

Alternative Treatments

The ICH guidelines[2][Sec.4.8.10(i)] require an explanation of "the alternative procedure(s) or course(s) of treatment that may be available to the subject, and their important potential benefits and risks." Most IRBs have not included the benefits and risks of alternative treatments. This is an area where many IRBs decide to limit their compliance with ICH. The IRB should consider whether the addition of these risks and benefits in consent forms will be useful to the subject or whether their inclusion will make the consent form longer, more confusing, and less effective.

Probability of Assignment to Each Study Arm in a Study

The FDA regulations[3][Sec.25(a)(1)] state that the consent form must include "a statement that the study involves research, an explanation of the purposes of the research, and the expected duration of the subject's participation, as well as a description of the procedures to be followed, and identification of any procedures which are experimental." The ICH guidelines[2][Sec.4.8.10(c)] state that, in addition, the informed consent should include "the trial treatment(s) and the probability for random assignment to each treatment." This difference can be addressed by including a description of each arm of the study in the consent form and including a statement about the likelihood of being enrolled in each of the study arms.

Compensation for Injury

The ICH guidelines[2][Sec.4.8.10(j)] require an explanation of "the compensation and/or treatment available to the subject in the event of trial-related injury" in all consent forms. The FDA only requires this information for research involving more than minimal risk.[3][Sec.25(a)(6)] In actuality, this difference is not that significant, as most drug studies are, in fact, greater than minimal risk and therefore require a compensation-for-injury clause.

Description of Subject's Responsibilities

The ICH guidelines[2][Sec.4.8.10(e)] require an explanation of "the subject's responsibilities." Often, this information is described in the section of the consent form that describes the research and the research procedures. However, some IRBs use a separate section of the consent form under the heading of "subject's responsibility" to address specifically the expectations regarding coming in for visits, maintaining diaries, and other such expectations. One of the unintended consequences of this approach is to make the consent form look more like a contract between two parties, and it may confuse subjects about their right to withdraw.

Statement of No Benefit

The ICH guidelines[2][Sec.4.8.10(h)] require an explanation of "the reasonably expected benefits. When there is no intended clinical benefit to the subject, the subject should be made aware of this." Many IRBs also customarily include this information now, and thus, compliance with this requirement should not pose any problems.

Prorated Payment in the Consent Form

The ICH guidelines[2][Sec.4.8.10(k)] state that "anticipated prorated payment, if any, to the subject for participating in the trial" must be included in the consent form. Although not an FDA regulatory requirement, prorated payment is addressed in the FDA Information Sheet entitled "Payment to research subjects,"[6] and it is common practice for IRBs in the United States to include this in consent forms.

Notification of Subject's Primary Physician

The ICH guidelines (Section 4.3.3) recommend "that the investigator inform the subject's primary physician about the subject's participation in the trial if the subject has a primary physician and if the subject agrees to the primary physician being informed." The FDA regulations and guidance do not address this issue. Some IRBs require a section in the consent form specifically addressing notification of the subject's primary physician, and providing the subject with a list of choices, such as contacting the primary physician, not contacting the primary physician, or stating that the subject does not have a primary physician.

No Direct Benefit Studies

This area is not specifically addressed in the FDA regulations. ICH states that "except as described in 4.8.14, a nontherapeutic trial (i.e., a trial in which there is no anticipated direct clinical benefit to the subject), should be conducted in subjects who personally give consent and who sign and date the written informed consent form."[2][Sec.4.8.13] Furthermore:

Non-therapeutic trials may be conducted in subjects with consent of a legally acceptable representative provided the following conditions are fulfilled:

(a) The objectives of the trial cannot be met by means of a trial in subjects who can give informed consent personally.

(b) The foreseeable risks to the subjects are low.

(c) The negative impact on the subject's well-being is minimized and low.

(d) The trial is not prohibited by law.

(e) The approval/favorable opinion of the IRB/IEC is expressly sought on the inclusion of such subjects, and the written approval/favorable opinion covers this aspect.

Such trials, unless an exception is justified, should be conducted in patients having a disease or condition for which the investigational product is intended. Subjects in these trials should be particularly closely monitored and should be withdrawn if they appear to be unduly distressed.[2][Sec.4.8.14]

The ICH requirements for inclusion of subjects in trials with no direct benefit are straightforward. To comply with ICH requirements, IRBs should ensure that subjects without the capacity to consent are not enrolled in nontherapeutic trials, except as described previously here.

IRB Responsibilities

Several differences exist between the FDA and ICH regarding the responsibilities and duties of the IRB.

Documents the IRB Must Review

The ICH provides a list of documents that the IRB should review.

The IRB/IEC should obtain the following documents: trial protocol(s)/amendment(s), written informed consent form(s) and consent form updates that the investigator proposes for use in the trial, subject recruitment procedures (e.g., advertisements), and written information to be provided to subjects, investigator's brochure (IB), available safety information, information about payments and compensation available to subjects, the investigator's current curriculum vitae and/or other documentation evidencing qualifications, as well as any other documents that the IRB/IEC may require to fulfill its responsibilities.[2][Sec.3.1.2]

Compliance with ICH requires reviewing all of the listed materials.

The FDA regulations do not specifically list in one place what documents an IRB should review. The FDA requires the IRB to review the consent form[4][Sec.109(b)] and "copies of all research proposals reviewed, scientific evaluations, if any, that accompany the proposals, and approved sample consent documents."[4][Sec.115(a)]

Review of Changes in Research

The ICH guidelines[2][Sec.3.3.7] state, "The IRB/IEC should [specify] that no deviations from, or changes of, the protocol should be initiated without prior written IRB/IEC approval"[2][Sec.4.5.3] and "Investigators . . . should document and explain any deviations from the approved protocol." Review of changes in research is required by the FDA regulations,[4][Sec.108(a)(4)] but this regulation historically was interpreted to apply only to changes in the research that affected all of the subjects, such as a change to the written protocol. Now, as a result of the ICH requirement, many sponsors and investigators are submitting protocol deviations and violations that occur in the course of the trial, such as missed study visits. The vast majority of these reports do not affect subject safety. In an effort to limit the IRB resources necessary to review all protocol variances that occur on a trial, IRBs may wish to establish a policy limiting the submission of protocol deviations and violations that have already occurred to those that have the potential to affect subject safety. The disadvantage of this approach is that it leaves the determination of the potential harm to subjects with the investigator alone.

Availability of Written Procedures and Rosters

The ICH guidelines[2][Sec.3.4] state, "The IRB/IEC may be asked by investigators, sponsors, or regulatory authorities to provide copies of its written procedures and membership lists." FDA regulations do not contain a similar disclosure provision. Many IRBs consider their membership roster as private information and are concerned that disclosure to sponsors may encourage attempts at inappropriate influence. Some IRBs have addressed this concern by disclosing the roster with the names deleted.

IRB Appeals Process

Although FDA regulations do not require an appeals process, the ICH does[2][Sec.3.3.9] by stating that "the IRB/IEC [will have] procedures for appeal of its decisions/opinions." A written appeals process is a good practice as long as it does not violate the FDA regulation that prohibits any other body or individual from approving a study that the IRB has disapproved.[4][Sec.112]

Conclusion

In the United States, compliance with the ICH E6 guidelines is voluntary for IRBs in that it is not a federal regulation. However, pharmaceutical sponsors often insist that the ICH requirements be met. IRBs have to assess their level of compliance and decide whether the changes in operations can be made without compromising subject protections or institutional values.

Investigators and institutions also must review the applicable sections of the ICH guidelines for duties and responsibilities required to be compliant. IRBs and institutions also need to define the applicability for their policies intended to address ICH requirements (i.e., if they apply only to clinical trials of drugs, to all studies, or some subset of studies).

References

1. International Conference on Harmonisation. A brief history of ICH. Updated July 1997. Access date 23 August, 2001.
   http://www.pharmweb.net/pwmirror/pw9/ifpma/ich8.html

2. International Conference on Harmonisation. ICH harmonised tripartite guidelines: E6 Guideline for good clinical practice, 1 May, 1996. Access date 23 August, 2001.
   http://www.ifpma.org/pdfifpma/e6.pdf

3. Code of Federal Regulations. Title 21, Chapter 1—Food and Drug Administration, DHHS; Part 50—Protection of Human Subjects. Updated 1 April, 1999. Access date 18 April, 2001. http://www4.law.cornell.edu/cfr/21p50.htm

4. Code of Federal Regulations. Title 21, Chapter 1—Food and Drug Administration, DHHS; Part 56—Institutional Review Boards. Updated 1 April, 1999. Access date 27 March, 2001. http://www4.law.cornell.edu/cfr/21p56.htm

5. Food and Drug Administration, DHHS. Good clinical practice: Consolidated guideline. *Fed Regist* 62(90):25691–25709, 1997.
   http://frwebgate.access.gpo.gov/cgi-bin/getdoc.cgi?db-name51997_register&docid5fr09my97-190

6. Food and Drug Administration. Information sheets: Guidance for institutional review boards and clinical investigators, September 1998. Access date 9 April, 2001. http://www.fda.gov/oc/oha/IRB/toc.html

7. Code of Federal Regulations. Title 45A—Department of Health and Human Services; Part 46—Protection of Human Subjects. Updated 1 October, 1997. Access date 18 April, 2001. http://www4.law.cornell.edu/cfr/45p46.htm

The Role of the Institutional Biosafety Committee: Human Gene Transfer Research

Michael B. Blayney

INTRODUCTION

Since 1976, the National Institutes of Health (NIH) has placed the authority, responsibility, and accountability for the safe conduct of recombinant DNA (rDNA) research on each host or sponsoring institution through its *Guidelines for Research Involving Recombinant DNA Molecules*. From the beginning, Institutional Biosafety Committees (IBCs) have been responsible for the review of rDNA research in compliance with the NIH Guidelines and the evaluation of potential risks to public health and the environment. Today, somatic gene transfer methods using rDNA (or DNA/RNA derived from rDNA) are being tested for their value as possible treatments for such maladies as cancer, cardiovascular disease, and diabetes.[1] Appendix M of the NIH Guidelines details the role that the NIH Recombinant DNA Advisory Committee (the RAC) and the local IBC play in approving and monitoring human gene transfer experiments. Please note the NIH Guidelines apply to research being conducted at or sponsored by institutions receiving NIH funds for recombinant DNA research, even if the particular gene therapy study is not NIH funded. The NIH Office of Biotechnology Activities website provides thorough information on this topic.[2,3]

Role of the IBC

Both the IBC and institutional review board (IRB) must ensure compliance with the requirements of applicable federal regulations. A significant lapse or oversight at any point within the research "compliance matrix" can have serious, lasting consequences. With human gene transfer studies, adequate institutional oversight is a significant internal challenge. These studies are complex and require: (1) proper staffing, (2) thoughtful organization, (3) timely exchange of information between IBC, IRB, and study sponsor, and (4) follow-up/recordkeeping.

Appendix M of the NIH Guidelines outlines the IBC's role in human gene transfer research. From a practical perspective, the adequate review and approval of a human gene transfer experiment requires a great deal of information. Many IBCs have important oversight relationships with other committees such as the IRB or Institutional Animal Care and Use Committee (IACUC). A comprehensive compliance review is critical in human gene transfer experiments since these studies inevitably involve several experts (some specially appointed), the timely exchange of information among committees, administrative oversight

by a qualified biological safety officer (BSO), and detailed recordkeeping. Adequate oversight and recordkeeping in human gene transfer experiments requires substantial time, resources, and personnel. As experience has proven, IBC, IRB, and IACUC responsibilities overlap—strengthening these ties ensures a more effective oversight process.

Recommended Information for the Review of Human Gene Transfer Experiments

1. Research protocol from the study sponsor
2. Investigator's brochure from the study sponsor
3. NIH correspondence: RAC review and supporting letters
4. FDA correspondence: Investigational new drug (IND) approval
5. A detailed standard operating procedure specific to the study

As mentioned in item 5, the development of a standard operating procedure (SOP) by the principal investigator (PI) of the study is critical. An adequate SOP details the receipt, storage, handling, preparation, and administration of the experimental agent. An adequate SOP also outlines the necessary contingencies for spills and exposure consultation. A well-written SOP includes the names, locations, and facilities involved—specific in all respects. Using information provided by the study sponsor, a detailed SOP makes the study "operational" and serves as a useful reference and training guide (as needed) for medical, nursing, housekeeping, and engineering staff. And finally, the BSO plays a critical role in the review and approval process and an even more critical role in study tracking, audit, and reporting to the IBC. The BSO represents the interests of the institution, oversees adherence to the NIH Guidelines, and is ultimately the final oversight authority. Most BSOs are members of the institution's environmental health and safety program.

Although the prescribed role of the IBC has remained constant, the implementation of the role of the IBC today is different than it was 30 years ago and promises to be different tomorrow. A thorough review of the websites[2,3] will help to ensure the local institutional system is appropriate and adequate.

References:

1. Lazo PA, Yunta M. Gene therapy using viral vectors: Strategy and design issues. In: *Viral Vectors: Basic Science and Gene Therapy*, Cid-Arregui A, Garcia-Carranca A (eds.) Natick, MA: Eaton Publishing/Bio Techniques Books. 2000.

2. National Institutes of Health. Office of Biotechnology Activities. Frequently Asked Questions about the NIH Review Process of Human Gene Transfer Trials. Available from: http://www4.od.nih.gov/oba/Rdna.htm and: http://www4.od.nih.gov/oba/RAC/RAC_FAQs.htm. Accessed 26 July, 2005.

3. National Institutes of Health. Office of Biotechnology Activities. "Frequently Asked Questions of Interest to IBCs." Available from: http://www4.od.nih.gov/oba/IBC/IBCrole.htm. Accessed 26 July, 2005.

Understanding the Food and Drug Administration's Investigational New Drug Process

Dale E. Hammerschmidt

INTRODUCTION

In 1962, the United States narrowly avoided a public health disaster when it failed to license a new drug, thalidomide, which had been on the market for several years in Europe, Britain, and Canada. By all reports, it was a wonderful sedative, with strong antinausea properties and almost no respiratory depression. It was finding wide use in treating "morning sickness" and pregnancy-related sleep disturbance, and its clearance in the United States would have been all but automatic. A Food and Drug Administration (FDA) official (herself ironically a Canadian) was unsatisfied that all was yet in order and delayed approval; in the time that followed, reports appeared of serious birth defects, most striking among them phocomelia ("flipper limbs"). The drug was not licensed in the United States; its marketing approval in other countries was withdrawn, and we now know it to be an inhibitor of the formation of new blood vessels. This near miss called attention to the lack of stringent protections against the potential dangers of new drugs, and the Food, Drug, and Cosmetic Act was amended to require evidence of efficacy and safety—as well as systematic reporting of adverse events and the informed consent of persons in studies of new drugs—before marketing approval could be granted. There have been numerous refinements to the process in the last 4 decades, and the current requirements are codified at 21 CFR 50,[1] 21 CFR 56,[2] and 21 CFR 312.[3]

The fundamental ideas underlying this process are straightforward, even if the details might sometimes be complex or confusing. In order that drugs being introduced to market are indeed acceptably safe and effective for their claimed indications, their evaluation must be carried out according to generally accepted principles of ethical propriety and scientific rigor; the evaluation must be overseen and subject to the scrutiny of the licensing agency, and on successful licensure, the advertising claims made for the drug must be limited to those that have actually been supported by data. The regulatory process for achieving these goals is a permitting system in which a sponsor planning to study a drug receives permission to do so after filing an investigational new drug application with the FDA; the application, the process, and the resulting permit are often known by the acronym IND. The permission granted is limited to the specific drug, the specific uses (indications) for which licensure is to be sought, and the specific evaluative study to be performed.

What Requires an IND?

The simplest example is that for which the process is named. An IND application must be filed when a sponsor wishes to test a newly developed drug to see whether its safety and efficacy are such that it can be approved for marketing. Remember, however, that the permission granted a successful IND applicant is very specific, as is the licensing approval that results. Thus, an IND is also required for studies of drugs that are already licensed if the intent of the study is to generate data that will lead to approval of a new advertising claim, a new clinical indication, or a new formulation of the product. Similarly, an IND (or an amendment to an existing IND) is required to add a new study design, a new patient group, or a new clinical indication to the evaluation of a product that is under study but not yet marketed.[3(Sec.2(a))]

What Does Not Require an IND?

If a drug is already licensed and approved by the FDA for marketing in the United States, it may be studied without an IND. However, there are conditions that must be met for this exemption to apply, some of which were previously implied.[3(Sec.(2b))] The study must not be one that is designed to change the approved indications, advertising claims, or labeling of the product. The study must not be one that changes dose, route of administration, or target population in a way that is likely to increase risk. The study is still subject to all of the usual requirements for institutional review board (IRB) oversight, and the study must not violate any of the FDA's rules about advertising and promotion of drugs.[3(Sec.7)] A simple example of an allowable study would be a postmarketing evaluation of a licensed drug to test whether its efficacy in ordinary clinical use is similar to that which had been found in carefully selected subject groups in Phase III trials.

Drug studies being done in animals do not ordinarily require an IND; however, if the results are to be used in support of the design of subsequent studies in humans, their quality and verifiability are important, and it is wise to follow the applicable FDA guidances.

Areas Where It Is Not Always Clear

Particular difficulty may be encountered when a drug is to be used on a single-patient basis, and there is no intent to develop the drug commercially. The wording of the context-setting regulation provides that the IND rules apply "to all clinical investigations of products that are subject to section 505 or 507 of the Federal Food, Drug, and Cosmetic Act or to the licensing provisions of the Public Health Service Act."[3(Sec.2),4(Sec.201etseq.)] Single-patient use will usually not satisfy the regulatory definition of "research"[5(Sec.102(d))] or of "clinical investigation,"[1(Sec.3(c))] and thus, it would appear to fail the applicability criterion. However, the specific definition of "clinical investigation" within the IND regulations is broader, including "any experiment in which a drug is administered or dispensed to, or used involving, one or more human subjects. For the purposes of this part, an experiment is any use of a drug except for the use of a marketed drug in the course of medical practice."[3(Sec.3(b))] A use of a nonmarketed drug in the course of medical practice would satisfy this definition of "experiment" and of "clinical investigation."

That creates several tensions, for which the resolution may be difficult or even contentious. Once such single-patient use expands to multiple patients, the likelihood of organized data gathering and contribution to generalizable knowledge increases. Thus, the activity creeps through a gray zone in the direction of research. Opinions (investigator, manufacturer, IRB, federal regulators) are likely to differ as to just when the line has been crossed. Moreover, there has been disagreement about the need for an IND for a use that is clearly research but does not have product licensure as a goal. Because the exemptions[3(Sec.2(b)(1))] specifically refer to a drug that is "lawfully marketed in the United States," they cannot be invoked for an unlicensed product. On the other hand, it is not clear that a drug not intended for marketing is subject to section 505 or 507 of the Food, Drug, and Cosmetic Act.

An additional tension relates to quality control. When a formal study is carried out under an IND, certain assurances are given, and there is a mechanism for the central reporting of adverse events. When an unlicensed agent is used on a single-patient basis and no IND application is filed, there is no mechanism for centralized adverse event reporting, and quality control may not be assured. IRBs have occasionally asked that investigators file IND applications specifically to bring an activity under federal scrutiny. This is an imperfect response, as the FDA may simply opine that an IND is not necessary, or an IND may be granted without careful examination of the quality controls that are in place.

In institutions in which such issues arise with any frequency, it is wise to establish institutional policies and procedures for dealing with them. For example, many academic centers now have research drug pharmacists and good laboratory practices facilities that can help a physician–investigator assure that the product being prepared meets the conventional standards for purity, stability, nonpyrogenicity, etc. Central data and safety monitoring may also be imposed for a center, even if it is not provided for on a national basis.

In circumstances in which it has been impossible to reach a confident decision as to the need for an IND, the FDA may be consulted directly.[3(Sec.2(e))]

"Off-Label" Use of Drugs

It is important to recognize that the approved labeling indications for a drug are marketing constructs as well as scientific ones. That is, a drug manufacturer must ask, "Is the market potential for this indication sufficient to justify the studies that would be necessary to obtain the corresponding approval?" From a business perspective, this decision must consider the size of the potential market, the quality of other competing drugs in that market, the advantages of the new product in that context, the likely profit per unit sold, the length of patent protection remaining to the new product, and the time and expense required to gain marketing approval for the proposed indication.

Often, even if the drug is a very good one for the indication under discussion, the answer will be, "No. We'll never recover our R&D costs before the patent runs out." In a more general sense, this type of consideration encourages a manufacturer to seek first the marketing approval that best combines ease of study and initial yield, and then to be very selective in seeking additional approvals. Even if a drug is the best possible therapy for a rare disorder, the profit potential may not be sufficient to make the manufacturer seek specific labeling approval for that use.

Often, it rapidly becomes clear that a drug has valuable uses beyond its approved indications. A treating physician may administer a drug for an indication other than the approved ones ("off-label" use) without regulatory barrier. That is, one may consider preliminary reports or the mechanism of action of a drug and decide that it is likely to work in a given situation—then go ahead and try it. Such use is specifically allowed without an IND;[3(Sec.2(d))] an IND is only required if such use is carried out in a systematic way with the intention of generating information of use in a licensing application.

Confusion may arise because the question "Is this research?" is distinct from the question "Is an IND required?" If a clinician uses a drug off-label in a systematic way with the intent to generate or contribute to generalizable knowledge, the regulatory definition of research with human subjects has been satisfied.[5(Sec.102(d))] Thus, IRB oversight and other protections will be required, even though an IND may not be. As a simple example, an allergist or pulmonologist may wish to compare two licensed drugs for their efficacy and ease of use in patients with asthma. A prospective, randomized, crossover trial is to be carried out. Publication is likely; however, no drug company is involved, and the use of the results in support of an advertising claim is unlikely. This is unambiguously research involving human subjects, but nothing about the study brings it under IND rules.

These distinctions are very important because they preserve the ability to use drugs clinically in difficult situations. If every off-label use were to be construed as research or if every off-label use were to require an IND, only patients with common and well-studied conditions would be candidates for treatment.

Outline of the Process

The overarching purposes of the IND process are to ensure the rights and welfare of study subjects and to ensure the quality and integrity of the data on which licensing applications are to be based. The former dominates the process in consideration of Phase I trials, whereas data quality questions become more important in later trials.[3(Sec.22(a))]

The process begins with the submission of a "notice of claimed investigational exemption for a new drug" by the sponsor. Typically, the sponsor is the drug manufacturer; it may be the clinician–investigator. Sometimes the manufacturer is the clinician–investigator, as when an intramurally developed drug enters clinical trials on its home turf. This application sets forth the background information establishing that the time is right to move into human studies, and it sets forth a fair amount of detail about the plan of investigation in humans. A detailed protocol for the first human studies and a complete investigators' brochure for them are typically made part of the initial application. Specific content guidelines are provided at 21 CFR 312.[3(Sec.23)]

The FDA then has 30 days to respond. For commercial IND applications, the response is typically a beginning of the dialogue to agree on what additional information may be needed or what modifications may be required in the plan of investigation or the information for researchers. In investigator-initiated INDs involving products of low risk, the response is often simply granting the request.

After approval has been secured, the described investigations may begin, but only in strict accordance with the protocols that have been accepted by the FDA. The approval is for a very specific course of study and is not a more general permission to study the drug. Carefully following the approved protocol is often one of the most important safety provisions of research. Individual study sites may not begin to enter subjects until appropriate local approvals are in place (including IRB approval).

The investigator and sponsor then have a number of record-keeping and reporting obligations that must be satisfied. Data must be kept secure and must be verifiable. Data must be monitored for safety issues as well as for study quality. Adverse events must be reported, both to the FDA and to IRBs. Changes in protocols must be submitted for approval, both to the FDA and to IRBs, and may not be implemented until approved by the IRB and reported to FDA, unless their purpose is to protect subjects from serious harm (e.g., by removing a newly recognized substantive risk). Annual progress reports must be submitted to the FDA, as must continuing review applications/reports to the IRBs.

Exactly how these responsibilities are divided depends a bit on the nature of the study. If it is a multicenter study with a commercial sponsor, the sponsor deals with the FDA and the local investigator deals with local regulatory matters, such as IRB oversight. If it is a single-site study and the investigator has been involved in developing the product, the same person may be dealing with both local and federal concerns.

Special Types of IND

There are two special categories of IND of which IRBs should be aware, even though neither is very common.

The first is what is known as a "treatment" IND.[3(Sec.34)] When antiretroviral drugs were first being developed, there was great concern (fueled by advocacy from groups of HIV-infected persons) that they be made available for treatment use as early as was feasible—recognizing that no therapy existed for HIV infection. Special rules were adopted to facilitate this, allowing the drugs to be used for treatment while Phase II studies were still underway. After initial enthusiasm, the use of such INDs has declined because most of the need is satisfied by the inclusion of compassionate-use arms in Phase III studies.

The second is a special class of IND for studies invoking the special waiver of consent for treatment studies in an emergency setting. Recognizing that "retrospective consent" and "passive consent" are oxymoronic, the Office for Protection from Research Risks and the FDA developed a set of rules under which therapeutic trials in an emergency setting could be done.[1(Sec.24)] These rules provided for "community consultation" in lieu of individualized consent and restricted the research to a very narrow context involving attempts to improve the care of very serious conditions under circumstances that precluded getting surrogate consent in a timely manner. One of the procedural safeguards put in place for such research was to require a special IND, even if the product under study were covered by another IND or were even licensed.[3(Sec.54)] In effect, it created a mechanism for the FDA to always have oversight authority for such research. IRBs should be aware that any time they are considering an application under subsection 24 of 21 CFR 50, a special IND application will be required.

Another Special Case—IND: Yes; IRB: No!

More common than the special provisions for waiving consent in the emergency care setting is the circumstance in which a treating physician wishes to use an experimental drug (or device) in a life-threatening situation and does not have time to get prospective IRB approval. The IND regulations provide an exception to the requirement for prospective approval for this scenario. To use an experimental agent under such circumstances, the following conditions must be met.[2(Sec.102(d))]

1. It must be a life-and-limb–threatening situation. Although the regulation says "life-threatening," the interpretation has generally been given that this may be limb threatening or merely likely to become life threatening if the customary delay for IRB approval were interposed.

2. There must be no standard therapy available. This may be true in an absolute sense, or standard therapy may be failing in this patient, or there may be contraindications to standard therapy, or there may be reason to believe that standard therapy will be ineffective or excessively dangerous.

3. There must be insufficient time for prospective IRB review. Typically, such requests involve drugs that must be started within hours or, at most, a couple of days. If more time is available, full IRB review—even if it means a special quorum call—is a better option.

4. There must be no preclusive regulatory barriers. This is seldom a limiting factor. Many of the drugs for which such requests are made are ones that are in Phase III trials and for which the manufacturer has a compassionate-use IND provision already in place. Moreover, in a genuine emergency, the FDA will often authorize release of the drug while an application for such an IND provision is still in preparation.[3(Sec.36)]

5. The concurrence of a physician uninvolved in the patient's care is often added to the list. This is a requirement for the waiver of consent in such situations, but it is not a strict requirement if the patient can give consent or if an appropriate surrogate consent giver is available.[1(Sec.23(a))] Nonetheless, it is a useful additional safeguard.

Such an exception may only be invoked once for a given drug at a given site[2(Sec.104(c))] (although operationally the possibility of an unexpected second need is recognized). The physician (now also an investigator) must report the use in writing to the IRB of local jurisdiction within 5 working days,[2(Sec.104(c))] and all of the record-keeping and reporting obligations of an investigator accrue to him or her. The physician also must be aware of the fact that this drug use is occurring in the absence of IRB approval; this may have implications for use of any data that result.

If the drug is a product of a commercial supplier, that supplier/sponsor will want assurance that the regulatory obligations will be complied with. That request often comes in the form of a request for an "emergency IRB approval" (an unfortunate misnomer). Many institutions therefore have a local policy that clinicians screen such requests with an IRB officer. That provides some assurance that the rules will in fact be satisfied, provides an entrée into the required oversight process, and allows the IRB to generate a letter to the sponsor indicating that the request has been screened and found to meet the regulatory criteria for exemption from the requirement for prior IRB review.

When Things Go Really Wrong

A sponsor may withdraw an IND at any time, with or without cause. The FDA may also terminate an IND under a number of circumstances. A clinical hold is a suspension of an IND, during which no new subjects may be enrolled, and subjects who have already been enrolled may only continue the study drug if it is clinically necessary for them to do so.[3(Sec.42)] This action may be taken when it appears that subjects are being exposed to greater risk than had originally been recognized; the IND—and the studies—are then often reactivated when appropriate adjustments in study design have been made. A clinical hold may also result if the researchers' qualifications are called into serious question or if the study design proves flawed in a way that precludes meaningful results.

More serious deficiencies may lead to termination of an IND. In that case, reactivation is not foreseen and the project is shut down.[3(Sec.44)] If the cause is clear and compelling danger to research subjects, this may be a rather precipitous action. If it is for problems in study conduct that do not place subjects at increased risk, the FDA will ordinarily notify the sponsor of the intent to terminate the IND and give the sponsor an opportunity to respond.

Tensions

The IND process often creates problems because it involves interface between groups of people who tend to be intelligent and sophisticated, but whose areas of sophistication and expertise may not agree. A few are important enough to mention here.

Local investigators often expect to be able to submit their manufacturer-sponsored protocols to their local IRBs and have smooth sailing. This is often not the case. Sponsors vary widely (and protocols from a single sponsor vary widely) in the quality and organization of the information they provide in the investigators' brochures. The quality of consent forms is also quite variable. Thus, it is sometimes easy and sometimes difficult to craft a successful IRB application from the materials provided.

It is often the local investigator's understanding that the protocol cannot be changed in response to IRB concerns, as it is often understood that the protocol provisions have been mandated by the FDA. Far more commonly, the IRB's concerns address something that the FDA has not mandated but has merely failed to disallow. In fact, the FDA depends on IRB review and is usually receptive to protocol amendments made in response to IRB concerns. The sponsor, of course, does not want to have 25 slightly different protocols in effect at its 25 active sites, and thus, it is in the sponsor's best interest to resist trivial changes and to try to implement uniformly those that address an important issue. The weaknesses in this part of the process are several. First, many protocols are not "vetted" by a demanding IRB before they go out. As a result, the process of critical IRB review is done piecemeal; the result may be nonuniform, and consensus about what is important builds agonizingly slowly. Second, the IRB's primary interaction is with the submitting local investigator. This is often someone who is clinically busy and does not want to spend a lot of time with administrative issues. It is also often someone who is not particularly knowledgeable about the regulations or FDA process and who knows little about the sponsor's actual reasons for any provisions that might be problematic for the IRB. IRBs, for their part, may or may not have expertise pertaining to an individual protocol before them and thus may or may not be able to help the local investigator find a resolution. The institutions where the research is to be conducted may see the whole issue primarily in terms of revenue flow and may try to encourage prompt IRB acceptance of sponsored research without carefully examining other dimensions.

A common example of this is the exclusion of women of childbearing potential from clinical trials of potential benefit to individual participants. Federal guidelines since 1994 have identified this as a justice concern that IRBs must address,[6] but many sponsors continue to have such exclusions in their protocols—presumably out of concern for liability risk exposure. Many investigators' brochures also do not have the necessary information to explain and defend such exclusions to an IRB (which is ironic, as many of them, in fact, turn out to be allowable). The local investigator may then go before the IRB, armed only with his or her understanding that the FDA has probably required the exclusion. Unfortunately, it may take several exchanges before the truth is known and avoidable delay has been substantial.

Another common example is the inclusion in sample consent documents of language that seems to set sponsor's liability limits. This is not allowable under FDA rules,[1(Sec.20)] DHHS rules,[5(Sec.116)] or International Conference on Harmonisation guidelines.[7(Sec.4.8.4)] Again, the poor local investigator is caught in the middle, as the IRB and the sponsor disagree about the allowability of a specific wording.

A major set of tensions centers about privacy and confidentiality with respect to study subjects and their medical records. The FDA has the authority to compare primary sources with case report forms to establish that the data on the case report forms are or are not correct (in the worst case, that the study subject does or does not exist). In clinical studies, such primary sources are often medical records. FDA regulations, in fact, require that consent forms for FDA-scrutinized research include the information that identifiable records may be audited.[1[25(a)(5)]] The sponsor does not have audit authority per se, but has the obligation to guarantee the integrity of data submitted to the FDA in a licensing application.[3[Sec.58(a),62(b)]] Therefore, the sponsor has a major interest in access to medical records, but the legal and ethical authority for such access is not automatically present. This tension is best resolved by a clear disclosure in the consent process that the quality assessment/assurance activities of the sponsor may include checking the subject's medical record to make sure that the tabulated data are correct. The details of this agreement may be problematic, as the easiest thing for the sponsor is to seek unfettered access or to seek study sites where few questions will be asked.

Conclusion

The ethical conduct of research with human subjects requires that the science be meritorious, that subject selection be equitable, that unnecessary risks be avoided, that risks and benefits be in reasonable balance, that those risks and benefits be examined independently by someone without a stake in the process, and that an information and consent process appropriate to the circumstance be employed. The IND process—supported by the more general FDA regulations for human subjects' protection—is an attempt to put those principles into practical (and auditable) form.

A fair number of rough spots exist, quite a few of which derive from something I like to term "regulatory autism." Autistic children find it difficult to imagine what another person may be thinking, even at the most basic level. That may be perceived as an exaggeration of a normal trait when one reflects on the difficulties in regulatory process. Sponsors may have trouble figuring out what is in the minds of their local investigators, the IRBs, and federal regulators. IRBs may have trouble figuring out what is in the minds of investigators, sponsors, regulators, and so on.

That being said, the regulations provide a framework in which compliance yields research that is usually credible and usually ethical. Better education of all parties to the process and more open exchange and dialogue among them could help ease or eliminate many of the tensions that persist.

References

1. Code of Federal Regulations. Title 21, Chapter 1—Food and Drug Administration, DHHS; Part 50—Protection of Human Subjects. Updated 1 April, 1999. Access date 18 April, 2001. http://www4.law.cornell.edu/cfr/21p50.htm

2. Code of Federal Regulations. Title 21, Chapter 1—Food and Drug Administration, DHHS; Part 56—Institutional Review Boards. Updated 1 April, 1999. Access date 27 March, 2001. http://www4.law.cornell.edu/cfr/21p56.htm

3. Code of Federal Regulations. Title 21, Chapter 1—Food and Drug Administration, DHHS; Part 312—Investigational New Drug Application. Updated 1 April, 1999. Access date 18 April, 2001. http://www4.law.cornell.edu/cfr/21p312.htm

4. 103rd Congress. Public Health Service Act (§201)—Title 42 US Code. Updated 1 January, 2001. http://frwebgate2.access.gpo.gov/cgi-bin/waisgate.cgi?WAISdocID52637221675101010&WAISaction5retrieve

5. Code of Federal Regulations. Title 45A—Department of Health and Human Services; Part 46—Protection of Human Subjects. Updated 1 October, 1997. Access date 18 April, 2001. http://www4.law.cornell.edu/cfr/45p46.htm

6. Mastroianni AC, Faden R, Federman D (ed.), Committee on the Ethical and Legal Issues Relating to the Inclusion of Women in Clinical Studies, Division of Health Sciences Policy, Institute of Medicine. *Women and Health Research: Ethical and Legal Issues of Including Women in Clinical Studies,* Vol. 1. Washington, DC: National Academy Press; 1994. http://search.nap.edu/books/030904992X/html/

7. International Conference on Harmonisation. E6 Good Clinical Practice. ICH harmonised tripartite guidelines: Guideline for good clinical practice. Updated 1 May, 1996. Access date 23 August, 2001. http://www.ifpma.org/pdfifpma/e6.pdf

Differences Between Department of Health and Human Services and Food and Drug Administration Regulations

Robert J. Amdur

INTRODUCTION

As discussed in Chapter 1-6, the Department of Health and Human Services (DHHS) and the Food and Drug Administration (FDA) have separate regulations related to research involving human subjects.[1–3] From the standpoint of institutional review board (IRB) policy and procedure, the two sets of regulations are similar such that in most situations an IRB that is in compliance with DHHS regulations will also be in compliance with those of the FDA and vice versa. However, regulations from these two agencies are not identical, and in some settings, there are important differences with which the IRB needs to be familiar.

Institutions that do not have an assurance of compliance with the Office for Human Research Protections must comply with FDA regulations when research involves the investigational use of drugs, biologics, or devices, regardless of the source of research funding. When an institution conducts research that is subject to both DHHS and FDA regulations, the process of IRB review must comply with both sets of regulations. For more information on when research is regulated by the DHHS or the FDA, see Chapter 1-6. A copy of selected DHHS and FDA regulations for protection of human subjects are provided in Part 11.

A comprehensive review of the differences between DHHS and FDA research regulations is presented in the Office for Human Research Protections Guidebook[4(Chap.IIB)] and in appendix E of the FDA Information Sheets.[5] In this chapter, discussion is limited to three areas that frequently generate discussion in the IRB community.

Emergency Use of a Test Article

In contrast to DHHS regulations,[1(Sec.116)] FDA regulations[3(Sec.104)] do not require prospective IRB approval for "emergency use" of a test article in specific situations. The DHHS requires IRB approval for all research that does not meet the regulatory criteria to be exempt from IRB review (see Chapter 4-1). DHHS regulations do not explicitly address the emergency use of an investigational article without IRB approval other than to say that they are not intended to limit access to emergency medical care.

IRBs at institutions with an OHRP assurance (see Chapter 8-2) frequently encounter the situation in which a physician wants IRB approval to use an investigational medication or device in a "compassionate-use" situation that does not constitute research. The usual scenario involves (1) a patient with a serious medical problem that is unlikely to respond to standard therapy, (2) a promising treatment involving a drug that is being studied at another institution under IND with the FDA, and (3) it is not desirable to transfer medical care to an institution where the investigational treatment is available. In this situation, a physician who does not have access to the desired treatment at his or her institution will call the study sponsor and ask for use of the investigational medication outside of the study setting. The sponsor will tell the physician that it will not provide the medication in question because FDA regulations do not permit the use of an investigational drug without IRB approval. The physician then asks their IRB to approve the use of the investigational medication on a "compassionate-use" basis—meaning in a manner that does not constitute research. The request for IRB approval is usually made on short notice because these situations usually involve an emergent or semiemergent medical condition.

A discussion of how an IRB should handle this situation is discussed in detail in Chapter 4-4. The bottom line is that there is a mechanism for managing this situation in a way that usually satisfies all concerned parties: the FDA, the DHHS, the study sponsor, the local physician, and the IRB. For the purpose of this discussion, it is sufficient to recognize that use of an investigational agent without IRB approval identifies a situation where DHHS and FDA regulations may differ.

IRB Management of Serious Adverse Event Reports

The management of serious adverse event (SAE) reports from multicenter clinical trials is one of the most important and controversial issues facing IRBs today. Most IRBs cannot afford to waste time with activities that do not meaningfully affect the protection of human research subjects. IRBs are confused about the regulatory definition of an AE. They are unsure of when an investigator is required to report an AE to the IRB, the timing of AE reporting, the procedure for IRB review of an AE report, and the relationship between the IRB and a data and safety monitoring board. Part of the problem is differences between DHHS[1[Sec.103(5),108,111(a)(6),116(b)(5)]] and FDA[2[Sec.108(b)(1)]] regulations related to the various components of this topic. A comprehensive discussion of the SAE reporting issue is presented in Chapter 7-3.

Explaining Access to Study Records in the Consent Document

An issue that is frequently overlooked by institutions that focus on DHHS regulations[1[Sec.116(a)(5)]] is the requirement by the FDA[2[Sec.25(a)(5)]] to include in the consent document a statement that the FDA may inspect a subject's medical record as part of a review of information pertaining to the research study. Although the DHHS has the right to inspect the records of studies that are subject to DHHS regulation, DHHS regulations do not require an explicit statement regarding review of study records in the consent document.

Conclusion

The DHHS and the FDA have separate regulations related to research involving human subjects. The two sets of regulations are similar such that in most settings the IRB that is in compliance with the DHHS regulations will also be in compliance with those of the FDA and vice versa. However, there are three main situations where the regulations differ in a way that affects IRB policy. These situations are the emergency use of a test article (the compassionate-use situation), the management of AE reports, and the explanation of access to study records in the consent document.

References

1. Code of Federal Regulations. Title 45A—Department of Health and Human Services; Part 46—Protection of Human Subjects. Updated 1 October, 1997. Access date 18 April, 2001. http://www4.law.cornell.edu/cfr/45p46.htm

2. Code of Federal Regulations. Title 21, Chapter 1—Food and Drug Administration, DHHS; Part 50—Protection of Human Subjects. Updated 1 April, 1999. Access date 18 April, 2001. http://www4.law.cornell.edu/cfr/21p50.htm

3. Code of Federal Regulations. Title 21, Chapter 1—Food and Drug Administration, DHHS; Part 56—Institutional Review Boards. Updated 1 April, 1999. Access date 27 March, 2001. http://www4.law.cornell.edu/cfr/21p56.htm

4. Penslar RL, Porter JP, Office for Human Research Protections. *Institutional Review Board Guidebook,* 2nd ed. 6 February, 2001. Access date 29 March, 2001. http://ohrp.osophs.dhhs.gov/irb/irb_guidebook.htm

5. Food and Drug Administration. Information sheets: Guidance for institutional review boards and clinical investigators, September 1998. Access date 9 April, 2001. http://www.fda.gov/oc/oha/IRB/toc.html

Veterans Administration Research Guidelines

Peter Marshall and Kathy Schulz

INTRODUCTION

The purposes of this chapter are to describe the additional regulatory and policy requirements that institutional review boards (IRBs) in the Department of Veterans Affairs (VA) must follow and to help individuals at non-VA facilities understand some of the additional guidance provided by the VA. The information provided in this chapter applies to VA IRBs* and affiliated academic institution IRBs that serve as the IRBs of record for VA facilities. (Although typically VA medical centers, VA facilities may also include VA health care systems or VA regional offices.) At VA facilities, the IRB is considered a subcommittee of the research and development (R&D) committee,[1(¶3)] which is responsible for all research conducted at the facility. The information provided here is excerpted from VA policy and guidelines and is intended to be educational; this chapter should not be used as a substitute for careful review of those policies.

VA Policy and Guidance

As described in other chapters, the "Common Rule" was developed as a joint effort of federal departments and agencies to standardize the rules for human subject protection.[2] For the Department of Veterans Affairs, the Common Rule is codified in 38 CFR 16, Protection of Human Subjects.[3]

Although some differences exist among the departments and agencies that were signatory to the Common Rule, the fundamental requirements and obligations are consistent. We learn more about the application of the federal rules and the commitments of institutions to protect human subjects under a federalwide assurance (FWA) elsewhere in this volume. What is important to remember here is that the Common Rule as codified by the Department of Veterans Affairs does not include Subparts B–D of the Department of Health and Human Services (DHHS) regulations (45 CFR 46), which describe additional protections for fetuses, pregnant women, human in vitro fertilization, prisoners, and children. Despite the omission of these sections in agency law, VA policy[1(¶5a(2))] requires that all facilities follow these sections under certain circumstances. All VA facilities conducting research involving human subjects (including research on human subjects tissue and data, where applicable) are required to hold an FWA.

The Veterans Health Administration (VHA) Handbook 1200.5,† which outlines the procedures for implementing 38 CFR 16, is the primary source of guidance concerning agency interpretation of the Common Rule for the protection of human subjects. Handbook 1200.5 applies to all research involving human subjects that is conducted by VA personnel on official VA time or in VA facilities (including approved off-site locations) regardless of the source of funding, if any.[1(¶4b)]

Funds and Personnel Management

The specific reference to funding source may be a cause of confusion to professionals outside the VA. In many ways, research funds are available to researchers at the VA just as they are at academic facilities throughout the nation (e.g., National Institutes of Health grants, foundation grants, pharmaceutical companies, and gifts) and are primarily intramural. In addition to these traditional funding sources, the VA receives funds for research through a specific research appropriation and provides research funds through an internal competitive grants program in support of its mission to contribute to the public health, emergency management, and socioeconomic well-being of our nation.[5] Unlike academia, however, the VA manages

---

*IRBs in VA facilities were previously referred to as "Subcommittee on Human Studies."[1(¶2)]
†Handbook 1200.5 was officially implemented on 15 July 2003, replacing VA Manual M-3, Part I, Chapter 9, which was last revised on October 30, 1992.[4]

the funds it receives through a variety of interrelated programs. Although a university or biotech corporation may have a single grants office that manages all funds, the VA has an internal grants management program for funds provided through the VA and in many cases works closely with an affiliated not-for-profit research and education corporation and often with the grants office at the affiliated academic institution, as well. Most VA medical centers also participate in a significant amount of unfunded research as a by-product of their residency and fellowship programs.

The not-for-profit corporations were created to facilitate the research and education programs at VA facilities. These corporations manage grants and funds from intramural sources, pharmaceutical companies, and gifts to further the research and education mission at the VA. They provide traditional grants and contracts support and often hire personnel to work on specific grants for investigators, as well as providing additional research infrastructure. They are managed by a board of directors that includes membership from the VA facility to which they are connected and the affiliated academic institution.

Education and Credentialing of Researchers

The research staff at many VA facilities is a complex mix of employees and volunteers. Some are federal (VA) employees; some are on the payroll of the not-for-profit corporation, and some are employed by the affiliated academic institution or are working part-time for two of these agencies. There are also individuals who volunteer to work at the VA, often to gain experience before completing an advanced degree. Without elaborating on the rules for managing these relationships, it is important to note that individuals who are not paid by the VA are required to submit to a federal background check (federal employees are required to pass a background check as a condition of employment) in order to obtain and maintain a "worker without compensation" or "WOC" appointment.

As of March 3, 2003, all individuals engaged in research at the VA are required to document annual completion of education modules and submit to verification of their credentials before they begin research activities. This includes investigators, research coordinators and research assistants, and members of the IRB and R&D committees. Facilities have been allowed to define "annual" on a 365-day period, a fiscal year, or a calendar year basis. The Program for Research Integrity Development and Education (PRIDE) (discussed later here) in the Office of Research and Development (ORD) has developed annual modules to meet the educational requirements.

Just as funds and personnel management may differ at the VA, interpretations of the Common Rule and the expectations of VA facilities engaged in research within the VA system may exceed the regulatory *de minimus* of the Common Rule. To understand these subtleties and how they may affect research at—or with—VA facilities, it is important to be aware of VA organization and definitions.

The FWA

All VA facilities involved in human subject research must apply through the VA's Office of Research Oversight (ORO) to the Office for Human Research Protections (OHRP) for an Assurance of Compliance. The facility must obtain this assurance before conducting any research[1[¶5a(2)]] involving human subjects. In addition, VA not-for-profit research and education organizations that manage funds for human subjects research must also hold an FWA, even though all research is conducted at the VA facility.

Institutional Official

The FWA required by the OHRP necessitates that the institution designate an institutional official (IO) who is responsible for ensuring the protection of human subjects who participate in research at their institutions by developing a Human Research Protection Program (HRPP) that has sufficient resources and support to comply with all federal regulations and guidelines governing human subject research. The IO is the individual legally authorized to bind the institution, typically is the signatory official for all assurances, and assumes the obligations of the facility's FWA. Within the VA, only the facility director is authorized to serve as the IO on the FWA.[1[¶3i]] At the affiliated not-for-profit research and education corporation, this is typically the chief executive officer.

Principal Investigator

A principal investigator (PI) is that individual who conducts a research project, under whose immediate direction research is conducted or who is the leader of a research program or team. Subinvestigators or co-investigators work under the general direction of the PI and may be involved in some or all aspects of the research project, including the design of the study, conduct of the study, analysis and interpretation of the collected data, and writing of resulting manuscripts. Pursuant to VA Guidance,[1[¶3n,t]] each of these individuals will be a VA employee either paid directly by the VA, appointed to work without compensation (WOC), or be assigned to the VA under the terms of an Intergovernmental Personnel Act.

Many facilities have developed a process by which an individual may attain PI status to ensure that only individuals who have met a standard set of criteria and/or experience are in a position to direct research at that facility. This is an institutional title (not unlike professor) that confers certain endorsements and expectations. Although PI status may allow an individual to apply for grants or submit regulatory applications (e.g., IRB, Institutional Animal Care and Use Committee [IACUC]) without a mentor, it does not allow research to be conducted without regulatory approvals in place. When a number of individuals collaborate on a project there will usually be one PI with overall responsibility for the project, even though several individuals on the study team have been granted "PI" status.

The R&D Committee

The R&D committee is charged with maintaining high standards for the research program at the facility and advising the IO on all aspects of the facility's research program.[6] The committee maintains a diverse membership, including representation from the dean's committee at the affiliated university (where one exists), clinicians, active VA researchers, statisticians, and ex-officio members representing the research office and institutional administration as well as a representative from the affiliated not-for-profit corporation. To carry out its charge and depending on the size of the local research program, the R&D committee may deliberate *en banc* on all issues or may appoint one or more subcommittees. R&D subcommittees often include the IRB, IACUC (animal use), biosafety, research integrity, budget, space, and others.

The VA R&D committee must approve all research (not only research involving human subjects) to be undertaken at the facility or using facility resources or personnel on VA time. The R&D committee, either independently or through established subcommittees, evaluates proposed research for scientific merit, applicability to the VA setting, qualifications of the investigators, and compliance with regulatory requirements.[7]

Although the Common Rule establishes the requirement of IRB review and ongoing approval of research involving human subjects, nothing in the rule prevents an institution from establishing additional requirements. Many (academic or private) institutions require informal approvals such as departmental sign-off on projects that will impact those departments. At the VA, the R&D committee fulfills its obligations to the IO to approve all research by providing an additional review of human subjects research. In other words, the R&D committee cannot waive the requirement for IRB review, nor can it approve human subjects research that has not received the approval of the facility's designated IRB. Research exempt from human subjects (IRB) review is nevertheless subject to review and approval by the R&D committee and may be subject to review by another of its subcommittees.[1[¶9d]] VA-approved research, therefore, is research that has been approved by the local R&D committee[1[¶3q]] and, in many cases, by one or more of its subcommittees.

Although many VA facilities have affiliated not-for-profit research and education corporations, these corporations are limited in scope, as we have outlined previously. VA personnel (some of whom may be WOC) conduct the research at the VA facility. This research is subject to the policies of the VA facility, including review and approval by the IRB designated by the VA as well as the local R&D committee.

VA IRB

VA policy requires each facility to designate an IRB of record in its FWA.[1[¶5a(3)]] The IRB selected by each facility will reflect the local needs of the facility and may be a VA-based IRB (either at the local facility or another VA facility) or an IRB(s) at the affiliated academic institution. VA policy prohibits the use of commercial IRBs.[1[¶5a(3)(g)]]

Facilities that choose to have an in-house, or VA IRB, will establish that committee pursuant to federal requirements and VA policies, not unlike an IRB formed at any other institution or academic center. Such an IRB will serve the needs of the facility at which it is established and is officially a subcommittee of the R&D committee. In some situations, a nearby VA facility may elect to use another VA's IRB as its IRB of record. In this instance, the facilities would have a Memorandum of Understanding (MOU) or other agreement outlining this relationship, and their FWAs would designate the role of the IRB for each facility.

IRB members in VA-based IRBs will be appointed by the facility director for a period of 3 years and may be reappointed indefinitely. The chair of a VA IRB will be appointed by the facility director for a term of 1 year and may be reappointed indefinitely.[1[¶6k,m]] When the facility relies on the IRB at the affiliated university, the R&D committee reviews the membership and performance of the IRB on an annual basis. If research involving a Food and Drug Administration (FDA)-regulated article is involved, a licensed physician will be included in the quorum.[1[¶7f(1)]]

Many VA facilities have affiliation agreements with nearby medical or dental schools. These agreements serve the intuitions in several ways and frequently permit sharing of personnel and/or resources. VA policies allow an IRB established by the affiliated medical or dental school to serve as the IRB of record for the VA facility. In order to use the affiliated medical school's IRB, the VA and the affiliate enter into a MOU or other written agreement that outlines the responsibilities of the VA and the affiliate.[1[¶5a(3)(b)]] The affiliate IRB will be expected to comply with the provisions of 38 CFR 16 and VA policy and guidelines (such as Handbook 1200.5) when reviewing and approving VA research.

The VA will provide two or more VA-salaried[8] (at least 5/8 full-time equivalent (FTE) individuals as full members of each affiliate IRB that reviews VA research.[1[¶5a(3)(a)]] These individuals must serve as full voting members on the IRB, reviewing all materials presented to the committee, not merely VA issues. At least one of these members must have scientific expertise and at least one of these members must be present during the review of VA research presented to the committee. Although not specifically required, a facility may wish to consider designating as one of its members a veteran or a representative of a legally recognized veterans' organization. In large programs, the VA may find it is not feasible to designate two members to each of the university's IRBs and may choose to limit review of VA research to one or two of the IRBs established at the university. In other words, if the university has six IRBs, the VA facility may not be able to identify 12 appropriate individuals to serve as full IRB members and may restrict review of VA research to two or three of the IRBs, for which they are able to provide appropriate members.

When the VA elects to use the IRB at an affiliated institution it is important to establish a strong working relationship between the IRB and the appropriate VA research staff. Routine meetings, membership on policy committees, participation on the R&D committee or other methods will help the institutions stay abreast of evolving expectations and ensure any necessary adjustments are made on a timely basis. At a minimum, the VA R&D committee will need access to IRB records, documentation of approval, and minutes of IRB meetings.[1[¶5a(3)(c)]]

A third type of VA IRB is a regional committee consisting of members from a number of facilities. This type of IRB would exist only to review limited studies that are designed to be done throughout a broad regional area, such as a VISN (Veterans Integrated Service Network, discussed later here), where routine IRB review would involve a number of individual IRBs and prove unrealistically burdensome. At this writing, such an IRB would require approval of both the ORD and ORO (see sections later here that describe ORD and ORO in more detail); facilities that may be interested in such a program should contact these offices for additional guidance.

Monitoring Safety

The data and safety-monitoring plan outlined in the protocol developed by the investigator is an important part of the IRB's review. This is especially important for studies that do not have or are not required to have a Data Safety and Monitoring Board or Data Monitoring Committee and are blinded, have multiple sites, enroll vulnerable populations, or employ high-risk interventions. The plan must, at a minimum, include procedures for reporting adverse events.[1[¶7a(6)]]

Exempt Research

All requests for exemption from human subjects regulations must be approved by an IRB chair or designee, or as outlined in facility policies, based on the exempt categories in 38 CFR 16.101(b). Decisions shall be made in a timely manner and communicated to the investigator as well as the IRB. Research found to be exempt from IRB review will, nevertheless, require review by the R&D committee before initiation and such research will then be included in the R&D committee's annual review of research projects.[1[¶8b]]

Vulnerable Populations

Research involving children or prisoners may not be conducted by VA investigators while on official duty or at VA facilities (including approved off-site facilities) unless a waiver has been granted by the Chief Research and Development Officer. Where a waiver has been granted, IRBs will ensure that all additional requirements are met as

described in the handbook.[1[App.D¶4]] Research involving in vitro fertilization or in which the subject is a fetus, in utero or ex utero (including human fetal tissue), may not be conducted by VA investigators while on official duty or at VA (including approved off-site) facilities.

Applicability of Policy

The VA includes the risk of loss of insurability among the other listed risks in category 38 CFR 16.101(b)(2)(ii).[1[App.A¶2b(2)]] The determination of exempt status for research and demonstration projects under category 38 CFR 16.101(b)(5) will be made by the VA Under Secretary for Health on behalf of the Secretary of Veterans Affairs.[1[App.A¶2e]]

Obligations of the Committees

Whether the IRB is VA-based or situated at the affiliated academic institutions, it is officially a subcommittee of the VA R&D committee. In the case of an affiliate IRB, the R&D committee is charged to review the IRB at least annually to ensure the IRB continues to meet the needs of the VA's HRPP.

The R&D committee (or designated subcommittee) will need to review most, if not all, of the materials submitted for IRB review to determine the scientific merit, qualifications of the investigator, and appropriateness of the research at the VAMC and for this reason may keep full duplicate files, particularly when the IRB is located at the affiliated medical school. The R&D can accept or reject the decisions of its' subcommittees, but cannot alter those decisions.[9] The committees can make recommendations or require changes to secure approval, but research cannot be undertaken until both the IRB and the R&D committee have approved it.

From time to time, an investigator may feel caught between the committees. For example, one of the R&D committee's responsibilities is to assure the scientific quality of research studies. At the same time, one of the criteria for IRB approval is that the risks to subjects are reasonable in relation to anticipated benefits to subjects and the importance of the knowledge that may reasonably be expected to result.[10] If the IRB approves the study but the R&D committee determines that it is not meritorious, the investigator will need to go back to the IRB for approval of a modification to secure the approval of the R&D committee.

Similarly, a study may have received full approval from both committees, only to have the IRB suspend research or take other action against the investigator. Because the R&D cannot overturn this decision, the study will be suspended at the VA. Despite the additional reporting requirements, which we discuss later, such a scenario serves to reinforce the necessity for strong communication between the IRB and the R&D committees.

IRB Records

Adequate IRB records must be maintained to document IRB activities. Minutes of an IRB meeting must be written and available for review within 3 weeks of the meeting date. After approval by the IRB members at a subsequent IRB meeting, the minutes may not be altered by anyone, including a higher authority.[1[¶7i(2)]] Complete (not redacted) minutes, whether from the VA or affiliate IRB reviewing VA research, are submitted to the R&D committee and maintained in the facility research office. The R&D committee reviews and acts on all IRB minutes regardless of whether the IRB is established at the facility or at the affiliate university.[1[¶7j(3)]]

HRPP Accreditation

As in any other institution conducting research involving human subjects, each VA facility so engaged has an active HRPP to ensure the protection of human subjects participating in research. Beginning in 2001, the VA contracted* with the National Committee for Quality Assurance (NCQA) to provide an independent review and analysis of the HRPP at each facility engaged in human subjects research.

Each facility is evaluated based on a written application and on-site survey by NCQA personnel. Sites with internal IRBs are evaluated on four criteria (institutional responsibility, IRB management, consideration of risks and benefits, and informed consent standards), whereas sites relying on outside IRBs (at another VA or the affiliated university) are reviewed on only one section of these standards (institutional responsibility) and their results are considered in conjunction with the accreditation score obtained by the IRB at the affiliate site. All VA IRBs must be reviewed by NCQA pursuant to the contract issued by ORD, whereas university IRBs may elect to be evaluated by the Partnership for Human Research Protection Accreditation Program, an NCQA affiliate, or the Association for the Accreditation of Human Research Protection Programs Inc.[11] University IRBs have the option to be reviewed by NCQA solely on the work done for the VA medical center; however, such a survey would not confer accreditation on the university, but only on the VA facility.

The initial contract for accreditation surveys was granted to NCQA for the period 2001 through 2005. Whether future contracts are awarded to NCQA, the Association for the Accreditation of Human Research Protection Programs (AAHRPP) or another agency cannot be predicted. Regardless of the mechanism, it is anticipated that the VA will continue to seek accreditation of its human subjects protection programs, just as it maintains accreditation for the animal research program, laboratory, and hospital services.

Informed Consent

Documentation of written informed consent for research is written on VA Form 10-1086, even when the IRB of record is at the affiliated university.[1[¶1d]] VA policy mandates the use of an approval stamp on each page of the consent document approved by the IRB.[1[¶7a(4)(a)]] The stamp is required only to reflect the date of the most recent IRB approval. In other words, a consent that is amended during an IRB approval cycle will show the date the amended version was approved. Facilities should carefully consider the wording on this stamp so as not to obligate reconsenting a participant if there are no changes to the consent language (i.e., at continuing review).

Witness to Consent

A witness "whose role is to witness the subject's (or the subject's legally-authorized representative's) signature" should sign and date the consent at the time of signing by the participant.[1[¶3a(2)(b)]] The role of this witness is limited to witnessing the signature, and this individual need not be present for the consent discussion. The consent document should clearly reflect the role of the witness (whether to the signature of the participant or to the entire consent process), particularly when the IRB or sponsor has mandated the use of a witness to the consent process.

Documentation of Medical Chart

VA medical centers typically provide both clinics and hospitals, often under one roof. Regardless of where patients are seen, the VA has a single system of records for medical care of its patients. Medical records are fully computerized and available at the bedside or in the clinic on a computerized patient record system. The IRB should determine whether it is necessary to document (flag) a patient's chart to note participation in research.[1[¶3c]] Flagging the chart places a warning on the opening screen to notify providers that the patient is participating in research and whom to contact to learn more about that research. Most facilities also have the technology to scan a copy of the informed consent for research (VA Form 10-1086) into the system. In some cases, it may not be in the patient's best interest to annotate the medical record regarding participation in research. Such circumstances might include research that involves no greater than minimal risk, only a single encounter, surveys, use of previously collected specimens, or situations where identification of the research may provide greater risk than the research itself.

Progress Notes

Good clinical practice includes carefully annotating charts with progress notes to document encounters. A progress note should include the name of the study, the person obtaining the subject's consent, a statement that the subject (or the subject's legally authorized representative) was capable of understanding the consent process, a statement that the

---

*The contract in place at the time of writing expires in 2005 and will be subject to rebid; whether future contracts are placed with NCQA or another agency cannot be predicted.

study was explained to the subject, and a statement that the subject was given the opportunity to ask questions as well as contact information of research personnel. If consent and enrollment occur at different times, an additional note should be added when the subject is enrolled (starts study interventions or treatment). The chart should also be annotated when participation has concluded.[1][¶3e]

Although it is not a requirement that progress notes be kept in the computerized patient record system (researchers may elect to document study files), consideration should be given to the potential for emergency access to research information. Discussion of the relative merits of record-keeping methods may assist the IRB in determining whether or not to require flagging the official chart for research participation.

Research-Related Injury

The VA policy regarding treatment of research-related injuries to human subjects is defined in 38 CFR 17.85. Treatment will be provided when the research was approved by the VA R&D committee and is conducted under the supervision of one or more VA investigators and will be provided, except in limited circumstances, in VA facilities. Injuries that result from an individual's failure to comply with study procedures are not generally covered. The consent form should include language explaining the VA's authority to provide treatment.[1][App.C¶2a(11)(a)]

Role of the Pharmacy

In the VA, all medications are stored in the pharmacy. This is especially true of research medications. Medications are dispensed by prescription and prescribing is limited to providers designated on VA Form 10-9012 (the Investigational Drug Information Record). Before a prescription can be filled, the pharmacist must have on file a copy of the approved protocol, the investigator's drug brochure, the signed VA Form 10-9012, and a copy of the executed consent document for the participant.[12] The pharmacist may serve as a member of the R&D or one if its subcommittees and should be consulted early in the approval process to ensure any pharmaceutical products can be managed by the research pharmacist as outlined in the protocol.

Participation of Nonveterans as Research Subjects

Nonveterans may be entered into VA-approved research studies only when there is an insufficient number of veterans available to complete the study. All regulations pertaining to the participation of veterans as research subjects, including requirements for indemnification in case of research-related injury pertain to nonveteran subjects enrolled in VA-approved research.[1][Sec.16]

Payment to Research Subjects

In general, VA policy prohibits paying subjects to participate in research. In certain circumstances, payment may be permitted with IRB approval.[1][¶12a,b] These include such situations as when the study is not directly intended to enhance the diagnosis or treatment of the medical condition for which the subject is being treated, and the standard of practice in affiliated or non-VA institutions is to pay subjects; participants at collaborating non-VA institutions in multisite studies are being paid at the rate proposed or for unreimbursed transportation expenses that would not be incurred in the normal course of receiving treatment.

Surrogate Consent

Enrolling individuals in research who are unable to consider participation and consent for themselves requires a careful, documented request by the researcher and review by the IRB. The research proposal should outline the circumstances for including individuals with impaired decision-making capacity and research should provide no significant risk and/or a reasonable probability of benefit to the subject. An IRB considering research involving incompetent persons should include as a member or consultant someone who has expertise in this area and should document the finding that only persons with impaired decision-making ability are appropriate candidates for the research being proposed.

Before seeking surrogate consent, the medical record must include a signed, dated progress note documenting the finding of incompetence. This may be based on a legal determination or on consultation with the service chief or Chief of Staff who determines that the individual lacks decision-making competency and is not likely to regain it in a reasonable period of time, or on consultation with a psychiatrist or psychologist if the incompetence is a result of mental illness.

Legally authorized representatives should be taken through a full consent process, including all information that would be provided to a participant. The surrogate should be reminded that his or her obligation is to try to determine what the potential subject would chose if she or he were competent, or if that is not possible, what is thought to be in the best interest of the subject. When possible, the researcher should explain the study to the subject, even though consent will be obtained from the surrogate. Under no circumstances may a subject be forced or coerced to participate in a research study.[1][¶11a]

Legally Authorized Representatives

The VA definition of legally authorized representative is expanded beyond that provided for in the Common Rule[13] but limits those who can serve as a surrogate for the purposes of enrolling another in research. A legally authorized representative includes not only a person appointed as a health care agent under a Durable Power of Attorney for

Health Care or a court-appointed guardian of the person, but also next of kin in the following order of priority unless otherwise specified by applicable state law: spouse, adult child (18 years of age or older), parent, adult sibling (18 years of age or older), grandparent, or adult grandchild (18 years of age or older).[1[¶3q]]

Retention of Records

Required records, including the investigator's research records, should be retained for a minimum of 5 years after completion of the study and in accordance with VHA's records control schedule, applicable FDA and DHHS regulations, or as required by outside sponsors.[1[¶7i]] It is important that VA facilities using the services of an affiliate IRB notify the IRB of this requirement or include it in the MOU. Some facilities have elected to collect the investigator's files at the conclusion of research and transfer them to a secure storage facility to ensure they are maintained for the required period.

Suspended Research

One can readily envision two situations that could result in a research suspension. The first involves a delay in continuing review (renewal) of approved research and the second a for-cause action taken by an oversight committee or agency.

Investigators should make every effort to secure timely renewal of approved research. It is the responsibility of the investigator, not the IRB or R&D committee, to monitor approval dates and submit applications for renewal in a timely manner. Unfortunately, errors do occur and approval may lapse. In this instance, no new subjects may be enrolled until the IRB and R&D committees have reviewed and approved the application for continuation. Continuation of previously enrolled subjects should be reviewed by the IRB chair in consultation with the chief of staff to determine what is in the best interest of the individual participants.[1[¶7g(2),g(2)(a),g(2)(d)]]

Research suspended for-cause is a very different matter. This involves an active determination by the IRB, R&D, or another agency (e.g., FDA, OHRP) that there have (or appear to have) been serious problems with the conduct of the research and it has become necessary to stop that research. In this instance, the immediate needs of participants should be reviewed with the IRB and the chief of staff as outlined previously here, no new subjects may be enrolled, and the IO and ORO (and often oversight agencies such as FDA and/or OHRP) must be notified as soon as possible.[14] Depending on the nature of the suspension, it may be necessary to review other research (i.e., studies conducted by the individual researcher and other research approved by the IRB) before concluding the case.

Tissue and Specimen Banking

As of the publication deadline, VA polices on tissue banking are limited to a November 2000 directive[15] and a memorandum from the Chief Research and Development Officer issued in March 2001.[16] A new handbook is in preparation and is unavailable for citation at this time. Readers are encouraged to contact the local VA research office or research compliance officer to determine policies in effect.

ORD

Located within VA Central Office in Washington, DC, the ORD is responsible for the overall policy, planning, coordination, and direction of research activities within VHA. The ORD oversees all VA R&D committees that are located within VA facilities.

The PRIDE is a specialized program within ORD responsible for training, education, policy development, and guidance related to human subjects protection throughout the VA.[1[¶3r]] The work of developing policies, guidance, education, and training is carried out by PRIDE groups such as the Guidance and Policy Center and the Center for Advice and Compliance Help.

ORO

Also headquartered in Washington, DC, the ORO advises the VA's Under Secretary for Health on all matters regarding compliance and assurance for human subjects protections, as well as animal welfare, research safety, physical security, and research misconduct.[17] Formerly known as the Office of Research Compliance and Assurance, the ORO manages the VA's FWAs and the MOUs addressing human research protection with affiliate IRBs. The ORO reviews accreditation reports for regulatory compliance, oversees investigations of alleged research misconduct[1[¶3s]] or suspension of research privileges, and may conduct routine reviews designed to review prospectively and systematically regulatory compliance of VA facilities conducting research. The reviews are consultative and directed at identifying issues of noncompliance and providing recommendations for correction as needed. Depending on the scope of and extent of noncompliance, ORO may require action plans and establish timelines for corrective action. If issues of noncompliance are identified that are harming patients or potentially likely to harm patients, ORO has the authority to conduct for-cause reviews and seek immediate remedial action when necessary.[18]

ORO has several regional offices to carry out its mission and assist local facilities with review and management of routine regulatory issues as well as allegations of noncompliance. Facilities are required to report[19] serious or continuing noncompliance with human subjects regulations; adverse events leading to IRB action; unexpected deaths of research subjects; for-cause suspension of research approval; changes in the FWA or MOU; and/or initiation of inquiries for research misconduct to their regional ORO office.

VISN

The VA is organized into 22 regional networks known as VISNs. Each has a local director and limited network staff. Although their role in research is limited, the networks allow sharing of resources between some of the larger facilities and their smaller neighboring facilities.

Community-Based Outpatient Clinic

The community-based outpatient clinics (CBOCs) are designed to provide general outpatient care in areas that are several hours away from VA medical centers. Each CBOC has an affiliated (parent) medical center that is responsible for CBOC operations. Although it is often necessary to transport veterans to the medical center for advanced procedures (e.g., colonoscopy), many routine procedures and clinic visits can be managed at the CBOC. Approval for research to be conducted at the CBOC would be secured at the parent medical center.

Conclusion

The protection of human subjects in the VA has, for the most part, the same regulatory basis as other facilities. The VA's obligations to our veterans, its national prominence, and a commitment to excellence have led to the development of additional policies and oversight procedures that may not be necessary in smaller programs. The VA employs a large number of IRB and research specialists and participates in internal and external education for its personnel and its professional colleagues. In this chapter, we have tried to outline the nuances of the VA's overall HRPP but acknowledge that policies change and each facility may have policies or procedures that are more stringent than those outlined here. If you have the opportunity to work with a VA site, we encourage you to contact the local facility, ORO, or ORD to learn more about the VA's HRPP.[20]

Disclaimers

Peter Marshall, CIP, was previously with the Louis Stokes Cleveland Department of Veterans Affairs Medical Center, Cleveland, Ohio. Currently, Peter Marshall supports the Office for Research Protections in the U.S. Army Medical Research and Materiel Command. However, this chapter was written by Peter Marshall in his private capacity. No official support or endorsement by the Department of Veterans Affairs, the Louis Stokes Cleveland Department of Veterans Affairs Medical Center, or the U.S. Army Medical Research and Materiel Command is intended or should be inferred.

Kathy Schulz, CIP, serves as the Human Research Compliance Officer and Administrative Officer for Clinical Research at the San Francisco Veterans Affairs Medical Center. This chapter was written in her private capacity; no official support or endorsement by the Department of Veterans Affairs or the San Francisco Veterans Affairs Medical Center is intended or should be inferred.

References

1. Veterans Health Administration Handbook 1200.5. *Requirements for the Protection of Human Subjects in Research.* Veterans Health Administration. 15 July, 2003. Available online from: http://www1.va.gov/vhapublications/publications.cfm?pub=2 Accessed 13 June, 2005.
2. Department of Health and Human Services. Federal policy for the protection of human subjects. *Fed Regist* 56(117):28003–28018, 1991.
3. Code of Federal Regulations, Title 38—Pensions, Bonuses, and Veterans' Relief, Part 16—Protection of Human Subjects. Available online: http://www.access.gpo.gov/nara/cfr/waisidx_98/38cfr16_98.html Accessed 13 July, 2005.
4. Veterans Health Administration. Requirements for the protection of human subjects in research. In *Manual M-3, Research and Development in Medicine*, Part I, General. 30 October, 1992.
5. DVA Strategic Goals. Available online: http://www1.va.gov/about_va/page.cfm?pg=1
6. VHA Manual M-3, Part I, 2.01 a (1).
7. Veterans Health Administration. Functions. In: *Manual M-3, Research and Development in Medicine*, Part I, General. Updated 25 October, 1985. Access date 10 April, 2001. http://www.va.gov/publ/direc/health/manual/030103.pdf Sec.3.01b(1)
8. January 7, 2005. Memorandum from Acting Chief Research and Development Officer and Chief Officer, Office of Research Compliance. Checklist for Use in Developing a Memorandum of Understanding (MOU) between a VA Facility and an Affiliated Medical or Dental School for Use of the Institutional Review Board (IRB), page 2, item 7a. http://www1.va.gov/oro/docs/Checklist_Developing_MOU_010705.pdf
9. VHA Manual M-3 Sec.3.01e.
10. 38 CFR 16 Sec. 111(a)(2).
11. VHA Directive 2003-065. "Accreditation of Human Research Protection Programs." 30 October, 2003.
12. VHA Manual M-2, Part VII, paragraph 6.03(a).
13. 45 CFR 46, Sec. 102(c).
14. Memorandum from Acting Chief Officer, Office of Research Oversight, titled "What to report to ORO memo: ACTION." 12 November, 2003.
15. VHA Directive 2000-043, "Banking of human research subjects' specimens." 30 October, 2003.
16. Memorandum from Chief Research and Development Officer "VHA Directive 2000-043: Banking of Human Research Subjects' Specimens." 28 March, 2001.
17. Public Law 108-170, December 6, 2003. www1.va.gov/oro
18. Memorandum dated 1 November, 2004, from the Chief Officer, Office of Research Oversight. "Announcement of ORO Initiation of Routine Reviews at VA Facilities Conducting Research."
19. Memorandum dated 12 November, 2003, from the Acting Chief Officer, Office of Research Oversight (ORO). "What to Report to ORO?"
20. U.S. Department of Veterans Affairs/Veterans Health Administration. Office of Research and Development. http://www1.va.gov/resdev/ and Office of Research Oversight. http://www1.va.gov/oro/

State Law

Sandra P. Kaltman and John M. Isidor

INTRODUCTION

The Code of Federal Regulations charges institutional review boards (IRBs) with the responsibility of evaluating proposed research in light of applicable law.[1[Sec.107(a)],2[Sec.107]] Understanding federal laws, regulations, and guidelines is not enough to satisfy that responsibility. Every state has its own statutes, regulations, and case law that may impose requirements on the research process that add to or are different from what federal law requires. A wide range of issues may be affected:

1. Age of consent
2. Capacity to consent/legally authorized representative
3. Children's assent
4. Informed consent
5. Genetic research
6. Confidentiality of medical records
7. HIV/STD reporting requirements
8. Laws about referral fees and recruitment methods
9. Laws governing clinical research
10. Laws governing IRBs
11. Laws about investigational drugs
12. Laws about vulnerable patients
13. Laws about medical practice and delegation of authority to perform procedures

Although some federal laws in essence "overrule" conflicting state laws, that is generally not the case with state laws relating to the research process. Those laws vary considerably from state to state. Here are some examples.

Age of Consent

Federal law defers to state law in determining the age of consent for participation in research.[2[Sec.402(a)]] In most states, a subject who is 18 years old is considered to have reached the age of majority, and, as an adult, may give consent on his or her own behalf to participate in research. However, this is not the case in every state. In Nebraska, the age of majority is 19 years old.[3] In Alabama, although the age of majority is also 19, state law permits a 14-year-old to give consent for medical treatment.[4] In other states, such as Rhode Island and South Carolina, a 16-year-old can give consent for most kinds of medical treatment.[5,6] Similarly, many states have laws that emancipate minors, allowing them to make health care decisions as adults. Therefore, in order to determine whether research sites are properly obtaining consent in studies involving teenagers, the IRB must be aware of the relevant state law.

Surrogate Decision Makers

Every IRB reviewing studies involving older patients needs to know who is legally authorized to give consent for an incapacitated adult patient to participate in the procedures involved in research. Unless a potential subject has signed a durable power of attorney for health care designating someone to make health care decisions on his or her behalf, there is surprisingly little uniformity in state laws regarding who may make such decisions.

In some states, such as Kentucky and Arizona, the statute describes a hierarchy of people who can make health care decisions. However, the hierarchies are not identical. In Kentucky, decisions can be made by a court appointed guardian, a spouse, an adult child, a parent, or the nearest living relative, in that order.[7] In Arizona, the hierarchy also includes the domestic partner of an unmarried person, a sibling, and a close friend.[8] Other states, such as Ohio, have no provisions at all for alternate decision makers.

This lack of uniformity in state law is further complicated by the fact that less than half of the states have laws or regulations that specifically discuss who can act as a legally authorized representative in giving consent for research procedures, as opposed to general health care treatment.[9] Again, among those states, there is little consensus. Some states, such as New Hampshire and Pennsylvania, require court permission for participation in research.[10] Others, such as Florida, permit a legally authorized representative to give consent if the research is approved by an IRB under federal human subject protection regulations.[11]

Thus, in order to determine whether a site is obtaining consents from those who are legally authorized to give it, the IRB must know the applicable state law.

Genetic Testing

When reviewing studies that include genetic testing, the IRB must be aware of state law, if any, relating to such testing. Some states have specific laws about informed consent and genetic research. Most require written consent and some, such as Louisiana and Nevada, require the use of a specific consent form whenever genetic testing is performed.[12,13] Some states give the subject the right to be informed of the results of genetic testing.[14] This appears to be the exception to the rule. The National Bioethics Advisory Commission suggested that research results in general should not be disclosed to participants unless exceptional circumstances exist, such as when the findings are scientifically valid and confirmed, the findings have significant implications for the participant's health concerns, and a course of action to ameliorate or treat these concerns is readily available.[15]

Confidentiality of Medical Records

The clinical research industry took notice when the HIPAA (Privacy Rule) regulations were implemented. Tremendous resources have been devoted to studying the regulations and their implications for those involved in clinical trials. However, what some fail to realize is that although generally the HIPAA regulations preempt, or take precedence over, state laws, there is at least one very important exception to that general rule. In the event that a provision of state law relating to the privacy of individually identifiable health information is more stringent than what is required under HIPAA, it is the state law that must be used.[16] This is the case in both California and Washington state.[17] In both California and Washington, there are specific laws that affect the validity of the HIPAA authorization form to use and disclose Protected Health Information.

Thus, it is important to determine whether state laws about confidentiality of medical records impose any requirements or protections beyond what HIPAA requires and, if so, to make certain that the state laws are followed.

Referral Fees

Although it is still an occasional practice to pay referral fees to those sending potential subjects to an investigator, this practice is unethical, violates the HIPAA Privacy Rule regulation, and in some states, puts an investigator's medical license at risk.[18] Other states have specific laws prohibiting fee splitting, including referral fees.[19]

Other Laws Relating to Research

Three states have enacted statutes or regulations specifically relating to the conduct of clinical research. In those states, Virginia, California, and Maryland, some of the questions about how laws relating to general medical treatment will be applied in the research setting have been answered.[20] For example, under the Virginia statute, a legally authorized representative cannot give consent to any research procedures if there is greater than a minimal risk to the subject as the result of participation in research.

Another area in which state laws specific to research are being developed is registration of clinical trials and/or publication of the results of clinical trials. Although it would seem to make sense to have a national registry for such information for the sake of consistency, at publication time, at least five states have pending bills describing as many different methods of reporting and compiling information about clinical trials.[21]

The Importance of Court Cases

Besides determining which state statutes and regulations are applicable, the IRB must also make efforts to be aware of court decisions that have an impact on research. Although there have not been many court cases involving clinical research, those that do exist shape the law in the geographic area they come from and can be used as examples in other geographic areas as well. They also demonstrate how a failure to understand the law can expose those involved in research to liability.

No Right to be "Treated with Dignity" in Research
In Oklahoma, subjects and their family members alleged injury arising from participation in a vaccine study for melanoma patients.[22] They claimed that federal regulations for the protection of human subjects had been violated; they also alleged a violation of their right "to be treated with dignity," which they asserted arose from the Declaration of Helsinki and the Nuremberg Code. The U.S. District Court for the Northern District of Oklahoma dismissed the case, finding that, under Federal law, there is no constitutional "right to be treated with dignity" for people who agree to be subjects in clinical research.[23]

Written Informed Consent Is Not Always Valid
When a patient with recurring Stage IV breast cancer did not survive her participation in a cancer research study, her husband sued the research center.[24] The U.S. District Court for the Western District of Washington agreed with

the subject's husband that the research center had not obtained the subject's valid informed consent because it did not tell her that the most important chemotherapeutic drug described in the informed consent was no longer available for study patients at the research center. This case reminds us that merely having the subject sign the informed consent is not enough to make the consent valid; the written consent and the verbal information given to the subject must contain everything that could be important to the subject's decision to participate.

Maryland Court Makes New Law

In 2001, Maryland's highest court considered a case in which parents alleged that their children had been injured by exposure to lead paint in rental housing in Baltimore.[25] A research institute affiliated with Johns Hopkins University created a nontherapeutic research program requiring some homes to have only partial lead paint abatement and providing for measurement of blood lead levels of children residing in these homes.

In a lengthy opinion, the court made three significant points. First, the court determined that a special relationship exists between a researcher and a subject. A breach of those duties can be a basis for a negligence claim. Moreover, the court stated that under certain circumstances, an informed consent agreement in a nontherapeutic research project could constitute a legal contract, the breach of which could also give rise to legal claims. Finally, in nonbinding dicta, the court noted that in Maryland, a parent or other surrogate cannot consent to the participation of a child or other person under legal disability in nontherapeutic research in which there is any risk of injury or damage to the health of the subject. This does not mean that research otherwise approvable under 45 CFR 46.406 or the parallel FDA regulations of 21 CFR 50.53 is impermissible in Maryland.

In response to public outcry over this case, in 2002, the Maryland legislature enacted House Bill 917, entitled "Human Subject Research—Institutional Review Boards." The Bill applies the requirements of 45 CFR Part 46 to all research conducted in Maryland, regardless of whether it is federally funded. It requires IRBs to make their minutes available to any person upon request, after redacting confidential information. It also empowers the Attorney General of Maryland to seek injunctive relief for violation of the federal regulations protecting human subjects.

Intraocular Lens in Illinois

In an Illinois case, a court of appeals found failure to inform a patient that an intraocular lens that was being implanted was investigational and therefore a failure to obtain informed consent. The investigator had altered the IRB-approved informed consent to delete any reference to the study as "investigational." The court noted the breach of the IRB's obligation to compare the consent signed by the subject with the IRB-approved consent. The court further found that a failure to obtain proper consent could be a "medical battery," meaning a wrongful use of force, or negligence under state law, entitling the patient to receive compensation for injury.[26]

The *Moore* Case in California and the *Greenberg* Case in Florida

A leukemia patient in a study claimed that he was harmed when the investigator failed to disclose his financial interest in using the subject's cells to develop an extremely valuable cell line. In 1990, the California Supreme Court found that in order to obtain proper consent an investigator must disclose personal and economic interests unrelated to the subject's health that might affect the investigator's medical judgment. The court found that failure to make such disclosures could entitle the subject to compensation.[27]

The same issue arose more recently in Florida, where families suffering from a rare genetic disease donated blood, urine, and tissue samples to a researcher who was attempting to identify the specific gene responsible for the disease.[28] Without the permission or knowledge of the families donating the specimens, the researcher applied for and obtained a patent for the genetic sequence he successfully identified. The researcher and the research institution with which he was affiliated then earned significant royalties based on commercial products developed using the patent. The Florida District Court ruled that this unconsented use of human tissue to develop commercial products could give rise to a claim for unjust enrichment. This case highlights the importance of making sure that informed consent documents are sufficiently detailed about possible future uses of tissue and data collected in a study.

A Promise of Free Medication

A U.S. Court of Appeals has found that an informed consent document is a contract that can require a sponsor to perform services for study subjects even after a clinical trial ends.[29] In this case, the informed consent stated that subjects would receive the study drug free for 1 year after the conclusion of the double-blind phase of the study if the study drug appeared to be effective. When the sponsor did not provide the free study drug, 18 subjects filed suit. The court found that the sponsor could be forced to provide the study drug because the informed consent was considered to be a binding contract between the sponsor and subjects.

As these cases illustrate, state law can provide the legal basis for litigation against parties involved in research. IRBs and their members could be named in lawsuits. The liability of IRBs and their members is the subject of Chapter 8-9 of this book.

Sources of Information About State Laws

Unfortunately, there are few websites you can check for a comprehensive listing of all applicable state laws.[30] Some of the federal government websites have information about federal law.[31] Possible resources about state law include attorneys experienced in health care law, the state department of health, the risk-management department of the institution where the research is being performed, or the sponsor or contract research organization's legal department. It is risky for an IRB to assume that it is someone else's job to know the law applicable to the studies it reviews. Unless the IRB is aware of and understands relevant law, it cannot discharge its responsibility under the federal regulations to evaluate research in light of that law.

Conclusion

Federal regulations require the IRB to review research in compliance with applicable state law. In some situations, federal laws overrule conflicting state laws, but this is generally not the case with state laws relating to the research process. The range of situations in which state law has important implications for local IRB procedures and determinations is wide and constantly evolving. This chapter explains the main areas where state law is likely to impose restrictions on research conduct that go beyond those discussed in federal research regulations. Understanding how and when to apply state law to the local IRB process will be an ongoing challenge for the IRB and research community.

References

1. 21 CFR Part 56—Institutional Review Boards. Available at: www.fda.gov/oc/ohrt/irbs/appendixc.html

2. 45 CFR Part 46—Protection of Human Subjects. Available at: www.nihtraining.com/ohsrsite/guidelines/45cfr46.html

3. Rev. Stat. of Neb. Ann. §43-2101 (2004).

4. Alabama Code, §22-8-4 (2004).

5. S.C. Code Ann. §20-7-280 (2004).

6. R.I. Gen. Laws §23-4.6-1 (2004).

7. Ky. Rev. Stat. §311.631 (2004).

8. Ariz. Rev. Stat. §36-3231 (2004).

9. *Guide to Good Clinical Practice*, Thompson Publishing; February, 2005, Newsletter.

10. N.H. Rev. Stat. §464-A:25(1) (2004); 20 Pa. Cons. Stat. Ann. §5521(d) (2004).

11. Florida Stat. Ann. §765.113(1) (2005).

12. Nev. Rev. Stat. Ann. Title 54. §629.171; §629.181 (2004).

13. La. Rev. Stat. Title 22 §213.7 (2004).

14. Tex. Rev. Civ. Stat. Title 132, Art. 9031.

15. National Bioethics Advisory Commission, Research Involving Human Biological Materials: Ethical Issues and Policy Guidance, Vol. 1, Report and Recommendations of the National Bioethics Advisory Commission (1999), at http://www.ntis.gov

16. 45 CFR §160.203 (2005).

17. CA. Civil Code §56:10 (2005); Wash. Rev. Code §70.02.030; 70.02.050 (2005).

18. Hawaii Rev. Stat. §453-8(a)(9) (2004); Ky. Rev. Stat. §311.597(4) (2005); Ohio Rev. Code §4731.22(B)(18) (2005); Tenn. Code Ann. §63-6-214(b)(1) (2004), and *Swafford v. Harris*, 967 S.W.2d 319, 321 (1998).

19. N. Mex. Stat. §61-6-15(D)(16) (2005).

20. Md. Health Code Ann. §13-2001 (2004); Va. Code Ann. §32.1-162.18(B)(2003); Cal. Health and Safety Code §24173 (2003).

21. Connecticut HB 5821; Hawaii HB 102; Maryland SB 289; Tennessee HB 81; Texas HB 1029.

22. *Robertson v. McGee*, No. 01-CV-60-C, 2002 WL 535045(N. Dist. Okla.)

23. Order dated 01/28/02.

24. *Berman v. The Fred Hutchinson Cancer Research Center*, No. CCC01-0727L (W.Dist. Wash.), Order Granting Plaintiff's Motion for Partial Summary Judgment on Informed Consent Claim, dated August 8, 2002.

25. *Grimes v. Kennedy Krieger Institute*, 782 A.2d 807 (Md. 2001); also found at www.law.uh.edu/healthlaw/law/StateMaterials/Marylandcases/grimesvkennedykreiger.pdf

26. *Kus v. Sherman Hospital*, 644 N.E. 2d 1214 (Ill. App. 1995).

27. *Moore v. the Regents of the University of California*, 51 Cal. 3d 120 (Cal. 1990).

28. *Greenberg v. Miami Children's Hospital*, 264 F. Supp. 2d 1064 (S.D. Fla. 2003).

29. *Dahl, et al., v. HEM Pharmaceuticals Corporation*, 7 F.3d 1399 (9th Cir. 1993).

30. *See* www.clinlaw.com and State-by-State Clinical Trial Requirements Reference Guide, Barnett International, 2004.

31. *See* http://www.firstgov.gov/Topics/Reference_Shelf.shtml#laws

Institutional Review Board Member Liability

Sandra P. Kaltman and John M. Isidor

INTRODUCTION

In these litigious times, institutional review boards (IRBs) may find their members or potential members concerned about being sued as a result of their board service. Although this concern may have seemed far fetched 5 years ago, today it is not unreasonable. Growing media attention and public concern about protection for subjects participating in clinical research are making it more likely that IRBs and their members could be named as defendants in lawsuits relating to clinical research. The purpose of this chapter is to explain the liability issue as it pertains to individual IRB members and IRBs as an entity within an organization.

Potential Plaintiffs

Research Subjects

Who might bring such lawsuits against IRB members? The most obvious potential plaintiff is a subject alleging injury as a result of participation in a study. In such a case filed in federal court in the Northern District of Oklahoma in 2000, eight subjects (or their estates) sued all of the IRB members of the University of Oklahoma Health Sciences Center in Tulsa as well as other IRB and university officials and investigators.[1]

The research study at issue involved an investigational vaccine for melanoma skin cancer. All of the study subjects had melanoma. They alleged that they were not informed about the risks of their participation, that the vaccine was unsafe, and the study design unsound. Regarding the IRB members, the plaintiffs alleged that they neglected their duties by failing to (1) examine the protocol design, (2) examine the qualifications of the investigator, (3) review the operation of the clinical trial, (4) assure the protection of the participants, (5) review proposed amendments, (6) approve advertisements, (7) ensure proper reporting, and (8) make sure the clinical trial comported with ethical standards. They also alleged that the conduct of the study violated the subjects' right to "be treated with dignity in the conduct of a clinical trial." The U.S. District Court for the Northern District of Oklahoma dismissed the case, finding that under federal law the plaintiffs did not have a valid cause of action. The court also found that there is no constitutional right to be treated with dignity for people who agree to be subjects in research studies.[2]

In a similar high-profile case, the family of Jesse Gelsinger filed suit against the University of Pennsylvania after the 18-year-old subject died several days after beginning a gene transfer study at the University of Pennsylvania.[3] The case was settled before trial. The lawsuit alleged that the defendants failed to give Mr. Gelsinger the opportunity to give informed consent by failing to describe adequately the risks of the study and overstating the potential benefits. Although the IRB members were not sued, the bioethics advisor to the IRB was included as a defendant in the lawsuit.

In another noteworthy case in which the adequacy of informed consent was a major issue, a class action suit was filed in federal court in Florida on behalf of thousands of pregnant women who had agreed to participate in various research studies.[4] Although the IRB was not named, the institution was. The lawsuit alleged that the written consent documents were too difficult for the subjects to understand. There was no dispute that the subjects had signed the appropriate consent documents or that the documents presented accurate information. The subjects did not claim that they or their babies suffered any physical harm. After 10 years of litigation and without the defendant hospital or investigators admitting any liability, the case was settled in 2000 for $3.8 million.

As part of the settlement, the University of South Florida agreed to require researchers to ask all pregnant women who are potential study patients about their highest level of education. The university also agreed to use standard readability tests when designing consent forms for studies involving pregnant women before submission of such consents to the IRB. These cases show how important a clear and readable consent form becomes if a lawsuit is filed.

People Denied Access to Research

Another type of possible plaintiff is a person who wants to participate in a trial but is excluded or whose participation is limited in some way. In one such case that was decided by the United States Court of Appeals for the Ninth Circuit, the plaintiffs alleged that the sponsor of the fibromyalgia study should be forced to provide the subjects with the study drug at no cost for 1 year after the study ended.[5]

The consent document stated that after the completion of the study, the subjects would receive the study drug for 1 year at no cost if statistical analysis showed efficacy compared with placebo. The sponsor tried to back out of the arrangement on the basis that the Food and Drug Administration (FDA) had rejected the investigational new device application, although allowing the next phase of the trial, an open label study, to go forward. The Court of Appeals found that the consent document created a binding contract and ordered the sponsor to provide the drug at no cost. Although the IRB was not sued, the case shows that dissatisfied subjects can use the courts to achieve their aims and that IRBs and their members could be included as defendants along with sponsors and investigators.

In a 2003 case filed in North Carolina state court, the plaintiff sued the sponsor, the contract research organization monitoring the study, the IRB, and the principal investigator.[6] The plaintiff alleged that he was allowed to enter into a psoriasis study despite not meeting the entry criteria and was assigned to placebo without being informed of the risks of placebo and how it might affect his psoriatic arthritis. Among the novel theories in this case, the plaintiff alleged that the IRB was in a fiduciary relationship with the subjects and therefore was obligated to act at all times in the best interest of the subjects. He also alleged that the IRB as a fiduciary of the plaintiff committed a constructive fraud on the plaintiff by not disclosing to him the risks of placebo, not disclosing a conflict of interest, and assuring him that his physical condition was curable.

The IRB moved to dismiss the claims against it that were based on the alleged existence of a fiduciary relationship. The IRB argued that the federal laws and regulations establishing IRBs do not create a special or fiduciary relationship between the IRB and the subject. The court agreed and dismissed those claims against the IRB, specifically ruling that the IRB did not owe a fiduciary duty to the subject as a result of the subject's participation in the study.[7]

The most likely type of legal claim a subject might assert against an IRB and its members is a negligence claim. In order to establish a viable claim for negligence, an injured subject would have to prove, by a preponderance of the evidence, that the IRB owed him/her a duty, that it breached that duty by failing to abide by the standard of care for IRBs, that the injury was caused by the IRB's breach of its duty, and that damages resulted.

A plaintiff might attempt to use 21 CFR 56 and 45 CFR 46 to show that IRBs have a legal duty to study subjects. Next, a plaintiff would have to prove that the IRB breached its duty in some way such as failing to provide a consent form with relevant risk information, or approving a protocol in which the risks to the subject were not minimized by the study design. The actions of the IRB would be compared with what a reasonably prudent IRB would be expected to do under the same or similar circumstances.

In order to establish that the subject's injury was caused by the IRB's actions or inactions, the plaintiff would have to show that the harm would not have occurred but for the actions of the IRB. This element of proof would be difficult because the IRB rarely has any direct contact with a study subject. Although a study subject could conceivably be injured as a result of interactions with an investigator or directly by the study product, an IRB could never be the sole cause of injury to a study subject.

Nevertheless, an IRB could be found to have a role in causing harm by approving unsafe study designs, inadequate consent forms or research involving unsafe products. Additionally, an IRB could be at risk if it allowed a protocol to continue despite safety information from the study that would require an IRB to withdraw approval.

Investigators

Investigators could also bring suit against IRBs and their members on a number of bases. Investigators who are not approved to conduct studies or whose approval is withdrawn by an IRB could allege that the IRB interfered with their business opportunities with sponsors or deprived them of their right to appeal their exclusion. If any information about denial of approval or withdrawal of approval is disseminated to others, except as part of a public record, the investigators could claim that they have been slandered or libeled.

In a Minnesota case, an investigator sued the University of Minnesota, its IRB, and the IRB members.[8] He sought to prevent them from disseminating information about the IRB's investigation into his conduct of a study in which questions had been raised by another faculty member as to whether consent had been properly obtained from non–English-speaking subjects. As a result of the controversy about the study, the investigator terminated it.

The IRB started an investigation, suspended the investigator's research privileges, and notified the FDA, which initiated its own investigation. The Federal District Court for the District of Minnesota found that barring the IRB from transmitting the results of its investigation would endanger the public, as well as hinder the IRB in its essential function of maintaining the integrity of institutional research on human subjects. The IRB was permitted to fulfill its own obligations in reporting the results of its investigation to the University and the FDA pursuant to the 21 CFR 56.[9]

The investigator also alleged that he should have had the opportunity to be present when the IRB took testimony from witnesses who criticized him and to cross-examine those witnesses who testified against him in the IRB investigation. The court held that the IRB had followed its own procedures in conducting the investigation. In addition, the investigator, unlike a defendant in a criminal case, did not have the right to be involved in all aspects of the IRB's investigation. As this case shows, it is important for an IRB to have procedures that comply with the federal regulations for handling problem investigators and to follow them.

Minimizing Exposure to Liability

In addition to following all of the regulatory requirements, IRBs and their members can take a preventive approach to limiting liability by using two methods: making certain that they have adequate general liability insurance and obtaining written indemnification from sponsors and clinical research organizations (CROs) with whom they work.

Every private IRB or institution should attempt to obtain general liability insurance that specifically covers all the functions of an IRB. The insurance should cover all IRB members and employees for all of the work they do for the IRB. If such coverage is in place at the time a claim is made or a lawsuit is filed against the IRB or its members, the insurance company should take over the defense of the case for the IRB. In addition, if a judgment is entered against the IRB or its members or a settlement is reached, the insurance company should pay the amount of the judgment or settlement up to the amount of the policy limits of the insurance.

Conclusion

IRB members should inquire about their IRB's insurance coverage and make certain they are covered for their IRB activities. In addition, members who have their own professional malpractice insurance, such as physicians, attorneys, and nurses, should check with their own carriers to see whether the scope of their own insurance includes their actions as IRB members. IRB administrators should be prepared for these questions and can seek assistance from legal counsel or a risk-management department in answering them.

The IRB should also ask all sponsors, CROs, and investigators involved in the protocols they work with to sign a written agreement to indemnify the IRB from all claims arising out of the IRB's work. This means that the sponsor, CRO, or investigator will assume responsibility for defending all claims and paying all costs, including judgments or settlements and attorney fees, connected with reviewing studies. In addition, IRB members can ask their IRBs and institutions to indemnify them from all claims arising out of their work as IRB members.

Although insurance and indemnity agreements cannot eliminate the threat of being sued, they can minimize the extent of exposure to potential liability. Indemnity agreements and insurance policies are critical protections. Legal counsel or a risk-management department can help by reviewing the agreements to make certain they are suitable for use in clinical studies.

References

1. *Robertson v. McGee*, No. CV00G0H(M)(N.D. Okla. 2000).
2. Order Dismissing Complaint, dated 01/28/02.
3. *Gelsinger v. Trustees of the University of Pennsylvania*, No. 000901885 (D. Penn. Sept. 18, 2000).
4. *Flora Diaz, v. Tampa General Hospital* No. 90-120-CIV-T-25B(M.D. Fla. 1996).
5. *Kristina Anne Dahl v. HEM Pharmaceuticals Corporation*, 7 F. 3d 1399(9th Cir. 1993).
6. *Hamlet v. Genentech*, No. 03 CVS 1161(Orange County, North Carolina).
7. Order dated July 29, 2004.
8. *James A. Halikas, MD, v. the University of Minnesota; the Institutional Review Board-Human Subjects Committee, of the University of Minnesota; and its members, 856 F. Supp. 1331* (D. Minn. 1994).
9. 21 CFR 56—Institutional Review Boards, also found at www.fda.gov/oc/ohrt/irbs/appendixc.html

Certificates of Confidentiality

Sandra P. Kaltman and John M. Isidor

INTRODUCTION

Although researchers generally do not disclose identifying information about subjects who participate in clinical research studies, there are circumstances under which investigators are required to make such disclosures. For example, if an investigator receives a valid subpoena from a court or administrative agency, he or she could be required to disclose records of a subject's participation in a study. Such records could include the subject's full name, address, and medical history.

In the 1970s, Congress realized that people were unwilling to participate in research involving certain sensitive issues, such as illegal drug use, unless their privacy was protected. This would mean that they could not be identified or possibly prosecuted as a result of participating in studies. As a result, Congress enacted a law allowing researchers to obtain Certificates of Confidentiality. These permitted them to protect the privacy of subjects by refusing to disclose their names and other identifying characteristics, even if asked to do so by courts or governmental agencies.[1] At least one court has upheld the validity of such certificates.[2]

The Partnership for Human Research Protection, one of the organizations that accredits human research protection programs, states in one of its accreditation standards that an IRB, when reviewing research, should consider whether a Certificate of Confidentiality should be obtained in order to protect subject privacy.[3]

How Do You Get a Certificate of Confidentiality?

Applications for federally funded research must be made to the agencies responsible for the funding. The Office for Human Research Protections (OHRP) does not issue Certificates of Confidentiality.[4] However, Certificates of Confidentiality are not limited to use in federally funded studies. The Food and Drug Administration accepts applications for Certificates of Confidentiality for research requiring an investigational new drug exemption.

Researchers may obtain Certificates of Confidentiality only if a determination is made that the research is of a sensitive nature and protection is necessary to reach the objectives of the research. The OHRP finds research to be sensitive if it involves collecting information that, if disclosed, could have adverse consequences for subjects, such as damage to their financial status, employability, insurability, or reputation.[4]

Other agencies may evaluate applications using different criteria. The National Institutes of Health uses a nonexhaustive list of sensitive research activities which includes collecting genetic information, information on psychological well-being of subjects, information on subjects' sexual attitudes, preferences or practices, collecting data on substance abuse or other illegal risk behaviors, and studies where subjects may be involved in litigation related to exposures under study (e.g., breast implants or occupational exposures).[5]

Limitations on Certificates of Confidentiality

The Certificate of Confidentiality does not apply to voluntary disclosure of identifying information by either a subject or an investigator. Therefore, even if a study is covered by a Certificate of Confidentiality, the subject may voluntarily disclose information about himself or herself. The investigator may also voluntarily disclose issues such as child abuse involving a subject or a subject's threats of violence to self or others. Subjects should be advised about the existence of a Certificate of Confidentiality, and the consent form should clearly outline the exceptions to the protection it offers.[4]

In addition, because the existence of a Certificate of Confidentiality does not prevent other types of intentional or inadvertent breaches of confidentiality, investigators and IRBs must make certain that adequate procedures exist to protect the confidentiality of identifiable private information that will be obtained in the research.[4] The Department of Health and Human Services (DHHS) personnel may request identifying information for purposes of performing audits, carrying out investigations of DHHS grant recipients, or evaluating DHHS-funded research projects.[4]

Mechanics of Certificates of Confidentiality

Applications must be made for particular research projects. Once obtained, a Certificate of Confidentiality is not transferable from one study to another.[4] In addition, if there are major changes in the protocol, the personnel responsible for the study, or the drugs to be administered, the issuing agency must be notified by the submission of an amended application.[4]

Confidentiality Certificates are effective from the date they are issued until the date of their termination. If the research will not be completed before the date the certificate expires, the recipient of the certificate must make a written application for an extension.[4]

Conclusion

Certificates of Confidentiality can serve to promote recruitment in studies requiring disclosures of sensitive personal information, and IRBs can suggest that investigators apply for them when appropriate. The website of the OHRP contains information about contacting different agencies to obtain Certificates of Confidentiality. As long as a certificate is in place when a subject enrolls in a study, the protection provided by the certificate is permanent. Information identifying that subject will never be disclosed unless it is volunteered by the subject or investigator.[4]

References

1. 103rd Congress, Public Health Service Act, 42 USC §241(d).
2. Court of Appeals of New York. *New York v. Newman,* 40 A.D. 2d 633, 672 (1973); 32 N.Y.2d 379; 298 N.E.2d 651. The United States Supreme Court refused to consider the case. *Cert. denied,* 414 U.S. 1163 (1973).
3. Partnership for Human Research Protection. Available at: http://www.phrp.org
4. Office for Human Research Protections, Guidance on Certificates of Confidentiality, 25 February, 2003; http://www.hhs.gov/ohrp/humansubjects/guidance/certconf.htm
5. National Institutes of Health. Available at: http://grants.nih.gov/grants/policy/coc/background.htm

Training Institutional Review Board Members

Jeffrey A. Cooper and Pamela Turner

INTRODUCTION

The Common Rule and Food and Drug Administration (FDA) regulations require that an institutional review board (IRB) "be sufficiently qualified through the experience and expertise of its members . . . to promote respect for its advice and counsel in safeguarding the rights and welfare of human subjects." [1][Sec.107(a)] Meeting this regulatory requirement requires initial and continuous training of IRB members. Institutions have been criticized for failing to provide training adequate to meet the needs of the IRB.

The IRB functions as a committee with a fund of communal knowledge. The regulatory requirement for IRB expertise applies to the entire IRB, not to each individual member. The regulations also note the requirement for experience, which in part can only be gained by serving on an IRB. Novice IRB members need to have a core understanding before participating in IRB functions, whereas more experienced members are expected to have a greater depth of knowledge. The regulations cited previously here also require that the IRB "shall be able to ascertain the acceptability of proposed research in terms of institutional commitments and regulations, applicable law, and standards of professional conduct and practice . . . if an IRB regularly reviews research that involves a vulnerable category of subjects, such as children, prisoners, pregnant women, or handicapped or mentally disabled persons, consideration shall be given to the inclusion of one or more individuals who are knowledgeable about and experienced in working with these subjects." Considering these requirements, three aspects of IRB-member training needs to be considered: (1) core knowledge required of all IRB members, (2) in-depth knowledge required of experienced IRB members, and (3) specialized knowledge required by specific IRB members.

Training for Core Knowledge Required of All IRB Members

Before participation in IRB review, IRB members should have an understanding of basic ethical principles, the regulatory requirements, and the mechanics of serving on the IRB. IRB staff may provide new IRB members with an orientation, may link new IRB members with an experienced IRB member as a mentor, or both. Regardless of the training method, all new IRB members should be provided with basic reference materials. Sources for these materials are listed, and some are reprinted in Part 11, *Reference Material and Contact Information*. All IRB members should receive and be familiar with a core list of guidance material. The following list should be modified to create a list of reference materials that matches the focus and scope of research reviewed by each IRB:

1. **Ethical Principles:** Nuremburg Code, Declaration of Helsinki, *The Belmont Report*
2. **Local Policies:** Federalwide assurances, IRB bylaws, institutional policies relevant to research, IRB standard operating procedures, investigator's manual
3. **DHHS Documents:** 45 CFR 46 DHHS Regulations, National Institutes of Health Policy on Inclusion of Women and Minorities, OPRR Report on Inclusion of Women and Minorities, National Institutes of Health Policy on Inclusion of Children, OPRR Report on Inclusion of Children, OPRR Compliance Activities: Common Findings and Guidance, Office for Human Research Protections (OHRP) IRB Guidebook, Research That May Be Reviewed Through an Expedited Review Procedure
4. **FDA Documents:** 21 CFR 50 and 56 (Basic FDA Regulations), 21 CFR 312 (FDA Drug Regulations), 21 CFR 812 (FDA Device Regulations), 21 CFR 10, 310, 314, and 320, FDA Information Sheets, Significant Differences in FDA and

DHHS Regulations for Protection of Human Subjects, Acute Care Waiver of Informed Consent reference, FDA Investigational Devices Exemption Manual

5. **Other Documents:** International Conference on Harmonisation Guidelines to Good Clinical Practice

At a minimum, all new IRB members should read *The Belmont Report* and be familiar with the basic applicable regulations governing the review of research by their IRB. Basic orientation can be conducted in one-on-one sessions or by videotape, Web-based presentations, or other formats. IRBs may also find it useful to use review checklists to guide new or experienced members in the review process.

Training for In-Depth Knowledge Required of Experienced IRB Members

All IRB members should have in-depth knowledge of the history and ethics of human subject protections and the regulations governing research in human subjects. A list of recommended topics follows:

History and Ethics

1. Ethical decision making (ethical theory, ethical principles, ethical rules, deductive and case-based reasoning, conflict, and incoherence)

2. History of research ethics (Nuremberg Code, Declaration of Helsinki, Public Health Service PHS policy, scandals such as the study of untreated syphilis in African American men, The National Commission on Biomedical and Behavioral Research, *The Belmont Report*)

3. *Belmont* principles (beneficence, respect for persons, and justice and derivative rules)

4. Applying research ethics to protocol review

5. Investigator–subject relationship (primary responsibility of investigator to protect rights, welfare, and safety of subjects)

6. Investigator–staff relationship (use of team management to maximize protection of subjects)

7. Current events (deaths of research subjects, recent research studies with questionable ethical basis, federal shutdowns of research, "hot topics")

8. IRB decision making (need for members to speak up and listen to minority views)

Regulations

1. Department of Health and Human Services regulations

2. FDA regulations

3. State and local regulations

Training Methods and Resources

IRB members can be provided with such training through a combination of resources. Less experienced members can be teamed with more experienced members in a mentor–trainee relationship. Information can be provided during a formal lecture series in an all-day session, distributed in small segments as part of each IRB meeting, or as part of a self-directed web-based, computer-based, or video-based teaching program. Members can participate in mock IRB review of hypothetical cases or actual papers with ethical issues. Members can be provided with articles from the literature relevant to IRB review. These articles can commonly be found in journals devoted to research ethics such as *IRB: A Review of Human Subjects Research* published by the Hastings Center, and medical journals such as the *New England Journal of Medicine*, the *Journal of the American Medical Association*, and the *British Medical Journal*. Over time, IRB members should be required to read all of the items in the reference materials.

Specialized Knowledge

Certain IRB members require specialized training. These members include the IRB chair and vice-chair, legal specialists, and advocates for populations served by the IRB such as prisoners, children, minority groups, non–English-speaking subjects, etc. These individuals should develop and maintain expertise beyond that of experienced IRB members. This expertise can be maintained through participation in regional or national meetings, participation in national discussion groups such as the IRB Forum, and review of publications. Publications with relevant literature include governmental publications such as OHRP and FDA guidance, reports of the National Bioethics Advisory Commission, books, and peer-reviewed literature.

Conclusion

IRB committee members must be trained to effectively conduct review of human subject research and protect the rights and welfare of human subjects. IRBs should consider training each member, appropriate to his or her level of expertise and experience, as a novice, experienced, or specialized member. Such training requires a multi-pronged approach that emphasizes initial and continuous training of all members.

Reference

1. Code of Federal Regulations. Title 45A—Department of Health and Human Services; Part 46—Protection of Human Subjects. Updated 1 October, 1997. Access date 18 April, 2001. http://www4.law.cornell.edu/cfr/45p46.htm

Investigator Training

Jeffrey A. Cooper and Pamela Turner

INTRODUCTION

The need for investigator training has become more apparent over the past several years, as indicated in a 1998 report published by the Office of the Inspector General. Investigators were found to have inadequate knowledge of their responsibilities in human subject research. Rules, based on the ethical principles of *The Belmont Report (Belmont)*, have been developed to guide investigators conducting human subject research.[1] The basic principles of *Belmont* include beneficence, respect for persons, and justice. The principle of beneficence requires that competent investigators design ethical research, protect human subjects from risk, and make continuing assessments of the risk/benefit ratio. The principle of respect for persons requires that researchers carry out the process of informed consent and protect subject privacy. The current Department of Health and Human Services (DHHS) regulations[2[Sec.103]] imply the need for investigator training by requiring that institutions assure the protection of human subjects in part through having competent investigators. Under Food and Drug Administration (FDA) regulations,[3[Sec.50]] sponsors are responsible for selecting qualified investigators and providing them with the information they need to conduct an investigation properly. However, there has been no uniform definition of the term *qualified*, and the process by which sponsors select and train investigators is highly variable. Because of the significance of the investigator's role in protecting human subjects, all institutional review boards (IRBs) are obligated to ensure that investigators conducting a research study are qualified to conduct the study, to uphold *Belmont* principles, and ensure compliance with the regulations and the requirements of the IRB in the approved protocol. The IRB may or may not need to conduct the actual training; however, in the current environment, investigator training commonly falls to the IRB. In this chapter, we outline the goals of training, discuss the methods available for training, summarize available resources, and provide information on how to implement investigator training.

Goals of Investigator Training

The ultimate goal of investigator training is to impart knowledge and understanding to an investigator that will result in behavior that protects the rights and welfare of research subjects. Proper training requires that investigators master four main objectives: (1) understand and apply the ethical principles underlying research; (2) put the rights, welfare, and safety of each individual enrolled in the research ahead of their professional, academic, financial, personal, or other interests; (3) meet organizational requirements and comply with all applicable federal, state, and local regulations; and (4) responsibly manage personnel involved in the research.

Understand and Apply the Ethical Principles Underlying Research

The *Belmont* principles form the basis for the protection of human subjects of research.[1] The first objective states that investigators should understand and apply these basic principles in research. Investigators should know what is involved within the study of ethics and see the ethical conduct of research as a virtue. They should be able to (1) carry out principle-based and case-based ethical decision making, (2) examine conflict and incoherence in research, (3) know the history leading to the formulation of the principles, (4) understand the relationship between the regulations and *Belmont* principles, and (5) apply those principles to protocol design and day-to-day practice of research.

Investigators should also be knowledgeable about recent history regarding subject deaths in research and unethical research.

Put the Rights, Welfare, and Safety of Each Individual Enrolled in the Research Ahead of Professional, Academic, Financial, Personal, or Other Interests

This is a corollary of the *Belmont* principle of beneficence and is described by some ethicists as a "moral fiduciary relationship."[4] Many investigators mistakenly consider their primary goal to be the execution of the protocol rather than the protection of their subjects. This objective identifies the need to manage conflict of interest and is required to maintain trust between investigators and subjects. We emphasize this objective because it has been neglected in the past.

Meet Organizational Requirements and Comply with All Applicable Federal, State, and Local Regulations

As part of this objective, IRBs should train investigators to do the following:

1. Design ethical research
2. Comply with federal regulations
3. Obtain IRB approval before implementing the research
4. Comply with IRB requirements
5. Implement approved research and obtain prior approval for modifications before implementing the change
6. Obtain and document informed consent/assent
7. Submit progress reports
8. Report unanticipated problems, injuries, and events
9. Retain records for required intervals

These obligations should be combined with other elements of appropriate data collection, documentation, and monitoring subsumed under the body of knowledge commonly referred to as "good clinical practice."

Responsibly Manage Personnel Involved in the Research

This objective requires that investigators understand that they are the leaders of a team of individuals responsible for the conduct of research. Investigators should ensure that the staff understands and acts according to the ethical principles governing research. As a team, it is paramount that they protect the rights and safety of research subjects and know and follow the policies and laws governing research. Investigators should ensure that the research team has adequate resources to carry out the research and that all personnel function as a team to ensure subject protection and regulatory compliance.

The issue of team management in research is important yet often overlooked. We and several other IRB administrators have found that many noncompliance investigations uncover a participant in the research, usually a research coordinator, who recognized the noncompliance issue, brought the information forward to the investigator, and was either brushed off or incorrectly assured that procedures were compliant. This is a well-described psychologic phenomenon known as the "response to authority" described in the ethically infamous Milgram Studies.[5] In the Milgram Studies, a principal investigator coaxed a participant to administer lethal electric shocks to a research subject, who was actually a member of the research staff (a confederate). Approximately two thirds of the participants delivered what they believed to be potentially lethal shocks to the confederate subject.

These authority relationships are common in research. They do not imply an authoritarian nature in the investigator, but rather an authoritative nature, or someone who is a respected leader with superior knowledge whom the staff looks to for guidance. The airline industry recognized in the mid-1980s that the authority position of the captain of the flight crew interfered with the functioning of the flight crew as a team to protect passenger safety. The airline responded with the implementation of crew training in "crew resource management."[6] This program is in part responsible for the dramatic improvement in airline safety in the past 15 years. The lessons of this program should be applied to the management of the research team and the leadership skills of investigators.

Training Methods

IRBs often view investigator training as an educational process wherein investigators gain knowledge from didactic teaching methods such as lectures, books, or computer-based training. However, this approach often overlooks two important issues. First, the goal of training should be to influence investigator behavior. In fact, the fundamental question of research ethics is "How ought researchers to behave?" Second, it is important to recognize that when it comes to professionals, education is often a relatively ineffective way to influence behavior. Therefore, in designing a training program, IRBs should consider a portfolio approach to improving investigator behavior and use multiple methods rather than relying on one particular method. There are five main methods for changing the behavior of professionals: performance feedback, rewards and penalties, participation in improving the process, administrative rules, and education. These methods are listed and discussed in decreasing order of effectiveness.[7]

Performance Feedback

The most effective way to influence a professional's behavior is through performance feedback. Auditing and monitoring are two methods of performance feedback commonly used by industry. We have implemented auditing and monitoring through a research quality assurance unit separate from the IRB. This separates the deliberative role of the IRB from its investigative functions, which may be perceived by investigators as intrusive. Auditing and monitoring are most effective when conducted as a collaborative learning experience. Generally, investigators want to be ethical and compliant, but often lack the objectivity to see their own shortcomings. When specific actions of noncompliance are pointed out and suggestions made for improvement of research operations, investigators are often very responsive.

Another form of performance feedback is to use monitored role playing and problem solving with group discussion, self-criticism, and feedback. This is the main method used for teaching crew resource management to commercial airline flight crews. Adding peer-based comparisons to performance feedback is often extremely helpful. Most investigators have a natural desire to excel, and when presented with data that show other investigators that have better outcomes, they often become highly motivated to improve their own practice. Peer-based feedback should be anonymous to protect the privacy of investigators.

Rewards and Penalties

The second most effective form of modifying investigator behavior is the use of administrative rewards and penalties. The FDA and the Office of Human Research Protections shutdowns of research represent an administrative penalty that has probably been a major influence on changing investigator behavior. The IRB's ability to bestow the right to conduct human subject research represents a powerful reward for investigators to participate in other training projects.

Participation in Improving the Process

The third most effective form of modifying investigator behavior is to involve investigators in improving the research process. To ensure built-in acceptance, whenever possible, encourage the input of investigators when planning any training program. They will often have specific needs, such as flexibility, or specific educational goals that can be accommodated in the design of the program.

Administrative Rules

Administrative rules, the mainstay of most IRB programs, do influence investigator behavior. Federal regulations, combined with local institutional policy, form the mainstay of these rules. Specific rules can be helpful in situations where issues of judgment or regulatory clarity arise. For example, institutions often develop administrative rules to determine what type of research is exempt from regulation or for prior clearance of emergency research, even though it is not required by regulation. Because investigators have different levels of knowledge, this is generally done to assure regulatory compliance. Institutions also will develop administrative rules for reporting adverse events because of the inconsistency and difficulty in interpreting various regulations. These administrative rules change behavior without the need to impart a high degree of knowledge and understanding on the part of investigators.

Education

Education represents the least effective method for changing physician behavior. Nonetheless, in many cases, education remains unavoidable in an effective training program. Investigators should have a core knowledge learned before conducting research. Even the implementation of administrative rules requires education to communicate the rules to all affected investigators.

Resources for Training

Numerous resources are currently available for training. These include books,[8] web-based training programs,[9] computer-based training programs,[10] lecture programs,[10] and independent consultants.[11,12] Each of these may need some customization to the needs of each IRB or institution. Most of these resources are educational, although independent consultants can provide help with performance feedback and establishing administrative rewards and punishments. The exact resources required will depend on an assessment of the internal strengths and weaknesses of each institution.

How to Implement Investigator Training

Successful implementation of an investigator training program requires more than having effective methods that lead to the desired behavioral objectives. For most investigators, the implementation of the training program represents a change from previous methods of doing business. Many investigators believe that they are too busy for further training, or they think they do not need it because they already have the knowledge required to conduct research. To change the mindset of these investigators requires understanding the principles of change management.[13] Effective change management involves three main steps. These steps will be required to implement a training program for research investigators.

Principles of Change Management

1. **Where and Why?** Create a compelling vision for the training program. Where will the training program lead? Why is it imperative that the training program be undertaken?

2. **Who and What?** Whom will the training program involve? What are the options for implementing the training program, and what are the preferences of the investigators?

3. **How and When?** What are the mechanics of the program? How will the training be conducted? What is the timeline for implementation?

Each step is best implemented with aggressive and repeated communication with investigators. We found that small, frequent "town meetings" with investigators in which a 10-minute presentation was made, followed by questions and answers, were very effective. The presentation was designed to explain the "where and why" of mandatory investigator training. The presentation explained the system of federal regulation of research, reviewed the recent enforcement actions of the DHHS and the FDA, explained our current training program, and emphasized that improved training was now an obligation of our DHHS assurance. We also acknowledged the negative perceptions of investigators and responded in order to minimize the impact of those negatives.

Investigators' Negative Perceptions of Training

1. **Unnecessary for Me.** We respond to the perception that training is "unnecessary for me" by emphasizing that the training actually is useful for every investigator.

2. **Not Enough Time.** Some investigators say that they do not have enough time to fulfill training requirements. We explain that training can be accomplished with a flexible time commitment.

3. **Unfunded Mandate.** Institutional officials and investigators may be concerned that ethical training is an unfunded mandate by the federal government. We explain that the recommended training program is inexpensive.

4. **Evaluations Are Unfair.** Investigators may be concerned that the focus of the training program or the evaluation of their performance in the training program is unfair. We respond that it is a self-directed training program that allows each investigator to focus on the areas that he or she is deficient in and to track progress personally.

Investigators' Positive Feedback

The town meetings were also an opportunity to explain to investigators the types of training programs initiated by other institutions, the options available to our institution, and to solicit feedback from investigators. This began the process of determining the "Who and What" in step 2. Several positive suggestions came out of those meetings and influenced the structure of the final program. For example, based on investigator suggestions we applied for and received category 1 American Medical Association continuing education credit. Several investigators believed that it was unfair to have to undergo training that would not be required of IRB members; in response, we asked IRB members to undergo the same training.

Notification of Investigators

After investigators are on board and accept the need for training and the method of training, final details need to be communicated clearly regarding the "how and when" step. We sent several direct communications to investigators; we also posted announcements in the medical center's weekly one-page newsletter. This step is important to minimize the number of investigators who claim that they were never notified about the training program or the implications associated with not completing the program.

Result of Change Program

In the end, our change program was very successful. We received many compliments from investigators about establishing a program that helped to educate them about the conduct of human subject research. The program has also increased the number of inquiries to the research office regarding regulatory compliance.

Conclusion

IRBs are now under a clear mandate from federal regulators to provide investigator training. Training currently focuses on education, but IRBs need to understand that the goal of training must be about behavior rather than just knowledge. Education is the least effective method to improve the behavior of investigators. IRBs have many resources available to them to accomplish training. However, IRBs should also understand that the greatest impediment to an effective training program is resistance on the part of investigators. They have to apply change management techniques in order to maximize the success of current and future training programs.

References

1. National Commission for the Protection of Human Subjects of Biomedical and Behavioral Research. *The Belmont Report: Ethical principles and guidelines for the protection of human subjects of research,* 18 April, 1979. Access date 22 March, 2001. http://ohsr.od.nih.gov/mpa/belmont.php3

2. Code of Federal Regulations. Title 45A—Department of Health and Human Services; Part 46—Protection of Human Subjects. Updated 1 October, 1997. Access date 18 April, 2001. http://www4.law.cornell.edu/cfr/45p46.htm

3. Code of Federal Regulations. Title 21, Chapter 1—Food and Drug Administration, DHHS; Part 312—Investigational New Drug Application. Updated 1 April, 1999. Access date 18 April, 2001. http://www4.law.cornell.edu/cfr/21p312.htm

4. McCullough LB. John Gregory (1724–1773) and the intervention of professional relationships in medicine. *J Clin Ethics* 8(1):11–21, 1997.

5. Milgram S. *Obedience to Authority.* New York: Harper Collins Publishers; 1983.

6. Industry Crew Resource Management. (CRM) Developers Group Web site, 2000. Access date 30 November, 2004. http://www.crm-devel.org/

7. Greco PJ, Eisenberg JM. Changing physicians' practices. *N Engl J Med* 329(17):1271–1273, 1993.

8. Dunn CM, Chadwick G. *Protecting Study Volunteers in Research: A Manual for Investigative Sites.* Boston: CenterWatch; 1999.

9. The Collaborative IRB Training Initiative (CITI) and the University of Miami. The Human Subjects Research Education Registration. Access date 30 November, 2004. http://www.miami.edu/UMH/CDA/UMH_Main/1,1770,4706-3,00.html

10. IRB 101 and 201 and Investigator 101 Training Programs. Boston, MA, Public Responsibility in Medicine and Research, 1999. Access date 30 November, 2004. http://www.primr.org/education/skill/irb.html

11. Impact Consulting Group. Access date 30 November, 2004. http://www.pwcglobal.com/

12. Price-Waterhouse-Cooper. Access date 16 April, 2001. http://www.pricewaterhouse.com/

13. O'Connor EJ, Fiol CM. *A road map for leading change: Energizers, barriers, and action steps. Culture Clash.* Chicago: American Hospital Publishing; 1997.

Accreditation of Human Research Protection Programs

Susan S. Fish

INTRODUCTION

Protection of human subjects has become a profession, both on an individual level and on an institutional level. Although there have been calls for peer review of institutional review boards (IRBs) since their inception, it is just now coming to fruition. This chapter discusses the history and reasons for accreditation in the human subjects protection field, describes the current status of accreditation, and discusses the implications for IRBs.

Background

Although protection of human subjects has been a keystone of clinical research for more than 50 years, thoughts of accreditation have only recently reached maturity. However, there have been calls for accreditation for more than 25 years. In 1978, the National Commission for the Protection of Human Subjects of Biomedical and Behavioral Research did more than issue *The Belmont Report* that gives us our ethical underpinnings for the conduct of clinical research. In their report, they also mentioned concern about requirements for the review of federally funded studies and the lack of requirements for review of all other studies. Such a double standard might suggest that IRBs are important only for meeting federal requirements rather than because of the nature of their work. Concerned about this apparent double standard, the National Commission in 1978 recommended that a program of peer-based site visits be undertaken.[1] They concluded that a full assessment of an IRB should be based on an examination of that IRB's performance in its particular institutional context and with its particular workload, membership, and procedures. The National Commission disbanded after its report was issued, and the President's Commission for the Study of Ethical Problems in Medicine and Biomedical and Behavioral Research was appointed. In 1981, the President's Commission decided to explore the possible benefits of IRB site visits to assess the qualitative aspects of the functioning of IRBs, suggesting that the site visits would be collegial and more educational in orientation than is typical of inspections or investigations. Two years later, the 1983 President's Commission Report included a chapter describing a study of IRBs, with the data having been gathered through peer-based site visits.[2] The report stated that site visits and a review process stimulate improvements at the institutional level. The Commission's site visitors were oriented more toward the goals and purposes of IRB review than toward technical conformity with regulatory requirements. The report then spent 12 pages discussing an accreditation model—in 1983, more than 20 years ago!

The Need for Accreditation

More recent reports from the General Accounting Office and the Inspector General's Office have also contained references to accreditation. The General Accounting Office in its 1996 report, *Scientific Research: Continued Vigilance Critical to Protecting Human Subjects*, stated that "little data exists that directly measures the effectiveness of human subject protection regulations." Thus, they suggested that protection of human subjects might be more than simply abiding by the regulations.[3] The Office of the Inspector General in 1998 issued a report entitled *IRBs—A Time for Reform* that recommended that all IRBs under the purview of the National Institutes of Health or OPRR (now the Office for Human Research Protections) and the Food and Drug Administration undergo regular performance-based evaluations. In addition, the evaluations were to be carried out in accord with the federal regulations.[4]

The lay press has had an equally important effect, continuing to highlight research activities as it has been doing for the past 30 or 40 years. For example, a cover story in the magazine *U.S. News and World Report* describes studies showing what appears to be a lack of informed consent by patients enrolled in cancer trials. This type of coverage in the lay press adds to the deterioration of the public's confidence and trust in the research effort. We must assure the public that its rights and welfare as research subjects are being protected, while we further the development of new diagnostic and therapeutic approaches to disease.

An Accreditation System

After more than 25 years of recommendations, why has the topic of accreditation only recently moved from discussion to action? First, the protection of human subjects has become a profession over the past 30 or so years. Public Responsibility in Medicine and Research is more than 30 years old, and Applied Research Ethics National Association is more than 20 years old. Applied Research Ethics National Association has developed a certification program for IRB professionals. Second, research has become more complex, and thus, it is more difficult to review studies and more difficult to design studies with risks minimized. In addition, it is more difficult to explain such complex studies to potential participants and, thus, more difficult for us to protect human subjects. Third, the patient empowerment movement has dramatically changed research. This movement is led mostly by HIV and cancer patient groups, and in some situations, subjects have become more like research partners than traditional research subjects. Finally, George Lundberg, the previous editor of *JAMA*, suggested "self-governance prevents legislation." There continues to be some suggestion that if we within the profession do not move forward on accreditation, then Congress may legislate such activities. Bills to increase regulatory oversight have been introduced into Congress every year for at least the last 5 years. For all of these reasons, and in order to help restore the trust of the public in the research effort, the beginning of the 21st century has been the right time to develop an accreditation system for programs of protection of human research subjects.

The Accreditation Programs: Similarities and Differences

To implement the accreditation program, two new organizations have been formed. The Association for the Accreditation of Human Research Protection Programs (AAHRPP) was born in 2000, from a beginning within Public Responsibility in Medicine and Research.[5] The Partnership for Human Research Protection (PHRP) was formed when the National Committee for Quality Assurance joined with the Joint Commission on Accreditation of Healthcare Organizations.[6] The National Committee for Quality Assurance had developed an IRB accreditation program for the Department of Veterans Affairs (VA) in 2001. That VA accreditation program was overhauled, and PHRP was born.

Both organizations strive to provide a process of voluntary peer review, as well as provide an opportunity for self-assessment. Each organization has a set of review standards that are publicly available on their respective websites. Both organizations focus on institutions within the United States. The AAHRPP states that organizations located in other countries may also apply. The PHRP states that it is currently developing a program for organizations that conduct research internationally. Both organizations have been active in providing guidance for

accreditation applicants and in providing education to the IRB community at large. Because human subjects protection is a shared responsibility, the accreditation process focuses on the entire program of protections, rather than just the IRB's processes and responsibilities. The accreditation standards are based on federal regulations. Both organizations offer accreditation for up to 3 years, with reapplication required after that time. Both organizations' fees may be seen as quite expensive if viewed as part of the IRB budget, but if seen as part of an organization's costs, they may be reasonable. There are many similarities between the AAHRPP and PHRP. However, it is their differences that distinguish them.

The AAHRPP describes five domains: institution, research review unit (including IRB), investigator, sponsored research, and participant outreach. Each standard has elements that describe how the standard is met. Although the standards are based on federal regulations and guidances, they go beyond the requirements of the regulations to encourage the development of "best practices" in protection programs. The applicant initially completes a self-assessment tool, which identifies inadequacies in the program, based on AAHRPP's standards. This allows the applicant to address inadequacies prior to application for accreditation. The AAHRPP also makes a preaccreditation consultation available. The application is submitted and reviewed, and a site visit occurs. There are over 70 site visitors who are volunteers drawn from the profession itself: IRB administrators, IRB chairs, institutional officials, and others affiliated with human subjects protection programs. Some come from institutions and organizations already accredited, whereas others are affiliated with organizations that have not yet entered the process. A list of site visitors can be found on the AAHRPP website. Accreditation results are confidential; the applicant may choose to make public the results of the accreditation process, and then AAHRPP will help publicize organizations that choose to make their status public. At the time of writing, there are 24 accredited human subjects protection programs listed on the AAHRPP website.

The PHRP also describes five areas in its standards: organizational responsibilities of the human research protection program, organizational responsibilities of the IRB, IRB structure and operations, consideration of risks and benefits, and informed consent. The process of assessment is similar in that there is a survey process that can allow the applicant to perform a self-assessment and address inadequacies identified. The survey is submitted as the application. Then there is an on-site survey conducted by PHRP surveyors. Surveyors are not identified on the PHRP website but are described as follows: a team of professionals active in the field of human research, with proven experience in human subject protections, and who have been individually and rigorously trained by PHRP. Accreditation results are not confidential; results of all surveyed organizations are listed, as well as a survey schedule of upcoming site visits. At the time of writing, there are nine accredited human subjects protection programs listed on the PHRP website.

Potential Benefits of Accreditation

The benefits of accreditation are just beginning to move beyond the theoretical, with a small but critical mass of organizations achieving accredited status. Many of the benefits still fall into the potential category. The most obvious benefit is that you can feel more confident that your organization is in compliance with the federal regulations and requirements after going through the accreditation process, both the self-assessment and the peer review. Accreditation does not mean that the FDA and the Office of Human Research Protections will not come knocking on your door, but your anxiety level may be lower if they do. The accreditation process requires an organizational approach, and this provides the IRB with opportunities to integrate and define an institution-wide human subjects protection program further. The peer-review process will help identify areas of excellence that can make the organization more competitive in many areas: attracting research funding, recruiting researchers, and recruiting subjects, to name a few.

Potential Costs of Accreditation

The most obvious cost is the application fee. The fee structures for both AAHRPP and PHRP are available on their websites. Less obvious, but possibly more costly, is the human effort necessary to prepare an application to either organization. Although this effort may decrease somewhat as more organizations become accredited and can share their best practices and helpful hints, many organizations have spent 6 to 12 months or more preparing an accreditation application. This results in time taken away from other improvements. Anecdotally, however, accredited organizations have said, "It was worth the effort."

Conclusion

By developing a set of performance standards and making these available to IRBs and human subject protection programs, the intent of accreditation is to help IRBs and human subjects protection programs do what they do better. The accreditation process is voluntary. An IRB, in conjunction with its institution and its researchers (its human subject protection program), has access to these performance standards. Self-assessment alone is a useful exercise and provides a framework to allow IRBs to determine where their strengths and weaknesses lie. If an institution's self-assessment is a positive one, it may decide that its program should apply for accreditation. The subsequent site visit will provide peer review and potential external validation of the self-assessment. In addition, the site visit will provide an outside source of new ideas for improvement and referral to other resources. If accredited, the IRB and its human research protection program can be identified to others as going beyond the federal regulations in protecting the rights and welfare of research subjects. It is hoped that this process of review—both self-assessment and peer review—will help to assure that the institutional value of protection of human subjects is instilled by the institutional official into all researchers and research staff. In addition, the IRB will have external, objective support for justifying the resources it needs to perform its important work.

References

1. National Commission for the Protection of Human Subjects of Biomedical and Behavioral Research. *The Belmont Report: Ethical Principles and Guidelines for the Protection of Human Subjects of Research*, 18 April, 1979. Access date 22 March, 2001. http://ohsr.od.nih.gov/mpa/belmont.php3

2. President's Commission for the Study of Ethical Problems in Medicine and Biomedical and Behavioral Research. *Implementing Human Research Regulations: Second Biennial Report on the Adequacy and Uniformity of Federal Rules and Policies, and of Their Implementation, for the Protection of Human Subjects.* March 1983.

3. General Accounting Office. *Scientific Research: Continued Vigilance Critical to Protecting Human Subjects.* GAO/HEHS-96-72. March 1996.

4. Office of Inspector General. *Institutional Review Boards: A Time for Reform* (OEI-01-97-00193). Department of Health and Human Services, June 1998. Access date 27 March, 2001. http://www.dhhs.gov/progorg/oei/reportindex.html

5. Association for the Accreditation of Human Research Protection Programs. Access date 22 June, 2005. http://www.aahrpp.org/

6. Partnership for Human Research Protections, Inc. Access date 22 June, 2005. http://www.phrp.org/

Certification of Institutional Review Board Professionals

Susan J. Delano, Sallyann Henry, and Gary L. Chadwick

INTRODUCTION

Certification is one part of a process called credentialing. It focuses on the individual and is an indication of current proficiency in a specialized field. It is a formal recognition that an individual has met the professional experience requirements and demonstrated understanding of a specific body of knowledge at a level sufficient to meet established standards. Certification is usually granted by a professional group and is a form of peer recognition rather than registration or licensure, which are legally mandated. Certification is not, however, an endorsement of particular individuals by the professional group, nor is it a guarantee of qualification to do a particular job.

Certification of persons who conduct research and are responsible for its review and monitoring have been discussed and supported at the national level by groups including the National Bioethics Advisory Commission and the Secretary's Advisory Committee on Human Research Protections.[1,2] In addition to institutional review board (IRB) professionals, research administrators and research monitors have well-established certification programs. Certification is increasingly being recognized as an important part of an effective human subjects protection program.

What Are the Benefits of Certification?

National certification of professionals involved in research assists the public, legislators, and sponsors by offering a standard for professional knowledge. It helps assure adherence to regulatory requirements, good clinical practices, and ethical principles. National certification enhances the employer's program and demonstrates support of professional standards.

For the individual, certification can provide a sense of professional accomplishment, enhancement of professional standing, and peer recognition. It identifies the individual as possessing technical expertise and demonstrates a commitment to professionalism. Certification may also serve as a valuable career tool by confirming value to current employers and by making one's resume more appealing to a prospective employer.

For a profession, certification can help to raise competency through the education and training in which individuals participate while preparing for initial testing and for renewal. It can also help set national standards of performance within the profession by analyzing the functions performed by professionals in the field, creating a "body of knowledge" based on these functions, and setting expectations for proficiency.

How a Certification Program Is Developed

In the credentialing process, many issues must be addressed, including who should be credentialed, what experience and qualifications are required, and what methods of credentialing and renewal will be used. Examinations must provide an objective measure of candidates' knowledge. Creating a valid examination process that will be respected by those in the profession and also by the community they serve is complex and includes a number of important steps.

The following describes an approach that has been used for the Certified IRB Professional (CIP) program. The CIP program is designed for individuals who have experience participating in and overseeing the daily activities associated with an IRB.

The first step in the process is establishing a credentialing board or council of experienced practitioners to oversee and develop the credentialing program. The council then develops and publishes the body of knowledge based on the skills and abilities needed for competent performance. Next, preliminary examination questions are written by a broad-based group of practitioners and edited by psychometric specialists. These questions are then reviewed by certified practitioners. Each question is considered to assess its accuracy, the correctness of the designated right answer, the incorrectness of the other answers (called distracters), and the clarity of the meaning of the question. Most importantly, this review evaluates whether each question deals with something that is directly relevant to the practice of the profession. Development of questions is an ongoing activity with new items continually required.

Draft examinations are then developed using questions that have gone through the review process. Each examination is reviewed by the council to ensure quality and ongoing validity. Each question is reviewed to ensure that it is currently relevant, accurate, and appropriate. The overall content of the examination is reviewed to ensure that it covers the material specified in the body of knowledge. A passing score is established based on sound psychometric standards.

How Do You Prepare for a Certification Examination?

Practicing the profession builds a base of skills and experience, but many candidates wish to polish that knowledge in preparation for a certification examination. As with any test, awareness of the content areas that will be covered is essential. The certifying organization provides a handbook for candidates, which includes the body of knowledge that will be covered and lists suggested references. For the CIP exam, it may be helpful to begin with basic regulatory documents and federal guidance documents. Other standard references and texts that are usually found in the IRB library, and Internet sources can be very useful. References that provide background and context to the subject area should be reviewed. For example, for IRB professionals, the history and the development of codes of ethics for human subjects research provide important background. Of course, consultation with professionals who are currently certified can be asked for advice on how to prepare.

Conclusion

A defining characteristic of a profession is a system of credentialing that indicates familiarity with a body of knowledge in a specialized field. The administration of an IRB has now reached a level of complexity and sophistication that makes it necessary and appropriate to have a meaningful certification process for IRB professionals. This chapter describes the general characteristics of a credentialing process and the details of the process that is currently used by the CIP program. Completing a high-quality credentialing program ensures that IRB professionals will share a core body of knowledge in a way that will improve the protection of research participants and facilitate productive interaction between all segments of the IRB community.

References

1. National Bioethics Advisory Commission. *Ethical and Policy Issues in Research Involving Human Participants.* Draft report. Bethesda, MD: U.S. Government Printing Office; 19 December, 2000. Access date 5 October, 2004. http://bioethics.gov/reports/past_commissions/nbac_human_part.pdf

2. Secretary's Advisory Committee on Human Research Protections, Meeting Minutes 29 March, 2004. Access date 5 October, 2004. http://www.hhs.gov/ohrp/sachrp/mtgings/mtg03-04/min0329.pdf

Preparing for a Food and Drug Administration Audit

Gary L. Chadwick

INTRODUCTION

The focus of this chapter is on Food and Drug Administration (FDA) inspections. The FDA operates a Bioresearch Monitoring Program, which conducts routine audits for institutional review boards (IRBs), and thus, IRBs are more likely to experience an FDA audit than one from other agencies. There are commonalities between audits, whether they are conducted by the FDA, the National Cancer Institute, the Joint Commission on Accreditation of Health Care Organizations (JCAHO), or any other entity.

The Audit Process

The FDA conducts audits of research to determine compliance with regulations and to verify the integrity of the data. Audits of IRBs determine compliance with the human subject protection regulations. Inspections are assigned by the Center for Drug Evaluation and Research, the Center for Biologics Evaluation and Research, or the Center for Devices and Radiological Health. Assignments to inspect IRBs are made for routine surveillance, for follow-up of complaints or concerns, and as part of the product approval process. The on-site audit is generally conducted by one or more field personnel from the local district office. Sometimes experts from FDA headquarters will accompany the field inspectors.

Ongoing Preparations

Readiness is the key to a good outcome. A phrase that you may hear at health care facilities is "survey-ready every day," referring to preparation for JCAHO audits. This phrase indicates that your policies and procedures are up-to-date and in order. Therefore, an audit is likely to show that you are operating correctly and that no major problems exist. Research institutions should strive toward continual readiness.

Conduct Internal Audits

A good way to assess readiness for an external audit is to conduct self-audits. The FDA has published a useful checklist in the FDA Information Sheets[1] that can be used for this purpose (available from the FDA website). Targeted internal audits are very helpful, especially if you think that you may have vulnerability in specific areas. It is always better to find something wrong yourself and fix it than to have someone else find it and put it in a report as a deficiency. When conducting self-audits, always document the audit activity both in the files reviewed and in a final report. If you find things wrong, the report should state what you have done, are doing, or are recommending to correct the problem. The report should be a useful tool both for the IRB and for institutional officials who have responsibility for the IRB.

Review FDA and Office for Human Research Protections Letters to Other Institutions

One of the best things you can do to anticipate inspection findings is to get copies of warning letters issued to other facilities. These letters are available to the public on the FDA's website.[2] The letters show what types of deficiencies are of concern. The Office for Human Research Protections (OHRP) also displays letters and cited deficiencies on its website.[3]

Maintain Adequate IRB Staffing

One of the major keys to successful IRB operation and therefore a good audit outcome is adequate staffing. The IRB function requires sufficient numbers of qualified personnel so that the review process operates in compliance, the necessary documentation is maintained, and the research is adequately tracked through the review cycle. Lack of staff and/or lack of qualified staff are a root cause of failure to pass an IRB audit.

IRB Written Procedures

Your written procedures along with the federal regulations will drive the inspection. The FDA does not accept an assurance of compliance document in place of written procedures. The FDA expects written procedures to describe how the institution complies with the regulations. The written procedures should be reviewed annually and updated as procedures and policies change. A revision log or at least a record of the revision dates on the title page is recommended. Again, this shows that you are keeping current and are in control of your program.

Notification and Preparation for Audit

Although the FDA may conduct an unannounced IRB inspection, usually they notify the institution by telephone in advance. By law, the FDA has the right to inspect at reasonable times with reasonable notice. For IRBs, reasonable notice is generally 2 to 3 days. Clinical investigators often get a notice a week or more in advance because the FDA does not expect that the investigator's office will be staffed and organized at the same level as is an administrative office such as the IRB.

FDA field inspectors will try to accommodate legitimate requests to postpone an audit (for example, if the IRB chair and administrator are both away at a training conference). Usually, only a couple of days' reprieve is acceptable.

Ask About Special Materials and Contact Numbers
After you confirm when the inspection will start (day and hour), ask how long the audit is anticipated to take so that you can make appropriate arrangements. It is also a good idea to ask whether there are any special materials or specific files the auditors would like to have available. Be sure to obtain contact information in case something comes up before the audit starts.

Alert Appropriate Institutional Authorities
As soon as possible after the notification call, you should alert the appropriate institutional authorities. Obviously, other IRB office staff, the IRB chair, and board members need to be alerted, as does the institutional official (IO) (the person who signed the institutional assurance document) and the chain of command. Collateral offices, such as the legal office and the grants management office, also may need to be informed.

Have Senior Officials Available
Any audit is important, but inspections from federal or state regulators are doubly so. The institution should prepare and respond as if the audit could shut down research at the institution (it has at some institutions). Senior officials should be available for interviews with the inspectors as well as quick consultations with the IRB staff during the audit. These senior officials need to understand and be able to articulate the importance of the function and the operation of the IRB within the institutional structure.

Have Files Organized and Readily Available
FDA audits are often linked to a specific study or studies. If you know in advance that a specific study is to be reviewed, be sure the clinical investigator and the sponsor are aware of the audit. They should ensure that their study files agree with the IRB files and that they are organized for the audit. Be sure that all the paperwork is in both files and that you can find all your study files. You may need to

get them back from reviewers or at least know who has the files and where they are.

Organize IRB Office Documents
The auditor will want to review the IRB written procedures; thus, put them on a special shelf in the room that will be used or on a cart if you will be using shared space. If you have not done so recently, it is a good idea to give the procedures a quick review just to be sure that nothing is out of date or missing. It is always a good idea to review copies of manuals and other documents that you will give to the investigator to make sure they are up to date and complete, with no pages or sections missing.

Prepare an Organizational and Personnel Chart
A table of organization (personnel chart) is very helpful for auditors. If the staffing pattern of the IRB and how the function fits into the institution's overall operations (reporting lines, etc.) are not part of the written procedures, this information should be provided as a separate document. Also, print out the IRB membership rosters for the past 3 or 4 years. The auditor will need these rosters to check against meeting attendance to ensure that a quorum was maintained at all meetings.

Organize the IRB Minutes
Gather the meeting minutes in a notebook or file and put them on the shelf or cart. Most auditors will want to see minutes for at least 1 year. Sometimes minutes for 2 or 3 years are requested; thus, be prepared. Again, check to be sure that the minutes are up to date. If the minutes are a couple of meetings behind, get them typed. If you have some that need to be approved and they will not be before the inspection, label them as "draft."

Prepare a Workspace for the Auditor
When selecting a workspace, do not put the inspector in the IRB workflow area. It is disruptive for both. In addition, the auditor may see you doing something that raises questions; problems have the tendency to crop up at the most inopportune moments. A private office or conference room is best. If you need to schedule an off-site room, keep it reasonably close to the IRB offices. For security, the space should be lockable, or the files and materials will have to be returned to the IRB office whenever the room is not occupied.

The workspace should be available for the full inspection time. Although most inspectors will accommodate some moving around because of a meeting or other need for the room, it is an inconvenience for them and it should be avoided if possible. The room you choose should have a table and comfortable chairs. Office supplies (e.g., stapler and paper clips) are not required, but are usually appreciated. The room should have space for three or four people to meet comfortably with the auditor.

Access to a Copy Machine
Auditors may be given unrestricted access to a copier if they will agree to make you copies of whatever they copy. Alternatively, you can make the copies they request and make copies for yourself, too. Either of these methods is

usually acceptable but should be agreed on at the beginning of the audit.

Access to a Telephone

Give the auditors access to a telephone. If they have a question and want to call someone about it, it is usually to your advantage for them to do so. FDA field investigators are generally not IRB experts, and thus, they may need to call headquarters to check on something unique to your site or to a study they are reviewing.

Commit Staff to Facilitate the Audit Visit

The time necessary for these preparations will be significant, and additional help may be needed to get things in order before the inspection starts. Everyone in the institution should realize the importance of having a good outcome, and thus, you should be able to draw on institutional resources. If you need to delay the protocol review process a couple of days to focus on the inspection, your investigators should understand. If you need to hire some temporary employees or reassign some personnel to help, your administration should support the expenditure and the conscription. The need for temps may be a sign that the IRB is understaffed.

During the inspection itself, the IRB staff and chair should plan on spending additional hours in the office. Time will be needed to prepare before the auditors arrive each day, and time will be needed at the end of each day for debriefing, finding requested information, and preparing notes, reports, or briefings. A short meeting with key institutional officials for debriefing and planning should be scheduled after the inspector leaves each day.

One person should be designated as the key contact for the auditor. This person will answer the inspector's questions and respond for the institution. Usually, this is the senior IRB administrator or the IRB chair.

The Inspection

Notice of Inspection (FDA Form 482)

When the inspector arrives, a "Notice of Inspection" will be given to the institution's representative (FDA Form 482). It contains the name of the inspector and the address of the inspector's district office. It also contains the preprinted standard terms of inspection. This form should be the first piece of paper put in the audit file, which is your record of the inspection.

Prepare a Notebook Containing FDA Correspondence

You should store your notes on the inspection and copies of all documents that the FDA inspector has copied in the audit file, folder, or notebook. It is very important to have exactly the same records that the FDA has taken so that you can accurately respond to any queries they might have later.

Review Documentation of the Auditor's Credentials

Along with presenting the Form 482, the inspectors will show you their credentials, verifying that they are from the FDA and that they have a legal right to have access to your records. In the unlikely event that the inspectors don't show their credentials, you should ask to see them. Remember that you are responsible for maintaining the security of your records. If you have any doubt about the legitimacy of the inspector's credentials or questions about the inspection procedures, you should call the district office listed on the Form 482.

The Orientation Presentation

After the inspector completes this identification and notification step and makes any introductory remarks about the audit, usually a brief orientation to your system is requested. This overview is given to the auditor by the most knowledgeable person or persons, usually the IRB administrator and/or the IRB chair. If there are unique aspects of your system or in how things are done, this is the time to explain them. This is also a good time to point out where the restrooms are and where the cafeteria and/or vending machines are located. If you normally have coffee or drinks and food available to staff, you may make it available to the inspectors, but providing such amenities is not required. In fact, FDA's conflict of interest rules prohibit acceptance of anything but light refreshments.

Request a "Mini Exit Review" at the End of Each Day

In the orientation presentation, you should ask for an update at the end of each day. This "mini exit review" helps to ensure that there are no surprises. This strategy often prevents being cited for something that was easily remediable. Some inspectors are uncomfortable with daily updates and if so, do not push it; they are not required to provide this service. Most will, however, and they usually appreciate the chance to clear their questions and problem areas. This also provides an opportunity for them to set the next day's agenda to facilitate gathering documents and scheduling people and rooms. It is a good idea to brief senior management after the daily exit interview and begin the planning for any necessary institutional corrective actions.

IRB Procedures, Membership Roster, and Minutes

Inspectors will always ask for the IRB written procedures, the IRB membership roster, and the IRB meeting minutes, so these should be ready beforehand. These documents will be reviewed and copied for forwarding to FDA headquarters. Note that the FDA does not accept an assurance of compliance document in place of written procedures. They are looking for your standard operating procedures, which are explanations of how you carry out the obligations and promises made in the assurance.

Study Files

Study files will be read by the inspector, and portions will be copied for later analysis. The review of study files usually comprises the majority of the audit. One of the best protective mechanisms for the site, if time permits, is to review the requested study files before they are handed over and place-mark (with tape flags or stickers) important letters and reports. This would include items such as the initial approval letter, continuing review approval letters, the current approved consent form, the protocol, progress reports, and communications with the investigator. This advance organization is intended to make it easier for the auditor and to be sure that the file is complete.

Record a List of Audit Interviews

At some point during the audit, the inspector will usually interview the IRB staff and the IRB chair to see how things actually work. They will compare the verbal explanations with how the functions are described in the written procedures. It is a good idea to keep a list of who meets with the inspector so that if questions arise later, you can go back to the source. Some institutions even keep notes on such interviews or conduct a postmeeting debriefing. These lists and notes should go into the audit file so that they are available when responding to later inquiries.

Observation of an IRB Meeting

If your IRB is scheduled to meet during the inspection, members should be prepared to have the auditor sit in. Not all inspectors will ask, but some will. General wisdom is not to offer if you are not asked, but some institutions may want to showcase their IRB if it is truly first-rate. Just remember the adage, "Whatever can go wrong, will go wrong—and at the worst possible time."

The Exit Interview

At the conclusion of the inspection, an exit interview will be conducted. You should gather the appropriate persons to participate. Such people would include the IRB administrator, the IRB chair, and the IO. Who attends should be guided by the tone of the daily summaries and by the scope of the responses that may be needed.

At the exit interview, you will be told what deficiencies were found. This may be just an oral summary, or they may be in writing on FDA Form 483. Basically, the Form 483, called the "Statement of Findings," is a blank page; anything can be written. Often, serious violations will be mixed in with lesser infractions. If a Form 483 is issued, usually each item that is listed will be reviewed. You should not argue with the inspector, however, it is appropriate to request clarification of items that you do not understand, and the inspectors should correct factual errors. Remember that inspectors may not be IRB experts, and sometimes they do misinterpret what they see.

If there has been an earlier indication from questions, comments, or the daily summaries that a major problem exists and if a preliminary plan for correction has been developed (as it should be), it can be offered. Remember that the Form 483 is only a preliminary finding—do not overreact. You should understand, however, why each observation was listed. Unless no Form 483 is issued, tell the inspector that you will send a written response in 7 to 10 days. This allows them to expect it so that they can include your response with their report.

The Establishment Inspection Report

After returning to the District Office, the inspector will write an "Establishment Inspection Report" or EIR, which contains both positive and negative observations. The EIR with all of the documentation collected from your site is sent to the FDA center that assigned the audit

for review and comment. If you have sent a letter in response to the audit, it will also be included.

Postinspection Activities

After the auditor leaves, review the audit notebook or file and ensure that copies of all documents that the inspector made and any staff notes that were taken are included. Write up the exit interview. (You can assign someone to take notes during the exit interview.) You should have a meeting with the appropriate institutional people to discuss the audit and to decide what needs to be corrected immediately.

The institution should develop a plan of correction and send it to the inspector's district office. The letter should be focused on those items that you can fix or have fixed. Send along any missing documents that you have found. You may dispute regulatory interpretations, especially if you know the inspector's interpretation is in conflict with agency guidance or even general wisdom. You can point out items cited on a Form 483 that are not based on regulations. (Having someone on staff who is an expert on the regulations is helpful.) Keep the tone of the letter respectful and factual.

Postinspection Letters and Response

Your institution will receive a letter from the FDA headquarters. Usually, the greater the FDA's concern (i.e., the longer the list on the Form 483), the faster the letter will arrive. The exit interview usually gives you some indication of the potential level of concern.

The FDA will expect the institution to have made progress on any major deficiencies by the time that you receive the postinspection letter from their headquarters.

The FDA's experts at the centers write the follow-up letters, and thus, argument about regulatory interpretation is rarely successful. Be very careful and sure of your position if you do choose to dispute items in these letters. Remember that everyone's goal is to ensure compliance and protection of human subjects.

A Voluntary Action Letter Versus a Warning Letter

The FDA issues two types of letters when deviations are found. Voluntary action indicated (VAI) letters simply ask for the correction of minor deficiencies found. If you receive a VAI letter, respond by explaining what you have done and/or what you are doing to fix the problem. Keep it short, but address all concerns raised in the FDA letter. This will usually close the process as far as the FDA is concerned.

Official action indicated (OAI) letters demand correction of what the FDA believes to be serious deficiencies and/or violations of the regulations. These letters are called warning letters. Often, they carry some type of sanction for the institution and its investigators.

Warning Letters

Warning letters must be taken very seriously. Explain how you have or will comply with any sanction. Explain what you have done and what you are going to do immediately to address the identified problems. Explain your long-range plans for ensuring that the problems stay fixed. Remember that the institution has had notice of the deficiencies since the time the Form 483 was issued, and thus, the FDA's letter should not be a complete surprise. Therefore, only having plans is not as acceptable as demonstrating progress; the institution needs to show reasonable action to correct deficiencies. The FDA will remain in contact with the institution until corrections are satisfactory.

After the deficiencies have been corrected and the case is closed, it is time to start preparing for the next audit. Keep the files and records up-to-date. Look for ways to improve IRB practices. Keep the staff and IRB members current by sending them to conferences and meetings.

Investigator Inspections

Investigator inspections are similar in format to IRB inspections. The FDA conducts two types of investigator inspections. These are called study-oriented and investigator-oriented inspections. (They used to be called routine and for-cause inspections.)

Study-Oriented Inspections

Study-oriented inspections are done at study sites that have participated in pivotal clinical trials. Pivotal trials are those that the FDA uses to approve drugs and devices for marketing. It is important that investigators let IRBs know when they are to be inspected because normally both the investigator and the IRB will be audited.

Investigator-Oriented Inspections

Inspections that are investigator oriented are usually the result of one or more reports of questionable behavior or of questions that have been raised. The FDA's suspicion index is raised for investigators who conduct studies outside of their specialty areas, conduct a large number of studies, enroll large numbers of subjects (especially in a short time), or have results that differ from the norm. Complaints from research subjects are taken very seriously by the FDA, and they usually result in at least a written inquiry if not a full audit.

Recently, an increasing number of investigator inspections have been triggered by sponsors reporting that they have concerns about the quality of the data received, or because the information flow is not sufficient for the sponsor to meet its obligations for reporting to the FDA.

Investigator inspections of either type usually focus on the review of research records for one or more specific studies. These records include source documents such as medical records, laboratory results, and tracings; case report forms; signed consent forms; IRB approvals; and other communications and correspondence. The FDA's watchwords for clinical investigators are "If it isn't documented, it didn't happen."

Inspection Activities

The actions that an investigator should take when notified of an FDA inspection are similar to those described previously here for an IRB audit. That is, the sponsor, institutional officials, and institutional offices—especially the IRB—should be notified. The investigator should ensure that records are complete and accessible. Again, a reasonable workspace should be provided, and key team members who participated in the research study should be available. It is critical for the investigator to be available during the inspection.

Resources

There are some resources available to IRBs and investigators to prepare for audits. The FDA publishes two documents as part of its *Compliance Program Guidance Manual*. "Compliance Program 7348.809"[4] is for use in IRB audits. The other is for clinical investigator inspections and is entitled "Compliance Program 7348.811."[4] Both are available by writing the FDA or visiting the FDA website. Guidance on operating an IRB and investigator responsibilities is available in the FDA Information Sheets.[5]

Conclusion

Although audits may not be fun, they need not be dreaded, especially if you are ready for them and know what to expect. Preparation and constant fine-tuning are keys to having a successful audit and a program that truly protects the rights and welfare of human subjects of research.

References

1. Food and Drug Administration. A self-evaluation checklist for IRBs. Updated 16 April, 2001. Access date 9 August, 2004. http://www.fda.gov/oc/ohrt/irbs/irbchecklist.html

2. Food and Drug Administration. Electronic freedom of information reading room, 12 March, 2001. Access date 9 August, 2004. http://www.fda.gov/foi/warning.htm

3. Office for Human Research Protections. OHRP compliance activities: Common findings and guidance, 10 July, 2002. Access date 7 August, 2004. http://www.hhs.gov/ohrp/compliance/findings.pdf

4. Food and Drug Administration. Office of Regulatory Affairs compliance references: Bioresearch monitoring, 21 February, 2001. Access date 1 August, 2004. http://www.fda.gov/ora/compliance_ref/bimo/7348_810/default.htm

5. Food and Drug Administration. Information sheets: Guidance for institutional review boards and clinical investigators, September 1998. Access date 4 August, 2004. http://www.fda.gov/oc/ohrt/irbs/default.htm

Preparing for an Office for Human Research Protections Site Visit

Thomas Puglisi and Michele Russell-Einhorn

INTRODUCTION

The Office for Human Research Protections (OHRP) has three statutory responsibilities under the U.S. Public Health Service Act: the administration of assurances, education, and compliance oversight. The OHRP conducts site visits in connection with the latter two responsibilities.

Education

The OHRP maintains a very active Quality Improvement Program (QIP) in addition to a number of other educational activities, including National Conferences and Community Forums. The OHRP's QIP "is intended to help institutions evaluate and improve the quality of their human research protections program."

The centerpiece of the QIP is a "Guided Self Assessment" through which an institution uses OHRP's Quality Assurance Self Assessment Tool to evaluate its human research protection program. The institution can then request a consultation with staff from OHRP's Division of Education and Development. The consultation can be held on-site or by video or audio conference, depending on the institution's preferences and OHRP's availability.

If the consultation is held on-site, it usually lasts for about a day and a half and includes interviews with the Assurance Signatory Official, research investigators, and the institutional review board (IRB) chair(s), members, and staff. Record reviews, a question and answer session, and an exit interview typically round out the visit.

The emphasis for this type of consultative visit is collegiality and constructive guidance.

Compliance Oversight

OHRP exercises its compliance oversight responsibility by conducting investigations of all credible allegations or indications of noncompliance that come to its attention. Corrective actions may be required under the institution's Federalwide Assurance or other assurance of protection for human subjects that each institution must maintain in order to conduct Department of Health and Human Services (DHHS)–supported human subject research.

The OHRP may receive information about possible noncompliance from a research subject or family member who has complaints about a research project, from a whistle blower who alleges noncompliance, from the funding agency, from institutional self-reports, via the media, or through review of the published literature.

In most cases, the OHRP is able to reach determinations regarding the alleged noncompliance and the institution's systemic protections for human subjects through an exchange of correspondence and review of relevant policies, procedures, and records. Corrective actions may or may not be required of the institution in connection with OHRP's determinations. In certain cases, however, the OHRP may need to conduct an on-site evaluation to determine whether noncompliance has occurred and whether specific or systemic corrective actions are warranted.

Most OHRP compliance oversight visits occur "for cause" within the context of an ongoing compliance investigation. However, the OHRP does from time to time conduct "not-for-cause" compliance oversight visits that have not been precipitated by a complaint or a report of possible noncompliance. For example, OHRP's site visit to Duke University in the late 1990s was a "not-for-cause" compliance oversight evaluation that was not precipitated by a prior complaint.

Compliance oversight visits are usually announced to the institution at least 1 to 2 weeks before OHRP's arrival. However, there is nothing that prohibits the OHRP from conducting unannounced site visits. If the circumstances of an OHRP inquiry suggested the need for an unannounced "surprise" visit, there is no doubt that the OHRP could and would exercise that option.

The Importance of Prevention

Any institution with a significant volume of DHHS–sponsored human subjects research will sooner or later experience an OHRP compliance oversight evaluation, perhaps including a site visit. The best strategy in preparing for such an event is to invest in long-term prevention. If the institution has maintained a strong, well-resourced human research protection program, it should be in a good position to deal with any compliance oversight evaluation or site visit. Proactive monitoring, adequate resources, and well-designed training programs all contribute to a strong system of protections capable of withstanding close scrutiny.

Thus, the preparation for an OHRP compliance oversight evaluation or site visit begins long before the investigation or site visit is announced. Perhaps the most common source of problems in the protection of human subjects is the institutional failure to maintain a well-resourced and well-trained IRB and to establish a culture in which all research investigators understand and take seriously their responsibilities for protecting human subjects.

The era is long past in which an institution can rely on an occasional memorandum to investigators about human subject protections and populate its IRB with untrained members supported by a clerical assistant. In today's world, it is critically important for the IRB to be supported by one or more certified IRB professionals who can provide expert advice and guidance to IRB members and investigators. Sufficient support staff must be provided to fulfill the IRB's growing record-keeping responsibilities. IRB members and research investigators must be well trained on a continuing basis.

One cannot overemphasize the importance of maintaining the knowledge and expertise of IRB members and staff through continuing education. The IRB chair, members, and professional staff should participate regularly in human research protection conferences sponsored by Public Responsibility in Medicine & Research and the Applied Research Ethics National Association, as well as in the regional workshops sponsored by OHRP and the local, regional, and national meetings sponsored by other groups. Regular participation in *The IRB Forum* and enrollment in the OHRP listserve are also important resources for staying up-to-date. Any institution whose IRB members and support professionals become isolated from the national IRB community runs the risk of maintaining an outdated program that will eventually get into regulatory trouble.

Responding to OHRP Compliance Oversight Investigations

The typical OHRP compliance site visit takes place within a compliance oversight investigation. It follows an OHRP inquiry to an institution concerning an allegation of noncompliance and receipt by the OHRP of the institution's response to the allegation. It is not uncommon for this initial exchange to be followed by additional questions from the OHRP and additional responses from the institution. The OHRP will schedule a compliance site visit if concerns about the allegation, and especially about the institution's systemic protections for human subjects, cannot be resolved through correspondence.

Just as the best strategy for avoiding an OHRP compliance investigation is to maintain a vigorous and well-resourced institutional program for protecting human subjects, the best strategy for avoiding an OHRP compliance site visit is to respond candidly and constructively to any OHRP compliance inquiry.

The OHRP's first step in evaluating an allegation of noncompliance is to present the allegation to the responsible institution and request that the institution investigate the allegation and provide the OHRP with a detailed report on its investigation, including appropriate documentation such as the IRB protocol file and other relevant records. At this time, the OHRP will also request copies of institutional policies and procedures for protecting human subjects.

After receipt of such a request, the institution should investigate the alleged noncompliance as thoroughly and objectively as possible. If the allegation is complicated or sensitive, it may be important to obtain the assistance of one or more external consultants in obtaining an objective analysis of the situation. At the same time, the institution should complete a self-assessment of its systemic protections for human subjects. Again, the assistance of external consults is often helpful in ensuring an objective assessment.

After the institution has obtained an objective understanding of the circumstances relevant to the allegation and an objective assessment of the adequacy of its systemic human subjects protections, it should report its findings to the OHRP in a straightforward and honest manner. If the allegation has been substantiated and/or if systemic deficiencies have been identified, the institution should present the OHRP with a detailed corrective action plan to address any shortcomings.

The OHRP's response to a candid and complete report of deficiencies accompanied by a substantive and detailed corrective action plan is inevitably positive. The OHRP has no authority to impose civil or criminal penalties for past noncompliance (although it will refer findings to other government agencies with such authority where appropriate). Rather, the OHRP's mission and authority focus on ensuring satisfactory protections for present and future human subjects. An institutional response that acknowledges past deficiencies and outlines a rigorous timetable for appropriate corrective action permits the OHRP to move on to other investigations at institutions where subjects may be at greater risk.

The Format for OHRP Compliance Site Visits

OHRP's compliance site visits are usually conducted by a team of two to five OHRP professionals and two to five external consultants. Consultants typically include at least one IRB expert (often an IRB chair and/or an experienced IRB administrator) and may include experts in particular scientific areas, depending on the nature of the allegation involved.

OHRP compliance site visits are usually announced to the assurance signatory official both orally (by telephone) and in writing (by letter) about 2 to 4 weeks in advance of the visit. If logistics permit, the OHRP occasionally invites the institution to choose from two sets of possible dates. More often, however, competing OHRP priorities and the limited availability of consultants preclude much flexibility as to the timing of the visit, and the institution must adapt to the dates announced by the OHRP.

When the site visit is announced, the OHRP will provide the institution with a tentative agenda and will request a complete list of all of the institution's human subjects research. This includes identification of the funding agency (if any), the initial IRB approval date, and the most recent date of continuing IRB review and approval. At 3 to 5 days before arrival, OHRP will request that the institution make available for on-site review the complete IRB files for 50 to 100 specific protocols that the OHRP has identified. In addition, the institution should be prepared for the OHRP to request additional files after the on-site record review has begun.

The OHRP will also request files for research that has been approved by the IRB under expedited procedures and for research determined by the institution to be exempt from IRB review requirements. The OHRP routinely requests the minutes for all IRB meetings held within 3 years before the site visit. In addition to IRB records, the OHRP may also wish to review specific research records, sometimes including relevant medical records of individual subjects involved in federally supported research. If such records are needed, the OHRP almost always notifies the institution in advance of its arrival on site.

An OHRP compliance site visit usually lasts between 3 and 5 days, depending on the size of the institution, the number of IRBs, and the complexity of the particular allegations of noncompliance. However, the typical OHRP compliance site visit begins with an introductory meeting with the assurance signatory official and any other officials deemed appropriate by the institution. It also includes at least 1 hour per day devoted largely to on-site review of IRB and research records and 1 day devoted to individual and/or group meetings with the IRB chair(s), members, administrator, and staff as well as selected federally supported research investigators and individuals relevant to any specific allegations that are under investigation. The goal of these meetings is to address both the allegations that precipitated the investigation and, more broadly, to achieve a thorough understanding of the institution's systemic protections for human subjects. The site visit concludes with an exit interview during which the OHRP summarizes its preliminary findings.

Except for the entrance and exit interviews, at which the assurance signatory official may include any number of appropriate individuals, the OHRP prefers that institutional observers are not present during its interviews with institutional personnel. Should institutional counsel wish to be present during these interviews, the institution should inform the OHRP before the site visit so that the OHRP can make the necessary arrangements with its own counsel.

The afternoon and evening before the exit interview are generally spent in executive session, during which the OHRP will reach and begin to document its determinations, including any corrective actions that may be necessary to ensure present and future protections for human subjects.

The determinations and required corrective actions are presented orally during the exit interview and formalized in a letter to the assurance signatory official within a few days after completion of the site visit. Alternatively, where immediate actions are needed to protect subjects' rights, welfare, or safety, the OHRP may issue its determination letter during the exit interview.

In either case, however, the OHRP's determinations are usually presented orally and explained thoroughly during the exit interview with the institution's assurance signatory official before the OHRP's departure at the end of the site visit.

Although the OHRP does not go out of its way to announce its determinations, institutions should understand that OHRP determination letters are available to the public under the Freedom of Information Act and are routinely posted on the OHRP website.[1] The OHRP will not comment to the media before issuing the determination letter. After the determination letter is released, the OHRP's comments are generally limited to explaining the meaning and significance of its determinations and any required corrective actions.

Surviving an OHRP Compliance Site Visit

An institution's first step after receiving notice of an impending compliance site visit should be to achieve an objective understanding of the quality of its institutional human research protection program. One effective strategy is to create a small but diversified task force, including individuals with authority to make decisions on behalf of the institution. The task force should develop the set of procedures that it will follow in reviewing the institution's system for protecting human subjects and, if appropriate, the specific allegation that precipitated the OHRP's investigation.

The OHRP has prepared and published on its website a document entitled "Compliance activities: Common findings and guidance."[2] Institutions should carefully review the issues described in this document and critically apply them to their own systems as a tool to identify systemic weaknesses and deficiencies. As indicated previously, it is often extremely beneficial to obtain the assistance of outside IRB experts to assist in this type of assessment. An assessment conducted solely by institutional personnel often lacks objectivity and exposes the institution to unrecognized risks that could be identified through a more unbiased assessment by recognized experts.

One important element that is often overlooked during institutional self-assessments is the existence of previous reports from government agencies that may be relevant to the institution's system for protecting human subjects. Many such agencies conduct audits or inspections of various aspects of federally supported or federally regulated research. Examples include Food and Drug Administration (FDA) inspections of clinical investigators; FDA IRB inspections; site visits to Department of Veterans Affairs (VA) facilities from the Office of Research Oversight; site visits to Department of Energy (DOE) facilities by the DOE Human Subject Protection Program; peer review evaluations from the National Institutes of Health funding components; and audits by National Cancer Institute Cooperative Groups.

Unfortunately, appropriate institutional officials are often not informed about the results of such evaluations. The institution should be certain to gather from all of its personnel and components every piece of correspondence and every report from every relevant government agency and monitoring organization. Far too many institutional officials find out about such materials during the exit interview at the conclusion of an OHRP site visit. At that point, it is too late for the institution to implement proactive, self-initiated corrective actions.

After the institution has conducted its own assessment, it should develop solutions and a detailed corrective action plan with timelines to implement those solutions. This kind of information can sometimes avert an extended shutdown of the institution's human subject research and can be incorporated directly into any required corrective action plan mandated by OHRP.

Managing the Logistics for an OHRP Site Visit

Many of the strategies suggested in Chapter 8-15 on FDA site visits are equally applicable to managing the logistics for an OHRP site visit. In addition, it is important for the institution to identify a responsible individual to assist the OHRP on administrative and logistical matters for the visit. The following are of particular importance.

Selecting a Work Site and Interview Rooms The OHRP prefers that a single, large conference room is reserved for its entire visit, including all meetings, interviews, and on-site executive sessions. The room should have a conference table and be large enough to accommodate the OHRP team and the largest institutional group to be interviewed.

Selecting Individuals to Be Interviewed The OHRP will provide a list of requested individuals, but with the OHRP's concurrence, the institution can sometimes add or substitute individuals of its own choosing.

Selecting Materials for Review The OHRP will provide a list of requested documents, but will be happy to review additional documents or materials that the institution wishes to provide.

Organizing Files The OHRP prefers that files are clearly labeled by IRB protocol number and the name of the principal investigator and that file contents are logically organized. Because the OHRP will request additional files after arriving, it is important that files are properly labeled, organized, and up-to-date on an ongoing basis.

Making Institutional Officials Available The assurance signatory official, the human protections administrator, and other institutional officials who have authority for the institution's system for the protection of human subjects (including those to whom the IRB reports) should be informed on a timely basis of all aspects of the site visit. In addition, they should be prepared to be available during the site visit as needed. If the assurance signatory official is not the institution's highest official, that official should be prepared to meet with the OHRP on request. The OHRP often requests such a meeting if serious deficiencies are determined to be jeopardizing the institution's systemic protections for human subjects.

Preparing Interviewees The institution should make sure that the institutional officials, IRB members and staff, investigators, study coordinators, and others who are going to be interviewed recognize the importance of their interviews. They should be instructed to be on time, but should be warned that meetings often run late and that they may need to stay later than anticipated. Institutions may assist interviewees in preparing for their meetings with the OHRP team, but they should never be coached in such a way as to provide less than accurate information. It is our experience that honesty and openness with the OHRP site visit team is in the long-term best interest not only of human subjects, but also of the institution itself.

Corrective Action Plans

As indicated previously, OHRP looks to the development of an institutional corrective action plan to resolve any weaknesses or deficiencies in the institution's system for protecting human subjects. A corrective action plan may be mandated by the OHRP after a compliance oversight investigation or compliance site visit in order to ensure protections for human subjects under an OHRP-approved assurance; an institution may voluntarily present a corrective action plan to the OHRP in response to self-identified problems or deficiencies.

In any event, a corrective action plan should be clear and succinct and should squarely address all identified deficiencies. It should make clear how the institution proposes to rectify any weakness and include a specific timetable for implementing each proposed action. Depending on the situation, corrective action plans often include bringing in outside expert consultants to help assess the effectiveness of existing human protection mechanisms; developing and conducting educational or training programs for IRB members or investigators; and/or assisting in designing and implementing improved policies and procedures.

The institution should consider the timetable for implementing proposed corrective actions very carefully. The OHRP is more interested in the quality and effectiveness of implemented corrective actions than in the speed of implementation. After being convinced that subjects are not routinely being exposed to unacceptable levels of risk, the OHRP often accepts corrective action plans that propose as long as 12 months for full implementation. However, the OHRP expects the institution to report and document meaningful progress at periodic intervals through the implementation period.

Finally, it is important to remember that the OHRP does not take actions for punitive purposes. Rather, the OHRP concentrates on ensuring present and future protections for human subjects. Indeed, the OHRP prides itself on assisting institutions that are genuinely concerned about strengthening their human subjects protection programs, and the OHRP professionals are always available to help institutions that self-identify problems and sincerely want to correct them.

Conclusion

Institutions that want to conduct research supported by the DHHS must file an assurance of protections for human subjects that is acceptable to, and approved by the OHRP. Institutions with OHRP assurances may be the focus of an OHRP site visit for the purpose of education and quality assurance or compliance oversight. This chapter has explained the mechanics of OHRP site visits with the emphasis on the things an IRB should do to avoid compliance problems. Preparing for and managing an OHRP site visit that is being done for compliance oversight requires planning, resources, and an understanding of specific steps to follow. This chapter provides IRBs with the information they need to interface with OHRP officials in a way that is likely to be productive from the standpoint of institutional function and research conduct.

References

1. Office for Human Research Protections. Compliance determination letters, 20 March, 2001. Access date 30 March, 2001. http://ohrp.osophs.dhhs.gov/detrm_letrs/jan2001.htm

2. Office for Human Research Protections. OHRP compliance activities: Common findings and guidance, 10 July, 2002. http://ohrp.osophs.dhhs.gov/references/findings.pdf

PART 9

Issues Based on Study Population

Vulnerability in Research

James M. DuBois

INTRODUCTION

It is no coincidence that the major events that led to the development of codes of research ethics and federal research regulations—the Nazi experiments with Jewish and mentally ill inmates, the Willowbrook trials with institutionalized children with mental retardation, and the Tuskegee syphilis study of poor and poorly educated African American men—all involved vulnerable participants. When our ability to protect ourselves is absent or diminished, we are more susceptible to both intentional and inadvertent harms. Whereas other chapters in this book examine the protections afforded to specific groups (such as pregnant women, prisoners, and children), this chapter explores the overarching concept of vulnerability and strategies for addressing vulnerability in research.

What Is Vulnerability?

The use of the term *vulnerable* in the context of research is different from its use in everyday parlance. Ordinarily, *vulnerability* simply refers to susceptibility to harm. In this sense, everyone is vulnerable because all human beings are capable of being harmed in many different ways. *The Belmont Report* refers to five basic categories of harm: social, economic, legal, psychological, and physical harms. Within each category there are radically different degrees of harm. For example, psychological harms may range from mild embarrassment to a psychotic relapse with significant resultant harms across all other categories: economic (e.g., lost employment), legal (e.g., being declared incompetent by a court), social (e.g., through stigma), and physical (e.g., through the side-effects of antipsychotic medications). Nevertheless, the concept of vulnerability in research has little to do with the kind or severity of harms. A survey of the work of advisory committees and regulations generally supports Levine's interpretation of vulnerability in research: vulnerable persons are "those who are relatively (or absolutely) incapable of protecting their own interests."[1(p.72)] Because the ongoing informed consent process is the main forum for self-protection in research, vulnerability pertains above all to threats to an individual's ability to grant voluntary, informed consent.[2,3]

To whom does this apply? That is, who counts as a vulnerable participant? There are two basic ways of answering this question. The first approach relies on group membership. It is the approach adopted by our current regulatory framework. The second approach analyzes the specific kinds of vulnerability that an individual may have. It is the approach advocated by the National Bioethics Advisory Committee (NBAC).

Current Regulatory Framework

Federal research regulations do not offer an exhaustive list of vulnerable populations. However, they mention nine populations by name: women, human fetuses, neonates, prisoners, children, persons with physical handicaps or mentally disabilities, and persons who are disadvantaged economically or educationally (45 CFR 46 and 21 CFR 56). *The Belmont Report* adds three populations to the list: racial minorities, the very sick, and the institutionalized.[4]

A group-based approach to addressing vulnerability has some advantages. First, it makes it easier to identify individuals as vulnerable. This in turn facilitates mandating and enforcing special protections. Additionally, cultural competence requires awareness of how members of a group share a common history or special characteristics that may affect attitudes and behaviors even if individuals vary significantly. Approaching vulnerability through the lens of community membership may facilitate the development of culturally and linguistically appropriate consent processes and protections.

Nevertheless, the NBAC identified several weaknesses to approaching vulnerability through the lens of group membership.[5] Such an approach may become unwieldy if we seek to craft special regulations for every group that may be vulnerable. For example, injection drug users, older persons, and undocumented immigrants may be vulnerable in some circumstances; nevertheless, no regulations currently exist to protect them. Moreover, it may be unnecessarily redundant because many groups require the same kinds of protections. A group-based approach also overlooks individual variation—some individuals may belong to more than one vulnerable group, and members of groups may be particularly vulnerable only to certain kinds of research harm. A group-based approach also chases a moving target because the status of groups changes with time; regulations tend to be too lumbering for such agile work. Finally, labeling groups as vulnerable can be stigmatizing or contribute to harmful stereotypes. For example, labeling persons with severe mental disorders as vulnerable may contribute to a stereotype that they are unable to provide informed consent, despite evidence that most individuals with depression or schizophrenia retain decision-making capacity.[6,7] In other cases, facile stereotypes of group vulnerability may distract from more common individual vulnerabilities. For example, a recent study of prisoners' decision-making capacity and motivations for entering into research found that decision-making capacity was more significantly impaired by cognitive factors than by environmental factors, although current regulations focus almost exclusively on the threats to voluntariness posed by incarceration and the subordinate relationships it creates.[8]

The NBAC's Analytical Framework

The NBAC recommended that institutional review boards (IRBs) adopt an analytic approach to vulnerability in research that bypasses many of the shortcomings of a group-based approach. An analytic framework inquires into the specific characteristics that individuals might have that would interfere with their ability to protect themselves in research particularly through the informed consent process. The NBAC identified six such traits.

1. *Cognitive or communicative vulnerability.* Participants may be insufficiently able to comprehend information, deliberate, and make or express decisions. This could be due to cognitive incapacity or due to circumstances, such as being presented with a consent form during a crisis or in a foreign language. This form of vulnerability may diminish a participant's ability to receive, understand, appreciate, and reason with information and to communicate a clear decision.

2. *Institutional vulnerability.* Individuals (e.g., prisoners or students) may be subjected to the formal authority of others. This increases the risk that participation will not be truly voluntary and that participants may be exploited or recruited solely for convenience.

3. *Deferential vulnerability.* Participants may be informally subordinate to another person. This could be due to traditional roles within a culture or society. For example, in some cultures, women may defer to their husband's wishes regarding participation, or some patients may routinely defer to the expressed or merely perceived wishes of their physician.[9] Again, this increases the risk that participation will not be truly voluntary and that participants may be exploited.

4. *Medical vulnerability.* Individuals may have a serious health condition for which there is no satisfactory standard treatment. This may lead to a perception that research offers the only hope and may contribute to difficulties weighing risks and benefits. Individuals may also suffer from the so-called therapeutic misconception in which research is mistaken for individually tailored therapy. This decreases comprehension and appreciation of risk and benefits.

5. *Economic vulnerability.* Individuals may lack access to adequate income, housing, or health care. When research appears to offer benefits that are badly needed and only available to the individual through research participation,

decisions may be unduly influenced and voluntariness compromised.

6. *Social vulnerability.* Some members of society may embrace stereotypes of participant groups or disvalue their interests, welfare, and contributions to society. This increases the risk of unfair treatment and stigmatization. For example, if a researcher stereotypes members of some groups as less intelligent, they may be given inadequate information during the consent process. Alternately, if researchers insufficiently value members of a group, they may be willing to subject them to a risk/benefit ratio that would not be acceptable to the general population.

If we apply this analytic framework to the subjects in the Tuskegee syphilis study (calling them participants would be insulting), we immediately recognize two important things. First, participants may have more than one kind of vulnerability: most subjects were vulnerable to some degree in every way described previously here except institutionalization. Second, the vulnerabilities of participants need to be addressed within the context of a specific protocol with a specific population; creating general rules for research with African American men would be stigmatizing and unhelpful.

Special Protections and Special Considerations

For better or worse, we currently have two different ways of identifying vulnerability in research—the group-based approach of federal regulations and the analytic approach advocated by the NBAC. These two approaches in turn yield different approaches to providing special protections or accommodations for vulnerable participants.

Current Regulatory Framework

Subparts B–D of the federal regulations (45 CFR 46 and 21 CFR 56) present special protections for only some specific populations: women, human fetuses, and neonates (subpart B); prisoners (subpart C); and children (subpart D). These special protections are discussed in other chapters in this book.

Apart from the specific protections enumerated for these groups, current federal regulations mention vulnerable populations in three places.

1. "If an IRB regularly reviews research that involves a vulnerable category of subjects, such as children, prisoners, pregnant women, or handicapped or mentally disabled persons, consideration shall be given to the inclusion of one or more individuals who are knowledgeable about and experienced in working with these subjects." (45 CFR 46.107(a)/21 CFR 56.107(a)).

This requirement is sufficiently vague that compliance cannot be measured. Some IRBs may do as little as "consider" taking action, whereas others have recruited mental health consumers, parents of children with severe illnesses, and representatives of vulnerable groups as members. There is some debate whether someone who merely is "knowledgeable about and experienced working with these subjects" is adequate because this does not ensure that the views or concerns of community members will be represented.[10]

2. IRBs shall determine that the "selection of subjects is equitable. In making this assessment the IRB should take into account the purposes of the research and the setting in which the research will be conducted and should be particularly cognizant of the special problems of research involving vulnerable populations, such as children, prisoners, pregnant women, mentally disabled persons, or economically or educationally disadvantaged persons." (46.111(a)(3)/21 CFR 56.111(a)(3))

This requirement reflects *The Belmont Report's* application of the principle of justice in section C.3. The authors of *The Belmont Report* were primarily concerned that vulnerable groups could be targeted for enrollment in a study due to their ready availability in research settings or because they are more easily manipulated as a result of their illness, institutionalization, or socioeconomic condition. Although this concern remains valid, IRBs need to consider balancing concerns. Because research may be beneficial to individuals and the communities that they care about, denying or hindering access to participation in the name of justice and protection may ironically create an injustice and harm individuals.[11] In recent years, we have seen a shift toward the inclusion of vulnerable or traditionally protected groups, largely in response to the activism of advocates for breast cancer and AIDS research.[12]

3. "When some or all of the subjects are likely to be vulnerable to coercion or undue influence, such as children, prisoners, pregnant women, mentally disabled persons, or economically or educationally disadvantaged persons, additional safeguards have been included in the study to protect the rights and welfare of these subjects." (46.111(b)/21 CFR 56.111(b))

On the one hand, this rule could be considered so vague as to be unhelpful. On the other hand, its vagueness creates space for ethical deliberation of the sort the NBAC recommends. Perhaps a more substantial limitation of this requirement pertains to the language of "safeguards" and "protection," for increasingly vulnerable communities are demanding not merely safeguards, but also justice and respect through inclusive processes.[12,13] IRBs might do well to shift from the language of "additional safeguards" to "accommodations" for vulnerabilities.

Although the Common Rule mentions vulnerable participants only in the three sections noted above, at paragraph C.1, *The Belmont Report* additionally states that "inducements that would ordinarily be acceptable may become undue influences if the subject is especially vulnerable." Once again, we see tensions between efforts to protect vulnerable participants and efforts to treat them beneficently and justly, for it is ethically questionable to offer less payment to vulnerable participants. Although the intention may be to reduce undue influence, the result may inequitable and may communicate a disvaluing of their time.[14]

Protections within an Analytic Approach

The analytic approach to vulnerability adopted by the NBAC yields a system of accommodations that is at once more general and more specific.

In contrast to current regulations, which focus on only three vulnerable groups in subparts B–D, the NBAC's analysis of vulnerability pertains to all groups, indeed to all individuals who might become participants in research. In this sense it is far more general.

However, insofar as an analytic approach allows researchers and IRBs to focus on the specific things that might hinder an individual's self-protection, it also allows for more specific and appropriate remedies. For example, consider research with participants who are at risk for cognitive or communicative vulnerability. Appropriate accommodations might include any of the following: formally assessing decision-making capacity; educating participants until they can demonstrate knowledge of consent information; obtaining assent from the participant and the permission of a surrogate decision maker; and involving a consent auditor or patient advocate to assist in explanations or to provide oversight.[15] In short, an analytic approach requires knowledge of best practices for accommodating specific vulnerabilities. However, much like optimal medical therapy is tailored to the individual, so too optimal accommodations are best provided by considering the needs of individual participants rather than mandating a specific practice for entire populations.

This is, of course, difficult to reconcile with the fact that IRBs are only presented with protocols and protocols describe populations not individuals. The solution is twofold. First, IRBs must embrace the concept of "being at risk for" a vulnerability. Not all patients with schizophrenia lack decisional capacity, but because cognitive impairments that affect capacity are more common among the population of people with schizophrenia than people without schizophrenia, they may be accurately described as "at risk." Second, IRBs need to address this heightened risk by empowering researchers to exercise discretion in determining when a specific accommodation is appropriate for an individual participant (e.g., when surrogate consent would be needed). In exceptional cases (e.g., protocols with very unfavorable risk/benefit ratios), a third party—e.g., a consent auditor or patient advocate—might be asked to make or advise on such determinations.

Because an analytic approach to providing accommodations for vulnerable participants requires knowledge of best practices, a growing number of people are calling for more empirical research on ethical issues in human research, which will generate evidence-based ethical practices.[16] As data become available, systems need to be created to disseminate best practices to IRB members.

IRB Deliberations: From Rule Following to an Ethical Analysis

IRBs are expected to implement the requirements of federal regulations in their review of research. However, in the review of research with vulnerable participants, the regulations are frequently sufficiently vague to allow ethical deliberation, and ethical deliberation is precisely what is needed. Regulations are focused above all on safeguarding or protecting individuals. Yet far more is at stake than the principle of nonmaleficence or the duty not to harm. Participants want research that respects them and takes into account their genuine needs and desires. Moreover, it is difficult to imagine a rule—however well intended—that cannot be harmful in at least some circumstances. As noted already, a rule excluding institutionalized individuals may unjustly exclude them from the benefits of research;[17] a rule limiting financial incentives in the name of avoiding undue influence may unfairly provide those in greatest need with the least compensation for their time and reinforce mistrust or resentment toward researchers.

Just as community consultation can improve IRB review,[18] so too community consultation and accommodations for vulnerable participants can improve the quality of research data. This fact should be emphasized as IRBs seek to build partnerships with investigators. Such partnerships are absolutely essential in research with vulnerable participants because typically only investigators are in a position to know what accommodations an individual needs.

Some have advocated for doing away with the concept of vulnerability and replacing it with "special scrutiny" practices in certain kinds of high-risk research.[19] However the concept of vulnerability cuts across risk levels and pertains to factors that limit an individual's ability to protect him or herself. Although it may be true that most people are vulnerable in one respect or another—not just those in a few select groups—it is also true that researchers ought to be keenly aware of the things that diminish an individual's ability to protect him or herself through informed consent. Whatever becomes of vulnerability as a regulatory concept, it will always have its place in the education of responsible and respectful researchers and reviewers.

References

1. Levine RJ. *Ethics and Regulation of Clinical Research*, 2nd ed. New Haven, CT: Yale University Press; 1988.

2. Weijer C. Research involving the vulnerable sick. *Accountability Res* 7:21–36, 1999.

3. Kipnis K. *Vulnerability in research subjects: A bioethical taxonomy*. In National Bioethics Advisory Commission (ed.). *Ethical and Policy Issues in Research Involving Human Participants. Volume II Commissioned Papers and Staff Analysis*. Bethesda, MD: National Bioethics Advisory Commission; 2001:G1–G13.

4. National Commission. *The Belmont Report: Ethical Principles and Guidelines for the Protection of Human Subjects of Research*. Washington, DC: Department of Health, Education, and Welfare; 1979.

5. National Bioethics Advisory Commission. *Ethical and Policy Issues in Research Involving Human Participants*. Bethesda, MD: National Bioethics Advisory Commission; 2001.

6. Appelbaum PS, Grisso T. The MacArthur Treatment Competence Study, I: Mental illness and competence to consent to treatment. *Law Hum Behav* 19:105–126, 1995.

7. Berg JW, Appelbaum PS. Subjects' capacity to consent to neurobiological research. In Pincus HA, Lieberman HA, Ferris S (ed.). *Ethics in Psychiatric Research: A Resource Manual for Human Subjects Protection*. Washington, DC: American Psychiatric Association; 1999:81–106.

8. Moser DJ, et al. Coercion and informed consent in research involving prisoners. *Comprehensive Psychiatry* 45:1–9; 2004.

9. Schneider CE. *The Practice of Autonomy: Patients, Doctors and Medical Decisions*. New York: Oxford University Press; 1998.

10. Campbell J. Reforming the IRB process: Towards new guidelines for quality and accountability in protecting human subjects. In Shamoo A (ed.). *Ethics in Neurobiological Research with Human Subjects*. Amsterdam: Gordon and Breach; 1997:299–304.

11. Kahn JP, Mastroianni AC, Sugarman J (eds.). *Beyond Consent: Seeking Justice in Research*. New York: Oxford University Press; 1998:xii, 190.

12. Dresser R. *When Science Offers Salvation: Patient Advocacy and Research Ethics*. New York: Oxford University Press; 2001.

13. Centers for Disease Control and Prevention. *Building Community Partnerships in Research: Recommendations and Strategies*. 1998.

14. Brody BA. Making informed consent meaningful. *IRB: Ethics & Human Research* 23(5):1–5, 2001.

15. National Bioethics Advisory Commission. *Research Involving Persons with Mental Disorders That May Affect Decision Making Capacity: Report and Recommendations*, vol. 1. Rockville, MD: National Bioethics Advisory Commission; 1998:88.

16. Sieber J. Empirical research on research ethics. *Ethics Behav* 4(4):397–412, 2004.

17. Pasquerella L. Confining choices: Should inmates' participation in research be limited? *Theor Med Bioethics* 23(6):519–536, 2002.

18. Freeman WL, Romero FC. Community consultation to evaluate group risk. In: Amdur RJ, Bankert EA (ed.). *Institutional Review Board: Management and Function*. Sudbury, MA: Jones and Bartlett; 2002.

19. Levine C, et al. The limitations of "vunerability" as a protection for human research participants. *Am J Bioethics* 4(3):44–49, 2004.

Research in Public Schools

Lorna Hicks

INTRODUCTION

The provisions of the Common Rule, Part A of 45 CFR 46, apply to all subjects, regardless of age or circumstance, including public school students. There are three direct references to children in the Common Rule, all of which identify children as vulnerable subjects. Although teachers, principals, school board staff, and the communities they serve are all concerned with the welfare of the children in their care, researchers and IRB members must be aware that there are vulnerabilities unique to school-based research.

This chapter will discuss some of those vulnerabilities and suggest issues to consider in the context of the criteria for institutional review board (IRB) approval of research as provided in 46.111. Subpart D of 45 CFR 46—Additional DHHS Protections for Children Involved as Subjects in Research, will be discussed as it relates to research in schools, with particular focus on identifying research that can and cannot be considered exempt under the provisions of the subpart. Finally, the Family Education Rights and Privacy Act and the Protection of Pupil Rights Amendment, regulations designed to protect the rights of children and their parents, will be summarized.

The Common Rule

Children's Vulnerabilities

The Common Rule identifies children as a vulnerable population that may need to be represented by a knowledgeable and experienced IRB member. The criteria for IRB approval of research, 46.111, notes that children are likely to be vulnerable to coercion and undue influence and that when considering equitable subject selection, researchers must take into account the purpose of the research and the setting in which it takes place.

Coercion and Undue Influence

46.111(b)

It is difficult, if not impossible, to eliminate undue influence in a setting in which more children's lives are orchestrate by adults and in which teachers are often important and, indeed, influential figures in children's lives. There are strategies, however, that may be used to increase the possibility that children will be comfortable making choices about research participation. For example, researchers can provide attractive alternatives to participation—not just time to do schoolwork—for children who do not want to participate in a study. They can enlist principals to help identify classrooms in which children are encouraged to make choices, as opposed to classrooms in which every student is expected to participate in the same activities. Consideration can be given to the powerful effects of peer pressure when recruiting adolescents.

When designing parental permission and child assent processes, researchers must bear in mind that parents and students might be concerned that if they do not participate in a research study there will be negative consequences. Responding to these concerns involves addressing them clearly and directly in the informed consent process. Parents might be reassured by statements such as this: "If you decide that you don't want your child to be in this study, it will not affect how the school treats your child." Also, parents and students may not feel entirely free to decline to participate in research if there is undue influence in the recruitment process. Parents might be unduly influenced if an invitation to participate in research comes from their child's principal, rather than from the research staff.

Equitable Selection of Subjects

46.111(a)(3)

Equitable subject selection, based on the ethical principle of justice, requires that the benefits and burdens of research participation be fairly distributed. In the school setting one implication of this principle is that every effort should be made to enroll those students who would most benefit from participation in a study—if there is the potential for direct benefit. The informed consent process is often an essential component for recruiting and enrolling such students.

Informed Consent

46.111(a)(4)

The consent paradigm for research with children requires that parents or legal guardians give permission for their children to become research subjects. The children, as appropriate for their developmental stage, provide assent.

As with all consent processes, the parental permission and child assent processes must include all of the information that potential participants need to make an informed decision. Permission and assent materials must be presented in the appropriate language and reading level and the voluntary nature of participation must be made clear.

Securing Parental Permission

One of the most confounding issues for researchers in the public schools is the difficulty of securing parental permission. Sending permission forms home is notoriously unreliable. The forms may never make it out of the students' backpacks or may end up in stacks of papers for busy parents to get to later. Parents may not be able to read the forms if they are not written in their native language. Without a high response rate, it may be impossible to obtain scientifically valid results or to assess intervention effects. It is possible that those families who already are burdened by poverty or lack of education are less likely to provide permission for their children to be involved in research that might provide some direct benefit to them. These may be the children that a researcher is most interested in understanding and most interested in helping.

There are strategies for improving response rates. If schools support research, they will encourage students to return parental permission forms with or without parental permission. Schools may allow researchers to reward students who return forms—again, with or without parental permission—with small gifts or allow them to bring pizza to a classroom with a particular response rate. Investigators may make use of publicly available directory information, as permitted by local school policy, to write and telephone parents, either as initial contact or follow-up. It may be possible under some circumstances to waive the requirement to secure parental permission.

Waivers of Parental Permission

46.116

The Common Rule provides four criteria for waivers of any or all of the elements of informed consent. The same criteria apply to waivers of parental permission (and also to child assent). In order to waive or alter any or all of the elements of informed consent, an IRB must find and document that all of the following criteria have been met:

1. *The research involves no more than minimal risk to the subjects.* "Minimal risk" means "the probability and magnitude of harm or discomfort anticipated in the research are not greater in and of themselves than those ordinarily encountered in daily life or during the performance of routine physical or psychological examinations or tests." Research with more than minimal risk would introduce risks not normally part of the daily experience of schoolchildren.
2. *The waiver or alteration will not adversely affect the rights and welfare of the subjects.* Some parental rights are defined by law. The Protection of Pupil Rights Amendment (PPRA), for example, may require written parental permission for research on sensitive topics. (See the discussion later here about PPRA.) However, neither "rights and welfare" nor "adverse affect" is defined in the regulations protecting research subjects. Investigators and IRBs must interpret what

these concepts mean in the local context through consultation with schools and communities. Some schools will not allow waivers of parental permission for any research because they believe parents have the right to know what their children are experiencing, particularly when the activities are not part of the curriculum.
3. *The research could not practicably be carried out without the waiver or alteration.* Inconvenience and expense are not acceptable factors in approving waivers. Scientific validity is. The requirement to secure permission, for example, may create large gaps in behavior sampling and diminished representativeness of the data.[1]
4. *Whenever appropriate, the subjects will be provided with additional pertinent information after participation.*

"Passive Consent" and Parental Notification

"Passive consent" has been used in school-based research in response to the difficulties of securing prior written permission from parents. The passive consent process involves notifying parents that research will take place and giving them the opportunity to state that they do not want their children to participate. The argument in support of passive consent is that if parents do not remove their children in response to the notification, they have provided permission. However, the passive consent process is *not* equivalent to informed consent. The provisions of the Common Rule require that parental or guardian permission for children to participate in research must be secured or waived in accordance with the four criteria provided in the regulations. Furthermore, on a practical level, sending notice does not mean that notice is received for a variety of reasons, including the parents' language and reading level.

The parental notification process can be used to provide parents with the option to remove their children from research, but *only* if the requirement for parental permission has been waived by an IRB. The notification can describe the study, provide contact information, and give parents the opportunity to enter into a consent process, even though the IRB has waived the requirement.

Child Abuse and Neglect

Some types of research have the potential to reveal child abuse and neglect. A study of at-risk students might do so; a study about teaching reading probably would not. If the potential exists, researchers must tell parents and older children during the informed consent process that the confidentiality they can provide is limited by their state's child abuse reporting requirements.

Assessing and Managing Risk

46.111(a)(1&2)

School-based research takes place in the context of a web of relationships—among students, between students and teachers, between parents and teachers, and so on—and care must be taken that those relationships are not put at risk in the research process.

Some of the risks in school-based research are familiar to IRBs, such as the risk of a breach of confidentiality. It is not uncommon for researchers to ask students to provide identifiable information about illegal activities, such as their use of illegal drugs. Standard confidentiality procedures can be adopted, including the use of certificates of confidentiality (http://grants2.nih.gov/grants/policy/coc/index.htm).

However, there are some risks in school-based research that are unique. For example, there is evidence that grouping high-risk adolescents for behavioral interventions can lead to peer contagion in which negative behaviors are reinforced.[1]

Another unique risk in school-based research is sometimes referred to as "educational harm." Diverting instructional time to research activities may constitute educational harm for some students; however, it is the role of the schools, not researchers, to determine when researchers may use class time. Educational risk directly related to research can occur if, for example, students find it difficult to resume learning activities after the research due to unsettling content or processes. Here, the researcher needs to take a role by providing a strategy to ease the transition back to learning. One way is to close potentially unsettling research activities with a positive activity.

Safeguarding Student Privacy

46.111(a)(7)
Public schools are, by definition, settings in which most of what happens is public knowledge. Nonetheless, there may be ways to safeguard student privacy. When appropriate, research can be designed so that the decision to participate can be kept private. For example, all students in a classroom can be given a folder, some containing research materials, others containing games or puzzles for children who are not research participants. In some schools, it is very common for children to be taken out of their classrooms for a variety of reasons. In a setting in which it is not the norm, researchers may need to come up with a mechanism for accessing students in a way that does not single them out from their classmates.

Subpart D of 45 CFR 46—Additional DHHS Protections for Children Involved as Subjects in Research

The applicability of Subpart D depends on the requirements of the federal sponsor and of the researcher's institution. Some federal research sponsors that have adopted the Common Rule have not also adopted Subpart D. For example, the Department of Education has adopted the subpart; the National Science Foundation has not. Thus, the National Science Foundation does not expect institutions to conduct research in accordance with the provisions of the subpart. However, institutions may choose to apply the provisions of the subpart to all research, regardless of the source of funding.

Subpart D identifies four categories of risk and associated benefits with corresponding consent requirements. Research in all four categories requires that adequate provisions be made for securing the assent of the children when, in the judgement of the IRB, the children are capable

of providing assent. Parental permission requirements vary by category. The majority of research in the public schools falls into one of two categories: (1) research with no more than minimal risk and (2) research with more than minimal risk and the prospect of direct benefit to the minor subjects. Such research requires the permission of both parents and review by the DHHS.

The remaining two categories involve research that poses more than minimal risk and no prospect of benefit to the children. One category includes research that may yield generalizable knowledge about the child's disorder or condition and requires consent of both parents. The other category includes research that may present an opportunity to understand, prevent, or alleviate a serious problem affecting the health or welfare of children. Such research requires Department of Health and Human Services review.

With regard to school-based research, other salient portions of Subpart D include (1) limits on the use of exemptions when children are research subjects, (2) the provision that waivers of consent and waivers of documentation of consent, as described in the Common Rule, are applicable to research with children, and (3) a provision for waivers of parental permission when is it not a reasonable requirement, for example, when the children are neglected or abused.

The Use of Exemptions in School-Based Research

The Common Rule describes six categories of research activities that, although they *do* meet the definition of research with human subjects, are *exempt* from the provisions of the Rule (46.101). These activities presumably pose little or no risk to the potential subjects.

As noted, Subpart D limits the use of exemptions for research involving children (for the complete text of the exemption categories, see Chapter 4-1, *Exempt from Institutional Review Board Review*).

The following activities with schoolchildren do not qualify for exemption under Subpart D.

1. Research involving surveys
2. Research involving interviews
3. Observation of public behavior when the researcher participates in the activities being observed

In contrast, the following research activities in public schools may qualify for exemption:

1. Research conducted in established or commonly accepted educational settings, involving normal educational practices, such as (1) research on regular and special education instructional strategies or (2) research on the effectiveness of or the comparison among instructional techniques, curricula, or classroom management methods

   It is important to take into account that the definition of a normal educational practice varies over time and from community to community. For example, many school districts have adopted programs designed to improve interpersonal skills, such as the widely used Second Step curriculum. In those schools, role playing to explore conflict resolution strategies may be considered a normal educational strategy.

2. Research using educational tests, unless the disclosure of identifiable information would create the potential for harm

3. Observation of public behavior in which the researchers do not participate in the activities being observed

4. Research involving the collection of study or existing data or records, if the data are publicly available or are recorded without identifiers

5. Some food and taste studies

Applying the Exemption Criteria in Accordance with Subpart D

The regulatory framework provided in the Common Rule is intended to provide a baseline for institutions to develop policies for protecting research subjects. The following examples illustrate how the exemption criteria would be applied in accordance with Subpart D when institutions have not further restricted the use of exemptions with children.

Example 1: Visual Vocabulary

A researcher is interested in implementing an elementary school art education curriculum designed to help students develop a visual vocabulary. The curriculum involves asking children to sort cards with reproductions of various Western artists as well as other activities. The curriculum has been used for over 15 years. The researcher is interested in adding some contemporary artists and those from other cultures to see whether there are any differences in the children's ability to make discriminations based on visual elements.

This research qualifies for exemption because it involves normal educational practices in a commonly accepted educational setting.

Example 2: Conflict with Friends

A researcher wants to ask fourth-grade students to respond to a written survey that includes hypothetical vignettes about handling conflict with friends.

It is possible that in some school districts this activity would be considered a normal educational activity and would thus qualify for exemption. If it is not considered normal educational activity, it would not qualify for exemption under Subpart D, which does not allow the use of exemptions for survey procedures with children.

Example 3: Recording Playground Conversations

Researchers studying peer rejection use wireless microphone audio systems combined with synchronized videotaping to record conversations among children on the playground. A focal child wears a small lightweight microphone. The transmission system can record audio information from as much as 300 feet away, thus allowing detailed recording of children's interactions in a natural large-group setting, unmediated by the close presence of adults.

Subpart D allows observations of children's public behavior to be eligible for exemption when the researcher does not participate in the activities observed. In this case, the researchers are not participating, so the deciding question is whether the children's behavior is public. The definition of private behavior in the Common Rule is "information about behavior that occurs in a context in which an individual can reasonably expect that no observation or recording is taking place." Although the children's conversations and private whispers occur in a public setting, the playground, they are arguably private information as they could not be observed without long-range recording devices. These devices are designed to hide the data collection process. Therefore, this research would not qualify for exemption. under Subpart D.

Student Educational Records

The Family Educational Rights and Privacy Act (FERPA) describes the process researchers must use to access students' educational records. FERPA requires schools to have written permission from a parent, or a student who is 18 or older, before releasing any identifiable information from a student's record. Information in school records may include religious affiliation, citizenship, disciplinary status, attendance, gender, ethnicity, grades/exam scores, test scores (e.g., the SAT), and progress reports.

Schools may disclose, without consent, "directory" information such as a student's name, address, telephone number, date and place of birth, honors and awards, and dates of attendance. However, schools must tell parents and eligible students that directory information is not protected, and they must allow parents and eligible students a reasonable amount of time to request that the school not disclose their directory information about them.

Search the term "FERPA" at the Department of Education's website www.ed.gov for the text of the regulation and guidance regarding its implementation.

Content of Surveys and Research-Related Instructional Materials

The Protection of Pupil Rights Amendment (PPRA), amended by the "No Child Left Behind Act" of 2001, gives parents some level of control over the content of third-party survey research and any instructional materials developed by researchers. The PPRA identifies eight sensitive topics and includes two provisions for parental review and approval of surveys and materials that include any of the eight topics. Each provision is associated with a Department of Education funding mechanism: (1) direct funding of a research program by the Department or (2) general school funding.

The eight topics are as follows:

1. Political affiliations or beliefs of the student or the student's parent

2. Mental and psychological problems of the student or the student's family

3. Sex behavior or attitudes

4. Illegal, antisocial, self-incriminating, or demeaning behavior

5. Critical appraisals of other individuals with whom respondents have close family relationships

6. Legally recognized privileged or analogous relationships, such as those of lawyers, physicians, and ministers

7. Religious practices, affiliations, or beliefs of the student or student's parent

8. Income (other than that required by law to determine eligibility for participation in a program or for receiving financial assistance under such program)

Research Funded Directly by Applicable U.S. Department of Education Programs

An "applicable program" means any program for which the Secretary of the Department has administrative responsibility as provided by law or by delegation of authority pursuant to law. If research is conducted under an applicable program, schools must obtain *prior written parental permission* before minor students are required to participate in any survey, analysis, or evaluation that reveals information about any of the eight sensitive topics.

Research in Schools Receiving Any Funding from the U.S. Department of Education

Under the "No Child Left Behind Act" of 2001, parents were given additional rights with regard to the content of surveys administered by third parties. School systems are required to develop and adopt policies that offer parents the right to inspect, on request, a survey created by a third party before it is administered to school students and the opportunity to remove their child from participation in third-party surveys containing one or more of the eight items described here. These parental rights apply in any school receiving general funding from the U.S. Department of Education.

As of this writing, new regulations for implementing the PPRA to include the provisions of the "No Child Left Behind Act" have not been published. This renders the existing PPRA regulations largely obsolete. Therefore, when research on one of the eight sensitive topics is not directly funded by the U.S. Department of Education, researchers may encounter three different school system policies for the implementation of PPRA. Schools may have no formal policy and make decisions on a case-by-case basis. They may require parental notification with the opportunity to opt out. Finally, schools may have a policy requiring active written parental permission for children to participate in the research.

Search the term "PPRA" at the Department of Education's website www.ed.gov for the text of the regulation and guidance regarding its implementation.

PPRA, FERPA, and Private Schools

If research is conducted under an applicable program of the U.S. Department of Education in a private school, the PPRA applies. A private school that does not receive any federal funding is not subject to the provisions of FERPA and PPRA.

Conclusion

Research in the public schools provides extremely valuable information, both in terms of improving educational outcomes for children and contributing to knowledge in areas of basic inquiry such as child development, developmental psychology, and educational psychology. Research in the schools requires the participation of school systems, teachers, and parents, as well as the researcher's institution, in order to meet our commonly held commitment to protect the children and adolescents who are the focus and at the heart of the research endeavor in the schools. This commitment requires bringing to the table the federal regulations for protecting children as research subjects. Because children exist in families and communities, research in the schools must respect community standards and the rights of parents with regard to their children's research experiences, as well as their values and aspirations for their children.

Reference

1. Dishion TJ, McCord J, Poulin F. When interventions harm: Peer groups and problem behavior. *American Psychologist* 54:755–764, 1999.

Suggested Reading

Asher SR, Paquette JA, Wentzel, KR, Gabriel SW. *Observing peer relations using a wireless transmission system: Ethical dilemmas and possible solutions.* Society for Research in Child Development, 2003 Biennial Meeting, April 24–27, Tampa, FL.

Koski G, Pritchard I. Students as research subjects. In: Post SG (ed.). *Encyclopedia of Bioethics*, Vol. 4. New York: MacMillan Reference; 2004:2469–2475.

Stanley B, Sieber J (eds.). *Social research on children and adolescents. Ethical issues.* Newbury Park, CA: Sage Publications; 1992.

Strike KA, Anderson MS, Curren R, van Geel T, Pritchard I, Robinson E. *Ethical standards of the American Educational Research Association: Cases and commentary.* Washington, DC: American Educational Research Association; 2002. (In particular, see Part II: Guiding Standards: Research Populations, Educational Institutions, and the Public.)

Selected Resources

Fordham University Center for Ethics Education (C. Fischer, Director): http://www.fordhamethics.org/casestudies.htm

Society for Research in Child Development: http://www.srcd.org/public.html

Phase I Clinical Trials in Healthy Adults

Cynthia S. Way

INTRODUCTION

Phase I clinical trials in healthy adults come early in the Food and Drug Administration's (FDA) New Drug Application (NDA) process, often on the heels of preclinical study data (testing in animals). The most common type of a Phase I clinical trial is known as a "first in human" research study. Other than predictors seen in the animal model and marketed drugs of the same class, first-time testing in humans is charting unknown territory. The primary purpose of these trials is to assess safety, with tolerability as a secondary purpose. Safety and tolerability are important to establish before conducting Phase II "proof of concept" research studies and Phase III "safety and efficacy" research studies.

Safety as an endpoint is a mainstay throughout all of the clinical trial phases of testing; however, baseline safety parameters are established in Phase I.

With some diseases, the FDA allows Phase I safety and tolerability testing to skip over the healthy adult population and go directly into the affected patient population (e.g., HIV, hepatic, renal, and oncology studies). This chapter does not address these types of Phase I clinical trials. For the purposes of this chapter, the term *Phase I* refers to clinical trials in healthy adults.

What types of Phase I clinical trials are there, and how are they designed? Who conducts Phase I clinical trials in healthy participants, and who are these healthy participants? What special considerations does an institutional review board (IRB) need to take into account when reviewing these types of research studies? I address these questions from my current perspective as Manager of Regulatory Support for Covance Clinical Research Unit, Inc., a global contract research organization (CRO). With over 15 years of experience working with IRBs (about one third of that time in Phase I research), I have come to appreciate and respect the unique contributions made to the drug development process by IRBs that review Phase I clinical trials and the participants they serve to protect.

Phase I Clinical Trial Designs

Phase I clinical trials are developed with preclinical study data in hand. The FDA regulates the amount of and types of preclinical testing to be done on an investigational compound, as well as the animal models to be used (rodent, rabbit, canine, nonhuman primate, or other). Preclinical studies provide answers to questions addressing toxicology safety (e.g., what does the drug or biological compound do to the physiology of the animal model?). Beyond the standard toxicology questions, *specialty* toxicology studies are conducted to answer questions about how the drug or biological compound affects genetic composition as well as reproductive systems. In addition, metabolism studies are conducted to learn how the animal model does (or

does not) metabolize, store, and excrete the drug or biological compound. Ultimately, bioanalytical methods are developed in preclinical studies to measure the levels of investigational compound in biological matrices.

A summary of the preclinical testing results is published in the Investigator's Brochure (IB). The IB is the primary source of information used to design Phase I "first-in-human" research studies.

The gold standard of Phase I testing is the randomized, double-blind, placebo-controlled, single-dose clinical trial. Variations from that design include single rising dose tolerance and multiple rising dose tolerance. Dose levels in these studies are extremely conservative, often hundreds of times lower than the amounts administered in preclinical testing. Rising dose tolerance studies administer increasing doses incrementally, with a washout period in between each dose group. Collaborative evaluation between the investigator and the sponsor determines whether to proceed to the next dose level.

Remember, the primary purpose of these research studies is to assess safety. Beginning at or close to a "no effect" level, far below the expected therapeutic level of the investigational compound, is the safest way to achieve this.

Pharmacokinetic (PK) and pharmacodynamic (PD) sampling are the cornerstones of Phase I studies. PK samples determine what the *body does to the drug* through biological sample collection and assay (e.g., blood, urine, and stool). Sometimes other biological samples are required as well, including saliva and semen. PD samples determine what the *drug does to the body* through tests and measurements such as ECGs, telemetry, psychometric testing, and vital signs.

There are other important clinical trial designs in Phase I as well. These studies are often conducted at the front end of the NDA process, but can also be conducted at any time along the way (e.g., simultaneous to Phase II and Phase III testing). Examples include mass balance (radiolabeled) studies, food effect studies, drug–drug interaction studies, and definitive QT interval studies.

Mass balance studies are known in preclinical testing as ADME studies (*absorption, distribution, metabolism, and excretion*). *Distribution* in the animal model is observed by dissection, and obviously, this step is not practiced in humans. By "attaching" a radioactive isotope (usually ^{14}C or ^{3}H) to the investigational compound, investigators are, however, able to see how it is *absorbed, metabolized, and excreted* in humans. Mass balance studies typically administer a single dose of radiolabeled investigational compound. FDA guidelines are followed regarding the allowable amount of radioactivity that can be attached to the investigational compound. Most mass balance research studies will administer far less than that amount, often making radiation exposure comparable to a couple of months of environmental background radiation.

Food effect studies are common in the NDA process. Ultimately, if the investigational compound gets to market, instructions on whether or not to take it with food will have come from this type of testing. Food effect studies are conducted to learn how food affects absorption, safety, and tolerability of the investigational compound when given in a "fasted" state and a "fed" state. The standard study design for the "fasted" state is to fast overnight before taking the investigational compound, as well as afterward for several hours. The standard study design for the "fed" state is to consume a high-fat meal, over a controlled period of time, just before taking the investigational compound. If the investigational compound is ultimately planned to be distributed in a powder form, it may be mixed in or sprinkled onto the food for consumption.

Drug–drug interaction studies are not required by the FDA in every NDA, but are common when the known therapeutic indication for the investigational compound dictates other drugs will most likely be administered simultaneously. These studies administer the investigational compound with other FDA-approved drugs in order to assess safety and tolerability of the combination(s).

Definitive QT interval studies are required by the FDA to answer the question of QT prolongation as it relates to cardiac safety. Frequent ECGs and Holter monitoring are essential to the conduct of definitive QT studies.

Conducting the Studies

The Phase I Research Unit

Phase I studies are generally conducted at stand-alone or specialty research units, often associated with a pharmaceutical company or a CRO. Most pharmaceutical companies contract with a CRO to conduct the clinical trial at the CRO's research facility on their behalf, although academic centers affiliated with a general clinical research center are also able to conduct Phase I testing.

A typical research unit will house multiple participants in one room and will offer access to common rooms for leisure time activities such as television and DVD players, billiards, books, puzzles, games, and/or Internet access. Nursing stations are part of the research unit, as are physical examination and phlebotomy rooms. Meals are served and eaten on the research unit in a dining room area.

Participants are required to wear identification at all times during a research study in order for staff to confirm their identity before study procedures. Doors in and out of the research unit are security monitored and alarmed. This keeps unauthorized visitors out and lets the research unit staff know whether a participant leaves. Participants are free to leave a research unit if they wish to discontinue being in a study—they are never locked in. However, having security monitoring and alarms helps a research unit know whether a participant has left without notifying the staff.

Any of the Phase I clinical trial designs discussed previously require that, for at least the majority of the clinical trial, participants must be confined to a research unit for two important reasons:

1. To monitor their health
2. To allow PK and PD sampling to be collected at protocol-driven specific time points

Safety

In this early phase of testing, it is in the best interest of the participants to be confined to a research unit (sometimes up to six or seven times the half-life of the investigational compound). Vital signs and ECGs around the clock are common safety measures employed during a clinical trial. "How do you feel?" is a protocol-driven question that is asked at multiple time points throughout the confinement in an ongoing effort to ascertain the well-being of the participant. All *adverse events* that occur are observed/reported and recorded in real time. Should a participant have a *serious and/or unexpected event*, medical care is always available on or near the research unit.

Sample Collection

The integrity of the clinical trial data relies on a controlled environment in which to collect frequent, consistent, and timely samples. It is not uncommon in a Phase I clinical trial to collect blood samples at half hour or hourly intervals for 24-hour periods or to have participants collect all their urine or stool during their participation. Diet is frequently controlled throughout the clinical trial, making sure that each participant eats the same amount or types of food. Some foods and most prescription, over-the-counter, or herbal preparations are prohibited in Phase I studies, as are nicotine, caffeine, and alcohol products because they can interfere with and/or confound PK and PD dynamics of the clinical trial data. Confinement on a research unit controls these aspects of the clinical trial.

Who Are These Participants?

The reasons why *patients* volunteer for Phase II and Phase III studies have been more widely discussed than the reasons that healthy adults volunteer for Phase I studies. For certain, many patients volunteer for Phase II and Phase III studies because of altruistic reasons. However, we also know that patients who may or may not benefit from participation in Phase II and Phase III clinical trials are, for better or worse, often driven by a hope that they will personally gain therapeutically from the research. Participants in a Phase I clinical trial, on the other hand, stand to gain nothing therapeutically, as they are not afflicted with any particular disease or disorder. There is no personal benefit to them, and yet there is often some risk incurred. That makes their interest and motivation all the more compelling. So who are they? The healthy adult participants who volunteer in Phase I studies are our friends, family, and neighbors. They come from all walks of life, and their reasons for volunteering vary. Some volunteer for purely altruistic reasons: to help humanity at large in its search for cures and treatments of the diseases and disorders that are a part of our world. Some volunteer with a loved one in mind, perhaps an uncle, a grandmother, or a child of a coworker that has a disease he or she hopes will be cured someday. By volunteering their bodies, if you will, they hope that perhaps they can be part of the solution to help people in need who are dear to them.

Many volunteer primarily because they are paid to do so. Payment for participating in Phase I research studies is allowed by the FDA, but amounts are not regulated *per se*. Each IRB overseeing a Phase I clinical trial is responsible for determining an appropriate stipend for participation (see IRB Considerations).

The examples of volunteering for altruistic reasons have more noble appeal to us as a society than volunteering primarily for money. However, if stipends were not offered, the number of altruistic participants would not be large enough to carry the day. Without the healthy adults who volunteer for Phase I testing, there would be no Phase II and Phase III testing. Still, IRBs must acknowledge and safeguard against participants who are less than truthful about their medical history or less than forthcoming about side effects they may experience during a clinical trial when it may affect their eligibility to be in a clinical trial or continue in a clinical trial (see IRB Considerations).

The Recruitment and Screening Process

Because the healthy participants sought for Phase I research studies are required to be generally healthy, recruitment cannot rely on an identifiable patient population (e.g., there is no doctor-to-doctor networking available in this arena of research from which to recruit participants). Recruitment of our friends, family, and neighbors usually begins with media advertisements (TV, radio, and print) and can even be found on the sides of city buses or on billboards. As stated in the FDA's Information Sheets, recruitment of participants begins the first step in the informed consent process.

Although Phase II and Phase III clinical trial recruitment materials must steer clear of promising medical benefits, Phase I clinical trial recruitment does not face that challenge, as participants must be generally healthy in order to qualify. It is important, however, to state the investigational nature of the clinical trial (e.g., research study) and to give enough qualifying parameters as to make inquiry meaningful. The content of advertisement should be straight to the point. A common advertisement may read as follows: "Participation needed in a research study; must be a healthy 18–55 year old, nonsmoking, male or female. One stay of 15 days with 2 outpatient visits. Up to $XXX will be provided. Contact XYZ if interested." A phone contact to the research unit will require the participant to answer questions about his or her health history. Subsequent to a satisfactory health history, dictated per protocol, the participant may be invited to come to the research unit for a screening visit.

Screening procedures for a standard Phase I clinical trial begins the next stage of the informed consent process. After consent is given, standard and customary medical procedures usually include a blood sample, a urine sample, an ECG, recording of vital signs, height and weight measurements, medical/medication history, and a physical examination. If a physical examination is not required by the protocol to be conducted at the screening visit, one will be required on clinical trial entry before administration of the investigational compound.

Blood and urine samples are provided in order to run laboratory tests such as a chemistry panel and a hematology panel. Other standard laboratory tests may include a screen for illicit drugs, HIV, hepatitis, or pregnancy. All laboratory testing must be within normal ranges (or deemed not clinically significant), with the exception of sponsor-approved deviations, to qualify for clinical trial entry. The goal of the screening tests is to establish baseline qualifications indicating a generally healthy adult who is not pregnant or taking illicit drugs.

IRB Considerations

IRBs that review Phase I clinical trials are held to the FDA's standards articulated in the Code of Federal Regulations (21 CFR) Parts 50 and 56, identical to all other

IRBs under the jurisdiction of the FDA, regardless of the phase of testing. However, as is noted previously in several instances, there are differences between Phase I and the later phases, thereby providing the IRB with a subset of unique considerations.

Benefits and Risks

There are no personal medical benefits to participating in a Phase I clinical trial. Although a research unit may offer the laboratory tests and physical examination results conducted at the screening visit as a "benefit," they should not be counted as a benefit when addressing this required element of consent in the informed consent process. The IRB should require a pointedly plain statement in the consent form indicating there are no medical benefits to participating in a Phase I clinical trial.

Risks and side effects may need to include those seen in animal studies, and this information should be clearly identified and communicated as such. Numbers of participants previously exposed to the investigational compound should be stated in the consent form, and if it is being given for the first time, this should also be stated, perhaps in more than one place.

In addition to listing the known risks and side effects of the investigational compound in the consent form, the IRB should require information indicating there may be unknown and long-term health risks, including risks to a fetus, associated with the investigational compound.

Alternatives to Participation

The one and only alternative to participation in a Phase I clinical trial is not to participate. IRBs should decide how to communicate this in the informed consent process in order to meet this required element of consent.

Language Level

Although complicating comprehension factors from an illness or disease are not present in healthy adults, as they may be in Phase II and Phase III research participants, the IRB must still consider approving a consent form that is free of medical jargon and is written at a grade level thought to be best understood by the general population from which the participants are recruited. Our family, friends, and neighbors have varying educational backgrounds. The IRB should consider approving a consent form written at or about the eigth-grade level (or lower) in an effort to invite maximum comprehension, even at the risk of "dumbing it down" to some.

Language

Participants in a Phase I clinical trial should, at a minimum, be able to communicate (speak and understand) in a language spoken at the research unit. Confinement of a participant to a research unit for a Phase I clinical trial who is not able to understand or be understood is not advisable, as it could pose inherent risks with regard to reporting adverse events and/or understanding the many study procedure requirements.

Additionally, literacy should not be presumed. IRBs should consider requiring participants to read aloud a section of the consent form to the person obtaining consent prior to signing the document. If a volunteer is not literate, a standard operating procedure should be in place at the research unit for presenting the consent form verbally in a *short form* format, as is allowed by the FDA.

Stipend Amounts

The IRB should not approve stipend amounts based on risk, as the extent of risk is typically unknown. Although it may be true that a first-in-human clinical trial could potentially pose more risk than a later stage clinical trial, there is no reliable way to ascertain risk to each and every participant. Often participants will receive only placebo, further complicating assessment of risk. IRBs should approve stipends that acknowledge the time and inconvenience incurred by participation, without presenting undue influence. Ranges may vary within the industry from $150 to $300 per study day. Some studies may require confinement to a research unit for up to 30 days or more. Thirty days of living away from home and/or absence from a job could dictate a stipend of up to $9,000.

IRBs should, and do, wrestle with the issue of comparatively high stipends, and the allure they may have to economically disadvantaged participants. It is known that some participants travel from research unit to research unit in order to exist primarily on stipends as a source of income and housing. The FDA is silent on the subject regarding this subset of participants; however, industry standards accept a minimum of a 30-day washout period between clinical trials. There is no industry-wide system, however, for tracking and sharing information on these participants, nor can we expect one to be developed easily without provoking alarm regarding personal autonomy and privacy infringements.

At a minimum, IRBs should address this issue by requiring a statement in the consent form, to be emphasized verbally during the consent process, indicating that "if you are not completely truthful with the study doctor or study staff about your past research study participation, your medical history and what medicines you take, you may harm yourself by being in this research study."

Financial Conflict of Interest

IRBs should require consent forms to disclose any financial conflicts of interest the investigators, as employees or consultants of a CRO or sponsoring company, may have. A statement in the consent form should be included to advise that the investigators are paid by the sponsor to conduct the research. It may be fair to also explain, when applicable, that the investigators do not have a financial interest in the long-term outcome of the research. The investigational compound that actually makes it to market will have been in the hands of many others long after the Phase I studies, and the ultimate outcome may not be known for a decade or longer.

Women of Childbearing Potential

Inclusion of women of childbearing potential (WOCP) is required by the FDA in the NDA process, but that does not imply an automatic requirement in the Phase I stage of the research. FDA and sponsors are often reluctant to include WOCP in the early testing phase, as teratogenicity outcomes are unknown at the outset. However, even though it will share concerns about teratogenicity, the IRB should require consideration of including WOCP where possible and be instrumental in the determination of adequate birth control requirements.

IRB Member Composition

IRBs that review Phase I research must adhere to the same composition requirements as all IRBs; however, added value can be obtained by recruiting both scientific and nonscientific members from the community at large, rather than from the CRO or sponsoring company affiliates. CROs and sponsors, because of their implicit for-profit business directives, can have the *appearance* of a financial conflict of interest. IRBs should consider membership that is primarily free of members with this perceived conflict. IRB members who are affiliated with the research can, of course, recuse themselves from voting where applicable. However, because of a possible perceived conflict of interest, not to mention complication of quorum requirements, IRBs should consider having members primarily from the local community.

Board Member Compensation

IRBs that review Phase I research studies may differ from those that review research affiliated with a medical center or an academic institution in that they are often paid a stipend. The stipend is usually monetary, but other incentives may be offered as well, for example, a meal or snack at each meeting, and/or mileage reimbursement. Stipend amounts will vary between IRBs, but should not be payment for research study approval, rather for research study review. Payment per protocol review can have the *appearance* of paying for approval; therefore, it may be advisable for IRB members to instead be given stipends on a per meeting basis.

Conclusion

Expertise in matters specific to the Phase I stage of research makes IRBs in this arena uniquely knowledgeable. Phase I IRBs and participants alike must consider their respective contributions within a "leap of faith" vacuum as the hope of cures and treatments for the diseases and disorders that medical science seeks to eliminate in the future. From this unique platform, serious attention should be given to both the potential value of and risks associated with this early phase of drug development. Diligent and thoughtful IRB oversight is critical to the well being of healthy adults participating in Phase I clinical trials.

Requiring Birth Control to Participate in Research

Bruce G. Gordon, Toby L. Schonfeld, and Ernest D. Prentice

INTRODUCTION

The inclusion of women in clinical research has been the source of much heated debate over the past 20 years, with legal (if not moral) consensus changing dramatically over this time. The specific regulations currently governing the inclusion of women (and in particular pregnant women) are discussed elsewhere in this book. In this chapter, we take as a given that the inclusion of women in clinical research is both morally and scientifically justified. With this as background, we briefly examine the ethical justification and the practical ramifications of the requirement for the use of contraception as a precondition for participation in clinical research.

Regulations and Guidelines Regarding Participation of Women in Research

The regulations pertinent to the inclusion of pregnant women in biomedical and behavioral research have been described in detail in other sections of this book. However, a brief reiteration is appropriate to understand the ethical and pragmatic basis for the following discussion of the requirement for contraception.

The mid-1970s saw a backlash against the biomedical research community, justified by the excesses of Tuskegee, Willowbrook, and other research misadventures and by the tragedy of thalidomide and diethylstilbestrol. In 1975, the Department of Health, Education and Welfare published regulations pertaining to research involving pregnant women (45 CFR 46 Subpart B), consistent with the recommendations of the National Commission for the Protection of Human Subjects of Biomedical and Behavioral Research. These regulations were based on a presumption of exclusion of pregnant women from research. This was followed in 1977 by Food and Drug Administration (FDA) guidelines for drug development that recommended that women of childbearing potential be excluded from Phase I (toxicity) and early Phase II (efficacy) trials of new drugs.[1] Although not mandated by these guidelines, investigators, sponsors, and institutional review boards (IRBs) tended to extend this policy to include all phases of drug development. There was little discussion at the time about potential benefits that might accrue to these women from participating or to the potential greater harm of subsequent use of these approved drugs in women on whom they had never been tested.

In the 1980s, attitudes began changing, in some measure because of the rise of AIDS and the benefits received by participants in trials of new antiviral drugs. Research began to be seen less as a burden and more as a benefit, and advocates for women's health lobbied vigorously for a relaxing of the protectionist rules and attitudes. In 1984, a Public Health Service task force found that the long-standing lack of research in women's health had compromised the quality of available information on diseases affecting women,[2] and in 1994, the Institute of Medicine (IOM) Committee on Ethical and Legal Issues Related to Inclusion of Women in Clinical Studies recommended that women should be enrolled as participants in clinical studies "in a manner that ensures that research yields scientifically generalizable results applicable to both genders."[3]

In 1993, the FDA issued "Guidelines for Study and Evaluation of Gender Differences in the Clinical Evaluation of Drugs," which articulated the agency's decision to reverse the 1977 policy that had barred most women from participating in the early phases of clinical trials.[4] In 1994, the National Institutes of Health issued "Guidelines on Inclusion of Women and Minorities as Subjects in Clinical Research," which stated that "women . . . must be included in all NIH-supported biomedical and behavioral research projects involving human subjects unless a clear and compelling rationale and justification establishes . . . that inclusion is inappropriate."[5]

In 2001, the Department of Health and Human Services published a final rule revising Subpart B.[6] Among the many changes to this regulation, the revised rule "institutes a policy of presumed opportunity for inclusion of pregnant women in research."

Ethical Rational for Requirement of Contraception

The ethical arguments regarding requirements of contraception mirror in part those used as justification for exclusion or inclusion of women from research; therefore, a review of these arguments is in order.

The most commonly cited rationale for the exclusion of women is the moral duty to avoid infliction of harm to a fetus. As Merton stated, the view is that "all women are always pregnable and therefore always pregnant."[7] Because the inclusion of women of childbearing potential carries a risk of causing fetal harm, these women should be excluded from research.

A counterargument is that this view is overly paternalistic. Researchers do not have the right to arrogate to themselves the determination of when participation in a protocol may create a greater risk of harm to the fetus than the chance of benefit. The judgment should be made by the pregnant (or potentially pregnant) woman. The principle of respect for persons would seem to demand that a woman of childbearing potential be allowed to make her own decision regarding participation. Nonetheless, there is precedent (in law, regulations and ethics) for protecting vulnerable populations, such as children, even when other parties (such as parents) are and should be responsible for this protection. The principle of respect for persons requires this protection, and the principle of nonmaleficence further impels us to at least "do no harm" to the fetus.

To a certain extent, the requirement for contraception can be seen as a compromise, allowing a practical, if not philosophic, resolution of this dilemma. The requirement for contraception serves to eliminate or at least attenuate the link between "pregnable" and "pregnant" and thereby eliminates (or reduces) the risk of fetal damage.

Another argument cited for exclusion of women is one of scientific rigor. Women and men are physiologically different, and thus, it is difficult or impossible to obtain "clean" data from gender-integrated trials. A similar argument can be made for excluding pregnant (and by implication, pregnable women) in that these women are physiologically different from women who are not of childbearing potential. As Merton stated, "The argument refutes itself: if the data obtained from a mixed population (men and women, or non-pregnant women and pregnant women) is so different from that generated by studying only one population, then how can it later be extrapolated to a real world with multiple populations? From the point of view of the women (or the pregnant women excluded) the data is not 'cleaner,' it is irrelevant."[7]

With the requirement for adequate contraception, pregnable women are no longer pregnant women, and the need to exclude them for scientific rigor is reduced. However, this solution is still not satisfactory because it skirts the issue of the scientific need to obtain data from pregnant women. This need was acknowledged in both the Public Health Service[2] and the IOM reports.[3] Indeed, Hall has argued that it is not only unethical but illegal to exclude pregnant women from clinical research.[8] Therefore, it could be argued that contraception is unethical because it leads to the exclusion of pregnant women.

Nonetheless, the requirement for contraception can be seen as a (partial) solution to the two main objections to inclusion of women in clinical research and as a way to minimize the risk to a fetus. However, practical concerns remain, some of which are addressed later here.

Practical Issues with Requiring Contraception

Consideration of "Risk" in Determining the Need for Contraception

As discussed previously here, we find the "scientific rigor" argument not compelling. The nonmaleficence argument is stronger, but still impacts on the autonomy of the women subjects. This impact is balanced in most cases by the need to protect the fetus from risk, but what if there is no risk to the fetus associated with a research protocol? Clearly, most studies involving therapeutic interventions such as drugs and medical devices carry some risk to the fetus (even if the magnitude of the risk is unknown). Still, there are drugs that are not shown to cause harm to the fetus (FDA category A drugs and some category B drugs). It would be difficult to make a strong case based on the nonmaleficence argument to require a woman of childbearing potential to use contraception if participating in a clinical trial where the only intervention is a drug of these classes. Similarly, it would be hard to justify a requirement for contraception for many nondrug studies if the interventions themselves are not risky to the fetus.

Adequacy of Birth Control

If there is adequate ethical justification for requiring contraception, then there appears an equivalent ethical requirement to assure that contraception is adequate (i.e., that contraception truly will eliminate or reduce the risk of fetal damage by eliminating or reducing the risk of pregnancy).

Various contraceptive methods have different failure rates, and these rates tend to vary according to age, race, ethnicity, marital status, and socioeconomic status.[3,9] Therefore, "adequate contraception" may be an elusive target, varying from population to population. Hormonal methods offer the advantage of low failure rate without the need to apply the technique before every episode of intercourse. However, hormonal contraceptives may interact with drugs being studied in clinical trials by affecting the pharmacokinetics or pharmacodynamics of the test drug. Alternately, and perhaps more concerning, it is possible that the drug being studied may interact in a manner that makes the hormonal contraception less effective. Barrier methods of contraception (especially multiple-barrier methods, such as condom or diaphragm, with spermicidal jelly) may be a better choice for drug studies, but compliance may be inferior.

Abstinence

Abstinence may be the ideal form of contraception, but probably only reasonable for very short-term studies. Nevertheless, many studies specifically exclude abstinence as an "adequate" form of birth control. Such an exclusion is ethically problematic, particularly among certain populations, such as nuns and lesbians (in the latter case, "abstinence" meaning refraining from sexual intercourse with men). Bush insists that "enrolling someone in a trial as a condition of their current sexual or religious belief is wrong.... If the [research] program treated nuns or lesbians differently from other women of childbearing potential, it would be invading their privacy and their rights to change their minds."[10]

In contrast, VandenBosch argued forcibly that "the criteria that exclude women who are not on birth control clearly fail to recognize and respect the values and personal choices of the female ... who has chosen abstinence. To include a [woman] who is taking oral contraceptives on the assumption that she can be relied upon to take that medication regularly to avoid pregnancy, but to exclude [one] who has chosen to abstain from sexual intercourse on the assumption that she cannot be relied upon to continue that behavior violates ... [the principle of respect for persons] ... which states to respect autonomy is to give weight to autonomous persons considered opinions and choices."[11]

Termination of Pregnancy

The IOM report recommends that pregnancy termination options be discussed as a part of the consent process in clinical studies that include unknown or foreseeable risks to potential offspring.[3] We concur with this recommendation in principle, although, clearly, implementation is difficult. Subjects and investigators alike are likely to have strong feelings regarding abortion, and state statutes may limit a subject's options. Nonetheless, a neutral, nonjudgmental discussion of this option is indicated at the time of initial consent to participate in the study.

Discussion of termination options at the time of enrollment in the research does not, however, imply that women should be asked whether they would terminate if they became pregnant. Asking such a question might be taken to be a suggestion on the part of the investigator or a requirement for participation in the research. Furthermore, and more importantly, we do not believe that a subject's stated intent to terminate a pregnancy is adequate justification to dispense with a requirement for contraception, and therefore, the answer is irrelevant. An intent to terminate is changeable and, properly, unenforceable and therefore does not serve to minimize risks to the fetus the way contraception would.

Adolescents as Research Subjects

Additional concerns arise when the participants in research are adolescents. Investigators must be particularly sensitive in discussions of sexual activity. Issues described previously here with regard to abstinence as a form of contraception are also pertinent to this group. VandenBosch makes an interesting point that "if the physician says the adolescent must be on 'acceptable' birth control to be in the study, the message may be interpreted as approval of sexual activity and disapproval of abstinence ... as 'unacceptable.'"[11]

Investigators and IRBs must be alert to risks of loss of confidentiality, particularly when discussing sexual activity and performing pregnancy tests. If this information is to be shared with parents (especially if required by state statute), then this should be stated clearly in the consent document and stressed to the adolescent prior to her enrollment in the trial. If the information is not to be shared with parents, Levine raises the concern that it might appear that the institution not only approves of deception but that it also collaborates with the adolescent in this deception, thus setting a poor example for the adolescent.[12]

Consent Issues

Several authors have discussed the information that should be present in the consent for women of childbearing potential who are involved in clinical trials. The IOM report recommends that "the informed consent process [should include] an adequate discussion of the risks to reproduction and potential offspring and, where appropriate, an adequate discussion of relevant considerations of birth control."[3] These discussions should, of course, include information regarding the risk of failure of various forms of birth control, although the IOM report further recommends that "the participant be permitted to select voluntarily the contraceptive method of his or her choice." Finally, the IOM report advised, "Pregnancy termination options be discussed as part of the consent process in clinical studies that pose unknown or foreseeable risks to potential offspring."[3]

Among other things, Halbreich and Carson suggested that the consent process include instructions for advising the investigator if pregnancy is suspected.[13] We concur, although we have been noting an increase in the number of clinical studies that include the "requirement" that women who become pregnant during a clinical trial be removed from the study and followed to determine the outcome of the pregnancy (often including assessment of the baby's health up to one year of age). Although the scientific rationale for this provision is clear and justifiable (though perhaps tainted by fears of litigation), we object strongly to this "requirement" as a violation of the subject's right to withdraw from or cease participating in the research. Our investigators and sponsors are informed that agreeing to this provision may not be a requirement for participation in the study. Women who become pregnant and are withdrawn from the study may be asked to allow this follow-up, but they are under no obligation to agree to it. Follow-up information may not be obtained without their express consent.

The extent to which consent forms actually include the information described previously here is unclear. Nolan and colleagues recently reported a survey of consent documents for studies conducted between 1994 and 1998 that involved drugs or radiation.[14] They examined whether consent forms discussed four broad categories of reproductive risk or fetal risk information: (1) reproductive/fetal risk, (2) mandatory pregnancy-related exclusion, (3) pregnancy prevention advice, and (4) pregnancy testing. They found that although many consent forms contained pregnancy-related exclusions (including anticipated pregnancy and breastfeeding), fewer contained information regarding the specific reproductive risk. Only a minority of consent forms mentioned methods to prevent pregnancy, pregnancy testing, or what subjects should do if they become pregnant during the study.

Model Policy

Our IRB has recently implemented a policy[15] standardizing the types of birth control that may be required of subjects of reproductive potential in an attempt to balance the competing ethical imperatives of minimizing risk of harm to the (potential) fetus and maximizing respect for the considered choices of the woman subject. This policy uses the FDA Use-in-Pregnancy categories[16] as thresholds for levels of required contraception.

In our policy, for research involving only drugs classified as category A (no risk to fetus), the investigator is strongly discouraged from requiring contraception because adequate, well-controlled studies in pregnant women have failed to demonstrate a risk to the fetus in any trimester of pregnancy. For research involving drugs classified as category B (no evidence of risk in humans but risk in animals), the investigator may require contraception, but is not obligated to do so. If the investigator does choose to mandate use of contraception, subjects participating in sexual activity that could lead to pregnancy are told they should use should use *one* reliable form of contraception while on study and for a specified number of months afterward. Reliable forms of contraception are defined as condoms (with spermicide), diaphragm or cervical cap (with spermicide), intrauterine device, or hormonally based contraception.

For research involving drugs classified as category C (risk cannot be ruled out) or category D (known risk to fetus), the investigator should mandate use of contraception for subjects participating in sexual activity that could lead to pregnancy. For category C, because of the unknown magnitude of the risk to the fetus, the investigator may require the use of either one or two forms of contraception; for category D, the subject and his or her partner should use *two* reliable forms of contraception.

Investigational drugs with no available data regarding the risk to the fetus are assigned to category C, as a middle ground between respecting subject autonomy and protection of the fetus. Placing investigational drugs in category B leaves the fetus too vulnerable to risk, whereas placing such agents in category D is too restrictive of the subject's autonomy.

As part of this policy, in order to secure consistency among protocols and consent forms, we also developed standardized language to be used in the risks section of the consent form. Any time contraception is required, the following statements are included in the adult consent form:

> It is possible that the medicines used in this study could injure a fetus if you or your partner becomes pregnant while taking them. You have already been told what is known about this possibility, and you are encouraged to ask further questions.
>
> You may want to discuss this with others before you agree to take part in this study. If you wish, we will arrange for a doctor, nurse, or counselor who is not part of this study to discuss the potential risks and benefits with you and anyone else you want to have present.

For category B, C, and D drugs the following is added:

> Because of the potential risks involved, you or your partner should not become pregnant while you are participating in this study, and you are strongly advised not to do so.
>
> If you are sexually active or become sexually active and can get pregnant or can get your partner pregnant, you must agree to use one [or two, for some category C and all category D drugs, as described in the text discussed previously here] of the following forms of birth control every time you have sex:
>   Condoms (male or female) with a spermicidal agent
>   Diaphragm or cervical cap with spermicide
>   IUD
>   Hormonal-based contraception
> The Investigator will discuss the risks and benefits of each of the different forms of contraception available to you in an effort to provide you with the information necessary for you to make a fully informed decision as to which form of contraception you will use. There is specific information available about the risks of each form of contraception and there is also information available about the "failure rates" of each form.
>
> By signing this and being in the study, you are agreeing to use the birth control methods listed above while you are on the study. Should you become pregnant while on this study, you must immediately notify the study personnel. The investigator will assist you in finding appropriate medical care. The investigator also may ask to be allowed to continue getting information about your pregnancy. You can refuse to provide this information.

Although there remain some difficulties with this policy (e.g., the validity of the FDA categories and the implication that the four model forms of birth control are of equivalent efficacy), this policy does address, at least implicitly, some of the concerns raised previously here.

The issue of nonheterosexual activity is addressed in that the policy only applies to subjects who are "sexually active . . . and can get pregnant or can get your partner pregnant." As nonheterosexual activity does not have the potential for conception, subjects are not required to use any birth control. Furthermore, because barrier methods of contraception are always an option, women who subsequently decide to engage in heterosexual activity need only use those noninvasive forms at the time of the sexual activity. These women would not be exposed to the risks of invasive birth control methods.

The issue of abstinence was also addressed implicitly by the requirement that every protocol allow for barrier forms of birth control. Because barriers are only used when engaging in sexual activity, subjects practicing abstinence can still agree to use these forms of birth control and not be required to undertake the risks associated with an IUD or hormonal contraception.

Conclusions

In summary, a requirement for contraception is probably justified (in many cases) as a compromise between the conflicting principles of autonomy and nonmaleficence. If contraception is required, there is an equivalent requirement for "effective" contraception, although the definition of "effective" varies between populations and studies. The informed consent process should address issues related to reproductive and fetal risk, contraception, and pregnancy testing.

Acknowledgments

Much of the material in the section "Model Policy" is drawn from another article, "Contraception in Research: A Policy Suggestion" in *IRB: Ethics and Human Research*, as cited later here.

References

1. U.S. Department of Health, Education and Welfare, Food and Drug Administration. General considerations for clinical evaluation of drugs. Publication No. HEW (FDA) 77-3040. Washington, DC: Food and Drug Administration; 1977.

2. U.S. Department of Health and Human Services, Public Health Service. Report of the Public Health Service Task Force on Women's Health Issues (Vol. II). DHHS Publication No. 88-50206. Washington, DC; 1984.

3. Women and Health Research. *Ethical and legal issues of including women in clinical studies* (Vol. I). In: Mastroianni A, Faden R, Federman D (eds.). Washington, DC: National Academy Press; 1994.

4. U.S. Department of Health and Human Services, Food and Drug Administration. Guideline for study and evaluation of gender differences in the clinical evaluation of drugs. *Fed Regist* 58(139):39406–39416, 1993.

5. U.S. Department of Health and Human Services, National Institutes of Health. NIH guidelines on the inclusion of women and minorities as subjects in clinical research. *Fed Regist* 59(59):14508–14513, 1994.

6. U.S. Department of Health and Human Services. 45 CFR part 46. Protection of Human Subjects, Final Rule. *Fed Regist* 66(11):3878–3883, 2001.

7. Merton V. The exclusion of pregnant, pregnable, and once-pregnable people (aka women) from biomedical research. *Am J Law Med* 19(4):369, 452, 1993.

8. Hall J. Exclusion of pregnant women from research protocols: Unethical and illegal. *IRB* 17(2):1–3, 1995.

9. Potter L. How effective are contraceptives? The determination and measurement of pregnancy rates. *Obstet Gynecol* 88:13S–23S, 1996.

10. Bush J. The industry perspective on the inclusion of women in clinical trials. *Acad Med* 69(9):708–715, 1994.

11. VandenBosch T, Ward B, Mattison D. A reappraisal of female adolescent participation in drug clinical trials. *IRB* 21(1):1–5, 1999.

12. Levine C. Commentary: Teenager, research and family involvement. *IRB* 3(9):8,1981.

13. Halbreich U, Carson S. Drug studies in women of childbearing age: Ethical and methodological considerations. *J Clin Psychopharmacol* 9:328, 1989.

14. Nolan M, Pressman E, Starklauf B, Gregory R. Consent documents, reproductive issues, and the inclusion of women in clinical trials. *Acad Med* 74(3):275–281, 1999.

15. Gordon B, Schonfeld T. Contraception in research: A policy suggestion. *IRB: Ethics and Human Res* 27(2):15–20, 2005.

16. Food and Drug Administration. Labeling and prescription drug advertising: Content and format for labeling for human prescription drugs. *Fed Regist* 44:37434–37467, 1979.

Research Involving Fetuses and In Vitro Fertilization

Ronald M. Green

INTRODUCTION

Biomedical research involving the human embryo or fetus raises a host of special concerns for institutional review board (IRB) reviewers. The embryo or fetus cannot consent to be a research subject. The fetus has a unique and inextricable relationship to the mother. The moral status of the embryo or fetus is a source of widespread disagreement. All of these considerations make embryo and fetal research one of the most controversial issues in our society.

Since the mid-1970s, beginning with the work of the National Commission for the Protection of Human Subjects of Biomedical and Behavioral Research, federal bioethics advisory groups have recommended a variety of regulations for the conduct of federally funded research affecting prenatal human life.[1] Many of these recommendations have attained the status of law and now form part of a complex body of regulations that must be taken into account by investigators working in this area as well as the IRBs that must approve and review their research. Many of these regulations have a sound moral basis. Others require IRB members to make difficult and controversial moral decisions. Some appear to be inconsistent with regulations in related research areas. This reflects the fact that regulations often incorporate one or another contested points of view from our ongoing social debates about the moral claims of embryos or fetuses.

Federal Regulations

Regulations governing research on embryos or fetuses can be classed into four broad categories: (1) research on the fetus itself, (2) research directed toward pregnant women or the condition of pregnancy (for which the embryo or fetus is an indirect subject of research), (3) fetal tissue transplantation research, and (4) research on the ex utero preimplantation human embryo or that uses human pluripotential stem cells (hPSCs) derived from such embryos.

These classes of research share at least five common features. First, they all presume some common definitions. The *fetus* itself is defined as "the product of conception from the time of implantation until delivery."[2[Sec.203(c)]] Implantation is confirmed through a presumptive sign of pregnancy such as missed menses or a positive pregnancy test.[2[Sec.203(b)]] *Pregnancy* is defined as encompassing "the period of time from confirmation of implantation (through any of the presumptive signs of pregnancy, such as missed menses, or by a medically acceptable pregnancy test) until expulsion or extraction of the fetus.[2[Sec.403(b)]]

Because implantation normally occurs before the end of the first week after fertilization, this definition differs from standard medical ones, which usually term the earliest product of conception as an embryo and define the fetus as coming into being only at the eighth week of pregnancy. It follows from the regulatory definition that the ex utero preimplantation human embryo (i.e., the embryo conceived through in vitro fertilization [IVF] but not yet or never transferred to a womb) is not covered by regulations pertaining to federally funded fetal research. In 1996, this perceived gap in regulations was closed when Congress adopted language found in the Dickey-Wicker Amendment to the Department of Health and Human Services budget bill.[3,4] This amendment, which has been reenacted in each subsequent year, prohibits federal funding of any "research in which a human embryo or embryos are destroyed, discarded, or knowingly subjected to risk of injury or death greater than that allowed for research on fetuses in utero" under existing federal regulations. Dickey-Wicker also offers a wide-ranging definition of the human embryo as "any organism . . . that is derived by fertilization, parthenogenesis, cloning, or any other means from one or more human gametes." Many individuals will have moral difficulties with a definition that affords parthenotes—egg cells that have been artificially stimulated to divide and cannot possibly develop beyond a few cell divisions—the same degree of research protection given to later fetuses. This is one consequence of the highly politicized process that has led to current regulations.

A second feature common to federal regulations in this area is the complexity of consent requirements. Because embryos and fetuses normally have male and female progenitors, the consent of both progenitors for any research is normally required. (Exceptions are embryos produced by somatic cell nuclear transfer [cloning] technology or parthenogenesis. Both types of organisms are defined as embryos under the provisions of current U.S. law.) However, the fact that the fetus resides inside the mother's body makes her position special. Not only is she often the most proximate individual to the fetus, her health or life can be affected by decisions in this research area. Federal regulations reflect this in their complex provisions for bypassing paternal consent in the case of some research protocols.

A third feature common to all regulations in this area is the effort to separate embryo or fetal progenitors from any medical or pecuniary advantages that research may offer. Donors of embryos or fetal tissues for research are prohibited from directing these cells or tissues to recipients (including relatives) who may benefit from transplants using them. Regulations also prohibit the provision of monetary or other inducements (such as free or discounted medical services) to embryo or fetal tissue donors or suppliers. This is consistent with the general discouragement of the sale of organs or body parts in this country, but it also reflects a special concern to prevent research from becoming an inducement to abortion or embryo destruction.

Fourth, constraints in current regulations seek to remove inducements to abortion or involvement in abortion procedures on the part of researchers. Regulations specify that individuals engaged in the research will have no part in any decisions as to the timing, method, and procedures used to terminate the pregnancy or in determining the viability of the fetus at the termination of the pregnancy. They also specify that "no procedural changes which may cause greater than minimal risk to the fetus or the pregnant woman will be introduced into the procedure for terminating the pregnancy solely in the interest of the (research) activity."[2(Sec.208)]

Fifth, and finally, there is a requirement pertaining to all of this research that appropriate studies on animals and nonpregnant individuals have been completed. This provision reflects the seriousness with which interventions affecting the human fetus or embryo are taken. It also poses an ongoing challenge to members of IRBs. Biological differences between animals or other human beings and developing human embryos or fetuses often recommend specific types of fetal or embryo research. Members of IRBs must determine when all "appropriate" alternative studies have been completed and when the step to fetal or embryo research may be taken.

Research Directed at the Fetus Itself

An IRB may approve research directed at the fetus in utero if (1) the purpose of the activity is to meet the health needs of the particular fetus and the fetus will be placed at risk only to the minimum extent necessary to meet such needs or (2) the risk to the fetus imposed by the research is minimal and the purpose of the activity is the development of important biomedical knowledge that cannot be obtained by other means.[2(Sec.208)] An example of the first purpose is the use of a new technique for fetal transfusion for Rh incompatibility; an example of the second is minor change in maternal diet or use of ultrasonography. As in pediatric and other human subjects research, minimal means that "the probability and magnitude of harm or discomfort anticipated in the research are not greater in and of themselves than those ordinarily encountered in daily life or during the performance of routine physical or psychological examinations or tests."[2(Sec.102)]

It is noteworthy that this standard for research on the fetus in utero is somewhat stricter than that which applies to research on children. Regulations permit research on children that represents no prospect of direct benefit to individual subjects and a minor increase over minimal risk if the intervention or procedure is likely to yield "generalizable knowledge about the subjects' disorder or condition which is of vital importance for the understanding or amelioration of the subjects' disorder or condition."[2(Sec.406)] Unless the mother's health is at issue, no such permission for a minor increase over minimal risk exists where research on the fetus is concerned.

Implicit in this strict standard is a refusal to distinguish between a fetus destined for abortion and one intended to be carried to term. At first sight, one might think it reasonable to permit some degree of increased risk to the fetus when pregnancy termination is in prospect and the fetus will die in any event. For example, the preabortion fetus might seem a suitable subject for research on whether a teratogenic drug passes through the placenta. However, endangering the fetus in such cases will either limit a woman's freedom to change her mind about abortion or will result in harm to the born child if she should choose to continue the pregnancy to term. The unacceptability of both of these alternatives recommends a standard of equal treatment of all fetuses with regard to risk. However, once this standard has been met, nothing prevents preferential use of fetuses intended for abortion in minimal-risk research.

The process of consent to such research is complex and may involve the IRB in difficult determinations and judgments. In all such research, the consent of the mother on behalf of the fetus is required. As a general rule, the father, as coprogenitor, is also required to consent on behalf of the fetus. However, there are three exceptions to this rule: (1) if the father's identity or whereabouts cannot reasonably be ascertained, (2) if he is not reasonably available, or (3) if the pregnancy resulted from rape.[2[Sec.208(b),209(d)]] The IRB has a limited role to play here in assisting investigators in determining when these conditions are met. It is usually sufficient for the IRB to ensure that the investigator obtains a statement about the applicability of one or another of these exceptions from the mother. No further assessment of the facts is required.

Research can also take place on the fetus ex utero after a spontaneous or induced abortion. In such cases, the fetus is judged to be viable if it is able to survive (given the benefit of available medical therapy) to the point of independently maintaining heartbeat and respiration. A viable fetus is treated by existing regulations as a premature infant and comes under the protections of regulations governing research on children. In general, a fetus that has not attained a gestational age of 20 weeks and does not exceed 400 grams in weight is judged to be nonviable. Independent medical assessment of nonviability is required when these limits have been exceeded. A nonviable fetus may be involved in research only if (1) its vital functions are not artificially maintained, (2) experimental activities that of themselves would terminate its heartbeat or respiration are not employed, and (3) the purpose of the activity is the development of important biomedical knowledge that cannot be obtained by other means. Until it is ascertained whether a fetus ex utero is viable, it may not be involved in research unless there will be no added risk to the fetus resulting from the activity, and the purpose of the activity is the development of important biomedical knowledge that cannot be obtained by other means or the purpose of the activity is to enhance the possibility of survival of the particular fetus to the point of viability.[2(Sec.209)]

The Fetus as an Indirect Subject of Research

Research on women who are pregnant necessarily implicates the fetus. Federal regulations specify that no pregnant woman may be involved as a subject unless either (1) the purpose of the activity is to meet the health needs of the mother and the fetus will be placed at risk only to the minimum extent necessary to meet such needs or (2) the risk to the fetus is minimal.[2(Sec.207)] In such cases, research may proceed only if the mother and father are legally competent and have given their informed consent. The father's consent is not required, however, if the purpose of the activity is to meet the health needs of the mother or if the three exceptions to paternal consent mentioned in connection with research directed at the fetus apply. In research undertaken to meet the health problems of a pregnant woman, her needs generally take precedence over those of the fetus,[2(Sec.207)] except, perhaps, where the health benefit to her is minimal and risk to the fetus is high.

Regulatory protections also apply to nonpregnant women of childbearing age. These regulations require that, when appropriate, subjects be provided "a statement that the particular treatment or procedure may involve risks to the subject (or to the embryo or fetus, if the subject is or may become pregnant) which are currently unforeseeable" as part of the informed consent process.[2[Sec.116(b)(1)]] In

such cases, IRBs may need to ensure that nonpregnant subjects are advised to avoid pregnancy or nursing for a time during or after the research. Furthermore, where appropriate, subjects should be advised to notify the investigator immediately if they become pregnant. In some instances, the potential risk may be sufficient to justify requiring that pregnant or fertile women either be specifically excluded from the research or studied separately.

These regulations raise several ethical questions for IRBs and for society as a whole. Research whose primary purpose is to meet "the health needs of the mother" can sometimes impose a difficult balancing decision on investigators. This is particularly true in cases where the health benefit to her is minimal and the risk to the fetus is high. IRB members are called on to determine just how much risk to the fetus is allowable to meet such needs. The very existence of this requirement, however, raises a larger question of whether the IRB is really the appropriate maker of this decision. Because a woman's health is at issue, some would ask why she should not have sole authority to determine the degree of risk to which both she and her fetus may be exposed.

Some have also questioned whether the fetal-protective nature of current regulations in this area does not evidence inherent discrimination and injustice. It has been pointed out, for example, that some substances have the potential to affect the genetic components of sperm and, through this, the health of any resulting child. Yet current regulations do not require investigators and IRBs to balance the health needs of fertile men involved in research against possible risks to their offspring.[5,6] It is also pointed out that current regulations have had a broad effect in reducing the amount of research done on women of childbearing age, preventing this group as a whole from benefiting from that research. The problem is compounded when drugs or procedures are then clinically used on women without the background of research results needed to test their efficacy or toxicity. Although members of IRBs must work within the framework of existing regulations, they should be aware of this ethical debate. They may also find that the debate impacts on their decision making when they must balance the requirement to protect potentially pregnant women while fulfilling the current federal mandate to include women in clinical trials and other studies.

A further complexity is posed by research aimed at improving our understanding of the process of pregnancy itself. Some studies in this area (e.g., a study of the physiological mechanisms initiating labor) are not directed at the health of either the mother or the fetus. Other studies, such as those examining the effects of maternal diabetes on a pregnancy, are directed at the health of both the mother and the fetus. In these cases, IRBs must determine how to categorize such research and which requirements apply. In general, unless the research is undertaken to meet the health problems of a pregnant woman or the fetus, the requirement of "minimal risk" to the fetus will apply, as will the paternal consent requirement (with its stipulated exceptions).

Fetal Tissue Transplantation Research

After the fetus is dead, its cells, tissues, organs, or placental material may normally be used in research with the consent of the mother and in accordance with any applicable state or local laws regarding such activities.[2(Sec.210)] However, special regulations apply to fetal cells or tissues intended to be used in transplantation research. This is another reflection of our ongoing social debates about abortion.

The important healing and curative potential of fetal tissue was recognized as early as 1928 when fetal tissue was first transplanted into patients suffering from diabetes. More recently, fetal neural tissue has been used, with mixed results, in the treatment of Parkinson's disease and other neurologic disorders as well as other conditions.[7] During the 1980s, there was substantial controversy about the ethical permissibility of such research. In 1988, a majority of the members of the Human Fetal Tissue Transplantation Research Panel concluded that permitting fetal tissue transplantation research under strict guidelines was "acceptable public policy."[8] However, because of resistance from then-President George Bush, this recommendation did not go into effect until 1993. In January of that year, President Clinton, in one of his first acts of office, issued an executive order permitting fetal tissue transplantation research. Subsequently, Congress passed this order into law in the provisions of the National Institutes of Health (NIH) Revitalization Act of 1993.[9]

In general, the relevant provisions of the NIH Revitalization Act seek to protect the donor of fetal tissue, ensure her free and informed consent, and reduce the likelihood that this research will offer her an incentive to abortion. The regulations also seek to prevent the emergence of a commercial market in cadaveric fetal tissues. To achieve these purposes, the act requires formal statements of consent or disclosure from the female donor, her attending physician, the researcher using fetal tissue, and the recipient of such tissue (donee). For example, the woman donating human fetal tissue must sign a statement declaring that the tissue is being donated for therapeutic transplantation research, the donation is being made without any restriction regarding the identity of individuals who may be the recipients of transplantations of the tissue, and the donation is being made without her (the donor) having been informed of the identity of those individuals who may be the recipients.

The attending physician must sign a statement declaring that the tissue has been obtained in accord with the donor's signed statement and that full disclosure has been made to her of (1) the attending physician's interest, if any, in the research to be conducted with the tissue and (2) any known medical risks to the donor or risks to her privacy that might be associated with the donation of the tissue and are in addition to the risks associated with the woman's medical care. In the case of tissue obtained as a result of an induced abortion, the attending physician's statement must also declare that the consent of the woman for the abortion was obtained before requesting or obtaining consent for donation, the abortion was conducted in accord with applicable state law, and no alteration of the timing, method, or procedures used to terminate the pregnancy was made solely for the purposes of obtaining the tissue.

The individual with the principal responsibility for conducting the research must sign a statement declaring that the individual is aware that the tissue is human fetal tissue donated for research purposes and may have been obtained as a result of a spontaneous or induced abortion or a stillbirth; that he or she has provided such information to other individuals with responsibilities regarding the research; that the researcher will require, before obtaining the consent of a person to be a recipient of a transplantation of the tissue, written acknowledgment of receipt of this information by the recipient; and that the researcher has had no part in any decisions as to the timing, method, or procedures used to terminate the pregnancy made solely for the purposes of the research.

Finally, an additional series of provisions of the NIH Revitalization Act declares it unlawful for anyone to solicit, acquire, receive, or transfer human fetal tissue for "valuable consideration" or as the result of a promise to the donating individual that the tissue will be transplanted into a recipient specified by such an individual or a relative of the donating individual.

It appears that these provisions, now in effect for over a decade, have calmed the fears of some individuals concerned that fetal tissue transplantation research might legitimize or increase the incidence of abortion. One sign of this is the fact that during legislative debates about stem cells, Representative Jay Dickey (R-Arkansas), one of the most outspoken opponents of research using stem cells derived from spare embryos remaining from infertility procedures (ES cells), was willing, within the protections of existing fetal tissue transplantation regulations, to permit research using stem cells derived from the gonadal ridge of aborted fetuses (so-called EG cells). However, it is not clear whether federally funded fetal tissue transplantation research or the use of cadaveric fetuses as a source of stem cells will continue to be permitted. In the first months of his first administration, President George W. Bush questioned any use of tissues from aborted fetuses in research.[10] Which direction he will eventually move remains to be seen.

Human Embryo Research

If the history of fetal tissue transplantation research is convoluted, that of research on the preimplantation ex utero human embryo is even more so. With the advent of IVF during the 1970s, the ex utero human embryo became available as a subject of research. The need to increase the efficiency of IVF procedures also provided an incentive to increase federal support for such research.

In the late 1970s, a special body, the Ethics Advisory Board (EAB), was formed by an act of Congress to review and provide guidance for federally funded research on the human embryo. In late 1979, the EAB issued its report containing a broad permission for such research under federal auspices, subject to guidelines and limitations indicated in the report and to be implemented by the board itself.[11] However, before the EAB's recommendations could be put into effect, there was a change in administrations. During the Reagan and Bush years, funding for the EAB and nominations to its membership were halted. The legal requirement of EAB approval of all such research and the absence of an EAB created a de facto moratorium on funding for embryo research in the United States. In 1993, the NIH Revitalization Act abrogated the requirement for EAB approval, freeing the NIH to support research in this area. To ensure ethical oversight, the NIH convened a special body, the NIH Human Embryo Research Panel, to provide recommendations for research guidelines. In September 1994, the panel issued its report, which was accepted by the Advisory Committee to the Director of NIH in December of that year.[12]

Among the Human Embryo Research Panel's recommendations was permission for the deliberate creation of human embryos for research purposes under certain restricted circumstances. This included circumstances when the research "by its very nature cannot otherwise be validly conducted" (as in research whose end point is fertilization) and when such embryos are needed "for the validity of a study that is potentially of outstanding scientific and therapeutic value."[12(p.44–45)] Within hours of the acceptance of the Human Embryo Research Panel report by the Advisory Committee to the Director of NIH, President Clinton issued a statement rejecting this recommendation and limiting permissible research only to embryos remaining from infertility procedures. Subsequently, the provisions of the Dickey-Wicker Amendment, which prohibits any research involving the destruction of human embryos, revoked even this qualified permission. Where federally funded research is concerned, therefore, current U.S. regulations treat research on embryos as a form of fetal research. Because possibly conflicting maternal health considerations do not appear to apply to research on the ex utero embryo, this means that IRBs may approve such research only if it represents no more than "minimal risk" for the embryo.

One consequence of the prolonged absence of federal support for human embryo research is the relegation of this research to privately funded fertility clinics that lack sufficient resources for such research or large, multicenter studies. This has contributed to the inefficiency of IVF and related procedures and accounts, in part, for their cost, often amounting to tens of thousands of dollars per treatment course. It has slowed research on birth defects caused by failures in embryologic development. Poorly researched infertility procedures also play a large role in the epidemic of premature births associated with current infertility treatments.[13]

Beyond the sphere of infertility medicine, the ban on federal funding for most human embryo research has recently become a source of controversy in other promising research areas. In November 1998, scientists at the University of Wisconsin and The Johns Hopkins University announced the creation of the first immortalized pluripotent stem cell lines (hPSCs).[14,15] The Wisconsin team, headed by James Thomson, used spare embryos remaining from infertility procedures for this purpose. These embryos were dissected; their inner cell mass of totipotent cells (capable of developing into virtually any bodily tissue) was removed and placed on a feeder layer to create a line of immortalized embryonic stem cells (ES cells). The Hopkins team, headed by John Gearhart, used tissues from the gonadal ridge of aborted fetuses (such stem cells are referred to as EG cells). Because the Thomson team's ES cell research required the destruction of embryos, it could not qualify for federal funding and was financed by private sources. The Gearhart team technically qualified for federal support because theirs was a form of fetal tissue research, but they did not seek it.

Many scientists view hPSCs as one of the most promising research areas in biomedicine today. These cells are undifferentiated, totipotent cells and are able to proliferate indefinitely in culture. After techniques for growing and redifferentiating such cells are developed, stem cell lines may be used to replace damaged cardiac tissue after a heart attack or repair now irreversible spinal cord injuries. Parkinson's disease, Alzheimer's disease, and diabetes are among the long list of conditions that might be cured by the ability to produce new bodily tissues.

In December 1999, the NIH issued draft guidelines specifying the conditions and restrictions under which it would support research using hPSCs. These guidelines rested on an NIH-solicited legal opinion that hPSCs are not themselves "embryos" within the meaning of the Dickey-Wicker Amendment and that research "utilizing" but not deriving hPSCs from human embryos does not constitute "research in which a human embryo or embryos are destroyed." This use-versus-derivation distinction was subject to criticism both by friends and opponents of federally funded stem cell research according to a report by the National Bioethics Advisory Committee advocating a broad permission for federal funding of both the use and derivation of ES cells. After a period of public comment, the NIH issued revised but roughly similar final guidelines on August 25, 2000.[16] Although they never went into effect, these guidelines remain one of the most developed bodies of thinking about ethical oversight for stem cell research.

The guidelines define hPSCs as "cells that are self-replicating, are derived from human embryos or human fetal tissue, and are known to develop into cells and tissues of the three primary germ layers." Research on such cells may be conducted "only if the cells were derived (without federal funds) from human embryos that were created for the purposes of fertility treatment and were in excess of the clinical need of the individuals seeking such treatment." The guidelines thus carry forth the prohibition begun with President Clinton's December 1994 intervention against any research using embryos that are deliberately created for research purposes. This prohibition is relevant to broad areas of stem cell research, including research on human therapeutic cloning. This involves the use of somatic cell nuclear transfer (cloning) technology to activate enucleated oocytes, which can then be dissected to produce immunologically compatible stem cells for the original cell donor/patient.[17] Although Great Britain's Human Fertilisation and Embryology Authority has been authorized to support this research, it remains off-limits for federal funding in this country. This is because the Dickey-Wicker Amendment defines even clonally activated eggs as "embryos" and prohibits their use in research in which they are destroyed, as is the case in stem cell research.

The NIH guidelines also applied to this area of restrictions found in fetal tissue research that were advanced to prevent the promise of research or its benefits from becoming an incentive abortion or embryo destruction. Thus, "no inducements, monetary or otherwise, [may be] offered for the donation of human embryos for research purposes." Fertility clinics and/or their affiliated laboratories must implement specific written policies against such inducements. There must be "a clear separation between the decision to create embryos for fertility treatment and the decision to donate human embryos in excess of clinical need for research purposes to derive pluripotent stem cells." To ensure that this is so by providing time for decision, only frozen embryos may be used as a stem cell source. Researchers or investigators proposing to derive or use human pluripotent stem cells in research should have no role in securing spare embryos for this research, and the attending physician for fertility treatment and researcher should not be one and the same person. As is true for fetal tissue for transplantation, donation of human embryos should be made "without any restriction or direction regarding the individual(s) who may be the recipients of transplantation of the cells derived from the embryo."

The guidelines specified that the consent for such research should include the following provisions: (1) a statement that the embryos will be used to derive human pluripotent stem cells for research that may include human transplantation research; (2) a statement that the donation is made without any restriction or direction regarding the individual(s) who may be the recipient(s) of transplantation of the cells derived from the embryo; (3) a statement as to whether information that could identify the donors of the embryos, directly or through identifiers linked to the donors, will be removed before the derivation or the use of human pluripotent stem cells; (4) a statement that derived cells and/or cell lines may be kept for many years; (5) disclosure of the possibility that the results of research on the human pluripotent stem cells may have commercial potential, and a statement that the donor will not receive financial or any other benefits from any such future commercial development; (6) a statement that the research is not intended to provide direct medical benefit to the donor; and (7) a statement that embryos donated will not be transferred to a woman's uterus and will not survive the human pluripotent stem cell derivation process.

Recognizing that the process of preparing stem cell lines may involve costs, the guidelines permitted payment for cell lines using federal funding as long as payment "does not exceed the reasonable costs associated with the transportation, processing, preservation, quality control, and storage of the stem cells." An assurance to this effect is also a requirement of IRB review.

Finally, the guidelines specified a series of research directions that are ineligible for NIH funding. In addition to prohibitions on the derivation of stem cell lines, the use of embryos deliberately created for research purposes, and somatic cell nuclear transfer (therapeutic cloning), they include "research in which human pluripotent stem cells are utilized to create or contribute to a human embryo;" "research in which human pluripotent stem cells are combined with an animal embryo;" and "research in which human pluripotent stem cells are used in combination with somatic cell nuclear transfer for the purposes of reproductive cloning of a human."

On August 9, 2001, in a public address to the nation, President George W. Bush announced the adoption of a national policy on stem cell research. This permits federal funding for research on cell lines developed (under private auspices) previous to that date. He thus adopted a conservative version of the use-versus-derivation position articulated earlier by the NIH (although not one that would permit the use of cell lines from embryos destroyed following the August 9 date). In the same address, the president also announced formation of a council "to monitor stem cell research, to recommend appropriate guidelines and regulations and to consider all of the medical and ethical ramifications of biomedical innovation."[18]

Many questions still remain unanswered. The council established by the president (The President's Bioethics Council) has never formally addressed the research-related issue of guidelines for stem cell research. Presumably, the donor requirements of the August 25, 2000, NIH guidelines govern NIH-funded research on the stem cell lines permitted under the president's August 9, 2001, policy. However, it is not clear that existing stem cell lines comply with all features of those guidelines. The NIH has stipulated that "in vitro research and research in animals using already derived and established human cell lines, from which the identity of the donor(s) cannot readily be ascertained by the investigator, are not considered human subject research and are not governed by the DHHS or FDA human subject protection regulations appearing at 45 CFR Part 46 and 21 CFR Parts 50 and 56."[19] As a result, IRB review is not required for such research. In March 2005, a committee of the National Research Council published recommended guidelines for all state or privately funded embryonic stem cell research.[20] Although these guidelines do not have the force of law, they are in the process of being adopted by some states and, in addition to the August 25, 2000, NIH guidelines, are a good reference point for those conducting privately funded research.

A further problem for federally funded research is the limited quantity and quality of these lines. Although the president spoke in August 2001 of 60 cell lines being available for research, by early 2005, only 22 such lines had been characterized and proved viable for research purposes. Furthermore, it has been shown that all of these lines are contaminated with molecules derived from the mouse cell feeder layers on which they were cultured. Because of problems of rejection, and transmission of murine viruses, this renders these lines largely unsuitable for human stem cell transplantation research.[21] These and other considerations suggest that the current federal policy on stem cell research may eventually come up for review, especially if research in the private sector or overseas realizes some of its promised benefits.[22,23] IRBs should remain alert to developments in this rapidly evolving area.

Conclusion

Research involving fetuses and IVF presents the IRB with a wide range of difficult regulatory and ethical questions. This chapter has presented the background information that IRB members, researchers, and institutional officials will need to establish policy related to this often complex and controversial area of research. Research involving stem cells is especially problematic as federal policy in this area is likely to undergo major changes over the next few years.

References

1. National Commission for the Protection of Human Subjects of Biomedical and Behavioral Research. Research on the fetus (DHEW (OS) 76–127) and Appendix: Research on the fetus (DHEW (OS) 76–128). Washington, DC: Government Printing Office; 1975.

2. Code of Federal Regulations. Title 45A—Department of Health and Human Services; Part 46—Protection of Human Subjects. Updated 1 October, 1997. Access date 18 April, 2001. http://www4.law.cornell.edu/cfr/45p46.htm

3. 104th Congress. Making appropriations for fiscal year 1996 to make a downpayment toward a balanced budget, and for other purposes. Public Law 104–99, Section 128; 110 Stat 34. 26 January, 1996.

4. 105th Congress. Omnibus consolidated and emergency appropriations for the fiscal year ending September 30, 1999, and for other purposes. Public Law 105–277; 112 Stat. 2681. 21 October, 1998. Access date 24 April, 2001. http://frwebgate.access.gpo.gov/cgi-bin/getdoc.cgi?dbname5105_cong_public_laws&docid5f:publ277.105.pdf

5. Merton V. The exclusion of pregnant, pregnable, and once-pregnable people (aka women) from biomedical research. *Am J Law Med* 19(4):369–451, 1993.

6. Charo RA. Protecting us to death: Women, pregnancy, and clinical research trials. *St Louis Univ Law J* 38(1):135–187, 1993.

7. Freed CR, Greene PE, Breeze RE, et al. Transplantation of embryonic dopamine neurons for severe Parkinson's disease. *N Engl J Med* 344(10):710–719, 2001.

8. National Institutes of Health. Human fetal tissue transplantation research: Report of the Advisory Committee to the Director. Washington, DC: The National Institutes of Health; December 1988.

9. 103rd Congress. National Institutes of Health Revitalization Act of 1993, 10 June, 1993. Access date 24 April, 2001. http://ohrp.osophs.dhhs.gov/humansubjects/guidance/publiclaw103–43.htm

10. Weiss R. Fetal cell research funds are at risk: Scientists fear curbs over abortion. *Washington Post*, A3, January 26, 2001.

11. Ethics Advisory Board. Report and conclusions: HEW support of human in vitro fertilization and embryo transfer. *Fed Regist* 44:35033–35058, 18 June, 1979.

12. National Institutes of Health. Report of the Human Embryo Research Panel, 27 September, 1994. Bethesda, MD.

13. Green RM. *The Human Embryo Research Debates: Bioethics in the Vortex of Controversy.* New York: Oxford University Press; 2001.

14. Thomson JA, Itskovitz-Eldor J, Shapiro SS, et al. Embryonic stem cell lines derived from human blastocysts. *Science* 282(5391):1145–1147, 1998.

15. Shamblot MJ, Axelman J, Wang S, et al. Derivation of pluripotential stem cells from cultured human primordial germ cells. *Proc Natl Acad Sci USA* 95:13726–13731, 1998.

16. National Institutes of Health. NIH Guidelines for Research using Human Pluripotent Stem Cells. *Fed Regist* 65: 69951, 21 November, 2000. Access date 7 May, 2001. http://www.nih.gov/news/stemcell/stemcellguidelines.htm

17. Lanza RP, Caplan AL, Silver LM, et al. The ethical validity of using nuclear transfer in human transplantation. *JAMA* 284(24):3175–3179, 2000.

18. President's statement on funding stem cell research. *New York Times*, August 10, 2001.

19. Office for Human Research Protections, Department of Health and Human Services. Guidance for Investigators and Institutional Review Boards Regarding Research Involving Human Embryonic Stem Cells, Germ Cells and Stem Cell-Derived Test Articles, March 19, 2002. Access date 4 July, 2005. http://stemcells.nih.gov/policy/guidelines.asp

20. Committee on Guidelines for Human Embryonic Stem Cell Research, National Research Council. *Guidelines for Human Embryonic Stem Cell Research.* Washington, DC: National Academies Press, 2005.

21. Ebert E. Human stem cells trigger immune attack. news@nature.com, 24 January, 2005. http://www.nature.com/news/2005/050124/pf/050124-1_pf.html

22. Normile D, Mann CC. Cell biology: Asia jockeys for stem cell lead. *Science* 307:660–664, 2005.

23. Holden C. U.S. states offer Asia stiff competition. *Science* 307:662–663, 2005.

Research Involving Pregnant Women

Angela J. Bowen

INTRODUCTION

Women have traditionally been protected from research risks, especially in early-phase studies. Women of childbearing potential were specifically excluded from participation in Phase I and II studies until new guidance was issued[1] that removed the need to preferentially exclude women of childbearing potential. This 1993 guidance also stressed the need for studies to be done to evaluate any sex- or gender-related differences in the response to study treatments. (These guidance documents unfortunately use *sex-related differences* and *gender-related differences* interchangeably, mirroring our cultural, political, and societal ambivalence in the use of these terms.) Later guidance documents to institutional review boards (IRBs) advised that they should "assure that women were not unreasonably excluded" from a protocol. This led many IRBs to devise systems to assure equal representation of women in all trials. The guidance did not anticipate that every protocol would have equal numbers of men and women, but simply aimed to assure that before approval some studies would be conducted in both sexes, thereby noting any differences of therapeutic significance.

The IRB process is ill equipped to determine whether enough women have been included in the evaluations of a new compound or device. The number of women already studied, or currently enrolled, is often not revealed in the protocol being reviewed, nor is the number planned into future studies. It is therefore appropriate that the study sponsor should assume the responsibility for determining if prior studies have adequately evaluated gender differences. From the standpoint of ethical standards, it makes no sense for the IRB to concentrate on the numbers of women enrolled in an individual trial.

Sex and Gender Differences

There are sometimes sex-dependent differences in pharmacokinetic and pharmacodynamic parameters. (*Sex dependent* denotes genetic, hormonal, reproductive, and physical differences.) There are likely to be gender differences in many areas of research, especially in the behavioral sciences. (*Gender differences* is used to describe the variability between men and women that is attributable to influences such as society, culture, or history.) These protocols should be carefully reviewed to ascertain whether one gender may have different risks, or receive different benefits, because of gender. Special protections may be necessary if increased risk or benefit is determined for one gender.

IRBs should recall that these guidance documents were developed in response to activist pressure to ensure that women had equal access to all things and to the pressure from these and other groups to ensure that drugs, biologicals, and devices were tested in all patient populations where they might be used. The historical practice had been to test compounds in normal young males through Phase II and, finally, in the general population, excluding pregnant women and children, in Phase III. After marketing, products were labeled with the indication that they had not been tested in pregnant women and children and, therefore, should be used with caution in these populations. This system was imperfect but did have the advantage that by the time the drug was marketed it had been through animal testing and the teratologic and mutagenic tendencies were well documented. Considerable generalizable knowledge was also accumulated before marketing under this system, thereby reducing the relative risk to pregnant women and their fetuses.

The original National Institutes of Health (NIH) regulations addressing research with pregnant women[2(Sec.207)] admonished that no pregnant woman could be involved as a research subject unless the purpose of the activity was to meet the health needs of the mother and the fetus was placed at risk only to the minimum extent necessary to meet such needs. This is still sound advice and should be weighed by the IRB in review of such research.

Although the FDA has urged IRBs to assist the agency in implementing changes and not to needlessly exclude pregnant women, the IRB's first responsibility is to the subject and not to social change.

Women of Childbearing Potential

One cannot discuss research in pregnant women without mentioning research in women of childbearing potential. It must be assumed that pregnancies will occur in this group regardless of the precautions advised. Thus, the IRB must evaluate the various safeguards that might be offered that would afford some increase in subject safety. Frequent pregnancy tests, "reliable" contraception, and abstinence are all recommended, with abstinence being the only choice one can really count on. Because reliable decision making in this age group is often not yet perfected, a strong warning about what to do in case unprotected intercourse occurs is highly recommended. The consent document should contain a clear warning about the possibility of birth defects if pregnancy should occur. In most cases, women of childbearing potential should not be included in trials if teratogenicity is likely. The risk of a malformed child far outweighs any possible societal benefit. Also, the risks of teratogenic compounds may be transferable between the sexes. A mutagenic compound may be given to a man who may impregnate a woman who is unaware of the risk. Some caution should be extended by the IRB to known consorts, where possible. When new information regarding risk becomes available during the course of the study, the consent document should be revised. Subjects may need to be contacted, and the IRB and investigator should consider narrowing the study inclusion criteria.

IRB Review of a Study Involving Pregnant Women

The investigator's brochure should be carefully reviewed by a physician IRB member to ascertain whether the appropriate animal studies have been completed and, if so, to evaluate the results. Look especially for fetal loss, deformities, low birth weight, and reduced survival, as well as any evidence of mutagenicity. If these studies have not been completed, research should not be commenced in pregnant women unless there is a clear therapeutic need or benefit to the mother or the fetus. In all cases, the risk to the fetus should be assessed and recorded in the minutes.

The protocol should be carefully reviewed for any opportunities to improve the risk/benefit ratio for both the mother and the fetus. In general, the later the term of the pregnancy, the less risk to the fetus. Therefore, if immediate intervention is not mandatory, delaying administration of the test article for as long as possible may be wise. The minutes of the IRB should clearly reflect that substantive thought and consultation, if necessary, have been given to protection of both mother and fetus. The protocol should be clear about what follow-up is planned for the pregnant woman up to and after delivery, although the research may be completed by then. Careful follow-up by the clinical investigator and consulting gynecologist can be recommended by the IRB. In no case should the investigator be the sole person to counsel or recommend termination of the pregnancy.

Be cautious in review that there is no added risk to the fetus as a consequence of the research and that, to the extent determinable, the possibility of survival of the fetus is enhanced by the research. Sometimes the research activity is directed at the fetus and not the mother. In such cases, the safety of the mother should be given primary attention.

The Consent Process

The consent document must clearly disclose all known risks of both the research article and research process, as well as how they compare with no intervention. When animal studies of reproductive toxicology and teratology have not been completed before initiation of clinical studies, the informed consent document becomes even more critical. The document must reveal, in simple terms, this lack of knowledge. If comparable compounds are available and are known or suspected to have deleterious effects on conception or fetal development, this should be included in the consent process and memorialized in the IRB minutes. Regular updates to the informed consent will be necessary as more complete information becomes available.

A considerable constituency believes that to exclude pregnant women from research until comprehensive reproductive toxicology testing is completed is to neglect them as a population. In any case, the pregnant woman must be fully informed regarding any reasonably foreseeable impact of the research on the fetus. As always, these controverted issues and their full discussion should be adequately recorded in the IRB minutes. If the father is known and available, his involvement in the decision should be encouraged, but not required.

The risks to the fetus and to the mother should be discussed individually so that it is clear who is at risk for what. If the father is available, he should be included in the consent process if the risk to the fetus is increased. If the mother's welfare is the primary concern, only her written consent should be required; however, having the father's agreement on behalf of the fetus is prudent. It is important to remember that the IRB can recommend and require additional protections beyond those already provided by the protocol. Consultation outside the research team can be beneficial to all parties.

Regulatory Issues

The Department of Health and Human Services amended its human subjects protection regulations in January

2001.[2] The final rule was published in the *Federal Register* on January 17, 2001, to become effective March 19, 2001. The rule supports all special protections for pregnant women and fetuses involved in research that have been in force since 1975. The rule aims to promote a policy of presumed inclusion for pregnant women in research. This inclusion will be accomplished by allowing the woman to be the sole decision maker to participate in research. This particular change replaces the old policy of presumed exclusion.

Paternal consent had been necessary under the previous regulations. This provision led to the exclusion of many women from protocols that were expected to have direct benefit to the pregnant woman. Fathers were often not known or were unavailable to give consent. Rape victims were an especially vulnerable class. The new regulation provides for autonomy in these situations:

Sec.207 (b) An activity permitted under paragraph (a) of this section may be conducted only if the mother and father are legally competent and have given their informed consent after having been fully informed regarding possible impact on the fetus, except that the father's informed consent need not be secured if (1) the purpose of the activity is to meet the health needs of the mother, (2) his identity or whereabouts cannot reasonably be ascertained, (3) he is not reasonably available, or (4) the pregnancy resulted from rape.

These changes in the regulations must be adhered to in the ongoing review of continuing projects funded under assurances with the Office for Human Research Protections; therefore, changes to consents and/or protocols may be necessary. Department of Health and Human Services regulations require that certain conditions be met before IRB approval when the research involves pregnant women.[3(Sec.203,204)] These regulations require that, when the board considers such research, it should ensure that all of the following conditions are met:

1. Where scientifically appropriate, preclinical studies, including studies on pregnant animals, and clinical studies, including studies on nonpregnant women, have been conducted and provide data for assessing potential risks to pregnant women and fetuses.

2. The risk to the fetus is not greater than minimal or any risk to the fetus that is greater than minimal is caused solely by interventions or procedures that hold out the prospect of direct benefit for the woman or the fetus.

3. Any risk is the least possible for achieving the objectives of the research.

4. The woman's consent or the consent of her legally authorized representative is obtained in accord with the informed consent provisions of 45 CFR 46, Subpart A, unless legally altered or waived.[2[Sec.101(i)][Sec.116(c),(d)]]

5. The woman or her legally authorized representative, as appropriate, is fully informed regarding the reasonably foreseeable impact of the research on the fetus or resultant child.

6. For children[2[Sec.402(a)]] who are pregnant, assent and permission are obtained in accord with the provisions of 45 CFR 46, Subpart D.

7. No inducements, monetary or otherwise, will be offered to terminate a pregnancy.

8. Individuals engaged in the research will have no part in any decisions as to the timing, method, or procedures used to terminate a pregnancy.

9. Individuals engaged in the research will have no part in determining the viability of a fetus.

The IRB should note that federal rules[3[Sec.202(e)]] define pregnancy as follows:

Pregnancy encompasses the period of time from the implantation until delivery. A woman shall be assumed to be pregnant if she exhibits any of the pertinent presumptive signs of pregnancy, such as missed menses, until the results of a pregnancy test are negative or until delivery.

Conclusion

Research involving pregnant women raises multiple important ethical and regulatory issues. Pregnant women are often vulnerable to exploitation and therefore require extra protections to ensure that research is conducted in an environment that allows all subjects to make informed and voluntary decisions about initial and ongoing research participation. This chapter explains the rationale for excluding pregnant women from research and the situations where the inclusion of this class of subjects may be appropriate. It is important for IRB members to understand the difference, in terms of criteria for IRB approval of research, between research that involves pregnant women and research that excludes women of childbearing potential.

References

1. Food and Drug Administration. Guidelines for the study and evaluation of gender differences in the clinical evaluation of drugs. *Fed Regist* 58(139):39406–39416, 22 July, 1993.

2. Code of Federal Regulations. Title 45A—Department of Health and Human Services; Part 46—Protection of Human Subjects, Subpart B, Additional DHHS Protections Pertaining to Research Activities Involving Fetuses, Pregnant Women, and Human In Vitro Fertilization. Updated 3 November, 1978.

3. Code of Federal Regulations. Title 45A—Department of Health and Human Services; Part 46—Protection of Human Subjects, Subpart B, Additional Protections for Pregnant Women, Human Fetuses and Neonates Involved in Research. Updated 13 November, 2001. Access date 11 March, 2005. http://www.hhs.gov/ohrp/humansubjects/guidance/45cfr46.htm#subpartb

Research Involving Children

Robert M. Nelson

INTRODUCTION

Research involving children requires careful attention to the additional regulatory provisions[1,2(Subpart D)] that are intended to protect children from being enrolled in research that exceeds a level of justified risk. The National Commission in *The Belmont Report* wrote about the "special provisions" for children that respect for persons requires, including "the opportunity to choose to the extent they are able" (i.e., assent), honoring dissent "unless the research entails providing them a therapy unavailable elsewhere," and "seeking the permission of other parties [e.g., parents] in order to protect the subjects from harm."[3] In addition, the National Commission also advocated "an order of preference in the selection of classes of subjects (e.g., adults before children)" as "a matter of social justice" based on the judgment that children ought not to bear the burdens of research unless absolutely necessary.[3] Finally, the National Commission discussed the scope of parental authority in enrolling a child in research, arguing that such decisions may be morally justified if either the research may directly benefit the child[1[Sec.405],2[Sec.52]] or the risks of participation in the research "are equivalent to normal risks of childhood"[4] (i.e., the concept of minimal risk).[1[Sec.404],2[Sec.51]] More controversially, the National Commission extended this notion of "normal" experience to permit parents to enroll children with a "specific disorder or condition" in some nonbeneficial research that "poses no significant threat to the child's health or well-being"[4] (i.e., no more than a minor increase over minimal risk).[1[Sec.406],2[Sec.53]] The concepts of minimal risk, minor increase over minimal risk, prospect of direct benefit, assent, and permission are the basis for the special protections for children.[1,2(Subpart D)] This basis rests on the moral foundation of respect for children, beneficence, justice, and the scope of parental authority.

This chapter reviews the issues that should be considered when an institutional review board (IRB) reviews research involving children, starting with the composition of the IRB and the general aspects of IRB review.

IRB Membership

Regulations[1,5[Sec.107]] require that if "an IRB regularly reviews research that involves a vulnerable category of subjects, such as children . . . , consideration shall be given to the inclusion of one or more individuals who are knowledgeable about and experienced in working with these subjects." Given that an IRB should also be "sufficiently qualified through the experience and expertise of its members," the simple addition of a pediatrician to an adult-oriented IRB does not create an IRB capable of reviewing pediatric research. In keeping with this concern, the Food and Drug Administration (FDA) guidance document on pediatric research requires that "there should be IRB/IEC members or experts consulted by the IRB/IEC who are knowledgeable in pediatric ethical, clinical, and psychosocial issues."[6] More concretely, the Institute of Medicine (IOM) recommends that an IRB "should have at least three individuals with . . . expertise in pediatric clinical care and research, the psychosocial dimensions of child and adolescent health care and research, and the ethics of research involving children" present as "members or alternates during meetings in which a research protocol involving children is reviewed."[7]

Exempt Research

Research involving children can be considered exempt from further IRB review in accord with the pertinent regulations.[1[Sec.101(b)(1),(b)(3)–(b)(6)]] However, the exemption for "research involving the use of educational tests (cognitive, diagnostic, aptitude, achievement), survey procedures, interview procedures, or observation of public behavior"[1[Sec.101(b)(2)]] cannot be used for research involving children unless the research involves only the "observation of public behavior when the investigator(s) do not participate in the activities being observed."[1[Sec.401(b)]] An

IRB should have a review process for determining exemptions that includes individuals with sufficient expertise in pediatrics to evaluate, for example, the normal educational practices that are used in "established or commonly accepted educational settings" for children.

General Criteria for IRB Approval

The Minimization of Risk

The general criteria for IRB approval must be considered in addition to the special protections afforded to children found in Subpart D. First, the risks to children in the protocol must be minimized.[1,5[Sec.111(a)(1)]] The IRB should consider the risks from the perspective of a child and not simply focus on the physical and economic risks. For example, the research area should be "child friendly" with an adequate play area and space for parents to remain with the child. Study-related laboratory samples should be obtained at the time of diagnostic testing whenever possible. With the growing number of pediatric drug studies, the IRB should be familiar with the various research design methods that minimize risk to the child. Examples include limiting research under some circumstances to pharmacokinetic and safety data, combining this approach with pharmacodynamic data, and minimizing the volume of blood withdrawn through the use of sensitive assays, pediatric-enabled laboratories, and population pharmacokinetic approaches.

A detailed explanation of these examples is provided in the FDA E11 guidance document.[6] First, "those conducting the study should be properly trained and experienced in studying the pediatric population, including the evaluation and management of potential pediatric adverse events." Second, "every attempt should be made to minimize the number of participants and of procedures, consistent with good study design." Third, data monitoring "mechanisms should be in place to ensure that a study can be rapidly terminated should an unexpected hazard be noted." The FDA E11 document presents a number of practical considerations "to minimize discomfort and distress." These include "personnel knowledgeable and skilled in dealing with the pediatric population and its age-appropriate needs, including skill in performing pediatric procedures; a physical setting with furniture, play equipment, activities, and food appropriate for age; . . . a familiar environment such as the hospital or clinic where participants normally receive their care; approaches to minimize discomfort of procedures, such as topical anesthesia . . . ; indwelling catheters rather than repeated venipunctures for blood sampling; [and] collection of some protocol-specified blood samples when routine clinical samples are obtained." Finally, given the difficulty at times of obtaining blood samples or placing an indwelling catheter, the IRB should consider limits on the number of "attempt[s] to obtain blood samples for a protocol and ensure a clear understanding of procedures if an indwelling catheter fails to function over time."[6]

Selection of Subjects

The IRB is required to assure that the selection of subjects is equitable, taking into account the "purposes of the research and the setting in which the research will be conducted."[1,5[Sec.111(a)(3)]] Children are at risk of being a population of convenience, especially for researchers recruiting from within their own places of employment and from their own colleagues. An IRB should have sufficient expertise to consider the risks of either coercion or undue influence from the perspective of a child, given the setting in which recruitment takes place. Finally, children should be included in research *only* if their participation is necessary to answer the scientific question being investigated.[4]

General Assessment of Risks

Before considering the special protections for children based on the category of risk and/or benefit, an IRB must first consider whether the "risks to subjects are reasonable in relation to anticipated benefits, if any, to subjects, as well as the importance of the knowledge that may reasonably be expected to result."[1,5[Sec.111(a)(2)]] As we shall see, Subpart D adds further specification to the reasonableness of risk by requiring either that (1) the risks are restricted for interventions or procedures that do not offer the prospect of direct benefit or (2) the potential benefits of the interventions or procedures included in the research are commensurate with the nonresearch alternatives. However, even minimal-risk research must be held to the standard of either anticipated benefits or knowledge gained in order to be approved by an IRB. In addition, the IRB should evaluate "only those risks and benefits that may result from the research" rather than the overall risks and benefits of therapies included in the research that the "subjects would receive even if not participating in the research." Using a "component analysis" of risks and benefits, a protocol that combines treatment and research could be judged as "minimal risk" based on the research component alone. These issues are discussed further later in this chapter.

Research Design

An IRB must evaluate the experimental design of a research protocol, including the sample size justification, in order to minimize risks and determine the reasonableness of the risks with respect to the knowledge to be gained. A protocol that cannot answer the research question posed should not be approved. A sample size that exceeds the number of children necessary to answer the research question exposes additional children to unnecessary risk and should not be approved. As explained in the FDA E11 guidance document,[6] a pediatric trial requires different efficacy endpoints based on considerations of the age and development of the subjects. In addition, a pediatric trial may need to evaluate any adverse impact on "physical and cognitive growth and development" along with "possible effects on skeletal, behavioral, cognitive, sexual, and immune maturation and development." An IRB that reviews research involving children must have the necessary expertise and experience to evaluate the unique (and necessary) features of pediatric research.

Expedited Review

Expedited review of research involving children can be conducted by an IRB in accord with the regulations.[1,5[Sec.110]] The only difference is in category 2 concerning the volume and frequency of blood draws that can be considered under expedited review procedures. For children, "the amount drawn may not exceed the lesser of 50 mL or 3 mL per kg in an 8-week period and collection may not occur more frequently than two times per week." This volume and frequency of blood draws does not establish an upper limit to what an IRB may approve using full-committee review. Neither does it establish an upper limit to what an IRB may consider minimal risk depending on the age, weight, and health of the child.

Special Protections for Children in Research

The regulations[1,5[Sec.111(b)]] require "additional safeguards . . . to protect the rights and welfare" of children involved in research as they are "vulnerable to coercion and undue influence." These special protections, found in Subpart D of 45 CFR 46 and 21 CFR 50, apply to all research subjects "who have not attained the legal age for consent to treatments or procedures involved in the research, under the applicable law of the jurisdiction in which the research will be conducted."[1[Sec.402(a)],2[Sec.50.3(o)]] The Children's Health Act of 2000 required that all research "involving children that is conducted, supported, or regulated by the Department of Health and Human Services (DHHS) be in compliance" with Subpart D,[8] with the FDA adopting the provisions of Subpart D, with the exception of Section 46.408(c), effective April 30, 2001.[9] The safeguards of Subpart D involve an additional determination by the IRB of the level of risk and the prospect of direct benefit presented by the proposed research. The IRB can approve research involving children only if it falls into one of three categories, provided that all of the criteria found in Section 111[1,5] are also fulfilled. The three categories are as follows.

1. Research presenting "no greater than minimal risk to children"[1[Sec.404],2[Sec.51]]

2. Research involving an intervention or procedure presenting more than minimal risk to children that offers the "prospect of direct benefit" or may "contribute to the . . . well-being" of the individual child[1[Sec.405],2[Sec.52]]

3. Research involving an intervention or procedure that presents only a "minor increase over minimal risk," yet does not offer any "prospect of direct benefit" or "contribute to the well-being" of the child[1[Sec.406],2[Sec.53]]

If an IRB cannot approve the research using one or more of these three categories, it must either not approve the research or refer it to the Secretary of the DHHS and/or the FDA Commissioner. The IRB should only refer the protocol for federal review if "the research presents a reasonable opportunity to further the understanding, prevention, or alleviation of a serious problem affecting the health or welfare of children."[1[Sec.407],2[Sec.54]]

Sections 405/52 and 406/53 can be considered a breakdown of the stipulation in Section 111 that the "risks to subjects are reasonable in relation to anticipated benefits, if any, to subjects, and the importance of the knowledge that may reasonably be expected to result." Research that presents greater than minimal risk (to be defined later) can only be approved if "the risk is justified by the anticipated benefit to the subjects,"[1[Sec.405[,2[Sec.52]] or the risk involved is only a "minor increase over minimal risk," and "the intervention or procedure is likely to yield generalizable knowledge about the subjects' disorder or condition which is of vital importance for the understanding or amelioration of the subjects' disorder or condition."[1[Sec.406],2[Sec.53]] For research to be approvable under Section 46.405/50.52, not only must there be a justifiable balance of risk and anticipated benefit, but "the relation of the anticipated benefit to the risk [must be] at least as favorable to the subjects as that presented by available alternative approaches." In effect, there must be "research equipoise" between the arm(s) of a trial and the alternatives available outside of the research. Whether one can consider a placebo arm under this category will be discussed later.

The concept of *research equipoise* refers to "the state in which genuine uncertainty exists [among the community of experts] regarding which intervention—experimental or control (including placebos)—is better."[10] In other words, neither the experimental nor control intervention is preferred. Existence of research equipoise "does not require numeric equality of intervention risks or potential benefits. Rather, research equipoise requires approximate equality in the risk/potential benefit ratios of the study and control interventions."[10] A Phase I pediatric oncology trial is usually considered under section Section 46.405/50.52, as the standard alternatives have been exhausted and the only remaining prospect for direct benefit may be the experimental intervention. "An experimental intervention may pose greater risk to participants than accepted practice, as long as it also offers the prospect of greater direct benefit to the participant and the relation between the risks and potential benefits falls within a range of equivalency to accepted practice."[10] Although a parent's decision to enroll a child in a Phase I oncology trial is difficult, many believe the decision may be justified provided that the alternatives of no further experimental treatment and palliative care are presented.

The provision for IRB review and approval of greater than minimal risk research that does not offer the prospect of direct benefit was one of the more controversial aspects of the National Commission's deliberations. One commissioner objected to the category, arguing that it unjustly exposed children with a "disorder or condition" to a level of risk, however minor, that was above that of a healthy child. Nevertheless, Section 46.406/50.53[1,2] allows for research that does not offer the prospect of direct benefit to the child enrolled in the research, provided that it is only a "minor increase over minimal risk," and additionally, the knowledge gained is of vital importance to understanding or ameliorating the child's disorder or condition. The ICH Good Clinical Practice Guidelines[11] also allows for nontherapeutic trials in children provided that the following conditions are met:

1. "Consent of a legally acceptable representative" is obtained.

2. The research objectives cannot be met using subjects capable of giving informed consent.

3. The "foreseeable risks to the subjects are low."

4. The "negative impact on the subject's well-being is minimized and low."

5. The "trial is not prohibited by law."

6. The IRB has approved in writing the inclusion of such children.

7. The research "should be conducted in patients having a disease or condition for which the investigational product is intended," unless otherwise justified.

It is a matter of interpretation whether a "minor increase over minimal risk" is the same standard as "the foreseeable risks . . . are low." In addition, Subpart D does not allow IRB approval of research presenting greater than minimal risk to healthy child volunteers (i.e., lacking a disorder or condition).[1[Sec.406],2[Sec.53]]

Interpretation of Minimal Risk and Minor Increase over Minimal Risk

Key to the interpretation of Subpart D is the definition of minimal risk and a minor increase over minimal risk, as it establishes the level of risk to which children may be exposed during the course of research that does not offer the prospect of direct benefit. *Minimal risk* is defined as "the probability and magnitude of harm or discomfort anticipated in the research are not greater in and of themselves than those ordinarily encountered in daily life or during the performance of routine physical or psychological examinations or tests."[1,5[Sec.102(i)]] The National Commission initially stipulated that this standard should be indexed to the lives "of healthy children."[4] However, the definition found in the current regulations does not include the phrase "of healthy children," perhaps out of concern that this would inappropriately restrict the types of research that could otherwise be performed. More recently, the IOM recommended that minimal risk should be interpreted "in relation to the normal experiences of average, healthy, normal children."[7] Even so, reasonable differences of opinion exist about the interpretation of minimal risk according to this uniform standard. In addition, minimal risk serves to anchor the concept of a minor increase over minimal risk, defined as "a slight increase in the potential for harms or discomfort beyond minimal risk."[4,7] The Children's Working Group of NHRPAC[12] provided a table listing the risk categorization of some common medical procedures as a first step in encouraging uniformity in IRB risk assessment.

The category of a minor increase over minimal risk is often essential to the analysis of a research protocol containing procedures that may or may not offer the prospect of direct benefit. For example, could one perform a bone marrow aspiration to obtain research information as part of an oncology treatment protocol if there was no prospect of direct benefit (i.e., no clinically relevant information

obtained at that same time)? Some would consider the overall risk and benefit of the protocol and find the research justified under Section 46.405/50.52.[1,2] However, consistent with Subpart D, others would evaluate the risks and potential benefit of the bone marrow aspiration independently of the overall treatment protocol using a so-called component analysis. As recommended by the IOM, "Institutional review boards should assess the potential harms and benefits of each intervention or procedure in a pediatric protocol to determine whether each conforms to the regulatory criteria for approving research involving children. When some procedures present the prospect of direct benefit and others do not, the potential benefits from one component of the research should not be held to offset or justify the risks presented by another."[7] Thus, the risk of the bone marrow aspirate performed solely to answer the research question must be limited to a minor increase over minimal risk and justified in relation to the potential to generate knowledge (i.e., 45 CFR 46.406; 21 CFR 50.53).[1,2] Accepting the argument in favor of a uniform standard of minimal risk, one could still allow a more relative standard of a minor increase over minimal risk provided that the research "intervention or procedure presents experiences . . . that are reasonably commensurate with those inherent in [the child's] actual or expected . . . situations."[1,2] In effect, only those interventions or procedures that are reasonably commensurate with a particular child's experience could be considered as a minor increase over minimal risk. "Research activities presenting such risks . . . to the children who would be the subjects of the research . . . would be considered normal for these children."[4]

Permission of the Parent(s)/Assent of the Child

The National Commission considered the commensurability of the research experience with a child's "actual or expected medical, dental, psychological, social, or educational" experience as supporting a child's ability to assent to and a parent's ability to permit the research. This requirement was explicitly added to the section referring to research presenting a minor increase over minimal risk (Section 46.405/50.53), as the commensurability of the research and nonresearch experience is implicit in the definition of minimal risk. A requirement that is common to all four categories of research (Section 46.404–407/50.51–54) is that "adequate provisions are made for soliciting the assent of the children and permission of their parents or guardians."

Parental Permission

Parental permission is treated in much the same way as informed consent, apart from some additional provisions found in Section 46.408/50.55. A *parent* (defined as "a child's biological or adoptive parent") or *guardian* (defined as "an individual who is authorized under applicable state or local law to consent on behalf of a child to general medical care") must agree to (i.e., permit) the child's participation in research.

For research protocols that do not involve an FDA-regulated product, all of the requirements of 45 CFR 46.116 concerning informed consent apply to parental permission, including the general and required elements. Similarly, the elements of informed parental permission can be modified or waived entirely in accord with Section 46.116(d). Documentation of parental permission is determined according to Section 46.117. For research protocols involving an FDA-regulated product, the process and documentation of parental permission must be in accord with Subparts B and D of 21 CFR 50. The elements of informed parental permission are the same. However, the only waiver of parental permission that can be considered is for emergent and life-threatening situations, either individually (Section 50.23) or as a group (Section 50.24). Of special note, the FDA did not adopt the provision under 46.408(c), which allows an IRB to waive parental or guardian permission if "a research protocol is designed for conditions or for a subject population for which . . . permission is not a reasonable requirement to protect the subjects . . . , provided an appropriate mechanism for protecting the children who will participate as subjects in the research is substituted, and provided further that the waiver is not inconsistent with federal, state, or local law." Many pediatric IRBs will waive the requirement for parental permission for research using adolescent subjects that involves medical procedures and treatment that the adolescent can consent to without parental knowledge, such as the use of contraceptives, treatment of sexually transmitted disease, treatment of alcohol and drug abuse, and so forth. Such a waiver does not appear to be available under FDA regulations, unless the IRB decides that the minor subject is not a "child" according to the regulatory definition.[2[50.3(o)]] Finally, there are some additional requirements for parental permission in Subpart D. "Where research is covered by Section 46.406/50.53 and Section 46.407/50.54 and permission is to be obtained from parents, both parents must give their permission unless one parent is deceased, unknown, incompetent, or not reasonably available or when only one parent has legal responsibility for the care and custody of the child."[1[Sec.408(b)],2[Sec.50.55(e)(2)]]

Child Assent

Assent is defined as "a child's affirmative agreement to participate in research."[1[Sec.402(b)],2[Sec.50.3(n)]] A child's passive resignation to submit to an intervention or procedure must not be considered assent. The National Commission recommended that the "assent of the children should be required when they are seven years of age or older."[4] However, the federal regulations do not specify any of the elements of informed assent and do not indicate an age at which assent ought to be possible. The assent process "should be developmentally appropriate given the ages and other characteristics of the children to be approached [and] provide opportunities for children to express and discuss their willingness or unwillingness to participate."[7]

An IRB is granted wide discretion in determining whether a child is capable of assenting and can waive the requirement for child assent if a child is not capable of assent; if the research offers a prospect of direct benefit not available outside of the research (thus falling under the scope of parental authority in overriding a child's desires); or given the same conditions under which parental permission can be waived. An IRB is granted wide discretion in determining whether and how a child's assent is documented. Finally, as a matter of both justice and respect for persons, efforts should be made to conduct research using children capable of assent before enrolling those less able to assent.

Choice of Control Group (Placebo Controls)

An algorithm for evaluating the ethics of placebo control is presented in Chapter 10-11. The circumstances under which a placebo control is appropriate are a matter of controversy. The Declaration of Helsinki states that "the benefits, risks, burdens, and effectiveness of a new method should be tested against those of the best current prophylactic, diagnostic, and therapeutic methods. This does not exclude the use of placebo, or no treatment, in studies where no proven prophylactic, diagnostic, or therapeutic method exists."[13] The FDA document on the choice of control group (E10)[14] argues that one can use a placebo control if withholding the known effective therapy would not result in "serious harm, such as death or irreversible morbidity in the study population." The FDA E11[6] document on pediatric trials does not discuss placebo controls. The World Medical Association added a clarification to the Declaration of Helsinki, stating that "a placebo-controlled trial may be ethically acceptable, even if proven therapy is available, . . . where for compelling and scientifically sound methodological reasons its use is necessary to determine the efficacy or safety of a prophylactic, diagnostic or therapeutic method; or where a prophylactic, diagnostic or therapeutic method is being investigated for a minor condition and the patients who receive placebo will not be subject to any additional risk of serious or irreversible harm."[13] The presence of a placebo arm in a clinical trial does not preclude the research from being considered under Section 46.405/50.52[1,2] as offering the prospect of direct benefit. If research equipoise exists, an IRB should consider the risks and potential benefits of the research from the perspective of the subject and evaluate the prospect of direct benefit without assuming the success or failure of the study intervention. Absent equipoise, the withholding of a known effective therapy from children enrolled in the research must present no more than a minor increase over minimal risk (and be approvable under Section 46.406/50.53).[1,2]

Approval by Federal Review Panel

Subpart D allows for the review and approval of research that is not otherwise approvable by an IRB provided that the research "presents a reasonable opportunity to further the understanding, prevention, or alleviation of a serious problem affecting the health or welfare of children" and "will be conducted in accordance with sound ethical principles."[1,2[Sec.46.407,50.54]] An IRB may refer the protocol to the Secretary of DHHS and/or the FDA Commissioner who, after consultation with a "panel of experts" and after "opportunity for public review and comment," may issue an approval for the research. Clearly, such a review panel can only discharge this responsibility if the referring IRB (1) has already determined that the research fails to qualify under 45 CFR 46[1[Sec.404,405,406]] and/or 21 CFR 50[2[Sec.51,52,53]]; (2) has determined that the research is potentially approvable under 45 CFR 46[1[Sec.407]] and/or 21 CFR 50[2[Sec.54]]; and (3) has provided the underlying documentation and rationale for both determinations. Since 2001, a number of protocols have been reviewed under this mechanism. In 2004, a permanent subcommittee of the FDA Pediatric Advisory Committee was established to review protocols referred under 21 CFR 50.54 and that involve both FDA regulated products under 21 CFR 50.54 and research involving children as subjects that is conducted or supported by the DHHS as specified in 45 CFR 46.407.[15]

Conclusion

Charged with reviewing the pediatric research regulations, the IOM "concluded that the federal regulations providing special protections for child participants are, in general, appropriate for children of different ages." "For the most part, the problems with the regulations relate to insufficient government guidance about their interpretation and implementation, shortfalls in data about implementation and compliance, and variability in investigator and IRB interpretations of the criteria for approving research involving children."[7] Over the past few years, there have been significant developments in the review and oversight of pediatric research that seek to address some of these problems, as reviewed in this chapter. An IRB that reviews research involving children needs to possess sufficient experience and expertise, needs to be familiar with the special protections afforded pediatric research subjects by Subpart D, and needs to be capable of both ethical, scientific, and regulatory analysis of research trials from a pediatric perspective. Just as it is inappropriate for an investigator to conduct research involving children without sufficient pediatric expertise, an IRB that does not have the necessary knowledge and skill to analyze a pediatric research trial according to the "sound ethical principles" embodied in Subpart D would not be in compliance with existing guidance regulations.

References

1. Code of Federal Regulations. Title 45A—Department of Health and Human Services; Part 46—Protection of Human Subjects. Revised 13 November, 2001. Access date 25 September, 2004. http://www.hhs.gov/ohrp/humansubjects/guidance/45cfr46.htm

2. Code of Federal Regulations. Title 21, Subchapter A—Food and Drug Administration, DHHS; Part 50—Protection of Human Subjects. Revised 1 April, 2004. Access date 25 September, 2004. http://www.accessdata.fda.gov/scripts/cdrh/cfdocs/cfcfr/CFRSearch.cfm?CFRPart=50

3. National Commission for the Protection of Human Subjects of Biomedical and Behavioral Research. *The Belmont Report: Ethical principles and guidelines for the protection of human subjects of research*, 18 April, 1979. Access date 25 September, 2004. http://www.hhs.gov/ohrp/humansubjects/guidance/belmont.htm

4. National Commission for the Protection of Human Subjects of Biomedical and Behavioral Research. Research Involving Children: Report and Recommendations. *Fed Regist* 43(9):2083–2114, 1978.

5. Code of Federal Regulations. Title 21, Subchapter A—Food and Drug Administration, DHHS; Part 56—Institutional Review Boards. Revised 1 April, 2004. Access date 25 September, 2004. http://www.accessdata.fda.gov/scripts/cdrh/cfdocs/cfcfr/CFRSearch.cfm

6. Food and Drug Administration. Guidance for Industry: E11 Clinical Investigation of Medicinal Products in the Pediatric Population (ICH), December 2000. Access date 25 September, 2004. http://www.fda.gov/cder/guidance/4099fnl.pdf

7. Committee on Clinical Research Involving Children, Board on Health Sciences Policy, Institute of Medicine of the National Academies. *Ethical Conduct of Clinical Research Involving Children*. Field MJ, Behrman RE (eds.). Washington, DC : National Academies Press; 2004. Access date 25 September, 2004. http://www.nap.edu/catalog/10958.html

8. 106th Congress. Children's Health Act of 2000, 17 October, 2000. P. L. 106-310. Access date 25 September, 2004. http://frwebgate.access.gpo.gov/cgi-bin/getdoc.cgi?dbname=106_cong_public_laws&docid=f:publ310.106.pdf

9. Food and Drug Administration, DHHS. Additional safeguards for children in clinical investigations of FDA-regulated products. *Fed Regist* 66(79):20589–20600, 2001. Access date 25 September, 2004. http://www.fda.gov/ohrms/dockets/98fr/042401a.htm

10. National Bioethics Advisory Commission. Ethical and Policy Issues in Research Involving Human Participants. Vol. I. Report and Recommendations. Bethesda, MD. August 2001. Access date 25 September, 2004. http://www.georgetown.edu/research/nrcbl/nbac/human/overvol1.pdf

11. International Conference on Harmonisation (ICH) Guideline for Good Clinical Practice E6. 10 June, 1996. Access Date 25 September, 2004. http://www.ich.org/MediaServer.jser?@_ID=482&@_MODE=GLB

12. National Human Research Protections Advisory Committee (NHRPAC). Final Report to NHRPAC from Children's Workgroup. Endorse 31 July, 2002. Access date 25 September, 2004. http://www.hhs.gov/ohrp/nhrpac/documents/nhrpac16.pdf

13. World Medical Association. *Declaration of Helsinki: Ethical Principles for Medical Research Involving Human Subjects.* World Medical Association, Inc.: WMA Policy. First adopted in Helsinki, Finland, in 1964. Revised October 2000; Note of Clarification on Paragraph 29 added by the WMA General Assembly, Washington 2002. Access date 25 September, 2004. http://www.wma.net/e/policy/pdf/17c.pdf

14. Food and Drug Administration. Guidance for Industry: E10 Choice of control group and related issues in clinical trials. *Fed Regist* 66(93):24390–24391, 14 May, 2001. Access date 25 September, 2004. http://www.fda.gov/cder/guidance/4155fnl.pdf

15. For details about the protocols reviewed, see the Children's Web page of the Office of Human Research Protections. Access Date 25 September, 2004. http://www.hhs.gov/ohrp/children/. For the Charter of the Pediatric Advisory Committee and Pediatric Ethics Subcommittee, see http://www.fda.gov/oc/advisory/OCPedsCharter.html. Access Date 25 September, 2004.Document5

Research Involving Adults with Decisional Impairment

Susan J. Delano

INTRODUCTION

Research involving adults with decisional impairment is not currently the subject of specific federal regulatory guidance. Federal research regulations provide that if an institutional review board (IRB) regularly reviews research involving a vulnerable category of subjects, the membership should include "one or more individuals who are knowledgeable about and experienced in working with these subjects."[1[Sec.107(a)]] The regulations also provide that "when some or all of the subjects are likely to be vulnerable to coercion or undue influence, such as children, prisoners, pregnant women, mentally disabled persons, or economically or educationally disadvantaged persons, additional safeguards have been included in the study to protect the rights and welfare of these subjects."[1[Sec.111(b)]]

Based on the work of the National Commission for the Protection of Human Subjects of Biomedical and Behavioral Research, which was created in 1974, the then Department of Health, Education, and Welfare in 1978 proposed specific additional regulations for research involving the "institutionalized mentally infirm." They were never adopted.[2(Chap.11)] Research involving subjects with decisional impairment has been the subject of extensive debate at the state and national level and is a component of the mission of the current Secretary's Advisory Committee on Human Research Protections.[3–5]

Who Are Adults with Decisional Impairment?

Adults who are decisionally impaired suffer from many different conditions that potentially affect their ability to reason and make sound choices. In the research context, this is most often considered in the context of a person's capacity to provide valid consent. The ability to provide initial or ongoing consent to research may be limited by a variety of problems associated with memory, understanding, and reasoning. For some, the impairment may be stable with little variation over time. For others, the level of impairment may fluctuate over time (e.g., a person with schizophrenia or a person who abuses drugs) or may progressively change over time (e.g., a person with Alzheimer's disease). It is also important to understand that capacity must be determined in relation to the specific task or decision-making circumstance. For example, a person may be capable of consenting to an interview but lack sufficient capacity to consent to a drug study.

The inclusion of decisionally impaired adults in research is an area of intense debate.[6] This is because, at the milder levels, these adults may be more vulnerable to coercion, and at more severe levels, they lack the capacity to provide informed consent, a basic legal and ethical requirement. For many, the issue of institutionalization is also a factor. Broad ethical concerns of justice, respect for persons, and beneficence are raised by the inclusion of decisionally impaired adults in research.

Protections for the Decisionally Impaired

The protections for this vulnerable population should be broadly applied to all decisionally impaired persons, regardless of the source of their impairment. A person impaired by a stroke, brain injury, or delirium secondary to renal failure or diabetes is entitled to the same level of protections as a person similarly impaired as a result of a mental illness such as schizophrenia or depression. With all such populations, however, care should be taken to distinguish between persons who are impaired and persons who have a condition that may cause impairment. For example, if a study involves persons with schizophrenia, the IRB should consider additional protections, as described in the following section. However, it would be incorrect to assume that all of the subjects will lack sufficient capacity to provide consent.

Issues That IRBs Should Consider

IRB Membership

If your IRB regularly reviews research involving adults with decisional impairment, your membership must include persons familiar with the nature of the disorders creating the decisional impairment and the concerns of the population. If your IRB does not regularly review this type of research, and your membership does not include this expertise, you must involve a consultant when reviewing studies involving this population.[1(Sec.107)] Depending on the amount and type of research you conduct with decisionally impaired subjects, multiple representatives may be appropriate.

Types of Expertise to Consider

1. Scientific/clinical expertise—Such expertise provides an understanding of the scientific/clinical aspects of the protocol and an understanding of the subject population (what burdens their condition imposes, what the treatment of their condition entails, what their living conditions are likely to be) and how the research is likely to impact them.

2. Patient/consumer representative(s)—These individuals will provide an understanding of the subject population and how the research is likely to impact them. These persons can also help tailor recruitment procedures to minimize coercion and enhance the consent process and content to maximize understanding and free choice.

3. Family member(s)—Family members can provide an understanding of the subject population and how the research is likely to impact them. These persons may act as advocates for the role of family members/friends (when approved by the proposed subject) in providing support to subjects in their decision making and monitoring research participation.

4. Advocacy group member(s)—These people can provide an understanding of the subject population and how the research is likely to impact them. They may also bring a broader perspective (e.g., National Alliance for the Mentally Ill).

Limits on the Inclusion of Incapable Subjects

Necessity of Involving Subjects Who Lack Capacity

A generally agreed on principle is that incapable subjects (persons who do not have sufficient capacity to consent) should not be involved in research that could be conducted with capable subjects. An exception to this principle is that an IRB may permit incapable subjects to participate in such research when it provides access to an important potential benefit, particularly one that is not otherwise available to the subjects. For example, the IRB may decide that it is appropriate to permit inclusion of incapable subjects in a study of a new drug if the subjects are intolerant of, or have not responded to, standard medications.

Debate Over Participation in Research that Does Not Offer a Prospect of Direct Benefit

This is the most intense area of debate, with the focus being on research that is more than minimal risk but not high risk. It is widely accepted that in the absence of a specific advance directive, authorizing participation in this type of research and surrogate consent, no incapable person should be involved in research that involves moderate or high risk when the research is not expected to benefit the person directly. Similarly, there is little debate about the authority of surrogates to consent to research involving no more than minimal risk. The remaining category, which generally equates to the "minor increase over minimal risk" category (e.g., magnetic resonance imaging with sedation, indwelling catheters for a short duration) in the children's regulations, has been directly endorsed, with surrogate consent and appropriate protections, by many groups such as the New York State Department of Health Advisory Work Group on Human Subject Research Involving the Protected Classes, the Attorney General's Research Working Group of the Office of the Maryland Attorney General, and Expert Panel Report to the National Institutes of Health: Research Involving Individuals with Questionable Capacity to Consent. The National Bioethics Advisory Commission's report on adults with decisional impairments includes recommendations that prohibit research involving more than minimal risk and no expected benefit except when the subject has previously created a specific advance directive, or the research is approved by a special federal panel.

Capacity

Capacity to provide consent is an essential component of valid consent.

Assessment of Capacity

For all research, regardless of the study population, the person who obtains the subject's consent must determine that the person has sufficient capacity to give it. In most cases, this assessment occurs as part of the discussion with the proposed subject about the study. The person obtaining consent evaluates the questions raised by the subject and the answers given to questions asked. The consent interviewer may only seek consent when he or she is satisfied that the person is capable of making the decision. Capacity is documented by the signature on the consent form of the person obtaining consent. (The person who obtains consent also documents, by his or her signature, lack of coercion and full disclosure.) When subjects are patients, a note should be written in the progress notes of their charts.

Based on the risk/benefit ratio of the study and the nature of the subject population, the IRB should consider the need for an independent assessment of capacity. The IRB may set qualifications for the person making the assessment, such as requiring a licensed clinical psychologist, psychiatric social worker, psychiatrist, or gerontologist. Generally, as the risks increase, the benefits decrease, the potential vulnerability of the subjects increases, and/or the likelihood increases that a person's capacity or lack of capacity will not be obvious, the requirements should become more stringent. The independent assessment of capacity should be documented by a formal note that is signed and dated. (A sample statement is shown in Figure 9.8.1.) When subjects are patients, a note should be written in the progress notes of their charts.

"I examined _____ on _____ for the purpose of determining whether he/she is
                    (name)   *(date)*

capable of understanding the purpose, nature, risks, benefits, and alternatives (including nonparticipation) of the

research, making a decision about participation, and understanding that the decision about participation in the re-

search will involve no penalty or loss of benefits to which the patient is otherwise entitled, for _____
                                                                                                        (investigation

_____ 's research project _____ .
       name)   *(title of project)*

On the basis of this examination I have arrived at the conclusion that

    (a)   this patient has this capacity at this time   [ ]

or (b)   there is a doubt about this patient's capacity at this time   [ ]

or (c)   this patient clearly lacks this capacity at this time   [ ]

[Statement must be signed and dated.]

Figure 9.8.1   Sample language for documentation of capacity

Standards for Capacity

The level of capacity required to consent varies according to the type and complexity of the decisions that are to be made. As the complexity and risks of the procedures increase, the required level of capacity should also increase. For example, the level of capacity needed to consent to a study involving a blood draw is less than the capacity required to consent to a placebo-controlled drug study. There are four commonly used standards of capacity:[7]

1. The ability to evidence a choice; that is, to communicate a yes or no decision. This standard is applicable to all risk/benefit levels.

2. The ability to understand relevant information, that is, the person can tell you what the research procedures involve and what the consent information includes (e.g., a right to withdraw). This standard is also applicable to all risk/benefit levels.

3. The ability to appreciate the situation and its likely consequences. The person can understand what research participation involves for him or her and what the likely outcomes are. He or she can apply the information to his or her own situation. This standard generally applies to all research involving more than minimal risk.

4. The ability to manipulate information rationally. This standard focuses on process, not outcome. For example, are decisions consistent with the religious, moral, and other beliefs of the person? This standard is critical at the most unfavorable risk/benefit levels.

Enhancing Comprehension

Enhancing comprehension increases the likelihood that a person will have the capacity to consent or to give a maximally informed assent. The process should be tailored to the specific population. Consider videotapes, photographs,

breaking down information into more easily understood components, repetition, and involving a family member, friend, or peer counselor. The IRB should also consider ways of ensuring that information about the study is provided to the subjects during study participation.

As part of the consent process, prospective subjects should be asked questions about the research to determine whether they recall and understand what has been explained.[8] Questions should be open ended, for example:

1. Can you tell me what will happen if you agree to take part in this study?

2. Will this study help you?

3. Can you tell me about the possible side effects of the study drug?

4. Do you have to be in this study?

5. Can you leave this study once it begins?

6. What will happen if you decide not to be in this study?

Education of the subject can occur during this process and should continue until the person understands the information and is able to provide correct answers.

Studies Involving Persons Who Lack Sufficient Capacity to Consent

If your IRB determines that it is appropriate to involve subjects who do not have sufficient capacity to consent, additional concerns arise.

Notifications to an Incapable Subject

To the extent possible, do each of the following:

1. Inform the subject about the study and seek his or her agreement to participate.

2. Notify the subject that he or she retains the right to object and can leave the study at any time.

3. Notify the subject in a sensitive way that he or she lacks the sufficient capacity to consent and provide an opportunity for the subject to contest the decision.

4. Explain surrogate consent procedures and options.

Surrogate Consent

Consider the proposed subject population. If it is likely that subjects will lose capacity during a study, they should be encouraged at the beginning of the study to appoint a surrogate. The surrogate will have the authority to consent to continuing participation, amendments to the study, and withdrawal from the study if the subject loses capacity.

For subjects found to lack sufficient capacity to consent, you should check with your legal counsel because the determination of who can provide surrogate consent for research is a matter of state law and varies from state to state. Although surrogate consent is routinely employed in research, as it is in clinical practice, the legal basis is often not clear.

Classes of Possible Surrogates

1. Surrogate appointed by the subject when fully capable (durable power of attorney, research advance directive, health care proxy). Although these surrogates are widely accepted, they have limited applicability, and such documents are rarely executed.

2. Court or court-appointed guardian with authority to consent to research. These are also widely accepted, but of limited use. Research is not generally contemplated when guardians are appointed. Unless the purpose of the research is to provide access to an experimental treatment, the stress and stigma associated with a court determination of a lack of capacity are seldom justified for research purposes.

3. Surrogate chosen by the subject when incapable of consenting but capable of choosing a surrogate. Individuals may lack sufficient capacity to consent to a complex study. However, they may have sufficient capacity to choose their spouse, adult child, friend, or trusted advisor to make decisions for them. The subject's capacity to choose a surrogate should be evaluated by an appropriately qualified person. The choice of a surrogate should be documented. (At least one witness who is independent of the research is recommended.) The surrogate should not be affiliated with the research or the institution. (This restriction should not apply if the surrogate is related to the subject by blood, marriage, or adoption.) Subject-chosen surrogates are generally accepted.

4. Family member (parent, spouse, adult child, adult sibling). This class of surrogates is used in practice every day, but with some legal uncertainty. Consent by family members is generally accepted for minimal-risk research and for research that offers a prospect of direct benefit. Family members are generally not permitted to consent to research involving higher risk and no expected benefit. Some disagreement exists about the appropriateness of family members as surrogates for research with no expected benefit and a minor increase over minimal risk.

5. Close friend. This class of surrogates recognizes nontraditional relationships. The use of close friends as surrogates has limited acceptance. In most states, there is currently no clear legal basis for their authority to consent to research.

Basis of Surrogate Decision Making

Research surrogates need to be informed about the study, its implications for the individual, and their role in providing initial and ongoing consent. Research surrogates also need to be informed about their responsibility for withdrawing a subject from participation when continuing participation is no longer consistent with the subject's known wishes or is no longer in the best interests of the subject.

The decisions of surrogates may be based on the preferred standard of substituted judgment, reflecting the views of the individual when he or she was capable. (The surrogate should consider known preferences, beliefs, and prior decisions about research.) Surrogate decisions can also be based on the best interests of the subject, when the views of the individual are not known.

Conclusion

Consent is an ongoing process. The research team should discuss participation with the subject, explaining procedures and obtaining continued agreement to participate as the study continues. Surrogates and, when appropriate, family members or friends should be kept informed about the subject's participation in the study. The subject should be asked for permission to involve family members or friends and may choose not to have them involved.

The IRB may add consent auditors to the consent process.[1[Sec.109(e)]] Their use is encouraged when the level of risk is high or when vulnerable subjects are involved in more than minimal risk research, particularly when there is no expected benefit to subjects. The IRB may also determine that a medical monitor should be appointed to review each subject's participation and recommend withdrawal from the study when clinically indicated. An expanded role has been proposed for data safety monitoring boards to provide information to IRBs during the course of a study.

The topics covered in this chapter and many other related topics are addressed in more detail in *Ethics in Psychiatric Research: A Resource Manual for Human Subjects Protection*, edited by Pincus, Lieberman, and Ferris.[9]

References

1. Code of Federal Regulations. Title 45A—Department of Health and Human Services; Part 46—Protection of Human Subjects. Updated 1 October, 1997. Access date 18 April, 2001. http://www4.law.cornell.edu/cfr/45p46.htm

2. Levine RJ. *Ethics and Regulation of Clinical Research*, 2nd ed. Baltimore, MD: Urban and Schwarzenberg; 1986.

3. National Bioethics Advisory Commission. Research involving persons with mental disorders that may affect decision making capacity: report and recommendations, December 1998. Access date 29 March, 2001. http://bioethics.gov/capacity/TOC.htm

4. National Institutes of Health. Research involving individuals with questionable capacity to consent: Points to consider, 5 January, 2001. Access date 29 March, 2001. http://grants.nih.gov/grants/policy/questionablecapacity.htm

5. New York State Department of Health. Report of the Advisory Work Group to the Commissioner of the Department of Health. Human Subject Research Involving the Protected Classes. December 1998. New York.

6. Michels R. Are research ethics bad for our mental health? *N Engl J Med* 340(18):1427–1430, 1999.

7. Applebaum PS, Grisso T. The MacArthur Treatment Competence Study: Mental illness and competence to consent to treatment. *Law Hum Behav* 19:105–126, 1995.

8. Wirshing DA, Wirshing WC, Marder SR, Liberman RP, Mintz J. Informed consent: Assessment of comprehension. *Am J Psychiatry* 155(11):1508–1511, 1998.

9. Pincus HA, Lieberman JA, Ferris S. *Ethics in Psychiatric Research: A Resource Manual for Human Subjects Protection*, 1st ed. Washington, DC: American Psychiatric Association; 1999.

Regulatory Issues of Research Involving Prisoners

Christopher J. Kratochvil, Ernest D. Prentice, Bruce G. Gordon, and Gail D. Kotulak

INTRODUCTION

Prisoners are considered a vulnerable subject population in need of additional protections. Institutional review boards (IRBs) overseeing research involving prisoners should be familiar with the federal and state regulations that apply to research conducted under their approval and oversight. Requirements may vary for research conducted in a federal prison versus a state facility and according to the source of funding. For the purpose of this chapter, however, only the Department of Health and Human Services (DHHS) regulations for the protection of human subjects who are prisoners are addressed.

Although no precise figures are available, it is likely that most of the research involving prisoners conducted in the United States is subject to DHHS regulations at 45 CFR 46.[1] These federal regulations include a subpart providing additional protections for prisoners who participate in research. It should also be mentioned that in 1978 the Food and Drug Administration (FDA) issued special regulations for research involving prisoners, but they were withdrawn. Thus, the current FDA regulations for the protection of human subjects, codified at 21 CFR 50, 56,[2,3] do not include any specific additional protections for research subjects who are prisoners. The FDA does, however, consider prisoners to be a vulnerable subject population for which the IRB must include additional safeguards.[3[Sec.111(b)]]

Historical Overview

Although medical experiments involving prisoners in the United States date back at least to the beginning of the 20th century, World War II was the impetus for a dramatic increase in the number of experiments performed in prisons.[4] With the war raging in both Europe and the Pacific, medical research to protect the lives of millions of American soldiers became an overriding goal. Society in general espoused the view that prisoners owed their country nothing less than participation in these worthy endeavors. Participation in research was cast as the prisoner's contribution to the war effort. Therefore, with little public scrutiny and, in many cases, willing cooperation of the inmates, the research proceeded apace. Prisoners participated in a wide range of experiments, including research on dengue fever, sandfly fever, gonorrhea, scurvy, malaria, gas gangrene, and studies of alternative sources of plasma.[5]

Some of the best known of these wartime prison experiments were the malaria studies conducted at Stateville Penitentiary in Illinois, which continued for 2 years and involved 400 prisoners.[6] During the 1946 Nuremberg doctors' trial, German physicians, accused of experimenting on concentration camp prisoners, offered the Stateville research as an example of similar experimentation in the United States.[7] Prominent American researcher and the prosecution's chief witness on American medical ethics, Andrew Ivy, defended the U.S. prison research program, stating that no American prisoner had ever been experimented on against his will. He also refused to concede that coercion was necessarily inherent in a prison environment. According to Ivy, as long as the consent of the subject was obtained, the research was based on animal experiments and was directed by qualified persons, then experimentation on prisoners was acceptable.[7] Indeed, the American Medical Association in 1948 endorsed these three principles.[8]

After the war, experimentation on prisoners in the U.S. continued unabated. The United States was one of a few countries in the world that persisted in using prisoners for research. In the 1960s, after the FDA mandated tests of new drugs on humans, large pharmaceutical companies turned to the penal system for a seemingly inexhaustible supply of "stable, long-term" subjects who were particularly valuable in Phase I drug and cosmetic testing.[9] The number of these subjects that fell ill or died as a direct result of these experiments was not insignificant.

In the late 1960s and early 1970s, as the public became aware of a series of ethically questionable studies, human subject research, in general, became an area of concern and distrust. In 1972, details of the then 40-year-long Tuskegee syphilis study were revealed in an exposé published in the *Washington Star* and subsequently in the *New York Times*.[10] Public outcry, largely mirrored in political circles, was immediate; it expanded to encompass concern over all research, especially that involving vulnerable populations such as prisoners. Both state and federal legislation were introduced to limit the use of inmates as research subjects, and state prison research programs were terminated in a large majority of the states. By 1976, the federal government announced the end of research in federal prisons.[11]

The Commissioner's Report

In 1978, the National Commission for the Protection of Human Subjects of Biomedical and Behavioral Research produced recommendations on prisoner research.[12] The Commission's report formed the basis for 45 CFR 46 Subpart C—Additional DHHS Protections Pertaining to Biomedical and Behavioral Research Involving Prisoners as Subjects.[1] Under these regulations, prisoner research continued, although clearly on a much reduced scale, particularly in the area of medical research. As a matter of fact, in the preamble to Subpart C, it is noted that most testimony before the commission opposed the use of prisoners in any medical research that did not offer direct benefit to the individual prisoner.[13] Clearly, the regulations were intended to provide a high level of protection. More recent events, however, have called into question the adequacy of these additional protections and the extent to which they are being used. In July and August 2000, the Office of Protection from Research Risks (OPRR) demanded the suspension of prisoner research at the University of Texas Medical Branch at Galveston and the University of Miami because it did not appear that Subpart C regulations were being followed.[14] In May 2000, the OPRR issued guidance to facilitate interpretation of the regulations in Subpart C, which was subsequently updated by the Office for Human Research Protections (OHRP) in May 2003.[15]

Application of Subpart C

It is important to note that 45 CFR 46, Subpart C, is only applicable to research involving prisoners which is funded by DHHS, conducted within DHHS (e.g., The National Institutes of Health), or conducted at an institution with a Federalwide Assurance (FWA) that commits to compliance with Subpart C. Subpart C is also applicable to prisoner research funded or conducted by the Central Intelligence Agency by Executive Order and the Social Security Administration by statute.

Definition of *Prisoner*

According to 45 CFR 46,[1][Sec.303(c)] "*Prisoner* means any individual involuntarily confined or detained in a penal institution. The term is intended to encompass individuals sentenced to such an institution under a criminal or civil statute as well as individuals detained in other facilities by virtue of statutes or commitment procedures which provide alternatives to criminal prosecution or incarceration in a penal institution, and individuals detained pending arraignment, trial, or sentencing." This includes situations where a human subject becomes a prisoner after the research has commenced.

One of the difficulties in the use of this Subpart C lies within the definition of "prisoner." Many of the current alternatives to incarceration were not even in existence at the time of the writing of Subpart C, such as house arrest with electronic monitoring. Additionally, although many others may not meet the definition of a prisoner per se (such as parolees or probationers, persons court-ordered to attend nonresidential treatment programs in the community, and those adjudicated to reside in halfway houses), all have impingements on their freedom and the potential for coercion. For these vulnerable subjects who may not be protected under Subpart C, they should be afforded additional protections under Subpart A in the charge to the IRBs to "be particularly cognizant of the special problems of research involving vulnerable populations" [Subpart A 46.111].

Composition of the IRB

An IRB reviewing prisoner research must be specially constituted.[1][Sec.304(a),(b)] The board must include at least one member who is a prisoner or a prisoner representative with the appropriate background and experience to serve in that capacity. Most IRBs, for obvious practical and logistical reasons, do not have prisoners as IRB members and, therefore, elect to use a prisoner representative. The representative should be someone with empathy for prisoners who can represent the concerns prisoners might have about a study but also have a close working knowledge of prison conditions and the life of a prisoner. Suitable candidates could be former prisoners, prison chaplains, or social workers who deal with prisoners or the families of prisoners. Individuals who are prisoner advocates may also qualify.

The IRB must include a prisoner or prisoner representative for any review of research involving prisoners, including initial review, continuing review, protocol amendments, and review of adverse events. If a human subject participating in an IRB-approved protocol becomes a prisoner after the research has begun, the principal investigator should promptly notify the IRB of the event. All research interactions, interventions, and obtaining identifiable private information about the incarcerated prisoner-subject must cease until the protocol and consent document are reviewed by the IRB again, with a prisoner representative present, and the requirements of Subpart C are satisfied.

The OHRP has provided guidance which allows one important exception, however.[15] "In special circumstances in which the principal investigator asserts that it is in the best interests of the subject to remain in the research study while incarcerated, the IRB chair may determine that the subject may continue to participate in the research until the requirements of subpart C are satisfied." Although burdensome, this rereview is necessary in order to reassess the risk/benefit relationship in light of the change in status of the subject. Unless the IRB reapproves the research for inclusion of prisoners, the newly incarcerated individual must be withdrawn from the study.

In the case of multisite studies, there is a need for advocates representing prisoners across all study sites. Sufficient knowledge of prisons at each site is necessary to help insure that the IRBs will be cognizant of potential risks and benefits of research conducted at all participating penal institutions. This speaks to the need for local IRB review in most cases, in order to make knowledgeable decisions regarding the ethics of specific protocols in specific locales.

Type of IRB Review

Per the requirements of 45 CFR 46,[1][Sec.101(i)] research involving prisoners may not be exempted under Section 46.101(b). In addition, the OHRP recommends that all prisoner research, even if technically expeditable under Section 46.110, should be reviewed by the full IRB with a prisoner or prisoner representative present at a convened meeting.[15] This suggestion is an acknowledgment that prisoners are a vulnerable subject population, and therefore, review by the full IRB is warranted from an ethical standpoint in order to obtain heightened scrutiny.

Types of Research Permitted

Only four categories of research involving prisoners are permitted under 45 CFR 46, Subpart C.[1][Sec.306(a)(2)]

Categories i and ii
Research that is not greater than minimal risk may be allowable[1][Sec.306(a)(2)(i),(ii)] if it consists solely of the following:

> (i) Study of the possible causes, effects, and processes of incarceration, and of criminal behavior, provided that the study presents no more than minimal risk and no more than inconvenience to the subjects; or
>
> (ii) Study of prisons as institutional structures or of prisoners as incarcerated persons, provided that the study presents no more than minimal risk and no more than inconvenience to the subjects.

Categories iii and iv
Research may be allowable under 45 CFR 46[1][Sec.306(a)(2)(iii),(iv)] if it consists solely of the following:

> (iii) Research on conditions particularly affecting prisoners as a class (for example, vaccine trials and other research on hepatitis which is much more prevalent in prisons than elsewhere; and research on social and psychological problems such as alcoholism, drug addiction, and sexual assaults) provided that the study may proceed only after the Secretary has consulted with appropriate experts including experts in penology, medicine, and ethics, and published notice, in the *Federal Register,* of his intent to approve such research; or
>
> (iv) Research on practices, both innovative and accepted, which have the intent and reasonable probability of improving the health or well-being of the subject. In cases in which those studies require the assignment of prisoners in a manner consistent with protocols approved by the IRB to control groups which may not benefit from the research, the study may proceed only after the Secretary has consulted with appropriate experts, including experts in penology, medicine, and ethics, and published notice, in the *Federal Register,* of his intent to approve such research.

IRB Classification of Research Under Subpart C

In the first two categories, (i) or (ii), the prospect of direct subject benefit is unlikely. The research, therefore, must present no more than minimal risk to the subjects. Research that falls within the second two categories, (iii) or (iv), has a higher prospect of offering the prisoner direct benefit. Thus, studies involving greater than minimal risk are permitted but may include a requirement for approval by the secretary of the DHHS after consultation with appropriate experts and publication of a notice of intent to approve in the *Federal Register.*

In deciding which category of research under Subpart C may be applicable, it is important for the IRB to recognize that the definition of minimal risk in Subpart C differs from that in Subpart A. Minimal risk is defined in Subpart C[1][Sec.303(d)] as "the probability and magnitude of physical or psychological harm that is normally encountered in the daily lives, or in the routine medical, dental, or psychological examination of healthy persons." This definition differs from that found in Subpart A[1][Sec.102(i)] in two respects. First, "harms" are specifically described as "physical or psychological." In nonprisoner research, IRBs consider a wide range of risks, representing the possibility of physical, psychological, social, economic, or legal harms. In Subpart C, however, only "physical or psychological harm" is mentioned. The reason for this limitation is not explained in the regulations. It is, therefore, unclear whether the implication is that only physical or psychological harms are relevant to prisoner research when deciding whether or not the risk is minimal. Certainly, social, legal, and economic risks are associated with some kinds of research involving prisoners and obviously must be assessed by the IRB. Indeed, such risks may be significant. Second, Subpart C specifies that the risk of harm must be relative to the "daily lives" of "healthy persons." Although the regulations offer no clarification, certainly the standard of minimal risk should not be based on the daily life of a healthy prisoner, for significant risk is often present within the prison environment. The reference to a healthy person implies an absolute standard, and IRBs should accordingly adopt a very conservative interpretation and application of the definition of minimal risk. Therefore, in the opinion of the authors, the threshold of minimal risk should be based on the daily lives of healthy, nonincarcerated individuals.

All category (iii) as well as category (iv) studies that involve assignment of subjects to control groups that may not benefit from the research require additional review at the level of the secretary of the DHHS. Unlike nonprisoner research, the IRB cannot consider a "prerandomization" benefit, that is, the chance of being assigned to the active arm, in determining the risk/benefit relationship in a category (D) study. Subpart C is more restrictive on this point. Each arm must, therefore, be analyzed separately in determining the prospect for direct subject benefit. This represents an additional protection for prisoners who participate in studies involving control groups where there may be limited prospect of direct subject benefit, such as a randomized clinical trial that uses a placebo control.

IRB Approval Criteria for Prisoner Research

As with all other types of human subject research, prisoner research must comply with the requirements of 45 CFR 46.[1(Sec.111)] Those requirements are as follows: the risks to subjects must be minimized; risks to subjects are reasonable in relation to anticipated benefits; the selection of subjects is equitable; informed consent is obtained and appropriately documented; the research plan makes adequate provision for monitoring the data collected to ensure the safety of subjects; and there are adequate provisions to protect the privacy of subjects and to maintain the confidentiality of data.

In addition to these general requirements, Subpart C provides specific protections for prisoners as research subjects, setting further conditions that must be satisfied before an IRB can approve a study. These seven requirements, which include appropriate categorization of the research, take into account the special circumstances of prisoners. They serve to minimize further the risks to subjects, help ensure that the prisoner will be able to give valid informed consent, and assure equitable subject selection. The following are the requirements specified:[1[Sec.305(a)]]

(1) The research under review represents one of the categories of research permissible under 46.306(a)(2).
(2) Any possible advantages accruing to the prisoner through his or her participation in the research, when compared to the general living conditions, medical care, quality of food, amenities, and opportunity for earnings in the prison, are not of such a magnitude that his or her ability to weigh the risks of the research against the value of such advantages in the limited choice environment of the prison is impaired.
(3) The risks involved in the research are commensurate with risks that would be accepted by nonprisoner volunteers.
(4) Procedures for the selection of subjects within the prison are fair to all prisoners and immune from arbitrary intervention by prison authorities or prisoners. Unless the principal investigator provides to the Board justification in writing for following some other procedures, control subjects must be selected randomly from the group of available prisoners who meet the characteristics needed for that particular research project.

(5) The information is presented in language which is understandable to the subject population.
(6) Adequate assurance exists that parole boards will not take into account a prisoner's participation in the research in making decisions regarding parole, and each prisoner is clearly informed in advance that participation in the research will have no effect on his or her parole.
(7) Where the Board finds there may be a need for follow-up examination or care of participants after the end of their participation, adequate provision has been made for such examination or care, taking into account the varying lengths of individual prisoners' sentences, and for informing participants of this fact.

Requirement (7)[1[Sec.305(a)]] is unclear in terms of how and to what extent the investigator, institution, or sponsor is responsible for providing care to both prisoners and parolees after their participation in research. Interpretation of this requirement is particularly problematic in clinical research on life-threatening illnesses such as cancer or AIDS where the patient is likely to need continued treatment, perhaps for a prolonged period and at considerable expense. For example, what does "adequate provision . . . for . . . care" mean? Does it mean that the prisoner or former prisoner who participated in the research must be provided free care for as long as necessary? In the absence of guidance from OHRP, it seems reasonable for an IRB to ensure adequate provisions are made for the care of subjects who suffer a research-related injury but not to extend the provision for treatment of an illness that predates the beginning of the study or is unrelated to the study.

DHHS Certification

After the IRB reviews prisoner research that is supported by the DHHS, the IRB must notify OHRP and (1) provide the name and qualifications of the prisoner representative, (2) provide a reasonably detailed description of the research, (3) document the category of research (i, ii, iii, or iv, per 45 CFR 46.306), and (4) document the additional seven protections required per 45 CFR 46.305. Research involving prisoners may not proceed until OHRP has reviewed the IRB's determination in accordance with 45 CFR 46, Subpart C, and concurs. When a category (i) or (ii) study requires the secretary of the DHHS to consult with a panel of experts before deciding whether a study is approvable, the OHRP acts on behalf of the secretary to convene the required panel. The OHRP has a standing panel to accommodate requests from institutions. If the research involving prisoners is not funded by the DHHS, the IRB need not notify the OHRP but should document in the record that the research has met all requirements of Subpart C. This may include, as necessary, appointment of a local review panel of appropriate experts to advise the IRB when the study is classified as category (iii) or (iv).

Participation in Research of Prisoners Who Are Minors

IRBs should recognize that when a research subject is both a prisoner and a minor, in addition to 45 CFR 46, Subpart

C, the board must also consider Subpart D— Additional DHHS Protections for Children Involved as Subjects in Research. The OHRP has issued specific guidance on this issue, suggesting that an adolescent detained in a juvenile detention facility would be considered a prisoner, and most likely subpart D would also apply.[15] However, if the minor is tried, convicted, and sentenced as an adult, then depending on state law, the prisoner may be constructively emancipated and can legally consent to participate in research. IRBs that choose to recognize constructive emancipation of an incarcerated minor should do so only after careful review of all considerations. This includes vulnerability of the minor, developmental age, and the fact that the rights of the minor's parents to direct the child's activities have been involuntarily subjugated to the state department of corrections. Clearly, involvement of such individuals in research requires close scrutiny, as a minor who is also a prisoner could be a highly vulnerable subject.

Protection at the Expense of Justice

Subpart C of 45 CFR 46 is obviously designed to protect the rights and welfare of prisoners who participate in research. Clearly, additional protection is needed. It is ironic, however, that although Subpart C protects the rights of prisoners, it also significantly restricts their right to participate in research. Although this population is vulnerable, it is of concern that the pendulum may have swung too far. Subpart C contains the only additional protections that require certification by the OHRP. The need for additional federal review of any placebo-controlled trials may well serve to limit access of prisoners to innovative research interventions. The result may be a paternalistic set of regulations that limit a prisoner's autonomy to decide to participate in and benefit from taking part in research. The principle of justice requires that both the benefits and burdens of research be distributed fairly. By denying prisoners the ability to make a decision as to whether they want to participate in research or by limiting their access to research, the basic principle of respect for persons may be violated. Thus, it is important to consider these principles as future regulations are established to "protect" prisoners from the risks of research.

Waiver for Epidemiological Research Involving Prisoners

One recent change to the regulations, which appears to be an acknowledgment of overly restrictive requirements, is the waiver for some epidemiological research involving prisoners.[16] Effective June 20, 2003, DHHS regulations 46.305(a)(1) and 46.306(a)(2) may be waived for DHHS to conduct or support "certain important and necessary epidemiological research on prisoners that presents no more than minimal risk and no more than inconvenience to the prisoner-subjects." This will allow prisoners to participate in epidemiological studies that focus on a particular condition or disease that might affect prisoners, as it could

any other members of the general population. Such research was not previously allowable as it did not meet any of the four categories of research permissible for prisoners, because it was not specific to prisoners and had no reasonable probability of direct benefit.

Secretary's Advisory Committee on Human Research Protections

Additional changes in the regulations addressing research involving prisoners may well be pending. The Secretary's Advisory Committee on Human Research Protections has been identifying and addressing many of the concerns with current regulations that have been discussed previously here. Specifically, issues such as research with individuals who have restricted liberties but do not meet the definition of a prisoner, expedited reviews, the role of local IRBs in multisite studies, follow-up care, and the definition of a control group are all being addressed.

Conclusion

Prisoners are clearly a subject population in need of additional protections. When reviewing research protocols involving prisoners, IRBs need to be acutely aware of the potential vulnerabilities of this group, as well as the current regulations in place to protect them. Although the protections may be in some cases overly restrictive, resulting in lost opportunities to benefit from research, they arose in an effort to protect a group that had been historically abused. Ongoing review of the regulations provides hope that a balance will be struck that allows prisoners access to the potential benefits of research, without being inappropriately subjected to potential risks, while keeping in mind the vulnerabilities of this population.

References

1. Code of Federal Regulations. Title 45A—Department of Health and Human Services; Part 46—Protection of Human Subjects. Updated 1 October, 1997.
2. Code of Federal Regulations. Title 21, Chapter 1—Food and Drug Administration, DHHS; Part 50—Protection of Human Subjects. Updated 1 April, 1999.
3. Code of Federal Regulations. Title 21, Chapter 1—Food and Drug Administration, DHHS; Part 56—Institutional Review Boards. Updated 1 April, 1999.
4. Hornblum AM. They were cheap and available: Prisoners as research subjects in twentieth century America. *Br Med J* 315:1437–1441, 1997.
5. Mitford J. *Kind and Unusual Punishments*. New York: Vintage Books; 1973.
6. Leopold NF. *Life Plus 99 Years*. Garden City, NY: Doubleday; 1958.
7. The Medical Case. Chapters 1–15. *Trials of War Criminals Before the Nuremberg Military Tribunals Under Control Council Law No. 10, Vols. 1 and 2*. Washington, DC: U.S. Government Printing Office; 1949.
8. Supplementary Report of the Judicial Council. *JAMA* 132(17):1090, 1946.

9. Hornblum AM. *Acres of Skin: Human Experiments at Holmesburg Prison.* New York: Routledge; 1998.

10. Jones JH. *Bad Blood: The Tuskegee Syphilis Experiment.* New York: Free Press; 1981.

11. Robinson RJ. Memorandum to the Office of the Commissioner (Food and Drug Administration document obtained via the Freedom of Information Act). 30 June, 1976.

12. National Commission for the Protection of Human Subjects of Biomedical and Behavioral Research. Report and recommendations: Research involving prisoners (DHEW (OS) 76–131). Washington, DC: Government Printing Office; 1976.

13. Department of Health, Education and Welfare. Additional protections pertaining to biomedical and behavioral research involving prisoners as subjects. *Fed Regist* 43(222):53652–53655, 1978.

14. Office for Human Research Protections. Compliance determination letters. Access date 4 January, 2005. http://www.hhs.gov/ohrp/

15. Office for Protection from Research Risks. OPRR guidance on approving research involving prisoners, 23 June, 2000. Access date 4 January, 2005. http://www.hhs.gov/ohrp/

16. Waiver of the Applicability of Certain Provisions of Department of Health and Human Services Regulations for Protection of Human Research Subjects for Department of Health and Human Services Conducted or Supported Epidemiological Research Involving Prisoners as Subjects. *Fed Regist* 68(119):36929–36931, 2003.

Research Involving College Students

Jennifer J. Tickle and Todd F. Heatherton

INTRODUCTION

Given that much research takes place in college and university settings, it is not surprising that college students are often participants in research studies. Indeed, some fields, such as psychological science, rely on college students as their primary research participants. Students are convenient, easy to recruit, and relatively inexpensive when compared with nonstudents. Although many of the issues related to research participation are the same for college students as other populations, there are two issues deserving special mention with regard to their research participation.

Coercion

College students are typically given the opportunity to participate in research in one of several ways: in exchange for course credit as part of a course requirement, in exchange for extra credit in a course, or in exchange for payment on a voluntary basis after recruitment. The Code of Federal Regulations[1(Sec.116)] states that an investigator should seek consent "only under circumstances that provide the prospective subject . . . sufficient opportunity to consider whether to participate and that minimize the possibility of coercion or undue influence." The central controversy about college student participation involves whether participation for course credit is considered coercive. For instance, in cases in which participation is linked to course requirements or credit, students may feel as if they have to participate in order to please the course professor. They may believe that their grades, potential letters of recommendation, or other opportunities in the department may be compromised if they do not participate in the research studies.[2(Chap.5)]

At the same time, research participation can be viewed as valuable for both the researcher and student participants. Research participation is a way for students to become involved in the learning process and to learn firsthand about the process of scientific research. Active learning by way of involvement is an effective way for students to acquire information. Therefore, the educational benefit of student participation in research should not be discounted.

Alternatives to Course-Required Research Participation

To decrease the potential for coercion with research participation for course credit, research departments can provide alternatives to participation that are comparable in time, effort, and fulfillment of course requirements. For instance, Gamble[3] and Cohen[4] have suggested such options as research papers (which can be comparable in time expenditure and educational benefit) or attendance at research talks given by department faculty (comparable in time, effort, and educational benefit) as alternatives to research participation. If alternative options cannot be offered, participants can at least be given a choice of studies in which to participate. Of course, as per federal standards,[1(Sec.116)] participants must be able to withdraw from participation in any study at any point without penalty. This means that even those participants who withdraw from a research study must receive full course credit for research participation. When evaluating research that involves course credit, the IRB should understand how course-related participation in a given department is structured and whether comparable options are offered in the place of research participation to help ensure the voluntary nature of that participation.[2(Chap.5)]

Recruitment Practices

Aside from actual course credit for participation, recruitment into research can be made less coercive with attention to the recruitment process itself. For instance, faculty and researchers can solicit participants more broadly, using sign-up sheets or general announcements rather than direct invitations to particular students. This reduces the likelihood of "undue coercion" by decreasing the influence of the faculty–student relationship and making the request less direct. IRBs should review all recruitment material to be sure the risks and benefits are not misrepresented and to be sure that participation for course credit is not presented in a way that is likely to be coercive.[2(Chap.5)]

Paying Students to Participate in Research

Rather than offering course credit for research participation, some researchers have funds to pay participants for their time. Paying research participants is discussed in several other chapters in this book. Payment, in the form of money, gifts, privileges, or other resources, can only be offered as a recruitment incentive, not as a benefit of participation. Therefore, payment for research participation must be commensurate with the time, effort, and discomfort involved in the research, as well as the risk of participating. Payment should not be so extreme as to unduly influence people to participate without considering the risks. Although explicit standards for the amount of incentive do not exist, IRBs should use reason when considering whether an investigator's plans for recruitment incentives seem excessive for a given study.[2(Chap.5)]

Some College Students Are Minors

One additional concern about using college students, particularly college freshmen, involves the age of the consent giver.[1(Sec.408)] Some college freshmen may be legal minors for whom parental consent is still needed. This is an issue to consider, especially if a college allows high-school students to take its courses. IRBs should remind researchers about the regulations and laws that relate to the need for surrogate (parental) consent to participate in research. IRB approval of research that targets college students should explicitly address the need for surrogate consent when appropriate.

Confidentiality

The second major concern of using college students as research participants, besides coercion, involves confidentiality. A variety of sensitive measures may be taken by researchers, ranging from medical information to ratings of self-esteem, depression, drug use, and so forth. Because of the close nature of many college environments, extra care must be taken to ensure participant confidentiality. For instance, data should be stored where access is restricted. If undergraduate research assistants are used for data collection, data coding, or data entry, they must understand the importance of the confidentiality of the data with which they are working. To help ensure confidentiality, all appropriate measures must be taken to keep participant names separate from data at all stages of the research process. IRBs should monitor this by requesting information about the process of data storage. Where possible, investigators should be encouraged to use code numbers to identify participants in the place of other more identifying information.[2(Chap.5)]

Conclusion

College students are not usually defined as a separate class of research participants from the standpoint of ethical standards or regulatory compliance. However, because research often takes place on college campuses and some categories of research specifically target the student population, it is useful to review the issues that IRB members, researchers, and institutional officials should consider when evaluating research projects that are likely to enroll college students. In this setting, coercion and confidentiality are the two most common areas of concern. This chapter discusses ways to minimize problems in each of these areas. An additional issue that is often overlooked is that some college students are minors. Research involving minors must comply with federal regulations and, often, state law that does not apply to research limited to adult participants.

References

1. Code of Federal Regulations. Title 45A—Department of Health and Human Services; Part 46—Protection of Human Subjects. Updated 1 October, 1997. Access date 18 April, 2001. http://www4.law.cornell.edu/cfr/45p46.htm

2. Penslar RL, Porter JP, Office for Human Research Protections. *Institutional Review Board Guidebook*, 2nd ed. 6 February, 2001. Access date 29 March, 2001. http://ohrp.osophs.dhhs.gov/irb/irb_guidebook.htm

3. Gamble HF. Case study: Students, grades and informed consent. *IRB: A Review of Human Subjects Research* 4(5):7–10, 1982.

4. Cohen JM. Extra credit for research subjects. *IRB: A Review of Human Subjects Research* 4(8):10–11, 1982.

PART 10

Institutional Review Board Issues Based on Study Design or Category

When are Research Risks Reasonable in Relationship to Anticipated Benefits?

Charles Weijer and Paul B. Miller

INTRODUCTION

The question "when are research risks reasonable in relationship to anticipated benefits?" is at the very heart of pressing disputes in the ethics of clinical research. Institutional review boards (IRBs) are criticized for inconsistent decision making, a phenomenon that may be traced in part to reliance on the vagaries of intuition to interpret federal regulation on acceptable risks and potential benefits.[1] Furthermore, the problem of acceptability of risks and potential benefits in research runs through a number of contemporary controversies, including the ethics of research involving placebo controls,[2] developing countries,[3] incapable adults,[4] and emergency rooms.[5] If IRBs are to be given clear guidance and if pressing ethical questions are to be addressed in a principled way, then a systematic approach to the ethics of risk in research is required.

A systematic approach to the ethical analysis of risks and potential benefits in research called "component analysis" has recently been developed.[6] Component analysis is built on the recognition that clinical research often contains a mixture of therapeutic and nontherapeutic procedures and that separate moral standards are required for each. It refines an approach originally developed by the National Commission for the Protection of Human Subjects of Biomedical and Behavioral Research in *Institutional Review Boards* and *The Belmont Report*.[7,8] As these documents informed the development of the Common Rule, component analysis is a needed explication of federal regulation. In its final report on research involving humans, the U.S. National Bioethics Advisory Commission endorsed component analysis, as have a variety of other commentators.[4,9,10]

In a recent flurry of articles, however, critics of component analysis have suggested that it is a flawed approach. It is argued that one of the core concepts of component analysis, clinical equipoise, conflates the ethics of clinical practice with the ethics of research.[11] It has also been argued that component analysis is misapplied to the ethical analysis of placebo controls.[2] Without engaging these criticisms directly, we would like to point out that it seems the critics have failed to appreciate how component analysis is supported by reasonable arguments. They have also failed to appreciate that it provides much needed guidance to IRBs on the ethical analysis of research risks and potential benefits and that it also offers the prospect of principled resolution of a wide variety of contemporary controversies. If component analysis does indeed meet these ends, then, even if flawed, one ought not to dispense with it until a more robust alternative is articulated.

Component Analysis Provides Clear Criteria for IRBs

The Common Rule instructs IRBs to ensure that "risks to subjects are minimized" and "risks to subjects are reasonable in relation to anticipated benefits, if any, to subjects, and the importance of the knowledge that may be reasonably expected to result" (45 CFR 46.111(a)(1,2)). Unembellished imperatives often provoke more questions than they answer. Which risks to subjects must be minimized? To what extent must they be minimized? Which risks and which potential benefits are to be considered in the reasonableness determinations? By what measure does one determine that risks are reasonable in relationship to benefits to subjects? By what measure does one determine

This chapter was originally published in *Nature Medicine* 10(6):570–573; 2004. Used with permission.

that risks are reasonable in relation to the knowledge that may result? In the absence of careful explication of these regulatory requirements, it is difficult to see how IRBs can effectively fulfill their mandate of protecting research subjects.[12]

Component analysis builds on the recognition that clinical trials often contain a mixture of interventions administered with differing purposes. Drug, surgical, and behavioral interventions are administered with therapeutic warrant; that is, they are administered on the basis of evidence sufficient to justify the belief that they may benefit research subjects. Other interventions, such as venipuncture for pharmacokinetic drug levels, additional imaging procedures, or questionnaires not used in clinical practice, are given without therapeutic warrant. They are administered solely for the purpose of answering the scientific question. As this distinction is morally relevant, IRBs must apply separate moral standards to their assessment of therapeutic and nontherapeutic procedures (Figure 10.1.1).

Therapeutic procedures must meet the ethical standard of clinical equipoise (Figure 10.1.1).[13] Clinical equipoise is

a research-friendly response to this question: "When may a physician offer enrollment in a clinical trial to his or her patient?" It provides that he or she may do so when the therapeutic procedures in a clinical trial are consistent with competent medical care. More formally, clinical equipoise requires that at the outset of a trial there exists a state of honest, professional disagreement in the community of expert practitioners as to the preferred treatment. Procedurally, the IRB does not make this determination by surveying practitioners. Rather, it scrutinizes the study justification, reviews relevant literature, and when required, consults with independent clinical experts. Clinical equipoise is satisfied if the IRB concludes that the evidence supporting the various therapeutic procedures is sufficient that, if were it widely known, expert clinicians would disagree as to the preferred treatment.

Nontherapeutic procedures do not offer the prospect of direct benefit to research subjects. When assessing risks associated with nontherapeutic procedures ("nontherapeutic risks"), the IRB must determine that two separate ethical standards are met. The IRB must determine that

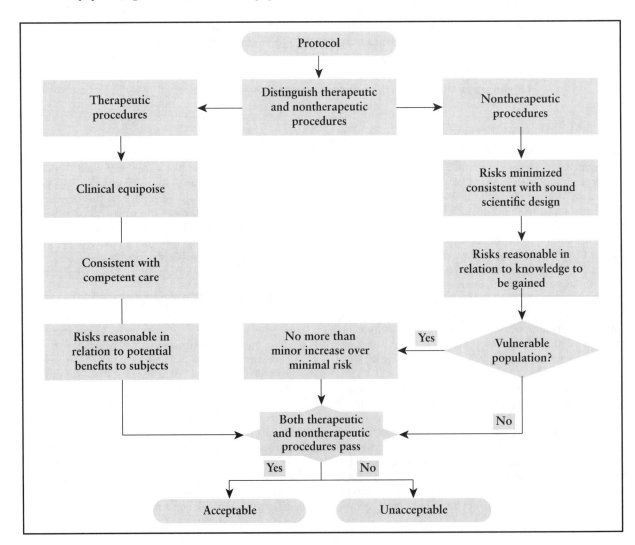

Figure 10.1.1 Component analysis of risks and potential benefits in research

nontherapeutic risks are, first, minimized consistent with sound scientific design and, second, reasonable in relationship to the knowledge that may be gained from the study (Figure 10.1.1). Procedurally, the IRB ensures that nontherapeutic risks are minimized by, where feasible, requiring the substitution of "procedures already being performed on the subjects for diagnostic and treatment purposes" (45 CFR 46.111(a)(1)(ii)). The IRB's determination that the risks of nontherapeutic procedures are reasonable in relation to knowledge requires that it judge the study's scientific value sufficient to justify risks to subjects. Because this judgment involves the appraisal of social priorities, community representatives must be included as fully participating members of the IRB.[14]

When research involves a vulnerable population, such as pregnant women, prisoners, or children, additional protection may be required. A threshold may be invoked limiting the nontherapeutic risks to which vulnerable subjects may be exposed (Figure 10.1.1). For children, nontherapeutic risks are limited to the standard of a "minor increase over minimal risk." In other words, a minor increase over the risks "ordinarily encountered in daily life" (45 CFR 46. 406(a), 46.102(i)). Procedurally, to determine whether the risks of nontherapeutic procedures fulfill this criterion, the IRB reasons by analogy.[15] It asks whether risks posed by nontherapeutic procedures are the same as those ordinarily encountered in daily life or are sufficiently similar to these risks (45 CFR 46.102(i)). Whether the referent for minimal risk ought to be the daily lives of healthy or sick children remains controversial.[16,17]

Research risks are reasonable in relationship to anticipated benefits when the IRB determines that the moral standards for both therapeutic and nontherapeutic procedures are fulfilled.

Component Analysis Enables Principled Resolution of Controversies

Component analysis provides clear criteria for IRBs to use in judging whether the risks of research are reasonable in terms of what might be gained by the individual or society. However, does it enable principled resolution of controversial issues in research that turn on evaluation of harms and benefits? Consider the four controversies cited previously here.

Placebo Controls

When is it acceptable to offer patients enrollment in a placebo-controlled trial in which they assume the risks of forgoing standard treatment? When applying component analysis, one must first determine whether the placebo control is a therapeutic or nontherapeutic procedure. It may be a combination of the two. A placebo control is at least a no-treatment control. A no-treatment control is the null case for therapeutic procedures, and it, along with therapeutic procedures in the experimental arm, must pass the test of clinical equipoise. According to clinical

equipoise, a no-treatment control is appropriate when there is no effective treatment for the condition of interest, the trial selectively enrolls treatment-resistant patients, the study is a test of an add-on treatment versus placebo in which all subjects receive standard treatment or treatment exists but "no treatment" is nonetheless consistent with competent medical care.[18]

Although there may be effective treatments for minor medical conditions, for example allergic rhinitis, mild dermatitis, mild hypertension, or baldness, a competent physician may nonetheless recommend no treatment for these conditions. The use of a placebo control for minor medical conditions is, therefore, unproblematic.[19]

Placebo controls may involve additional interventions administered for scientific purposes, for example, sugar pills, saline injections, or sham surgical interventions. These interventions are administered with the purpose of simulating, as closely as possible, factors in the treatment context not directly related to the therapeutic properties of the experimental intervention. These are nontherapeutic interventions and the risks associated with them must be minimized and deemed reasonable in relationship to the knowledge to be gained. In many, perhaps most, placebo-controlled trials, the risk of the nontherapeutic intervention (e.g., the sugar pill) is close to zero. When the placebo control involves interventions posing greater risk, such as saline injections or sham surgery, it is more difficult to justify. The IRB must ask whether the scientific ends of the study can be met with less risky interventions. Are the risks counterbalanced by the importance of the knowledge to be gained? Because the use of a no-surgery control arm presents a less risky alternative and because the risks posed by sham surgery may in some cases be serious, these moral requirements pose substantial obstacles to the ethical use of sham surgical controls.[20]

International Research

For clinical trials in developing countries, is the care to which subjects are entitled determined by local or international standards? Consider the controversy over clinical trials comparing short-course zidovudine to placebo for the prevention of perinatal transmission of HIV in sub-Saharan Africa and Thailand. The ACTG 076 regimen was the gold standard in developed countries[21] but was not used in these trials. Critics argued that the novel regimen ought to have been compared to ACTG 076 and that the failure to do so set up a double standard for research in developed and developing countries.[22] Defenders responded that no treatment was available in developing countries and that ACTG 076 was an unaffordable and impractical treatment alternative in this setting.[23]

In component analysis, both short-course zidovudine and the no-treatment control are therapeutic interventions that must satisfy clinical equipoise. Does clinical equipoise allow the control treatment to be determined by local standards? Angell argues that it does not and that the trials are unethical.[24] Crouch and Arras disagree and their reasoning seems convincing.[25] They remind us that the fundamental purpose of a clinical trial is the resolution of disagreement as to the preferred treatment. In other words, the aim of a trial is to alter clinical practice. Crouch and Arras stated, "Because clinical trials are responsive to and centrally concerned with the realities of clinical practice, it is crucial for the clinical trialists to take the study context into account when designing and conducting such studies."[25] Keeping in mind the pragmatic purpose of clinical trials, clinical equipoise seems to permit a trial design that asks "whether the shorter AZT regimen is safe in these populations, and, if so, whether the demonstrated efficacy is large enough, as compared to the placebo group, to make it affordable to the governments in question."[25]

Incapable Adults

Should incapable adults be included in clinical trials? If so, to how much risk should they be exposed by interventions performed solely for the sake of science? Regulations for the protection of incapable adults in research were first proposed in 1978 but were never implemented.[26] Repeated calls for additional protections for incapable adults have gone unheeded. The Common Rule requires that IRBs be "particularly cognizant of the special problems of research involving vulnerable populations," including incapable adults, and ensure that "additional safeguards have been included in the study to protect the rights and welfare of these subjects" (45 CFR 46.111(a)(3), 46.111(b)). IRBs are given no guidance, however, as to what additional safeguards are required. Thus, the central problem remains "designing appropriate protections for persons with mental disorders who participate in . . . research . . . while providing the opportunity to obtain the potential for benefit that may arise from . . . participation."[12]

It is cogently argued that the failure to address this problem through specific regulations runs the risk of both stymieing needed research and failing to protect incapable adults involved in research.[4] A failure to distinguish between therapeutic and nontherapeutic procedures in the ethical analysis of harms and benefits leads to "a situation that could exploit vulnerable subjects in the pursuit of knowledge" (p. 1391).[4] Component analysis is identified as essential to the protection of incapable adults. Incapable adults are vulnerable for the same reason that children are: they are not able to protect their own interests through informed consent. Thus, although specific protections for the complex and diverse population of incapable adults may at points differ from the protections currently afforded children, "regulations governing pediatric research provide a model" for developing protections for incapable adults. This implies that a threshold ought to be invoked limiting the nontherapeutic risks to which incapable adults may be exposed (Figure 10.1.1).

Emergency Research

Under what circumstances, if any, may clinical trials in emergency medicine enroll subjects who are incapable of providing informed consent and for whom no proxy decision maker is available? Debate as to what protections ought to be afforded to subjects in emergency research is premised on the assumption that it poses more than minimal risk. "Deferred consent" was invoked for a number of studies in the 1980s but was rejected by the Office for Protection from Research Risks because one cannot logically consent to a procedure that has already been performed.[27,28] As a result, emergency research came to a halt until complex regulations permitting the waiver of consent were implemented (21 CFR 50.24). These regulations fail to distinguish between therapeutic and nontherapeutic procedures and link the permissibility of risk to severity of illness by requiring that risks in the aggregate be

> Reasonable in relation to what is known about the medical condition of the potential class of participants, the risks and benefits of standard therapy, if any, and what is known about the risks and benefits of the proposed intervention or activity (21 CFR 50.24).

In this novel requirement, the level of permissible aggregate risk is linked to the severity of the patient's condition. This opens the door to exploitation, as it allows sicker patients to be exposed to higher levels of risk solely to meet scientific ends.

Component analysis has been applied to the problem.[29] Component analysis ensures, through the proper application of clinical equipoise, that the sum of risks and potential benefits of therapeutic procedures in a clinical trial are roughly similar to that which a patient would receive in clinical practice. The incremental risk posed by research participation, therefore, stems from nontherapeutic study procedures. Thus, a risk threshold such as minimal risk can only be sensibly applied to nontherapeutic procedures. The emergency room context generally limits nontherapeutic research interventions to chart review, additional history and physical examinations and recording data collected from monitoring equipment—all procedures that arguably pose no more than minimal risk to subjects. As the absence of a proxy decision maker renders emergency subjects relatively more vulnerable than children or incapable adults, a more restrictive risk threshold such as minimal risk *simpliciter* may be appropriate.

Critics Must Articulate a Robust Alternative

To our knowledge, component analysis is the only systematic elaboration of the entailments of the ethical principle of beneficence for IRB review of human subject research. It is supported by arguments that are, at first sight, reasonable. As we have seen, component analysis provides IRBs with much needed and clear criteria for the ethical analysis of research benefits and harms. Furthermore, it enables principled resolution of a variety of pressing problems in the ethics of research. Even if component analysis turns out to be a flawed approach—and we by no means grant that it is—it would continue to possess a social imperative in the sense that IRBs and policy makers require a systematic approach to make effective and consistent decisions. These facts seem to impose, therefore, a special burden on the critics of component analysis. If component analysis is to be overthrown, critics must articulate a robust alternative.

To be tenable, an alternative approach to the ethical analysis of risks and potential benefits must protect research subjects, allow clinical research to proceed, explain how physicians may offer trial enrollment to their patients, address the challenges posed by research containing a mixture of interventions, and define ethical standards according to which the risks and potential benefits of research may be consistently evaluated.

Consider, for example, Miller and Brody's recent suggestion that clinical equipoise be abandoned and that "an alternative framework for the ethics of clinical trials is needed."[11] They state that their "alternative framework provides accurate ethical guidance concerning clinical research" (p. 26).[11] With regard to the ethical analysis of risks and potential benefits in research, their alternative approach, stated in its entirety, is this: "Favorable risk–benefit ratio. Risk–benefit assessment of research protocols ultimately comes down to a matter of judgment" (p. 27).[11] Although we agree that judgment is required, this framework fails to provide the promised guidance. Indeed, it does not meet any of the five tenability requirements mentioned previously here. Miller and Brody's alternative does not provide clear criteria to IRBs and seems unlikely to enable principled resolution of contemporary controversies.

Conclusion

Optimal protections for research subjects require that substantive and procedural requirements flowing from fundamental ethical principles be elaborated and adopted. Component analysis represents the only systematic approach to the ethical analysis of risks and potential benefits in research. It is supported by reasonable arguments. Furthermore, it provides clear criteria for IRBs to use in judging whether the risks of research are reasonable in terms of what might be gained by the individual or society. Finally, it allows for the principled resolution of moral issues that turn on the evaluation of harm and benefit in research. If critics are to mount a successful assault on component analysis, they must acknowledge these accomplishments and articulate a robust alternative.

Acknowledgments
The authors are grateful to C. Heilig at the Centers for Disease Control and Prevention for preparing Figure 10.1.1. This work was supported by a Canadian Institutes of Health Research Investigator Award and Operating Grant (C.W.) and a doctoral fellowship from the Social Sciences and Humanities Research Council of Canada (P.B.M.). C.W. is a Visiting Scholar at the Department of History and Philosophy of Science at the University of Cambridge and Visiting Fellow at Clare Hall, Cambridge, UK.

References
1. Shah S, Whittle A, Wilfond B, Gensler G, Wendler D. *JAMA* 291:476–482, 2004.
2. Emanuel EJ, Miller FG. *N Engl J Med* 345:915–919, 2001.
3. Angell M. *N Engl J Med* 337:847–849, 1997.
4. Karlawish JH. *N Engl J Med* 348:1389–1392, 2003.
5. Valenzuela TD, Copass MK. *N Engl J Med* 345:689–690, 2001.
6. Weijer C. *J Law Med Ethics* 28:344–361, 2000.
7. National Commission for the Protection of Human Subjects of Biomedical and Behavioral Research. *Institutional Review Boards: Report and Recommendations* (DHEW Publication [OS] 780008), Washington, DC; 1978.
8. National Commission for the Protection of Human Subjects of Biomedical and Behavioral Research. *The Belmont Report: Ethical Principles and Guidelines for the Protection of Human Subjects of Research* (DHEW Publication [OS] 78-0012). Washington, DC; 1978.
9. U.S. National Bioethics Advisory Commission. *Ethical and Policy Issues in Research Involving Human Participants* Bethesda, MD: U.S. National Bioethics Advisory Commission; 2000:69–95.
10. Emanuel EJ, Wendler D, Grady C. *JAMA* 283:2701–2711, 2000.
11. Miller FG, Brody H. *Hastings Cent Rep* 33:19–28, 2003.
12. U.S. National Bioethics Advisory Commission. *Ethical and Policy Issues in Research Involving Human Participants* Bethesda, MD: U.S. National Bioethics Advisory Commission; 2000:13.
13. Freedman B. *N Engl J Med* 317:141–145, 1987.
14. Freedman B. *IRB* 9:7–10, 1987.
15. Freedman B, Fuks A, Weijer C. *Hastings Cent Rep* 23:13–19, 1993.
16. Kopelman LM. *J Med Philos* 25:745–764, 2000.
17. Miller PB, Weijer C. *IRB* 22:6–10, 2000.
18. Freedman B. *IRB* 12:31–34, 1990.
19. Weijer C, Glass KC. *N Engl J Med* 346:382–383, 2002.
20. Weijer C. *J Law Med Ethics* 30:69–72, 2002.
21. Connor EM, et al. *N Engl J Med* 331:1173–1180, 1994.
22. Lurie P, Wolfe SM. *N Engl J Med* 337:853–856, 1997.
23. Varmus H, Satcher D. *N Engl J Med* 337:1003–1005, 1997.
24. Angell M. *N Engl J Med* 337:847–849, 1997.
25. Crouch RA, Arras JD. *Hastings Cent Rep* 28:26–34, 1998.
26. Department of Health, Education and Welfare. *Fed Regist* 43:53950–53956, 1978.
27. Fost N, Robertson J. *IRB* 2:5–6, 1980.
28. Ellis G. *Office for Protection from Research Risks* 93–3, 1993.
29. McRae AD, Weijer C. *Crit Care Med* 30:1146–1151, 2002.

Internet Research: A Brief Guide for Institutional Review Boards

Jeffrey M. Cohen

It is clear that the Internet will be used more and more in conducting human subjects research. Such research is not limited to the social and behavioral sciences, but is increasing in the biomedical sciences as well (see the *Journal of Medical Internet Research*, http://www.jmir.org/). Research on the Internet presents new concerns to some of the traditional human subjects issues: risk/benefit, informed consent, participation by minors, and confidentiality. Investigators are going to have to provide technical information on how they will deal these issues, and institutional review boards (IRBs) are going to have to have sufficient expertise to ask the right questions and evaluate the information provided.

Several sources are available that discuss the advantages, disadvantages, and ethical concerns of Internet research.[1,2] This chapter provides a guide to IRBs reviewing Internet research.

Types of Research Activities on the Internet

Three types of research activities are conducted on the Internet:

- Recruiting subjects over the Internet
- Observation of Internet activity
- Collecting data over the Internet

Recruiting Subjects Over the Internet

The use of the Internet to recruit subjects presents similar issues as with any other recruiting tool; the IRB needs to review information presented to subjects. Not only does the IRB need to review the text of the recruitment, but it also has to examine the context in which the recruitment takes place (e.g., posting a message on a newsgroup or creating a website to recruit subjects). When the web is used to recruit subjects, the IRB must see an example of what the prospective subjects will see (i.e., a "screen shot").

Observation of Internet Activity

Observation of Internet activity usually involves such activities as gathering information about the use of the Internet and recording user information or users' comments. Examples include having the participant observe an online discussion group, using "cookies" to track websites visited, or asking visitors to a website to provide demographic information. The human subjects issues involved in this type of research generally involve consent/disclosure issues, as well as issues of privacy and confidentiality.

Gathering Data Over the Internet

This type of research generally involves having subjects submit data, for example, survey data, over the Internet and presents the most serious human subjects concerns. As in the other types of Internet research activities, the investigator needs to indicate how subjects' consent will be obtained and their confidentiality protected. Of particular concern with this type of research is the potential participation by minors, which issue investigators must address in their IRB protocols.

Human Subjects Issues

Risk

There are two sources of potential harm to subjects from research: harm resulting from participation in the research (e.g., acute emotional reactions to certain questions) and harm resulting from breach of confidentiality. Although most research conducted on the Internet is relatively innocuous, some research may involve the potential for adverse psychologic reactions by subjects. Because there is generally no direct contact with subjects participating in research over the Internet, it may be difficult or impossible to deal with individual subject reactions. In addition, although there are mechanisms to provide debriefing material to online subjects, it is difficult to ensure that they actually access the materials. As a result, some sensitive research may not be appropriate for the Internet. A breach of confidentiality is the primary source of harm in most Internet research and is dealt with later here.

Benefit

Conducting research on the Internet raises concerns about the reliability and validity of the data. This can be the result of skewed subject populations because of differences in access to computers, the ease with which subjects can mislead investigators, or difficulty in preventing multiple submissions. Research that results in unreliable or invalid data can have no benefit and, therefore, no risk is justified.

Consent

Informed consent and the documentation of informed consent are two of the most troublesome issues in Internet research. There are mechanisms for obtaining informed consent in Internet research, but documentation of consent is more problematic. Under the regulations,[3[Sec.116]] informed consent involves presenting the potential subjects with the required information and obtaining their voluntary consent to participate. One mechanism for doing this is familiar to everyone who downloads software from the Internet. Before downloading or installing the software, the individual is presented some sort of license agreement text and must check off "I agree" before they can proceed. A similar procedure can be used for Internet research. The required information may be presented to the subjects who must check off "I agree" before they participate in the research. Particularly for research posing minimal risk, this would satisfy the informed consent requirement of the regulations. For some less innocuous research, additional safeguards may be required to ensure that the subjects actually read the information before proceeding may be required.

Some Internet research may qualify for a waiver of informed consent if it meets the regulatory criteria for a waiver.[3[Sec.116(d)]] These criteria include minimal risk; the waiver does not adversely affect the participant's rights or welfare, the research could not practicably be carried out without the waiver and, where appropriate, participants are debriefed.

As previously noted, documenting the consent is more of a problem. The procedure described previously here would not satisfy the regulatory requirements for documentation of informed consent.[3[Sec.117]] The regulations require written, signed documentation of consent, unless waived by the IRB. Because the technology for digital signatures is not yet widely available, there is no way to obtain documentation of consent over the Internet.

Not all research, however, needs documentation of informed consent; IRBs can waive the requirement for documentation of consent when the regulatory criteria for a waiver are met.[3[Sec.117(c)]] When documentation of consent is required, investigators can have subjects submit a signed consent form (which can be downloaded) and send them a password to gain access to the research pages.

In any event, investigators must indicate to the IRB how they plan to obtain consent from subjects. The IRB must decide if its consent procedures are adequate and meet the regulatory requirements.

Participation by Minors

Another major area of concern in Internet research is the participation by minors in the research. The basic problem is that, even for research not intended for minors, it is difficult to ensure that minors are not participating. Because investigators cannot be sure that minors are not participating, it must be assumed that they will participate, and if so, parental permission is generally required.

The IRB has the authority to waive the requirement for parental permission,[3[Sec.408(b)]] and where the research qualifies for such a waiver, no additional safeguards for minors are required. Either minors can participate without permission or participants could be required to state that he/she is over 18 years of age. Where parental permission is required, investigators can use passwords as was described in the section on informed consent. To screen out minors completely from the research, investigators can take advantage of Internet monitoring software (SafeSurf and RSACi ratings) or use adult check systems. Because no system can guarantee that minors are not participating, some research may not be appropriate for the Internet.

Privacy and Confidentiality

Privacy and confidentiality are often lumped together by IRBs. They are, however, separate concepts and have different implications for the review of Internet research. Privacy refers to individuals' right to have control over access to themselves and their information, whereas confidentiality refers to how information that is obtained from individuals is protected.

Privacy

With regard to Internet research, privacy concerns most often arise in research on Internet activity and generally relate to whether such activity is identifiable and constitutes public or private behavior. In order to meet the regulatory definition of research, the investigator must be obtaining "identifiable, private information."[3[Sec.102(f)]] Although participants in Internet activity usually use pseudonyms (screen names, handles, etc.), this does not mean that they are anonymous. Although not publicly linked to actual names, individual identities can often be "readily ascertained" (e.g., using a search engine), thus meeting the regulatory definition of identifiable information. In addition, within online communities, a person's online identity may be as important to them as their actual identity, and thus, online identities may need to be protected as much as actual identities.

Although a great deal of online activity is open to the public, federal regulations base the definition of "private information" on the subjects' "reasonable expectation of privacy." Thus, the determination of privacy is more complicated than it seems. In many situations (e.g., chat rooms), participants expect privacy and do not expect their activity to be studied by researchers. This might be considered a reasonable expectation of privacy and should be considered by the IRB.

Confidentiality

As stated previously here, the primary source of risk in Internet research is an inappropriate breach of confidentiality. The risks of breach of confidentiality are not limited to Internet research, but the fact that most data collected in Internet research is electronic makes the evaluation of this risk more problematic for IRBs.

Obviously, anonymity provides the strongest confidentiality protection; however, anonymity of data obtained over the Internet is not as easy to achieve as it may seem. Data transmitted via e-mail cannot be anonymous without the use of additional steps. Almost all forms of e-mail contain the sender's e-mail address. In order to maintain anonymity, the research must use an "anonymizer"—a third-party site that strips off the sender's e-mail address. Data submitted over the web can only be anonymous if software is used to store the information directly in a database without identifiers; otherwise, identifiers are attached to the data. Web servers automatically store a great deal of personal information about visitors to a website and that information can be accessed by others. If investigators are going to claim anonymity for data obtained over the Internet, then they are going to have to explain how they are obtaining that anonymity and IRBs are going to have to evaluate the adequacy of those procedures.

After an investigator obtains identifiable information, then concerns are raised about data security. There are two potential sources of breach of confidentiality with electronic data—inadvertent disclosure and deliberate attempts to gain access to research data (hacking). The use of computers and the Internet to obtain, store, analyze, and communicate research data increases the likelihood of inadvertent disclosure of that data. Incidents of computers with sensitive research data being stolen and of identifiable research data being inadvertently sent to entire listservs have occurred. Although there have been no recorded incidents of hacking research data, it is not inconceivable that others could have an interest in obtaining valuable research data.

Technology can provide reasonable security but cannot guarantee absolute security. The use of controlled access privileges, firewalls, encryption, and limited Internet access on computers, as well as adequate physical security for computing equipment, can help protect against security breaches, but all systems have vulnerabilities and cannot ensure security. The level of security should be directly related to the sensitivity of the data and the likelihood of outside interest in the data. Investigators and IRBs should do a risk analysis to determine the appropriate level of security for the data.[4] The best protection for highly sensitive data is "defense in depth"—multiple layers of security. However, because it is impossible to guarantee absolute data security over the Internet, some extremely sensitive research may not be appropriate for the Internet.

Conclusion

The review of Internet research presents a challenge for IRBs. As has been described, the technology introduces additional concerns to the issues that the IRB must consider before approving a protocol. IRBs must require investigators to provide technical information on how they are going to deal with these issues. That means that the IRB will have to know what questions to ask in order to obtain the appropriate information. Then the IRB will then have to evaluate the information provided by the investigators to determine whether the measures that are being taken are adequate and comply with the regulations. This means that the IRB will need considerable technical expertise. IRBs are going to have to find that expertise either within their membership or from outside experts who can provide consultation.

References

1. Kraut R, Olson J, Banaji M, Bruckman A, Cohen J, Couper M. Psychological Research Online: Report of Board of Scientific Affairs' Advisory Group on the Conduct of Research on the Internet. *American Psychologist*;59(2):105–117, 2004.

2. Ethical and Legal Aspects of Human Subjects Research in Cyberspace, American Association for the Advancement of Science, November 1999. Access date 21 February, 2005. http://www.aaas.org/spp/dspp/sfrl/projects/intres/main.htm

3. Code of Federal Regulations. Title 45A—Department of Health and Human Services; Part 46—Protection of Human Subjects. Revised 13 November, 2001. Access date 21 February, 2005. http://www.dhhs.gov/ohrp/humansubjects/guidance/45cfr46.htm

4. Acker T. Securing Sensitive Data in a Research Environment: A Case Study. Access date 21 February, 2005. http://www.giac.org/practical/GSEC/Tim_Van_Acker_GSEC.pdf

Qualitative Social Science Research

Dean R. Gallant and Alan Bliss

INTRODUCTION

Not all research in the social sciences is laboratory-based experimental work. There is a long tradition of qualitative research by anthropologists, ethnographers, sociologists, survey researchers, psychologists, and others whose observations are typically conducted outside the laboratory. The purpose of their research is often to develop hypotheses rather than to test and validate them in controlled studies. Methods include observation (including participant observation), questionnaires or surveys, interviewing, or review and analysis of existing data. Because of the potential range of activities involved, qualitative research in the social sciences can present special problems for institutional review boards (IRBs), investigators, and the subjects themselves.

When Does Qualitative Research Require IRB Review?

Some regulatory guidance is available—but not much. Because the Common Rule focuses largely on quantitative procedures primarily in the biomedical area, such as experimental protocols, hypothesis testing, and controlled studies, many aspects of the regulations are a poor fit for the circumstances of qualitative research. It is no surprise that IRBs struggle as they try to apply these regulations to ethnographic studies, focus groups, or oral histories. With regard to oral histories, in October 2003, the Office for Human Research Protections (OHRP) revised its construction of the Common Rule. Most oral history interviews are not conducted for the purpose of developing generalizable knowledge; therefore, the OHRP considers that it no longer meets the regulatory definition of research as articulated in 45 CFR 46. The circumstances of certain interviews, however, continue to suggest the need for informed consent on the part of the interviewee, which we discuss later here.

The Common Rule[1][Sec.102(d)] defines research as "a systematic investigation . . . designed to develop or contribute to generalizable knowledge." How can IRBs decide when qualitative research meets this test? Criteria for defining research intent are the subject of Chapter 4-3. The key is to focus on the intent of the researcher. Collecting information for a biography would not warrant IRB review because the intent is to assemble information particular to a specific individual. Contrast this with the participant–observer who travels for a year with a nomadic community to study their way of life. Here the intent is to study and illuminate the common—that is, generalizable—aspects of their behavior. In general, IRB review may be required if human subjects are involved and the researcher's intent is to generate insights about phenomena that are themselves the actual topic of inquiry (i.e., the knowledge is generalizable, as opposed to person-specific, knowledge).

With that said, some research is exempt.[1][Sec.101.b(2)]

[Research is exempt if the only procedures involve] the use of . . . survey procedures, interview procedures or observation of public behavior, unless:

(i) Information obtained is recorded in such a manner that human subjects can be identified, directly or through identifiers linked to the subjects; and

(ii) Any disclosure of the human subjects' responses outside the research could reasonably place the subjects at risk of criminal or civil liability or be damaging to the subjects' financial standing, employability, or reputation.

Types of Risk

Participants in medical protocols can risk death or disabling injury. This is not so in qualitative social science research, where the risks are typically of a different order of magnitude. Most subjects in such research are healthy volunteers; however, they nevertheless can face real risks, and it is the investigator's responsibility to ensure that those risks are minimized. Possible risks include the following:

1. Breach of confidentiality, whether actual or potential
2. Violation of privacy, even when confidentiality is assured

3. Validation of inappropriate or undesirable behaviors of subjects, perhaps based on misunderstanding of the researcher's intent

4. Presentation of results in a way that does not respect (or agree with) the subjects' interests

5. Possible harm to individuals not directly involved in the research, but about whom data are obtained indirectly (secondary subjects), or who belong to the class or group from which subjects were selected

6. Harm to subjects' dignity, self-image, or innocence as a result of indiscreet or age-inappropriate questions in an interview or questionnaire

In practice, of course, many of these risks overlap, and disentangling them into separate categories must be done somewhat arbitrarily. With the exception of the last item mentioned previously, the risks faced by subjects during participation are ordinarily negligible. They are simply being observed or asked to talk about their everyday lives much as they might do with a friend over a cup of coffee or a glass of beer. It is more likely that risks will emerge after participation is completed. Let us consider some examples.

Breach of Confidentiality

Subjects routinely share the stories of their daily lives with friends and colleagues. However, typically, a researcher collects information with the hope of publishing the results—if not necessarily attributing the subjects' comments directly (as a reporter might do), then at least revealing the cumulative knowledge gained from the research inquiry. If identities are poorly disguised, whether from others or from the participants themselves, subjects can risk embarrassment or more serious harms.

A classic example is *Small Town in Mass Society,*[2] in which Arthur J. Vidich and Joseph Bensman report in great detail on the private lives of citizens of a small town in upstate New York. One of the authors lived in "Springdale" for 2 years and collected extensive information about the townspeople's public and private lives. Names were disguised in the book, but individuals' identities were all too obvious to the subjects themselves—and their neighbors—and the hard feelings and debate that followed the book's publication testify to the problems of conducting clandestine participant observation.

Data need not be revealed to cause problems. Even if their participation was voluntary, subjects may have second thoughts or worry about possible release of sensitive personal information, as in the case discussed later here.

Violation of Privacy

Privacy refers to a state of being free from unsanctioned intrusion. Ordinarily, individuals have a right to privacy (i.e., control over the extent, timing, and circumstances of sharing information about themselves with others). Violation of this right, although not necessarily a direct harm, contradicts *The Belmont Report's* principle of respect for persons.

In the mid-1960s, Laud Humphreys, a sociology graduate student at Washington University, conducted a study of men who frequented "tearooms" (public restrooms where strangers met for impersonal sex). Most of his subjects had no idea that he was a researcher. Humphreys served as a "watchqueen" and would cough or otherwise signal to warn participants of the approach of police or others. He secretly noted the license plate numbers of many subjects and through the Registry of Motor Vehicles obtained their names and addresses. A year later he arranged for these subjects to be added to a city-wide health survey and, in disguise, visited their homes to collect extensive personal information about them.

His 1970 book, *Tearoom Trade,*[3] won the C. Wright Mills Award from the Society for the Study of Social Problems. Nevertheless, many colleagues and members of the press roundly criticized Humphreys for violating the privacy of his subjects, despite the acknowledged fact that the subjects' behavior took place in a public space, and even though Humphreys (who was sympathetic toward his subjects) took scrupulous pains to keep identifiers separate from his data and destroyed all names soon after his data collection was complete.

Validation of Bad Behavior

Some research may unintentionally reinforce undesirable characteristics of research subjects. An investigator interviewing members of clandestine militant groups in a war-torn country worried about his ability to collect good data, thinking that subjects would be unwilling to reveal their "secrets." However, to his surprise, and perhaps dismay, subjects reported that this interest from a faculty member at a major research institution gave an imprimatur of legitimacy to their anarchistic efforts! Another investigator studying recreational drug use among teens quickly learned that it was necessary to develop a relationship of trust with his subjects, including being able to talk with them without criticizing their drug-taking behavior. A nonjudgmental relationship like this, with a senior researcher at a prominent university, can have the unhappy effect of persuading subjects that their behavior is acceptable—if not fascinating—to wise adults. In such cases, it may be appropriate for the IRB to discuss its concerns with the investigator to help narrow the gap between strict scientific objectivity and responsible social values.

Presentation of Results

A sociologist studying a multilevel marketing organization, although frank with his subjects about his role as a researcher, came to unflattering conclusions about the company's techniques and its effects on recruits. How should he balance his personal obligations to those who shared their experiences with him with his professional responsibilities as a social scientist to report the truth as he observed it? Did he owe his subjects any special consideration if publication of his results—although neither a violation of confidentiality nor libelous—reflected poorly on individuals associated with the organization? At what point does "objectivity" cross the line to "betrayal," and how can the IRB help the investigator steer away from that line? Some researchers allow their subjects to review portions of research reports that refer to them directly, but this is not always practical or even possible if results are aggregated.

Risk of Harm to Others
Federal regulations specifically enjoin the IRB from considering the potential harmful effects of research results on society.

> The IRB should not consider possible long-range effects of applying knowledge gained in the research (for example, the possible effects of the research on public policy) as among those research risks that fall within the purview of its responsibility.[1][Sec.111(a)(2)]

Nevertheless, when research deals with controversial topics, discussion of such risks will inevitably surface at IRB meetings, and members may feel strongly that legitimate knowledge to be gained from a study could be interpreted wrongly or be publicized with mischievous intent. In such cases, it may be appropriate for one of the investigator's colleagues on the IRB to mention, offline, the concerns that were raised, but it is not proper for such concerns to affect IRB deliberations. Interestingly, there is no parallel prohibition from consideration of research benefits; investigators and IRBs routinely consider the value of new knowledge to society when balancing risks and benefits.

Are possible harms to secondary research subjects—that is, individuals who do not themselves participate in the study, but about whom the investigator obtains information via interview or other hearsay means—an appropriate area of concern for the IRB? In December 1999, the OPRR cited failure to obtain informed consent from secondary subjects as a finding in a letter of suspension of IRB authority.[4] Oral historians and genetics researchers, among others, reacted promptly, insisting that extension of this regulatory interpretation would effectively halt much of their research, as they could not possibly obtain informed consent from everybody about whom they indirectly received information. As of this writing, the question is unresolved, but the OPRR (now the OHRP) has not rescinded its interpretation, and thus, IRBs should at least consider whether special consideration should be given to secondary subjects in studies where primary informants provide information about others. Oral histories that are no longer covered by the Common Rule, however, would also seem to be relieved of this regulatory interpretation on the grounds that generalizable knowledge is not the purpose of information being collected from primary subjects or about those concerning whom data is collected only incidentally.

Direct Harm to Subjects
A researcher asking youngsters questions about a range of sexual behaviors or the use of inhalants or illicit drugs will likely encounter parents who insist the research is "robbing the children of their innocence." Unfortunately, if the survey is not sensitively designed, the parents may be right. Harms from inappropriate instruments are not limited to children. Interviews of adults that include a range of questions about illegal or immoral behaviors may be demeaning or insulting. The IRB should ensure that the researcher understands enough about the potential subject population to minimize the chance of harming or needlessly offending them. Administering surveys in person allows investigators to judge whether certain avenues of questioning are appropriate for an individual subject. Reviewing surveys and questionnaires with representative community members (or parents, for surveys of children) may reveal sensitive or problem areas that can easily be fixed before the survey goes out to the field.

Special Considerations

There are several other issues for IRBs to attend to when reviewing qualitative research.

Respect for Subjects' Privacy
As many of the previous cases indicate, respect for subjects' privacy is essential, yet this simple advice is not always easy to follow. Humphreys' tearoom research demonstrated that public spaces can be the site of very private behaviors. Another example is Internet chat rooms, which often operate with the expectation of privacy even though they are accessible to anybody with a computer and a connection to the web. Is the right to privacy absolute even when behaviors are only relatively private? Should a false sense of privacy be respected? These are thorny issues for investigators and IRBs, and the answers are not at all obvious. See the thoughtful paper on ethical issues raised by research in cyberspace, based on a 1999 conference sponsored by the American Association for the Advancement of Science.[5]

Informed Consent
Although the content and issues may differ, informed consent is no less important in qualitative research than it is in clinical research. However, much qualitative research is exploratory, and the areas of inquiry may not be apparent even to the research team. How then can subjects truly be informed? Prior information about risks, insofar as they are known or can be anticipated, cannot be withheld. However, if the range of possible risks is potentially very large, how can an investigator present accurate information about the study in a manner that will not simply frighten subjects away? One strategy is to sustain the consent process throughout the course of a subject's participation. As new data are acquired and the researcher's overall knowledge of risks expands, subjects can be reminded that participation is voluntary, and their understanding of the risks and benefits of participation can be refreshed. This process should not be used to mask risks or to lure subjects into a relationship with the investigator before they fully understand the consequences, but it can help them develop an understanding of the research and the context of their role in it. Their continued participation is then based on active awareness of emerging developments.

Distortion of Subjects' Behavior
The simple presence of participant observers may lead to distortion of subjects' behavior. (This can be considered a more general expression of the experimenter effect, where the actions of the experimenter inadvertently influence subjects' performance on a task.) In, *When Prophecy Fails* (1956),[6] a small group of people who believed that the end of the world was at hand, eventually had to acknowledge

the uneventful passing of the doomsday hour. The group of believers was infiltrated by several observers who, merely by their interest, reinforced the authenticity of the group's cataclysmic expectations. The authors (Festinger, Riecken, and Schachter) discuss at length how the research team's presence did not contaminate the validity of their observations, but nevertheless admit that their actions were not without effect on the believers. Even straightforward observation or interviewing can prompt subjects to behave unnaturally—and occasionally to their detriment—if they try to mold their behavior to what they imagine to be the researcher's expectations. This is especially likely when the researcher is viewed as a higher status individual or when subjects are children. Minimizing the possibility of such distortions while maintaining an ethically defensible position on the boundary between unobtrusive and surreptitious can be a challenge. Chapter 6-5 is devoted to a discussion of research in which subjects are intentionally deceived in order to study human behavior.

Reportable Situations

Much qualitative research deals with sensitive topics and looks deeply into subjects' daily lives. As a result, investigators can encounter reportable situations such as evidence of child or elder abuse or neglect or the likely prospect of harm to self or others. In most states, investigators have a legal obligation to report such situations to appropriate authorities. Researchers who are at all likely to uncover reportable situations must be prepared for that possibility. Appropriate consultation should be available if the researcher is not a trained clinician with relevant clinical experience. A strategy for alerting subjects to the need for reporting is essential; depending on the nature of the study and the subject population, this can involve mention of the reporting requirement as part of the informed consent process, or a more ad hoc procedure when the likelihood of reportable situations is small. The IRB should consider the adequacy of the investigator's plans and may want to seek counsel from experts in the field.

In the case of an oral history interview of a subject in a sensitive position, it is appropriate for the IRB to require an informed consent document, recent reinterpretation of oral history practice under the Common Rule notwithstanding. Examples could include an interview conducted with a prison inmate or with a person confronting terminal illness.

Certificate of Confidentiality

Whether or not a researcher is studying behaviors likely to yield information about reportable situations, subjects' reputations, relationships, employability, or legal status may be threatened by disclosure of identifiable information. The law does not recognize any automatic privilege for social science researchers; data are vulnerable to subpoena or other official inquiry. If identifiers must be retained (for longitudinal studies, or where subjects are videotaped or audiotaped, as for an oral history) and if the research deals with very sensitive topics, it may be appropriate to seek a certificate of confidentiality to protect against compelled disclosure—by federal, state, or local authorities—of

identifying information. Certificates of confidentiality can be granted by the federal funding agency on application and are also available to investigators without federal funding. These certificates do not prohibit the investigator from disclosing information (and, in some states, confidentiality certificate protections are overridden by mandated reporting requirements), but they do provide a measure of protection for research subjects that would not otherwise be available.

Conclusion

Despite the many concerns detailed here, we should not forget that most research subjects are competent, autonomous adults and—absent willful deception by the investigator—can usually judge for themselves the degree to which they choose to reveal information about their personal lives and actions. It is not the IRB's responsibility to eliminate risk, which is often an inherent component of research on sensitive topics. However, the IRB may and should counsel the investigator on how to present the purpose and methods of the research to subjects in such a way that they can understand why they might want to participate in the study and can make an informed, intelligent decision about any risk that their participation may entail. Qualitative research is, in essence, a kind of dialogue with its own special vocabulary; like all dialogues, it depends in large measure on shared understanding and common courtesy.

Following is the text of a policy statement that was developed by the Oral History Association and the American Historical Association in consultation with the Office for Human Research Protections. This policy applies to oral history that takes place within an institution that has filed a multiple project assurance with OHRP. As one of the seventeen federal agencies that have signed on to the Common Rule, the Department of Health and Human Services deals most directly with the type of clinical research that the federal regulations were originally intended to cover, and its concurrence with the policy statement should set the way for a uniform interpretation by other federal agencies.

Application of the DHHS Regulations 45 CFR 46, Subpart A to Oral History Interviewing

Most oral history interviewing projects are not subject to the requirements of the Department of Health and Human Services (DHHS) regulations at 45 CFR 46, subpart A, and can be excluded from institutional review board (IRB) oversight because they do not involve research as defined by the DHHS regulations. DHHS regulations at 45 CFR 46.102(D) define research as "a systematic investigation, including research development, testing and evaluation, designed to develop or contribute to generalizable knowledge." The Oral History Association defines oral history as "a method of gathering and preserving historical information through recorded interviews with participants in past events and ways of life."

It is primarily on the grounds that oral history interviews, in general, are not designed to contribute to "generalizable knowledge" that they are not subject to the requirements of the DHHS 45 CFR 46 and, therefore, can be excluded from IRB review.

Although the DHHS regulations do not define "generalizable knowledge," it is reasonable to assume that the term does not simply mean knowledge that lends itself to generalizations, which characterizes every form of scholarly inquiry and human communication. While historians do reach for meaning that goes beyond the specific subject of their inquiry, unlike researchers in the biomedical and behavioral sciences, they do not reach for generalizable principles of historical or social development, nor do they seek underlying principles or laws of nature that have predictive value and can be applied to other circumstances for the purpose of controlling outcomes. Historians explain a particular past; they do not create general explanations about all that has happened in the past, nor do they predict the future.

Moreover, oral history narrators are not anonymous individuals, selected as part of a random sample for the purposes of a survey. Nor are they asked to respond to a standard questionnaire administered to a broad swath of the population. Those interviewed are specific individuals selected because of their unique relationship to the topic at hand. Open-ended questions are tailored to the experiences of the individual narrator. Although interviews are guided by professional protocols, the manner in which an individual interview unfolds simply cannot be predicted. An interview gives a unique perspective on the topic at hand; a series of interviews offer up not similar "generalizable" information but a variety of particular perspectives on the topic.

For these reasons, oral history interviewing, in general, does not meet the regulatory definition of research as articulated in DHHS 45 CFR 46. The Office for Human Research Protections concurs with this policy statement, and it is essential that such an interpretation be made available to the many IRBs currently grappling with issues of human subject research.

Acknowledgments

Thanks to Donald A. Ritchie, of the Oral History Association, and Linda Shopes, of the American Historical Association, for collaborating in the development of this policy, and for disseminating it to practitioners and concerned others.

References

1. Code of Federal Regulations. Title 45A—Department of Health and Human Services; Part 46—Protection of Human Subjects. Updated 1 October, 1997. Access date 18 April, 2001. http://www4.law.cornell.edu/cfr/45p46.htm

2. Vidich AJ, Bensman J. *Small Town in Mass Society; Class, Power, and Religion in a Rural Community*. Garden City: Doubleday; 1960.

3. Humphreys L. *Tearoom Trade: Impersonal Sex in Public Places*. Chicago: Aldin Publishing; 1970.

4. Office for Human Research Protections. *Dear Colleague Letters, 20 March, 2001*. Access date 30 March, 2001. http://ohrp.osophs.dhhs.gov/dearcoll.htm

5. American Association for the Advancement of Science. Access date May 2001. http://www.aaas.org/

6. Festinger L, Riecken HW, Schachter S. *When Prophecy Fails*. Minneapolis: University of Minnesota Press; 1956.

Ethnographic Research

Elisabeth Smith Parrott

INTRODUCTION

There is no question that the authors of the Nuremberg Code, *The Belmont Report*, the Declaration of Helsinki, and, indeed, the federal regulations did not have ethnography in mind when they composed guidelines to govern the conduct of human subjects research. Although ethnography is one of the oldest qualitative methods of gathering data,[1] it has only recently come to be examined under the bright light of institutional review board (IRB) review. Researchers have been guided by the ethics statements of professional organizations, such as the American Anthropological Association.[2] Traditionally, the ethics review of ethnographic studies has come in the form of funding sources and departmental review. Although these sources of review are not impartial, in this discipline, such reviewers are probably more aware of the overall state of being of research participants than many other research fields. Compulsive self-examination is a feature of most ethnographers, even today, and although IRB review is new to this research environment, the values of beneficence and respect for persons have been an important part of many ethnographies. Although the worth of IRB review is indisputable, applying regulations that mainly refer to medical procedures and behavioral interventions to the ethnographic process can be a bewildering task.

Rooted in the social sciences—particularly anthropology and sociology—ethnography concerns itself with the lived experience of a population. As Hammersley and Atkinson wrote,

> In its most characteristic form [ethnography] involves the ethnographer participating, overtly or covertly, in people's daily lives for an extended period of time. They are watching what happens, listening to what is said, asking questions—in fact, collecting whatever data are available to throw light on the issues that are the focus of the research.[1]

In recent years, ethnography has sprouted up as the investigative method of choice in an ever-widening array of fields: medicine, education, geography, music, and other fields beyond the more traditional applications in the social sciences. In medical settings, particularly psychiatry, it is used to create a broader understanding of the impact of illness and subsequent medical intervention than usually supplied by formal outcomes analysis. Ethnography is employed by researchers at all levels and disciplines, from students (both in fulfillment of classroom assignments and independently) to health care practitioners, public health officials, educators, and social scientists.

Given the varied application of the technique, as well as the diversity in the backgrounds of ethnographic researchers, it is not surprising that IRB review of ethnographic research presents a unique set of challenges. It is not always immediately clear what path the course of approval should follow for ethnography research. Depending on the focus of the research and the plans for reporting the data, the study might be eligible for exemption or might best be examined in the setting of the expedited committee. In rare cases, ethnographic proposals require the rigors of full-committee review. It takes skill, experience, and most importantly, unhurried dialogue with the researcher to determine the appropriate level of review.

The first section of this chapter examines various institutional approaches to ethnography review. Then we discuss methods for preparing ethnographers for IRB review, assessing risk in ethnographic proposals and determining the review status of a study. Next comes a discussion of the three categories of ethnography review: exempt, expedited, and full-committee review. From there we examine the review process and the role of advisors and consultants. We end the chapter with discussions of variations to the informed consent process, the use of audiotaping, videotaping, and still photography, the review of research involving vulnerable populations, and finally, international research.

Institutional Approaches to Ethnography Review

Perhaps the greatest obstacle to painless review of ethnographic research is the lack of familiarity that most IRBs have with this type of research. Some institutions create IRBs dedicated to social science research that become very familiar with the issues surrounding ethnographic fieldwork. Many institutions, however, see few ethnographic proposals and approach them with uncertainty. Such institutions often rely on consultants on a case-by-case basis for help and advice in examining the unique ethical issues surrounding ethnography review.

The very decision to review ethnographic research can be confusing. Sometimes ethnographic proposals do not seem to describe a formal examination of a population with the intent to publish. Such studies may lead the IRB to reason that the federal definition of research—"a systematic investigation, including research development, testing and evaluation, designed to develop or contribute to generalizable knowledge"[3[Sec.102(d)]]—will not be met. Using this argument, some institutions have decided that most undergraduate projects do not meet the criteria for research and therefore fall outside the purview of the IRB. However, before reaching this conclusion, the institution must carefully assess its mission and the institutional agreement with the Office for Human Research Protections.

Other institutions acknowledge that, although some undergraduate ethnography research may not meet the federal definition of research, the process of IRB review is educational to students and worthwhile in that it prepares future researchers for the ethical conduct of research. A policy of reviewing all undergraduate research also enables an institution to monitor student research and ensure that harmful proposals do not move forward.

At all levels of review, it is the role of the IRB to ensure that risks to subjects are minimized: "(i) by using procedures which are consistent with sound research design and which do not unnecessarily expose subjects to risk."[3[Sec.111(a)(1)]] The message here is that risks should not be undertaken lightly, for the sake of curiosity or for the fulfillment of an academic exercise, no matter how advanced the level. The typical ethnographic proposal does not purport to change public policy or even change the lives of the ethnographer's participants, although this may be an unintended consequence of the research. Rather, the goal of such research is to gather information about the human condition in order to understand better the complex ways in which people and populations function. Ethnography often functions as the equivalent of basic science: studying human behavior for the sake of knowledge itself.

However fundamental a social science ethnography is, there are situations where proposed research is clearly legitimate and others where the research design clearly does not warrant intrusion on participants' lives. For example, an ethnographic project evaluating the impact of a job-training program for individuals with severe mental illness could clearly benefit participants and society as a whole. In contrast, an undergraduate proposal seeking to document the sexual habits of fellow students in order to fulfill a classroom assignment probably introduces more risk than it is worth. A submission such as this presents a good opportunity to educate researchers about sensitivity in social science research and provide guidance in developing a less sensitive proposal for review.

Advising Ethnographers

The review process for such seemingly innocuous studies often involves a great deal of researcher education about the need for IRB review, the rationale for and methods of removing identifiers from data, and the process of obtaining appropriate informed consent. Because the data collection process associated with ethnography meets the federal definition of minimal risk—that is, the ethnographer himself has no plans to intervene with life as it happens—it may appear that IRB review is of little value. However, the risks associated with recording data and writing the ethnography may be significant. Ethnographers, particularly undergraduates and those working in fields that do not routinely interact with the IRB, often need to be educated about these risks and the role of IRB review in planning and implementing ethnography.

The process of determining review status often begins with the informal submission of a research protocol or summary. However, even before considering individual proposals, it is essential that the IRB educate the research community at large about the need for ethics review for all research involving human subjects. Researchers must also understand that the IRB has the authority to make the final decision regarding the review status of a project.

Providing researchers with a detailed list of questions, including definitions for such key terms as anonymous, confidential, identifiable information, can help prevent misunderstandings in the review process. Responding to a set of core questions relevant to ethics review may be helpful to ethnographers and the IRB alike. Points to cover include the following:

1. Methods for the identification and contact of potential participants. Researchers should describe how potential participants might refuse participation. If appropriate, contact letters, advertisements, or phone scripts should be written and submitted for IRB review.

2. A description of the topics under investigation. The researcher should assess the sensitivity of the inquiry and explain whether participants' answers may be embarrassing or put them at risk for criminal prosecution. Surveys, questionnaires, telephone or interview scripts, and letters must be reviewed before use.

3. Methods for recording data. This should include plans for recording or removing participants' identifiers and for protecting the confidentiality of participants.

4. Plans for obtaining informed consent.

5. Plans for the participation of minors, if appropriate. In addition, plans for obtaining parental consent and the consent of relevant institutional authorities, such as school principals and teachers, should be considered.

Planning for informed consent is often a fruitful way both to gather information about the research project and educate researchers about their project's risks. Training researchers about the required elements of informed consent is essential. The IRB may supply a template for consent documents and information sheets as well as samples of such documents for ethnographic projects. Researchers should be encouraged to submit draft documents to the IRB for feedback and informal review prior to comprehensive IRB review of the study as time allows.

These aspects of study participation are of particular importance to participants of any population:

1. The purpose of the research

2. A description of what participation will entail and the duration of the study

3. A description of the risks and benefits of participation

4. An explanation of how data will be recorded and information about the use and preservation of audio or videotapes

5. A lay discussion of the anonymity or confidentiality of data, including measures to safeguard data, publish data, etc.

6. A description of any financial considerations, including costs and/or payments to participants

7. Contact information, including the title and institutional affiliation of the researcher and his or her advisor (if appropriate)

Finally, it is important to emphasize to researchers, particularly inexperienced researchers and students, that anything can happen in the field. Researchers should bring concerns, complaints, and adverse events to the attention of the project advisor and the IRB immediately.

Assessing Risk

As with any research proposal, the first task at hand is to determine risk status. The federal regulations state, "Minimal risk means that the probability and magnitude of harm or discomfort anticipated in the research are not greater in and of themselves than those ordinarily encountered in daily life or during the performance of routine physical or psychological examinations or tests."[3][Sec.102(i)]

At first glance, it may seem that all ethnographic research meets this definition for minimal risk, as by definition ethnography observes life as it happens, with no planned

interventions and few interruptions. IRBs, particularly those that mainly review biomedical research, come to expect that risk to participants is introduced in the process of collecting data during procedures such as the administration of an experimental drug or a surgical procedure. In contrast, although the data collection phase of ethnography may present risks to participants, such as when a conversation becomes emotionally difficult for a participant or institutional authority figures request access to field notes, for the most part, the risks of data collection are minimal (Frederick Erickson, Ph.D., personal communication dated October 17, 2000).

It is worth noting that study termination is one period of the data collection phase that presents considerable risk in many research settings (Hoyt Alverson, Ph.D., personal communication dated July 25, 2001). If participation observation has been successful, then by definition the departure of the ethnographer generates feelings of loss in the community. In many cases, participants lose a trusted friend, someone who listened to them, treated them impartially and respectfully, participated in daily life, and perhaps even supplied money, food, transportation, or labor to the community. From the very beginning, ethnographers need to plan ahead for the termination of research, taking into account the characteristics and needs of the study community. Moreover, plans for ending the research should be discussed with participants at the initiation of the study and regularly throughout the period of data collection.

Perhaps the most widely recognized risks of ethnography are encountered when the researcher writes and publishes the data. It is in this situation, when an ethnographer reports back to the research participants (which in the case of applied institutional ethnography may involve hospitals, schools, or other fixtures of community life), that the potential arises for wider reaching harms. Potential harms range from embarrassment to administrative or even legal action in response to data that have been revealed. Therefore, it is important that in their review of proposals and their education of investigators IRBs focus on this aspect of the research plan (Frederick Erickson, Ph.D., personal communication dated October 17, 2000).

The other characteristic of ethnography that affects its potential for harm is that, by definition, ethnographic techniques prohibit the researcher from controlling what happens in the field. Because the ethnographer's role is to observe rather than direct or limit the actions or narrative of the participant, it is critical that the ethnographer consider every aspect of life that could possibly be affected in the field. Thus, the emotional, social, and political ramifications of asking questions, reporting observations, and sharing conclusions with others outside of the research population must be examined comprehensively at the time of initial review.

The impact of reading an ethnographic account of oneself should not be underestimated. Individuals, or in fact entire communities, may be disturbed by the way they are represented in ethnographies. After publishing her ethnography of psychiatric clients, anthropologist Sue Estroff recalls being called in the middle of the night by a former research participant.

> The voice I heard was almost chanting in rage and anguish. There was ridicule, too, and precision cuts at my fast-fading concepts of myself as a kind, careful, and just ethnographer. She had asked for a copy of the book I had written about her and the others. I gave it to her as a gift. She had just read what I had written about her ten years before. She was wounded by images of herself in the past—psychotic, rambling, wise, and charming. I had exploited her, used her, misunderstood everything and was unmasked now, she said. Not the bright, "liberal," sympathetic researcher I claimed to be, but worse than the others for my self and other deception. Furthered my career, made a name for myself, all at her expense. How could you? (By now I was asking this silently, along with her.) How could you come see me again, spend the whole day with me, like a friend, pretending to understand, to like me?
>
> The facts were not in dispute—their public presence and meaning, and my commentary were. Seeing the now non-sensical notes she wrote when psychotic, seeing herself at that bewildered time on the printed page were somehow intolerable. She chanted on in howling pain and anger; nothing I said made any difference. I was shaking by now, desperate to intervene, to break the grip of the agony now swallowing both of us. Could we meet and talk it over? No. I never want to talk to you again. Could I please explain what I had written, place it in the broader concept of the book? Had she read the rest of it? No. No. Was there anything I could say or do to help? No. Please, would she accept my apology? No. She hung up. I called back. Don't ever bother me again. I apologized once more. She hung up again.[4]

Although she had signed a consent document, participated in the research freely, was not identified in the publication, and was aware that Estroff intended to publish, the participant did not anticipate how disturbing it would be to read an intimate, public account of her mental illness.[4] Responses such as these are to some degree unavoidable. However, the example teaches us that the way ethnography is reported and shared with the research community allows for harm to the research participants for an almost indefinite period of time.

In this way, ethnography review teaches us to think broadly. For example, if presented with a proposal to elicit family histories from a community of people, we may find ourselves asking a range of tough questions: Is it likely that this research format will lead the participant to reveal intimate details of family life unanticipated by the researcher? If so, how can reliving difficult memories affect the participant? Is the researcher prepared to respond sensitively to a distraught informant? Will the researcher be able to maintain professionalism should informants reveal unanticipated information that may be shocking or disturbing? How will risks to confidentiality and reputation be minimized? When researchers propose to observe cultural activities, we find ourselves asking how the presence of an outsider could inhibit or harm the participants. What happens if participants feel ashamed, humiliated, or violated by the presence of an observer? Who provides consent for the researcher to observe a group? If an individual refuses to participate in the research, should the project be canceled, or is it possible to work around one member of a group?

Revisions to the Research Plan

To complicate matters, it is not uncommon for an ethnographic project to change direction during the data collection process.[1] In fact, researchers may approach the IRB for approval of a study with very little idea of what the ultimate research focus will be. They may simply wish to find an interesting population and see where the process of participant observation takes them. Although it is natural for ethnography to evolve in the field, IRBs should require researchers to define their field questions and research methods as specifically as possible at the time of initial review, including plans for adapting to changes in the field setting (Frederick Erickson, Ph.D., personal communication dated October 17, 2000).

Of course, once the research is underway, researchers should communicate with the IRB about revisions to the research environment, the focus of the project, or the study procedures.

Category of Review

Designation of Exemption

After we determine that a study meets the definition of minimal risk, how do we determine which level of review is appropriate? Studies involving minimal risk face two options: (1) designation that they are exempt from further IRB review or (2) review by expedited committee. Despite the wide and varied application of ethnographic techniques, much of this type of research meets the criteria for exemption.[3][Sec.101(b)(2)]

> Research involving the use of educational tests (cognitive, diagnostic, aptitude, achievement), survey procedures, interview procedures, or observation of public behavior, unless (i) information obtained is recorded in such a manner that human subjects can be identified, directly or indirectly through identifiers linked to the subjects; and (ii) any disclosure of the human subjects' responses outside the research could reasonably place the subjects at risk of criminal or civil liability or be damaging to the subjects' financial standing, employability, or reputation.

These criteria allow for the exemption of innocuous studies, that is, studies in which participants are to be interviewed about or observed doing things that are not sensitive or potentially damaging. Such studies may be designated exempt regardless of whether identifiers are recorded. Presumably, this regulation also allows for the exemption of studies in which some sensitive topics may arise but in which absolutely no identifiers are recorded (i.e., the information is anonymous).

Ethnographic studies including minors cannot be designated exempt except in cases that would have to be called "nonparticipant observation," a rare situation in ethnography.

> . . . the exemption at 46.101(b)(2) for research involving survey or interview procedures or observations of public behavior does not apply to research covered by this subpart [concerning the participation of minors], except for research involving observation of public behavior when the investigator(s) do not participate in the activities being observed.[3][Sec.401(b)]

The determination of exemption requires a careful and forward-thinking process. If researchers describe their data as anonymous, we must be sure that identifying information will not be recorded at any time over the course of the study. For these purposes, a researcher who writes down the names of participants during the data collection phase of the research or keeps a list of participants' addresses for the purpose of following up with them but then creates aliases in the writing and publishing phase of the study, does not meet these criteria for anonymous data. Although not foolproof, one extra step in confirming the minimal-risk status of a study is to cite the federal exemption to the researcher and ask her or him (and the advisor, as appropriate) to confirm that the project meets the federal criteria.

As discussed previously here, ethnographic research often evolves in the field. Sometimes changes are made to the research that affect its exempt status. When notifying a researcher (and in the case of student researchers, the advisor as well) that a project has been designated exempt, it is best to explain the reason and conditions for the exemption (citing the federal regulation and providing a lay translation, if needed). At this time, the researcher should also be informed that if changes are made to the project that affect its exempt status, prospective IRB review and approval of the revisions is required.

Finally, it is also important to be mindful of topics that are not sensitive themselves, but might be closely affiliated with or lead to sensitive disclosures. When there is any doubt about the sensitive nature of the study, expedited review is the best option.

Expedited Review

The benefit of expedited review to the IRB is that thorough review of a study can take place without sending the study to the full committee. The idea behind expedited review is that two or three IRB members (regular members and/or alternates) who are familiar with the field of study and the ethnographic method may conduct a detailed review of the proposal. They will confer about it informally (in person, by phone, or by e-mail) and make a decision regarding approval. The reviewers often include the IRB chair and/or IRB administrator, if he or she is a voting member of the committee. Consultants may be used at this level to assess the adequacy of the research design and provide the IRB with detailed information about the research setting. At the reviewers' discretion, the study may be sent to the full committee for further review. The expedited process saves time for researchers, as the wait for review is usually shortened, and for the IRB as a whole, as the full-committee workload is reduced.

Ethnographic research very clearly falls under expedited review.[3[Sec.110 (a)(7)]]

Research on individual or group characteristics or behavior (including, but not limited to, research on perception, cognition, motivation, identity, language, communication, cultural beliefs or practices, and social behavior) or research employing survey, interview, oral history, focus group, program evaluation, human factors evaluation, or quality assurance methodologies.

Like the exempt category, expedited review is appropriate for studies that meet the federal definition of minimal risk. In terms of ethnographic research, the distinction between the categories of exempt and expedited review lies in the way research data are recorded and in other peripheral factors, such as the inclusion of minors. The expedited review regulation[5] allows for the recording of information that could identify a participant (such as name, address, voice or video recording, or still photography), unless "identification of subjects and/or their responses would reasonably place them at risk of criminal or civil liability or be damaging to subjects' financial standing, employability, insurability, reputation, or be stigmatizing, unless reasonable and appropriate protections will be implemented so that risks related to invasion of privacy and breach of confidentiality are no greater than minimal" (i.e., no greater than those encountered in daily life).

Full-Committee Review

Where there are significant risks (i.e., risks that exceed those encountered in daily life) involved, such as when the purpose of a study is to study illegal activities, full-committee review is needed. At this point, risk/benefit ratios may be difficult to assess. By definition, ethnography is a largely observational process; the main potential benefits to a participant are the possible psychologic benefits associated with "telling one's story." The potential benefits to society may also be somewhat vague, or at least not as clear as for some of the intervention-based studies that IRBs usually consider.

IRBs are required to determine that

Risks to subjects are reasonable in relation to anticipated benefits, if any, to subjects, and the importance of the knowledge that may reasonably be expected to result. In evaluating risks and benefits, the IRB should consider only those risks and benefits that may result from the research. . . . The IRB should not consider possible long-range effects of applying knowledge gained in the research (for example, the possible effects of the research on public policy) as among those research risks that fall within the purview of its responsibility.[3[Sec.111(a)(2)]]

The instructions not to consider the long-term ramifications of the research simplify the review of ethnographic risks but complicate the review of potential benefits. It is reassuring that we are not being asked to assess every possible negative effect a study might have in the distant future. This guidance, however, also instructs us not to count as benefits the long-range potential improvement in public policy that may result from ethnographic research.

The risks of this research method may be subtle. Remember that ethnography generally does not place participants at risk during the data collection phase. Rather, risks are introduced as the data are shared, with the participants themselves as well as with outsiders (Frederick Erickson, Ph.D., personal communication dated October 17, 2000).

The potential breach of privacy associated with this process is the most pressing review issue. Therefore, ethnographic research on certain topics, such as communities of illegal drug users, introduces significant risk. Participants who use illegal drugs may not do or say anything in the presence of the ethnographer that they would not do or say otherwise, and of course, they are at risk of being arrested by virtue of their behavior at any time, regardless of the ethnographer's involvement. However, the fact that their illegal behavior is documented does present risks additional to those they face in ordinary life.

Even when an IRB is well prepared to review ethnography, the consideration of a study involving significant risk can be a difficult and controversial process. Ultimately, a decision regarding approval will rest on the scientific validity of the study and the protections to participants built into the data collection process, the informed consent process, and the training and preparation of the researcher.

The Review Process

The key to reviewing ethnographic research is to ask for complete study information from researchers. It is critical that the IRB receive comprehensive descriptions of the following five aspects of the research plan:

1. The training and preparation of the researcher
2. The research environment
3. The participants' backgrounds
4. The questions that will be asked of participants or the general structure for gathering information
5. Plans for analyzing, storing, sharing, and publishing data

Of equal importance to the review process is the expertise of the IRB and the availability of appropriate advisors; thus, the IRB's understanding of its own capabilities is also critical.

In addition to submitting a response to core IRB questions outlined previously here, it is useful for researchers to submit comprehensive research protocols (such as those submitted for funding) if they exist. Reviewing the full protocol enables the IRB to check for discrepancies and confirm that the project designated "exempt" or "approved" by the IRB is identical to the funded project. Occasionally a researcher will state that a project does not record identifiers, for example, but then describe plans for photographing participants in the research plan. Educating researchers before the submission of proposals will help prevent misunderstandings in the review process, and a comprehensive review of project materials will enable the IRB to pick up on any persistent discrepancies.

Use of Advisors and Consultants

At our institution, we have learned that the key to appropriate review is bringing in not only the expertise of the IRB, but also the expertise of advisors to the researchers and consultants to the IRB in the researcher's field of study. As with all review, the trick is to combine the regulatory knowledge of the IRB staff with the field expertise of IRB reviewers. We accomplish this in two ways: first by relying on researchers' advisors to prepare students for the field and second by seeking out the review of experts to supplement IRB review when needed.

For example, when requesting a research summary from an undergraduate, we ask the student's advisor to confirm that the advisor has discussed the ethical issues surrounding human subjects research in the proposed research setting with the student researcher. We also routinely cite the federal regulation permitting the exemption or expedited approval of a study to the student and advisor. Their confirmation that the proposed research satisfies the regulations, although not sufficient for approval, helps to ensure that we have all understood the risks of the research in the same way.

At institutions where the emphasis of review is on biomedical research, administrators may need to look beyond the usual circles of reference in order to obtain expert ethnographic review. Social scientists experienced in ethnographic research are best able to guide the IRB in conducting a comprehensive review. Provided that an institution has social science departments, the chairpersons of the anthropology or sociology departments are often willing to help an IRB locate an appropriate consultant. When social scientists are unavailable, such as when ethnography is proposed in a medical setting, representatives from psychiatry may be well suited to work with the IRB in identifying special areas of concern.

Variations to the Informed Consent Process

As the saying goes, "Informed consent is a process, not a form." The process of informed consent refers to the discussions, review of written study materials (including consent documents and information sheets), and any other means by which the potential participant learns about the research setting. The term *informed consent* does not refer to the consent document alone. In fact, it rejects the notion that it is possible to obtain true informed consent simply by providing informants with a written statement about the research.

Here, too, in preparation for informed consent, ethnography tends to buck IRB convention. Researchers routinely balk at being asked to provide consent documents to people they plan to observe over the course of daily life, in large part because asking for signed consent emphasizes the ethnographer's outsider status, a feature that ethnographers actively try to minimize (Frederick Erickson, Ph.D., personal communication dated October 17, 2000).[1] It makes the casual conversation with a policeman on the street, the chance interview with the jazz singer in a club at 3 a.m., and the playful game of hide-and-seek with a child on an oncology unit into a formal research experience requiring federal oversight.

Federal regulations allow for the modification of standard consent procedures under certain circumstances. The waiver of signed consent is the variation to the informed consent process most readily permitted. Documentation of informed consent may be waived when the IRB finds

(1) That the only record linking the subject and the research would be the consent document and the principal risk would be

potential harm resulting from a breach of confidentiality. Each subject will be asked whether the subject wants documentation linking the subject with the research, and the subject's wishes will govern; or (2) That the research presents no more than minimal risk of harm to subjects and involves no procedures for which written consent is normally required outside of the research context.[3][Sec.117(d)]

This section of the regulations addresses two situations where documentation of consent may be waived. The first is when identifying information will not be recorded and the participant wishes not to be linked to the research. The second is when the research meets the criteria for minimal risk and does not involve any activities for which someone would ordinarily be required to sign a consent form. It is this second case that waives the requirement for documentation of informed consent for many ethnographers.

From time to time, researchers request that the requirement for informed consent itself be waived in full or in part. Sometimes it is impossible for ethnographers to obtain informed consent from each participant, particularly when participant observation, as opposed to interviewing, is the main source of data. The federal regulations permit the waiver of informed consent as follows.

An IRB may approve a consent procedure which does not include, or which alters, some or all of the elements of informed consent or waive the requirements to obtain informed consent provided the IRB finds and documents that (1) the research involves no more than minimal risk to the subjects; (2) the waiver or alteration will not adversely affect the rights and welfare of the subjects; (3) the research could not practicably be carried out without the waiver or alteration; and (4) whenever appropriate, the subjects will be provided with additional pertinent information after participation.[3][Sec.116(d)]

Although a bit more complicated to document, the criteria outlined previously here are widely applicable to minimal-risk ethnography. Indeed, the third criterion addresses the impracticality of obtaining consent in the setting of participant observation. When considering a waiver of this kind, the IRB documents that the researcher has met the federal criteria for a waiver. This documentation may be included in the reviewer's notes. It may also be helpful to document the researcher's confirmation of the criteria allowing a waiver.

Audiotaping, Videotaping, and Still Photography

Ethnography often makes use of audiotaping, photography, and videotaping technology. Researchers' plans for recording data should receive prospective IRB review and be included in the informed consent process. Plans to destroy, share, or archive the recordings should also be discussed with the IRB and with study participants. If a researcher chooses to archive recordings but obscure the identities of participants in publication (as is often the case), then plans for protecting the confidentiality of the original study records must also be addressed.

Occasionally, although researchers prefer to record or photograph participants, they state that they could carry out their research without such recordings. In these cases, participants should be provided with an opportunity to consent or decline to consent to recordings. This may be assured by providing separate signature sections or check boxes within the consent document for participants to consent or decline the recording.

Vulnerable Populations

Populations that are considered protected in the federal regulations, including prisoners, mentally incompetent persons, pregnant women, and children (including wards of the state), regularly participate in ethnographic research. The review of research involving prisoners should be conducted in compliance with the special protections outlined for this group.[3(SubpartC)] Regulations also explain how to obtain informed consent for the participation of mentally incompetent persons.[3][Sec.102(c)] Pregnant women are permitted to participate in ethnography research with no additional protections:[3][Sec.207(a)(2)] "No pregnant woman may be involved as a subject in an activity covered by this subpart unless . . . the risk to the fetus is minimal." Even when there may be significant risks to the pregnant participant, such as when the topic of the research is illegal behavior, the risk of ethnography to the fetus is minimal.

Children

Although children are not often the focus of ethnographic research, it is not unusual for them to be included in studies, particularly those originating in the social sciences or other disciplines where a cultural group of diverse ages is to be examined. Even when a study simply proposes participation observation that may include minors, it is important to remember that the federal regulations regarding the participation of minors apply.[3(SubpartD)] For these purposes, children are defined as "persons who have not attained the legal age for consent to treatments or procedures involved in the research, under the applicable law of the jurisdiction in which the research will be conducted." Subpart D requires parental consent until the participant reaches the legal age to consent personally, as specified by local law. Waivers to the documentation of informed consent and the informed consent process itself are permitted as described previously here.

From time to time, ethnography is proposed for use among a population of children. Such studies require the consent of a parent and the consent of the institutional authority. In a setting such as a school or hospital unit, teachers and health care providers may also need to provide consent. In addition, the IRB is instructed to ". . . determine that adequate provisions are made for soliciting the assent of the children, when in the judgment of the IRB the children are capable of providing assent. . . ."[3][Sec.408(a)]

With a description of the research setting and the age and maturity of the minor participants, the IRB can determine whether or not it is appropriate to obtain assent. If the IRB chooses to require minor assent, it must also specify how such assent is to be documented.[3][Sec.408(e)]

Research in Foreign Countries

Research proposed to take place in foreign countries can generate additional questions during IRB review. Assurance that the appropriate foreign authorities have reviewed the project and that the informed consent process is conducted appropriately, given the foreign population, is critical. Many times in international research, obtaining a signature for a consent document can be problematic, if not impossible. When researchers work with populations of illiterate persons, even a brief information sheet may be useless. In such cases, the IRB must focus on the training of the researcher and the plans for obtaining informed consent orally. As Frederick Erickson of UCLA explains, "In cross-cultural research—especially overseas but also here in U.S.—the cultural notion of individual volition and consent may not apply in the setting being studied. Thus, written consent from village elders and oral assent from others may be more culturally appropriate than elaborate written consent documents for everybody. And if an IRB is willing to be true to the 'spirit of the law' that is fine, but if they are hung up on the 'letter of the law' they can impose consent conditions that are unreasonable" (Frederick Erickson, Ph.D., personal communication on October 17, 2000).

If an IRB sets out to review international research without knowledge of the region where the research will take place, consultants can provide invaluable help. A brief summary proposing participation observation in a mining town in rural South America, for example, may appear innocuous to the IRB, but put the researcher and study participants in grave danger due to the political issues surrounding a mining community. A reviewer with expertise in the cultural and political issues of the region will be able to spot potential risks far more comprehensively than the average IRB.

Finally, in addition to helping the IRB understand issues specific to the region of study, consultants can verify that consent documents and information sheets have been accurately translated.

Conclusion

An IRB is most effective when it maintains an open dialogue with the research community and works with researchers to facilitate the conduct of ethical research. At times, ethnography can stretch the system, requiring thoughtful consideration of the intent of the federal regulations and the use of consultants in order to make sense of the ethical issues raised by each unique study. Because ethnographic research involves so much face-to-face, unstructured interaction between researchers and participants, the review process offers a unique opportunity not only to monitor and modify this type of qualitative interaction but, more importantly, to teach researchers how to estimate the risks of their work and understand the impact of their work on the participant community. Becoming aware of these issues is a central part of good ethnography regardless of the specific field of study. In this way, the IRB steps into the larger research process to benefit the community of ethnographers as well as the community of participants.

References

1. Hammersley M, Atkinson P. *Ethnography: Principles in Practice*, 2nd ed. London: Routledge; 1995.

2. American Anthropological Association. Access date 27 August, 2001. http://www.aaanet.org/

3. Code of Federal Regulations. Title 45A—Department of Health and Human Services; Part 46—Protection of Human Subjects. Updated 1 October, 1997. Access date 18 April, 2001. http://www4.law.cornell.edu/cfr/45p46.htm

4. Estroff SE. Whose story is it anyway? Authority, voice, and responsibility in narratives of chronic illness. In: Toombs SK, Barnard D, Carson RA (eds.). *Chronic Illness: From Experience to Policy (Medical Ethics Series)*. Bloomington, IN: Indiana University Press; 1995:78–104.

5. Office for Protection from Research Risks, NIH. Protection of human subjects: Categories of research that may be reviewed by the Institutional Review Board (IRB) through an expedited review procedure. *Fed Regist* 63(216):60364–60367, 9 November, 1998. http://ohrp.osophs.dhhs.gov/humansubjects/guidance/63fr60364.htm

Health Services Research

Ann Barry Flood

INTRODUCTION

Health services research involves the development of new knowledge and the application of existing knowledge for the improvement of health care and its delivery. While much of this research focuses on care delivered in organizational settings, this field also embraces the need to look at the health care for regions, market areas, and the population as a whole—that is, for users and nonusers of health care—in order to examine and improve access, quality, and cost-effectiveness.

Most would agree that health services research is not "a discipline." In recent years, academic programs have emerged to offer graduate-level training specifically in health services research, outcomes research, or the evaluative clinical sciences. Nevertheless, the majority of researchers in this field have had disciplinary-based training in the social sciences (principally economics, political science, psychology, public health, and sociology) and/or clinical training (principally medicine or nursing).

The field has emerged over the past three decades, shaped by two aspects of the multidisciplinary nature of the research. First, because of the diverse nature of the training of most practitioners in this broad field of research, many perspectives have developed regarding the most appropriate methods and most important questions. Second, because of the complexity and breadth of the basic content area and the array of methodological approaches required to study these phenomena, the cross-disciplinary approaches of health services research strengthen our ability to understand and assess health care and health policy.

AcademyHealth, the premier professional organization for this field, and the Agency for Healthcare Research and Quality (AHRQ), the lead federal agency charged with supporting this research, have a similar vision of this field.[1,2] Basically, it is to improve health care by conducting or sponsoring research designed to improve the quality of health care, reduce its cost, improve patient safety, decrease medical errors, and broaden access to essential services. AHRQ defines this research to include generating evidence-based information on health care outcomes (quality and cost, use, and access) with the intent to help health care decision makers make better-informed decisions and improve the quality of health care services.

Why Health Services Research Challenges the IRB

The multidisciplinary nature of health services research, the focus on groups or systems rather than individuals, and the pragmatic intent to inform policy makers, practitioners, and administrators often make it difficult for institutional review boards (IRBs) to determine how best to evaluate and monitor health services research projects. The overlap in methods with the social sciences, public health, and epidemiology is such that many issues related to human subjects protection are described elsewhere in this book. Problems involving research conducted in multiple sites or focused on vulnerable populations, such as racial or gender differences in health or receipt of health care, are also addressed elsewhere but clearly apply to health services research. Similarly, health services research can involve international comparisons and can necessitate deception in informed consent (such as when studying the impact of placebos or compliance with therapeutic recommendations, where the subjects' behavior or outcomes of interest may be negated by true informed consent). These categories are also addressed in Chapters 6-5 and 10-11, but the reader is reminded that they may apply to health services research as well.

In this chapter, we frame the discussion about human subjects protection by examining the nature of research designs in health services research, focusing in particular on the multidisciplinary and long-term nature of the work, its frequent location within organizational settings, its dependence on clinical data sources, and its pragmatic intent to improve health care. We discuss the implications for four key areas of human subjects protection: (1) issues of safety and balance between risks and benefits of participating in research, (2) the right to privacy and confidentiality of records of health and health care that are not generated by and for research, (3) the right to confidentiality of records generated solely as a consequence of participating in research, and (4) the right to choose to participate in research.

Health Services Research as a "Social Experiment"

The notion of conducting a systematic experiment in health services research, where a defined population is randomly (or at least systematically) assigned to receive alternative treatments for purposes of informing policy, sounds so radical that one might think it to be politically unfeasible in the United States. Yet, to a large degree, such experimentation is carried out in many guises all the time.

Medicare offers multiple examples. The initial implementation of the program, coupled with mechanisms to provide additional support for poor elderly, created profound changes in our health care system, not only with respect to enhancing access to care, but also fundamentally altering the payment sources for medical education and helping to ensure that medical education would be hospital-based in its orientation. Since then, numerous modifications such as the implementation of a prospective, lump-sum payment system for hospitals in the 1980s, a resource-based form of reimbursement for services by physicians in the early 1990s, a major reduction in payments for home health care in the late 1990s, and Health Savings Accounts and prescription benefits in the early 2000s are all social experiments that affect hundreds of health care organizations, thousands of providers, and millions of beneficiaries.

Similarly, states are encouraged by the federal government to serve as laboratories to implement major social policies such as universal coverage for health care, especially for children. Nearly every state has a waiver from the federal agency that administers Medicare to carry out variations in services provided, such as using disease management programs for people with specific kinds of chronic diseases. Several sites were funded in 2005 to carry out experiments to reward providers for providing high-quality care.

Quality improvement experiments are also carried out in many levels of health care organizations. Prior to these more systematic managerial attempts to study and improve the processes of care and its delivery, quality assurance, and utilization review efforts were regularly carried out in health care organizations. Managed care techniques, ranging from introducing tiered copayments for prescriptions or provider visits to physician profiling to monitor the cost-effectiveness of individual providers' care, also have been widely introduced by insurers or health care organizations.

Major funding foundations such as the federal government or private foundations regularly solicit proposals for demonstrations and evaluations of new policy initiatives such as strengthening hospital nursing or implementing medical home models for children with special needs.

Despite the potential for profound impact on people's lives and the vast numbers of resources and people involved, most of these social experiments do not fall under the purview of IRBs unless they are funded by grants and/or performed by people other than those employed by the government or the organizations charged with implementation—and are classifiable as "research" with the intent to be generalizable.

When should human subjects protection be addressed formally in such social experiments and what are the special considerations? For purposes of illustrating the particular issues of concern for IRBs, we next discuss five types of social experiments in health services research: (1) the "true" social experiment, (2) the "natural" experiment, (3) research for follow-up of patients who refuse to be randomized in randomized clinical trials, (4) feasibility and demonstration studies of health-services tools, and (5) management/quality improvement efforts in health care organizations or systems.

The True Social Experiment

The true social experiment is a research project with a design that involves explicit and voluntary enrollment of people into an experiment with randomized or systematic assignment to experimental models. In health services research, these alternative models generally require subjects to agree to be assigned to different types of payment or organizational systems for a substantial period of time and to comply fully with the requirements to remain enrolled and as assigned during the study. As with randomized clinical trials, these experimental models assume that there is no evidence to confirm that one model is substantially superior to another. However, in the social experiment, there is no definitive treatment protocol and no mechanism to try to control for differences in routine provision of care in the alternatives.

The RAND Health Insurance Experiment is a classic example of this type of research.[3] Conducted in the 1970s, it involved the assignment of approximately 2,000 nonelderly families to insurance plans that varied in the price of health services that the individual families would subsequently experience. A primary research goal was to examine the impact of financial incentives for the patient on health care utilization and outcomes. There were several key human protection issues faced in the course of designing and evaluating this study:

1. In informing prospective subjects to be recruited into the study, how should the long-term potential advantages and disadvantages of participation be framed? In this particular study, participation—irrespective of which program they were assigned to—appeared to be advantageous financially

for all participants and offered them a guarantee for several years of a minimum level of insurance that was not otherwise available. Here, the financial incentives that were integrally important to the experimental design were also seen as potentially coercive for inducing participation because the offer tended to sound "too good to be true." The researchers used three techniques to address these concerns. First, they created statements about insurance alternatives that were substantially clearer and simpler than all those available in the market. Second, they offered a variety of local contacts for information and to legitimize the research effort. Third, they pledged confidentiality of all data, including questionnaires and utilization.

2. How can incidental and unintended impact be anticipated and minimized? For a variety of design issues, the researchers chose to enroll a family unit rather than an individual. One of the subsequent complex sets of issues was what to do with family units that changed over the course of the study. One issue was how to handle the database for families that divided into smaller units. Ironically, the experiment also became a kind of endowment for enrollees in the study to use to allow access to the experiment to their new spouses.

3. Confidentiality of data. Because of the numbers of types of data, the length of the study, and the requirement for the data to be linked, confidentiality of data was difficult to ensure. The researchers used subcontractors to maintain a list of current addresses and names, to monitor changes in addresses or family composition, and to carry out linkages. The RAND researchers had a separate set of identifiers for their database but did not have names and addresses. When the RAND group needed to link other databases to their own, the subcontractor, who did not have access to all datasets, performed the linkages.

4. Burdens of participation. The RAND group monitored the burdens of enrollees, both to try to minimize dropout through corrective responses and to learn what enrollees disliked most. Interestingly, among the 15% who considered dropping out, the most frequent issue named was the complexity and difficulty of filling out forms. However, the most sensitive and disagreeable information to provide was not related to health or mental health; people were most reluctant to provide financial disclosures to the researchers.

The Natural Experiment

The natural or administrative experiment is a design that is commonly used when it is impractical for scientific, political, and/or economic reasons to conduct a true social experiment. Basically, the design calls for taking advantage of naturally occurring administrative or policy changes in order to study their impact. Examples of this in health services research include these studies of the following: (1) mortality in hospitals after a physician strike, (2) practice style changes after a major redesign of financial incentives for physicians in a group practice, and (3) financial and health impact following closures of hospitals.

In many cases, the databases to be used for the research are collected for other purposes, and the research involves historical or case-control comparisons of secondary datasets. Here, the issues of human subjects protection are primarily whether researchers should have access to the data and whether the data can be provided so that it is without identifying information.

However, these experiments can be designed so as to involve prospectively collected data and survey data. In these situations, the issue for human subjects is not whether they are offered a choice to participate or have any harms or benefits associated with being in the natural experiment (as that is occurring outside of the context of research). Instead, it is whether they are at risk for being evaluated systematically for changes in their performance or behavior. Here, humans to be considered in the research database typically include patients, individual providers, and staff responsible for organizational performance.

Preference-Based Trials: Research for the Follow-up of Patients Who Refuse to Be Randomized in Randomized Clinical Trials

In randomized control trials, patients must agree to be randomized into one of the treatment arms being evaluated. Typically, an important issue is to control for any differences in quality of care by instituting strong protocols for what actions should be taken, with little or no room for negotiating variations based on patient preferences.

Example

In an ongoing study being conducted in several hospitals, patients are being told about two basically equivalent alternatives for treatment of low back pain, one involving surgery and one essentially without an active intervention. Subjects are invited to join the randomized arm, but if they refuse because they would prefer to exercise a choice, they are invited to participate in the preference-based arm of the study instead. Such patients have follow-up in the same way as patients in the randomized arm.[4]

The primary reason for follow-up of patients who do not agree to be randomized is to examine whether choice appears to influence outcomes. The human subjects issues for this type of trial are essentially identical to those involved in a randomized control trial. However, this design raises an interesting issue for human subjects protection. If patients' willingness to participate in randomized control trials is intricately tied to their basic willingness to forego choice, it suggests that there may be a serious bias in recruitment of patients to randomized control trials. It also suggests that the basic design of the gold-standard clinical experiment prevents many people from participating in clinical research who would otherwise like to do so. The underlying ethical issue is this: "Is there a right to participate in such research?"

Feasibility and Demonstration Studies of Health Services Tools

With the increased attention to evidence-based medicine and systematic collection of data for monitoring outcomes comes the development of a variety of health services research tools such as several health outcomes tools approved by the Scientific Advisory Committee of the Medical Outcomes Trust,[5] patient acuity measures such as the APACHE scores for intensive care, and mortality prediction scores for surgical patients.[6] Many of these measures have undergone or will undergo rigorous research to examine their reliability and validity under a variety of circumstances. At the same time, whether for-profit or not, many of these tools are copyrighted and some are not open for scrutiny by the scientific community of the assumptions and evidence on which they are based.

In regard to human subjects protection, these developments—paralleling those in profit-based firms such as the drug industry or durable medical equipment companies—raise issues about the importance of financial disclosure regarding the current and future intended uses of the tools. Although the issues may be far more controversial and potentially profitable for research in genetic engineering and clinical product development, health services research has parallel conflicts of interest. It shares a need to address a fundamental issue for human subjects: When the research for which people are volunteering is primarily intended to fine-tune a tool for proprietary use, should there be a different standard of risks and benefits and disclosure for subjects?

Management/Quality Improvement Efforts in Health Care Organizations or Systems

This issue has already been touched on but is mentioned again in this context because of its fundamental importance to the issues of human subjects protection in health services research. When and how should human subjects issues be raised when the research efforts are primarily aimed at improving a system of care, and may not be designed to be generalized or reported outside of an institution? There have been many recent articles on this subject, attesting to the disagreement about whether and when IRBs should be involved and whether other mechanisms should be in place to ensure human subjects protection if risks are substantial.[7-11] Most commentators seek to balance concerns about avoiding overburdening IRBs with unnecessary oversight with concerns about overlooking serious and uninformed potential harm for patients. Solutions proposed range from identifying criteria that *should* trigger an IRB review to setting up alternative review committees to deal specifically with quality improvement projects. Evidence in support of the need for a more neutral evaluation comes from a study that found systematic differences between judgments of human subjects protection issues made by quality improvement managers, IRB directors, and journal editors. This study suggested that quality improvement officers may underidentify appropriate concerns.[12]

The most recent federal directive to the AHRQ is to study the systems of care that have given rise to an alarming number of medical errors and issues regarding patient safety. These concerns, coupled with increased attention to quality improvement techniques in health care, underscore the importance for IRB members and the processes of human protection to become better informed about who and what needs protecting. Defining issues too narrowly can defeat some of the most important charges to the IRB: to protect patients from ill-considered projects, to ensure that safety and risk/benefit ratios are monitored

and appropriate—but not to undermine efforts to improve quality of care and hold institutions and systems accountable for ensuring it.

Conclusion

This chapter has illustrated some of the reasons why health services research often challenges the IRB system. Health services research projects are often multidisciplinary in nature, focus on groups or systems rather than individuals, and are conducted with the pragmatic intent to inform policy makers. Health services research can involve international comparisons and can necessitate deception in informed consent (such as when studying the impact of placebos or compliance with therapeutic recommendations, where the subjects' behavior or outcomes of interest may be negated by true informed consent). In most cases, the main issue for the IRB to evaluate for a health services research project is confidentiality of the medical record and other forms of health information. The information presented in this chapter helps IRBs, researchers, and institutional officials to make informed decisions about ethical standards for the design and regulation of health services research projects.

References

1. AcademyHealth. What is Health Services Research? Access date 18 Feb, 2005. http://www.academyhealth.org/about/whatishsr.htm

2. Department of Health and Human Services. Agency for Healthcare Research and Quality. Quality Research for Quality Health Care. Access date 17 Feb, 2005. http://www.ahrq.gov/about/qr4qhc/qr4qhc-1.htm#contents

3. Newhouse JP. *Insurance Experiment Group. Free for All? Lessons from the RAND Health Insurance Experiment.* Cambridge, MA: Harvard University Press; 1993.

4. North American Spine Society Board of Directors. Spine Patient Outcome Research Trial (SPORT): Multi-center randomized clinical trial of surgical and non-surgical approaches to the treatment of low back pain. *The Spine Journal;* 3:417–419, 2003.

5. Medical Outcomes Trust. Generic and Condition-Specific Instruments. Access date 20 Feb, 2005. http://www.outcomes-trust.org/instruments.htm

6. French Society of Anethesia. 13th World Congress, Paris 2004. Scoring systems for ICU and surgical patients. Access date 20 Feb 2005. http://www.sfar.org/s/article.php3?id_article=60

7. Casarett D, Karlawish JHT, Sugarman J. Determining when quality improvement initiatives should be considered research: Proposed criteria and potential implications. *JAMA;* 283:2275–2280, 2000.

8. Bellin E, Dubler NN. The quality improvement-research divide and the need for external oversight. *Amer J Public Health;* 91:1512–17, 2001.

9. Lo B, Groman M. Oversight of quality improvement: Focusing on benefits and risks. *Arch Intern Med;* 163:1481–1486, 2003.

10. Nerenz DR, Stoltz PK, Jordan J. Quality improvement and the need for IRB review. *Q Manage Health Care;* 12(3):159–170, 2003.

11. Diamond LH, Kliger AS, Goldman RS, Palevsky PM. Quality improvement projects: How do we protect patients' rights? *Amer J Medical Quality;*19(1):25–27, 2004.

12. Lindenauer PK, Benjamin EM, Naglieri-Prescod D, Fitzgerald J, Pekow P. The role of the Institutional Review Board in quality improvement: A survey of quality officers, IRB chairs, and journal editors. *Am J Med;* 113:575–579, 2002.

Epidemiology/Public Health Research

Marjorie A. Speers

INTRODUCTION

Public health research spans the spectrum of scientific study. It includes scientific questions directed at understanding biological processes, behavior, and social interactions, as well as a wide range of interventions. Likewise, the methods used in public health research are as wide ranging as are research questions that are addressed. Because ethical issues of concern to institutional review boards (IRBs) regarding specific methods, such as the use of existing data or surveys, are covered in other chapters, the focus here is on a few key issues of importance to IRBs when they consider public health research, specifically epidemiological research.

Research Versus Practice

One of the more confusing and sometimes time-consuming issues facing IRBs regarding studies addressing a public health problem is whether the study is public health research or public health practice. Making this research determination is important for both moral and practical reasons. First, if the activity is research, then it must be reviewed by the IRB to ensure that the individuals participating in the research are adequately protected, the research is ethically justifiable, and it meets all the federal requirements for human research. On the other hand, if the activity is not research, then the IRB has no legal or regulatory authority to direct the activity. Second, given that IRBs are heavily burdened by the huge volume of studies that are research, they should not unnecessarily spend their time reviewing and monitoring activities that are not research and often for which there are other systems of protection (i.e., state laws regarding confidentiality protection or informed consent). It could be ethically inappropriate for an IRB to interfere with public health practice, especially in an urgent situation.

Definition of Research

The definition of research in the federal regulations is "a systematic investigation, including research development, testing, and evaluation, designed to develop or contribute to generalizable knowledge."[1][Sec.102(d)] Deciding whether a public health activity is research or practice is not easy because systematically collecting and analyzing data from individuals are essential functions of routine public health practice. In addition, scientific methods are often used in public health practice, adding to the confusion about whether the activity is research or practice. Moreover,

because the profession of public health deals with populations, the distinction between using individuals or groups is also not helpful in deciding whether an activity is practice or research.

There is limited guidance and scientific literature addressing the difficulties in classifying public health activities as research or practice. In 1999, the Centers for Disease Control and Prevention developed a document, "Guidelines for defining public health research and public health non-research," that provides guidance in classifying public health activities as research or practice.[2] In addition, in its report *Ethical and Policy Issues in Research Involving Human Participants* (2001), the National Bioethics Advisory Commission suggests that not all public health activities are research but did not expand much beyond the definition in the federal regulations or the Centers for Disease Control guidance.[3] The same confusion and questions still exist today.

Data Collection Techniques

Looking at methods or data collection techniques is instructive to the IRB that must decide whether the activity is research because public health practice and public health research activities both rely on the use of the same systematic procedures. For example, a case-control study design can be used to determine the risk factors in an outbreak investigation whose sole purpose is to bring the disease under control, but this is not research. Yet, the case-control design is routinely used in epidemiology to study disease etiology, and the study is research.

Thus, the IRB is forced to look at the researcher's intent in conducting the activity and ultimately the design of the activity. Public health practice activities are carried out with the primary intention of preventing or controlling disease or injury and improving health or improving a public health program or service. These activities are generally undertaken in such a manner that were some type of action necessary it could be initiated. Many argue that it is difficult to determine intent; however, several questions can be posed by the IRB to the researcher that will help in making the determination. The IRB can ask the researcher directly whether the activity is intended to generate new knowledge that will contribute to the scientific literature (i.e., that revises or improves on an existing principle, theory, or knowledge). In addition, the IRB might ask whether the activity is intended to directly benefit a population or group of individuals. The IRB can ask the researcher how the data will be used. Specifically, is there an intention to publish or present the results to the scientific community? Intention to publish or present results does not always imply that the activity is research. As part of their civic responsibilities, federal, state, or local government officials are obliged to publish results in government documents or share results with other public officials. This type of publication or presentation of data does not make the activity research. Perhaps another way to frame this question to the researcher is to ask whether the study would be conducted if the results could not be published in a scientific journal. If the answer is no, then the activity is research. Ask about the expected validity of the data, or look at the protocol. Often, data collected for public health practice purposes have limited validity or generalizability beyond the population being studied. For example, an estimate of disease prevalence in a particular county is meaningful to and has validity for that county, but it is not necessarily meaningful or valid for other counties either in that state or nationwide. Data generated from research activities should have validity that relates to our general understanding of a problem or situation.

Determining Research Intent

Often, a local IRB is not alone in making a determination about whether an activity is research. Sponsoring agencies will, and under federal regulations should, make a determination of whether an activity is research.[1(Sec.101)] Unfortunately, sponsoring agencies are not consistent in their interpretation of the regulations: The same activity might be classified as research by one agency and as nonresearch by another. Moreover, more than one local institution may be involved in the research, in which case each IRB often weighs into the decision of whether the activity is research. In the latter case, it becomes important for IRBs to talk to each other and resolve IRB issues up front.

Classifying a study as research or nonresearch becomes even more challenging when the study involves multiple components. For example, an evaluation component might be added to a disease reporting system (e.g., cancer registry) to determine how completely the reporting system is identifying cases. In this case, the ongoing disease reporting system is not research, but the evaluation component might be. When studies involve multiple components, IRBs should make an individual determination for each component regarding whether it is research.[2]

Privacy and Confidentiality

Much of the research conducted in public health does not involve invasive procedures. Instead, it involves the use of existing data (e.g., analysis of tissue samples, medical records, secondary analysis of databases) or surveys (or interviews) of individuals. Harms that may occur as a result of the research are mostly related to threats to privacy and breaches in maintaining confidentiality. Far too often these types of risks are overlooked by researchers and IRBs. Regulatory guidance regarding privacy and confidentiality is limited to the directive that IRBs may approve a research study only when they have judged that the study contains adequate protections for privacy and maintains confidentiality.[1[Sec.111(a)(7)]]

IRBs need to understand fully the concepts of privacy and confidentiality and their applications in research. Privacy and confidentiality are often incorrectly believed to be the same thing. Although the concepts are related, they address different issues. Privacy refers to a state of being of individuals. Individuals have information about themselves, and privacy refers to the ways in which researchers access information from individuals.[4] Privacy is influenced by culture, individuals' particular social situations, and the nature and context of the research.

Threats to Privacy

An individual's privacy is respected when the researcher seeks informed consent, but informed consent alone does not ensure that one's privacy interests are protected. To avoid threats to privacy, IRBs should consider all the factors involved and procedures intended to be used to obtain information from the research participant. Although it is not possible to list all the factors and procedures here, the IRB should at least look at the following:

1. What types of harms are likely to result from participating in the study? Examples of harm might include worry, irritation, fear, embarrassment or self-doubt, arrest, stigmatization, or unemployment.

2. What type of information is being gathered? Is it sensitive or associated with a stigmatizing condition (e.g., drug addiction)? Are there cultural norms that may influence participants' willingness to share the information?

3. How will the information be gathered? What procedures will be used? Do the procedures reduce risk of embarrassment or other psychologic or social risk if the information is sensitive (e.g., using a written questionnaire as opposed to a face-to-face interview if the questions are sensitive)?

4. What procedures will be used to ensure that participants can refuse to participate in general or refuse to answer a question?

5. In surveys, are interviewers of the same ethnicity, gender, socioeconomic status, or age as participants?

Confidentiality Protection

Confidentiality protection relates to the way in which data that can be linked to individuals are handled and used. Protection of confidentiality begins with the understanding between the research participant and the researcher about how the participant's data will be handled and with whom it will be shared.[5] In this sense, confidentiality is related to privacy because it involves informing the participants about how the data will be managed and shared and seeking their approval during the informed consent process. Thus, there are two aspects to confidentiality: how the data will be managed and with whom the data will be shared.

IRBs should carefully review the data management plan for the study and determine whether any of the proposed procedures might cause a breach in maintaining confidentiality. Such procedures include transmitting data, creating or eliminating linkages between the data and identifiers, data storage, and plans for long-term use or destruction.

IRBs should also review other study procedures that might influence confidentiality, such as the method by which participants will be paid or recontacted for follow-up. For example, using checks to reimburse participants for costs associated with participating in the study may create an unnecessary link between the participants and the study.

Finally, IRBs should review the study to determine with whom identifiable data will be shared and whether this information is clearly communicated to the prospective participants during the informed consent process. The review should include consideration of voluntary disclosures to others as well as the potential for compulsory disclosures. IRBs need to be aware of state and local privacy and confidentiality laws regarding mandatory reporting requirements (e.g., reports of child abuse) as well as federal reporting requirements (e.g., Food and Drug Administration regulations related to the use of investigational new drugs). Local IRBs should consult with their institutions' general counsel or contact their state attorney general's office regarding relevant state law.

Informed Consent

In some cases, applying the federal regulatory requirements[1(Sec.116,117)] for seeking informed consent and documentation of the informed consent process can be problematic in public health research. In surveys, the requirement that documentation of the informed consent process is a signed written consent form sometimes seems inappropriate (e.g., written consent for a telephone survey) or overly burdensome (e.g., a survey involves no more than minimal risk and the consent form is longer than the list of survey questions). The federal regulations do not provide much flexibility to IRBs in determining the type of documentation or the need for it. A signed written consent form is the only form of acceptable documentation.[1(Sec.117)] Yet, there

are other forms of documentation that could serve the same purpose as a signed written consent form, such as using a witness, audiotaping or videotaping the consent process, using an audit process, or randomly recontacting a sample of the participants.

The federal regulations allow the documentation requirement to be waived if one of two criteria can be met: (1) the only record linking the participant to the research is the consent form and the principal risk is breach in confidentiality, or (2) the research presents no more than minimal risk of harm and involves no procedures for which written consent is normally required outside the research context. Whereas the application of the first criterion is straightforward, the application of the second criterion to surveys is unclear. IRBs should work with researchers to waive the requirement for signed written consent forms when another method of documentation that is more appropriate to the research context can be used.

Conclusion

Epidemiological and public health research can raise some special issues for IRBs. IRBs that review a substantial amount of public health research should consider having public health professionals as members. It may also be useful to the IRB to have a member from either the state or local health department or to build a relationship with the health department for consultative purposes.

References

1. Code of Federal Regulations. Title 45A—Department of Health and Human Services; Part 46—Protection of Human Subjects. Updated 1 October, 1997. Access date 18 April, 2001. http://www4.law.cornell.edu/cfr/45p46.htm

2. Centers for Disease Control and Prevention. Human subjects research: Guidelines for defining public health research and public health non-research, 14 March, 2001. Access date 20 March, 2001. http://www.cdc.gov/od/ads/opspoll1.htm

3. National Bioethics Advisory Commission. Ethical and Policy Issues in Research Involving Human Participants (draft report). Bethesda, MD: U.S. Government Printing Office. Updated 19 December, 2000. Access date 20 March, 2001. http://bioethics.gov/pubs.html

4. Boruch RF, Cecil JS. *Assuring the Confidentiality of Social Research Data*. Philadelphia: University of Pennsylvania Press; 1979.

5. Institute of Medicine, Committee on the Role of Institutional Review Boards in Health Services Research Data Privacy Protection. Protecting data privacy in health services research. Washington, DC: National Academy Press, 2000. Access date 20 March, 2001. http://www.nap.edu/html/data_privacy/

Survey Research

J. Michael Oakes

INTRODUCTION

This chapter considers human subject protection issues in biomedical, biobehavioral, and public health surveys (hereinafter called health surveys). Surveys are the most common method of data collection, used in both clinical trials and observational epidemiological investigations. They are too often viewed as benign, posing no or only minimal risk, by both survey researchers and institutional review boards (IRBs). This view is incorrect. The risks associated with information that may be discovered in survey studies may be every bit as serious as the physical risks associated with an investigational drug or medical device.

In most cases, the risks posed by survey research involve privacy and/or confidentiality. Two distinguished survey researchers wrote, "When all the rationales and justifications for its use have been stripped away, the . . . survey is ultimately an intrusion into the private lives of individuals."[1] Included are the risks of harm or loss (e.g., disclosure of private medical problems or sexual preference), inconvenience (e.g., boredom, frustration), psychological risk (e.g., insult, trauma), and social (e.g., embarrassment, rejection), economic (e.g., loss of job, credit, insurance), and legal (e.g., subpoena, fine) risk.

The objective of this chapter is straightforward. I aim to help IRB chairs, administrators, and members improve their reviews of health survey research protocols. To this end, a brief background is given to put the method in perspective, and the federal regulations regarding survey research are highlighted. The unique aspects of survey research an IRB may wish to consider are sketched, including the use of real-world examples from the IRB I serve. Finally, specific and practical recommendations for reviewing and monitoring survey research are offered.

Background

Because there are many variations on the theme, it is important to be clear on what a survey is. The *IRB Guidebook* defines *survey studies* as those designed to obtain information from a large number of respondents through written questionnaires, telephone interviews, door-to-door canvassing, or similar procedures.[2]

In other words, a research health survey involves a systematic and standardized approach to data collection through questioning a sample of individuals, households, or organizations. This definition includes in-person, mail, telephone, Internet, and other such surveys. Excluded are related techniques of focus groups, semistructured interviews, and observational analysis, although many of the issues discussed herein apply.

Department of Health and Human Services Regulations Related to Survey Research

General IRB responsibilities related to privacy and confidentiality are addressed in 45 CFR 46.

1. Criteria for IRB approval of research.[3][Sec.111(a)(7)] "When appropriate, there are adequate provisions to protect the privacy of subjects and maintain the confidentiality of data."

2. General requirements for informed consent.[3][Sec.116(a)(5)] "A statement describing the extent, if any, to which confidentiality of records identifying the subject will be maintained."

3. Revised criteria for expedited review of research.[4] "Research not meeting these criteria must undergo full board review."

The word *survey* is mentioned four times in 45 CFR 46, twice under the exemption clause (Section 46.101), once in a footnote referring to the children's section (i.e., Subpart D), and once in the exemptions section of the children's section itself.

In 45 CFR 46,[3][Sec.101] which outlines what research is and is not covered by the statute, Subsection (b) reads as follows:

(b) Unless otherwise required by Department or Agency heads, research activities in which the only involvement of human subjects will be in one or more of the following categories are exempt from this policy:

2) Research involving the use of educational tests (cognitive, diagnostic, aptitude, achievement), survey procedures, interview procedures or observation of public behavior, unless:

   (i) information obtained is recorded in such a manner that human subjects can be identified, directly or through identifiers linked to the subjects; and

   (ii) any disclosure of the human subjects' responses outside the research could reasonably place the subjects at risk of criminal or civil liability or be damaging to the subjects' financial standing, employability, or reputation.

3) Research involving the use of educational tests (cognitive, diagnostic, aptitude, achievement), survey procedures, interview procedures, or observation of public behavior that is not exempt under paragraph (b)(2) of this section, if:

   (i) the human subjects are elected or appointed public officials or candidates for public office; or

   (ii) Federal statute(s) require(s) without exception that the confidentiality of the personally identifiable information will be maintained throughout the research and thereafter.

The most important section[3][Sec.401(b)(2)] means that survey research is exempt from IRB oversight unless identifying information is collected and the disclosure of such information may cause harm to the subjects. Some distinguished commentators suggest the "and" preceding point (ii) means that most survey research is beyond the scope of IRB review. Shelton, for example, argues that it is not enough that risk is hypothetically possible, but that risks from survey information must be readily significant and appreciable for research to be covered by an IRB.[5] However, Shelton discounts the ease with which links between databases can increase risk. It no longer takes much effort to merge databases from any number of sources and discover new information about subjects, placing them at risk. This is especially true when researchers recruit subjects from the same neighborhoods, clinics, or businesses, as is typically the case. Subject protections will be maximized by placing less weight on the risks from disclosure and more on whether the data are identifiable. Although de-emphasizing the requirement of "appreciable risks from disclosure" means that few health surveys will enjoy exemption status, as noted later here, this should not inhibit the conduct of survey research to a meaningful degree.

Subpart (b)(3) goes on to say that research on elected officials and research that enjoys strict federal confidentiality protections are both exempt from IRB review. Also exempt are surveys on groups, organizations, and associations, which are called *establishment surveys*. The reason for this is that organizations are not human subjects and thus 45 CFR 46 does not apply. IRBs should be aware, however, that in order to learn who filled out the questionnaire, many establishment surveys query the characteristics of the respondent himself or herself. Such questions may preclude the exemption. Except for the footnote referring to it, the other place the word survey appears is in Subpart D, "Additional Protections for Children." Here the regulations[3][Sec.401] say that the survey research exemption applicable to adults does not apply to children.

Research Design

Just as with other research designs and methods, IRBs must evaluate the quality of the design of survey studies. A poorly designed survey study will yield little useful information and thus poses (minimal) risks without benefits, rendering the proposal unworthy of IRB approval.

There are many design issues specific to survey studies; in fact, too many to comprehensively discuss here. Interested readers are encouraged to review Bickman and Rog,[6] Aday,[7] Rossi, Wright, and Anderson,[8] McDowell and Newell,[9] Dillman,[10] Fink,[11] Fowler,[12] Lehtonen and Pahkinen,[13] and Henry.[14] In addition to these texts, major journals publish methodological articles on survey research.

Response Rates

To assess the quality of a survey protocol, IRBs must have a general understanding of the term *response rate*. *Response rate* refers to the proportion of potential participants who complete the survey after being contacted about enrolling in the study.[7] If a survey contacts 402 eligible respondents but only 376 complete the questionnaire, the response rate is 94%. Response rates are important to survey studies because a low response rate means that many targeted subjects refused to participate. This is troublesome because it is unlikely that those who refused are statistically identical to those who participated, and this bias may render the entire study useless.

There is no hard rule on what constitutes an acceptable response rate, but the closer to 100% the better. Expected rates vary by survey mode (in-person, mail-back, and telephone), with in-person achieving the highest. Although it seems that many survey researchers hold out 70% as a target value, mail-back studies of physicians may be as low as 40%, whereas studies of a rare cancer may require 90% response to be meaningful. Response rates for federally funded national health surveys conducted in person have ranged from 85% to 95%.[7] Remember this: To avoid bias, nonrespondents must not be systematically different from respondents in terms of characteristics that are important to the study.

Sampling and Coverage Errors

Sampling errors result from collecting data on only a subset of subjects on a sampling frame, which is merely a list of potential subjects. Although related to response rate, sampling errors can be precisely calculated with statistical formulas and may be of interest to IRB members or consultants with statistical experience. Coverage error results from excluding potential subjects from a sampling frame. IRBs may look at whether investigators convincingly show that the group of potential subjects who are targeted are the same as the individuals in the list that will be used to contact them. It may be useful for the IRB to inquire whether those eligible subjects who refuse to participate in the survey are not expected to be systematically different from those that agree to participate. Again, this is no minor detail, as poorly executed sampling plans have indirectly harmed thousands through the promulgation of poorly evaluated health policies.[15] A related IRB issue is the probable equitable recruitment of underrepresented members of society, such as racial minorities, women, and, in some cases, children.

Recruitment

The recruitment of subjects for survey research is no less important than any other aspect of study design. It is important for IRBs to remember that a study that involves a no-risk survey is still unethical if the recruitment practices violate the IRB's ethical standards.[2]

Consider this real-world example. Although some would consider it standard operating procedure to contact a list of subjects that a physician-group or laboratory identifies as having elevated cholesterol, others would take issue with this proxy consent and consider the contact an invasion of privacy that was potentially burdensome and coercive to subjects. Experience suggests that problems will occur if potential subjects receive recruitment letters when (1) subjects have not explicitly given their physician-group permission to release information about them for research purposes or (2) subjects are not aware of the condition that caused them to be contacted—hypercholesterolemia in this example. Although many more troubling cases may be imagined, more mundane cases must not be overlooked. The point is that just because a survey protocol appears benign does not mean its recruitment procedures do not harm human subjects.

A related recruitment issue stems from efforts to get a disposition on each subject. Survey researchers define disposition as a code indicating whether the survey has been completed, whether the subject actively refused (i.e., saying, "I do not want to be in the study and do not call me again"), whether the subject simply refused (i.e., saying, "I am too busy now"), or whether the subject was never contacted. In this era of mass marketing, survey study designers may plan to make 10 calls to a given telephone number or send three or four questionnaires to a house before coding the subjects as "unavailable." Moreover, subjects who hem and haw before saying no may be recontacted and converted to completing the survey by more experienced interviewers. That skilled interviewers ably convince subjects to participate raises the potential for coercion. IRBs must balance the needs of survey researchers, who want to generate credible results, and the needs of the subjects, who deserve privacy and freedom from harassing phone calls and mailings.

Call scripts document how study representatives interact with subjects, and they are the first item to review if there is a question of coercion or harassment. One mechanism to prevent recruitment problems is to separate temporally the announcement of a study and recruitment for it. Providing a mechanism (800-number or self-addressed postcard) for prospective subjects to say that they do not want to be contacted may be appropriate is some cases.

Informed Consent

Standards for informed consent in survey research are no different than for research that does not involve a survey.[3[Sec.116(a),(b)]] In many cases, researchers will request IRB approval with the understanding that informed consent will be obtained but not be documented in writing. Department of Health and Human Services regulations provide for the waiver of documentation of informed consent in two situations that frequently apply to survey research.[3[Sec.117(c)]]

An IRB may waive the requirement for the investigator to obtain a signed consent form for some or all subjects if it finds either:

(1) That the only record linking the subject and the research would be the consent document and the principal risk would be potential harm resulting from a breach of confidentiality. Each subject will be asked whether the subject wants documentation linking the subject with the research, and the subject's wishes will govern; or

(2) That the research presents no more than minimal risk of harm to subjects and involves no procedures for which written consent is normally required outside of the research context.

In cases in which the documentation requirement is waived, the IRB may require the investigator to provide subjects with a written statement regarding the research.

It is important that researchers understand that this waiver does not mean that subjects may be enrolled in research without giving full and voluntary informed consent. It simply means that written documentation of consent is not required. It may be useful for IRBs to remind survey researchers of the evidence that fully informed subjects respond to questions with the most candor.[16,17]

Surrogate Surveys

An ethically challenging aspect of survey research concerns surrogate, proxy, or what others might call "indirect" surveys. Surrogate surveys elicit information from one person about another. Classic examples include husbands reporting information about their wives, adult children surveyed about their aging parents, or teachers about their students. It is essential that IRBs and researchers understand that there are often two subjects in these kinds of studies: the person responding to the survey and the person who is the subject of the survey. The full level of ethical protections and consent requirements applies to both subjects.

Botkin[18] reads 45 CFR 46 narrowly and argues that the person who is the primary subject of the survey (e.g., the wife in a study where the husband provides personal information about his wife) is a research subject only if names and other identifying information are collected. He goes on to say that even if an IRB determines that the primary subject is a research subject, a waiver of consent (not just documentation of consent) is usually justified. Botkin correctly recites the justifications for a waiver, but his arguments do not apply to many situations.[18]

In my experience, most health survey questions are sensitive to someone. Although small compared with other medical interventions, the degree of risk should be determined by each subject, not the researcher. Being an experienced survey statistician, I believe information coded for the "father" or "daughter" of an identified (primary) subject makes the surrogate data identifiable. If an employer gets unauthorized access to the survey data of an employee and then, through coded and linked data, discovers her husband is HIV positive, it is not a big leap to infer that the primary subject herself is at least at greater risk for HIV, if not positive herself.

As a result of these concerns, the IRB that I serve on is more conservative than Botkin, and insists that investigators get informed consent from both primary and surrogate subjects when a breach in confidentiality could result in meaningful harm. In some cases, it is impractical or impossible to get consent from all subjects who are at risk from survey information. Survey projects that do not meet the appropriate ethical standards should not be approved by the IRB.

Psychological and Social Harm
It is unclear whether or not a question, or set of them, can harm someone. More systematic research is required. Anecdotally, a January 2001 query of IRB professionals via the web-based IRB Forum (formerly MCWIRB) revealed several cases where survey questions, in and of themselves, appeared to harm study subjects.

1. Three weeks after answering the questionnaire for a cancer study, a man in his early 20s committed suicide, leaving a note stating that until he answered the questionnaire he did not really realize all of the experiences he had missed.

2. A survey researcher was investigating attitudes toward rape. When filling out the questionnaire, several subjects became visibly emotionally distressed and asked the investigator for help.

3. A study involving adolescents with emotional difficulties included a few questions about sexual preference. One subject interpreted the questions as if the researcher were suggesting she or he was a homosexual. The subject became very upset, attacked the researcher, and had to be restrained.

It is common for health surveys to include items about mental health status (e.g., depression), previous sexual abuses, illicit and prescription drug use, and physical disabilities. These questions are of a sensitive nature, and they may (1) provoke emotional responses by subjects and (2) place respondents at risk for discrimination, recrimination, or other harms—even physical ones. IRBs must balance the need to study difficult questions in vulnerable populations with their mandate to ensure the protection of human subjects.

Arguments that subjects are aware of the risks and thus a review of questions is not necessary may not withstand empirical scrutiny. Survey researchers are well trained to ask easy, noninvasive questions first in order to build rapport with subjects. Then, often gently, the more difficult questions are asked. This funneling technique is useful for survey researchers because respondents become more and more willing to answer tough questions after rapport is built. The problem is that once subjects begin to express their feelings, attitudes, and opinions—and because talking about oneself can be therapeutic, they often do—their ability to withdraw at any time may be practically forestalled. People want to appear consistent and cooperative and will thus continue to answer questions when

they otherwise would not. Although IRBs must be sure not to cripple the research enterprise, the ultimate definition of sensitive rests with the subject, not the investigators.

Even more generally, sensitive questions may be difficult to recognize. Health surveys will typically include questions on income, age, race, and gender. Although ostensibly benign, when coupled with responses about drug use, sexual behavior, or say, mental illness, these linked responses may result in inappropriate stigmatizations of groups of individuals. For example, a survey study that finds Hispanic or Asian men to have a greater propensity for domestic violence may inappropriately create a social stigma that affects the entire Hispanic American or Asian American community. The point is that even seemingly benign questions may pose critical risks and thus deserve close IRB scrutiny. In focusing strictly on protecting human subjects, IRBs should ensure that subjects understand the potential for social risks prior to participation.

Privacy and Confidentiality

Confidentiality is different from privacy. Survey data deserve as much attention to confidentiality as any other data, including genetic markers. Rights to confidentiality may be distinguished from rights to privacy by noting that confidentiality implies that consented surrendered information must be used only in the negotiated and disclosed manner, whereas privacy implies that no consent for information is granted. Beauchamp and Childress make the point:

> An infringement of X's right to confidentiality occurs only if the person to whom X disclosed information in confidence fails to protect the information or deliberately discloses it to someone without X's consent. By contrast, a person who without authorization enters a hospital record room or computer data bank [and views or records information] violates rights of privacy.[19]

Assuming that researchers have been authorized to collect and use a subject's information, survey research raises several more or less unique confidentiality issues. The *IRB Guidebook* makes this point:

> In most research, assuring confidentiality is only a matter of following some routine practices: substituting codes for identifiers, removing face sheets (containing such items as names and addresses) from survey instruments containing data, properly disposing of computer sheets and other papers, limiting access to identified data, impressing on the research staff the importance of confidentiality, and storing research records in locked cabinets.[2]

Because research suggests most respondents do not believe their answers will be kept confidential, it is incumbent on researchers and IRBs to regain or establish this trust. Pursuant to trust, the most important IRB issue with respect to nonanonymous (survey) data is the linking file.[20] A linking file is usually an electronic data file that contains each respondent's identifying information and the respondent's unique study identification number. Unless there are special reasons not to—such as when investigators are using computer-aided telephone interviewing (CATI/CAPI) computer systems to collect the data—this file should be the only place where subject identifying information is stored. Access to this file should be limited to only those who literally need access. The IRB should insist that the data file is encrypted, as computers may be hacked or physically stolen. All data files containing survey responses or any other information should be expunged of identifying information. Only the unique study identification number should be used. If CATI/CAPI systems are used to collect data, appropriate file deletion procedures should be enforced when the collection is complete.

Cryptic identifiers are easy for statisticians and computer programmers to assign to each person. They may simply be some combination of first and last name letters, birth dates, and, say, zip codes. Jane Smith, born on July 6, 1967, and living in Longmeadow, MA, may thus have the code JASM766701106, which will almost certainly be unique for linking and analytic purposes. More advanced methods are also easily implemented.

Compensation

The tension between the need to recruit and retain research subjects and the obligation to protect them from coercive interests makes compensation one of the most difficult and debated topics in applied bioethics. The *IRB Guidebook* pointed this out:

> Federal regulations governing research with human subjects contain no specific guidance for IRB review of payment practices. One of the primary responsibilities of IRBs, however, is to ensure that a subject's decision to participate in research will be truly voluntary, and that consent will be sought "only under circumstances that provide the prospective subject . . . sufficient opportunity to consider whether or not to participate and that minimize the possibility of coercion or undue influence" [Federal Policy §46.116; 21 CFR 50.20].[2]

Dickert and Grady sketch four objections to monetary compensation: (1) that the promise of money leads to undue inducement, (2) that only the economically disadvantaged will participate, rendering unequal benefits to the wealthy, (3) that paid subjects may care only about money and not about credible scientific results, and (4) that subject payment changes the investigator–subject relationship into a commercial one.[21] However, the authors admit that payment is probably here to stay and may be ethically justified. Accordingly, they go on to outline three approaches to payment: (1) the market model, where subjects are paid so as to attract and keep them; (2) the wage-payment model, where subjects are paid a standardized (unskilled labor) wage for participating; and (3) the reimbursement model, where subjects are reimbursed for expenses. Dickert and Grady ultimately advocate for the wage-payment model on the grounds that it is most egalitarian and should yield the least chance for coercion.[21]

Because the level of risk and effort is generally less than that encountered in biomedical studies, the question of compensation for health surveys is often overlooked in the bioethical literature. However, health surveys do raise some more or less unique questions about compensation.

For example, how much compensation, if any, should an investigator offer in a study of homeless drug or alcohol addicts who will only be interviewed once? What form should the compensation take: cash, food, or clothing? Anonymity is breached if payment is by check. When should the payment be made? Before or after completion of the survey? Must all questions be answered to receive a "completion bonus?"

In an effort to improve response rates, survey researchers have worked on the compensation problem. IRBs may use empirically generated survey research results in their deliberations about respondent compensation. Clearly, the potential for coercion is reduced when between $1 and $5 is included up front, as opposed to promises of payment when some task is complete. Evidence suggests, however, that this may be sufficient to gain the required response rates.

Conclusion

This chapter argues for continued, if not more vigorous, IRB review of health survey protocols. IRBs must balance the demand for research and the advancement of knowledge with the risks surveys pose. Although usually not the same level of risk posed by surgical, pharmacologic, or device trials, because surveys are ubiquitous, even marginal ethical infractions can cause aggregate harm. Given the wide use of surveys in all research domains, the impact of survey harms may be large. Accordingly, all protocols (even clinical trials) that employ survey methodologies should be reviewed by survey researchers at least. When reviewing survey research studies, IRBs should obviously consider all the regulations and obligations of 45 CFR 46, as well as those found in *The Belmont Report*, the Nuremberg Code, and the Declaration of Helsinki. Concerns raised in other kinds of reviews should also generally apply to survey research protocols.

In addition, IRBs may consider the following unordered summary points:

1. All survey protocols should be reviewed by an IRB official to determine exemption or expedite status. Proper assessment requires reviewing the entire protocol, including recruitment, contact, and analysis procedures.

2. Although it offers the maximum protection, few health surveys can be anonymous.

3. Survey research involves identifying information if subjects may be identified at any point in the study, including the recruitment of subjects or payment by check.

4. Surveys of prisoners and other vulnerable populations must be reviewed by the full IRB.

5. Reviewing recruitment protocols and scripts is integral to the protection of subjects.

6. Written consent documents may not be necessary, but the informed consent process is.

7. With projects that involve primary and surrogate subjects, the IRB should require that all subjects are afforded the full level of protections.

8. Nonresponse bias must be minimized or eliminated.

9. High response rates often require multiple subject contacts, but subjects should be protected from harassment.

10. The formatting and layout of the questionnaire influences response rates in a small way.

11. Pretests are almost essential, and good ones require significant resources.

12. Compensation is helpful, but evidence suggests sending $1 to $5 before the questionnaire is sent is sufficient and unlikely to be coercive.

13. Evidence suggests lotteries do little to improve survey response rates.

14. Linking files should be kept separate from response data and protected by limited access and encrypted methods.

15. Unless they gather information about respondents (i.e., human subjects), establishment (i.e., organizational) surveys are exempt.

16. IRBs should consider how survey studies are concluded. After expressing experiences and emotions, subjects are particularly vulnerable and deserve continued protection and sensitivity.

Acknowledgments

This chapter was improved by the comments and criticisms of several colleagues and friends. I thank Cheryl Caswell, Samantha Dunn, Kevin Smith, Joan Sieber, and Andre Araujo, as well as the entire institutional review board at the New England Research Institutes. Special thanks to members of the MCWIRB.ORG listserve who willingly shared their thoughts and opinions. I remain indebted to Professors Peter H. Rossi and Andy B. Anderson for their detailed comments on this paper, as well as their training more generally. The usual caveats apply.

References

1. Fox JA, Tracy PE. *Randomized Response: A Method for Sensitive Surveys.* Beverly Hills: Sage Publications; 1986.

2. Penslar RL, Porter JP, Office for Human Research Protections. *Institutional Review Board Guidebook,* 6 February, 2001. Access date 29 March, 2001. http://ohrp.osophs.dhhs.gov/irb/irb_guidebook.htm

3. Code of Federal Regulations. Title 45A—Department of Health and Human Services; Part 46—Protection of Human Subjects. Updated 1 October, 1997. Access date 18 April, 2001. http://www4.law.cornell.edu/cfr/45p46.htm

4. National Institutes of Health. Protection of human subjects: Categories of research that may be reviewed by the Institutional Review Board (IRB) through an expedited review procedure. *Fed Regist* 63(216):60364–60367, 1998.

5. Shelton JD. How to interpret the federal policy for the protection of human subjects or "Common Rule" (Part A). *IRB: A Review of Human Subjects Research* 21(6):6–9, 1999.

6. Bickman L, Rog DJ. *Handbook of Applied Social Research Methods.* Thousand Oaks: Sage Publications; 1998.

7. Aday LA. *Designing and Conducting Health Surveys: A Comprehensive Guide,* 2nd ed. San Francisco: Jossey-Bass Publishers; 1996.

8. Rossi PH, Wright JD, Anderson AB. *Handbook of Survey Research.* Orlando: Academic Press; 1983.

9. McDowell I, Newell C. *Measuring Health: A Guide to Rating Scales and Questionnaires,* 2nd ed. New York: Oxford University Press; 1996.

10. Dillman DA. *Mail and Internet Surveys: The Tailored Design Method,* 2nd ed. New York: John Wiley & Sons; 2000.

11. Fink A. *The Survey Handbook.* Thousand Oaks: Sage Publications; 1995.

12. Fowler FJ. *Improving Survey Questions: Design and Evaluation.* Thousand Oaks: Sage Publications; 1995.

13. Lehtonen R, Pahkinen EJ. *Practical Methods for Design and Analysis of Complex Surveys,* Revised Edition. New York: John Wiley & Sons; 1996.

14. Henry GT. *Practical Sampling.* Newbury Park: Sage Publications; 1990.

15. Hartley SF. Sampling strategies and the threat to privacy. In: Sieber JE (ed.). *The Ethics of Social Research: Surveys and Experiments.* New York: Springer-Verlag; 1982:167–189.

16. Singer E. Informed consent: Consequences for response rate and response quality in social surveys. *Am Soc Rev* 43(12):144–162, 1978.

17. Loo CM. Vulnerable populations: Case studies in crowding research. In: Sieber JE (ed.). *The Ethics of Social Research: Surveys and Experiments.* New York: Springer-Verlag; 1982:105–126.

18. Botkin JR. Protecting the privacy of family members in survey and pedigree research. *JAMA* 285(2):207–211, 2001.

19. Beauchamp TL, Childress JF. *Principles of Biomedical Ethics,* 4th ed. New York: Oxford University Press; 1994.

20. Turner AG. What subjects of survey research believe about confidentiality. In: Sieber JE (ed.). *The Ethics of Social Research: Surveys and Experiments.* New York: Springer-Verlag; 1982.

21. Dickert N, Grady C. What's the price of a research subject? Approaches to payment for research participation. *N Engl J Med* 341(3):198–203, 1999.

Research Involving a Medical Device

Erica J. Heath

INTRODUCTION

Although charms and talismans to prevent or cure disease have been used from ancient times, there was rarely any more than anecdotal proof as to their safety or efficacy. Along with other machinery, by the mid-1900s it became easier and cheaper to manufacture, distribute, and advertise devices on a large scale. After a brief history, this chapter describes the major components that distinguish the device regulations from the drug regulations, issues raised in clinical investigations of devices, and finally, the very critical and central role that institutional review boards (IRBs) play in the regulation of medical devices.

History

As is often the case, the congressional mandate to regulate devices followed several publicized scandals—lead poisoning of infants from lead nipple shields, women harmed by pessaries that punctured the uterus, and various prophylactics that failed.[1] In 1938, Congress granted the Food and Drug Administration (FDA) the authority to seize misbranded devices to protect people from "fraudulent claims." Multiple seizures were made, but little could be accomplished because of the very limited mandate. For example, in the late 1940s, Dr. Dinshah Ghadiali sold the Spectrochrome,[2] a 1,000-watt lamp in a cabinet with colored glass slides, purported to cure diabetes, cancer, tuberculosis, and syphilis. It sold for $90 with much literature. The FDA made multiple seizures and initiated criminal actions. In the mid-1960s, the FDA began an action to seize the Diapulse, a heat-generating device marketed for 121 therapeutic claims with no data for any. The court case was lengthy, with an injunction being issued in 1972.

By the late 1960s, the FDA was concentrating on the safety of medical devices, but without any additional mandate beyond seizure for misbranding, their task was difficult. In fact, in several cases—a nylon ligature[3] and a cardboard antibiotic sensitivity test[4]—they successfully argued that devices were drugs in order to regulate them. For other devices, such as the Dalkon shield, intraocular lenses, and cardiac pacemakers with serious defects, such arguments were unsuccessful, and the devices could not be regulated.

In 1969, the Department of Health, Education, and Welfare (now the Department of Health and Human Services) formed a medical device study group chaired by Dr. Theodore Cooper. The Cooper Committee studied the problems, the range of kinds of devices, and the medical device business environment and published their findings and recommendations. Among the recommendations they proposed were (1) the classification of devices according to the amount of regulation needed, (2) peer review of new devices with a specific view toward protection of potential patient users, and (3) review efforts in proportion to potential harms.

The next FDA commissioner, the same Dr. Cooper, had little trouble implementing the Cooper Committee recommendations, culminating in the Medical Device Amendments of 1976.[5] A new unit called the Bureau of Devices (now known as the Center for Devices and Radiologic Health [CDRH]) was formed within the FDA. Concepts forged for regulation of devices differ significantly from drug regulations that were their precursor:

1. Devices were defined and distinguished from drugs.
2. Three classes of devices were identified based on the need for regulatory control.
3. Several routes to market were defined.
4. Several types of exemption were allowed for investigational devices.
5. Decisions external to the FDA were allowed concerning which devices posed enough risk to merit submission to the FDA for prior review.

One good review of the history of device regulations is the 1976 Report by the House Committee on Interstate and Foreign Commerce;[1] it can be found in a 1976 Food and Drug Law Institute publication. A second resource, which is far more fun, is the Museum of Questionable Medical Devices now located at the Science Museum in

Minneapolis. Many of the devices on display in the museum can be seen at their website.[2]

Definition of a Medical Device

An elementary feature distinguishing drugs from medical devices is that one can interact chemically with the body, whereas the other cannot. This, however, leaves a large intermediate territory. The second element is that a medical device is a device that is being studied or promoted for a medical purpose.

Combination devices[6] such as pumps or patches delivering drugs might be classified as either drugs or devices depending on which part is investigational. As this decision makes a substantial difference in the requirements that must be met to go on the market, it is a core element in sponsor strategy. On December 24, 2002, an Office of Combination Products (http://www.fda.gov/oc/combination/) was formed within the FDA.

In vitro diagnostic test kits (IVDs) are medical devices http://www.fda.gov/cdrh/oivd/regulatory-overview.html[7][Sec.809] Their regulatory status depends on their intended use. When they are used for a medical diagnosis, an IVD is of IRB interest. Nonmedical laboratory use generally is not of IRB interest. Radiologic products that introduce energy are regulated as devices.

Code of Federal Regulations— Medical Device

All of the regulations about medical devices are found in the Code of Federal Regulations, Title 21, Part 800 through Part 1050.[7] The most critical section to IRBs are 21 CFR 812.2, 812.3, and 812.66. In many ways, the device regulations are similar to the drug regulations. However, because of their uniqueness and their history, several important distinctions are made.

Classification of Devices[7][Sec.862,892]

In 1976, the FDA identified about 1,100 device manufacturers responsible for about 8,000 devices on the market, none of which had been reviewed for safety or effectiveness. Although most of those devices were not known to have caused any harm, a literature search for the Cooper Committee found 10,000 injuries over 10 years with 751 fatalities.

The Medical Device Amendments of 1976 established three classes for devices reflecting the level of regulation thought to be required to establish that a device was "safe and effective" and the control required to maintain this assurance. In practice, the levels of risk and control are generally equivalent. Over the next decade, all of the 8,000 or so devices that had been on the market as of May 26, 1976, were classified into classes I, II, or III within 16 specialty groups.[7][Sec.862,892]

Class I—General Controls

Many devices need very little regulation to assure that they are safe and effective. Basic controls such as those on manufacturing and claims were expected to be sufficient. (Examples include crutches, band-aids, cast components.)

Class II—General Controls Plus Special Controls

The largest device category, this encompasses those device types that could be considered to be safe and effective if they met class I restrictions and if there were some additional standards according to the kind of device. Examples of devices include magnetic resonance imager and methyl methacrylate for cranioplasty.[7][Sec.882.5300] The special controls might include special labeling requirements, additional performance standards, or the addition of postmarket surveillance.

Class III—General Controls Plus Premarket Application

This class most resembles the traditional IND-to-NDA track of drugs. Class III devices are the most interesting ones for IRBs. These are devices about which there is insufficient information to determine that they are safe and effective. Any "new" devices (i.e., they are not substantially equivalent to any prior device) about which there are few or no data are automatically class III.

One hundred seventeen preamendment devices that were determined to be in class III were allowed to remain on the market without demonstrating safety or efficacy with the caveat that, at any time, the FDA could ask for a submission of clinical data. This has been done in several cases. Because data on intraocular lenses were requested before the final device regulations were published, they had their own regulation. Silicone gel breast implant data were requested in April 1991, causing manufacturers to create large adjunct and core studies to gather information on a product already being marketed.

Registration and Listing[7][Sec.807]

Device manufacturers must register all their manufacturing facilities. This registration allows the FDA to conduct manufacturing inspections. Manufacturers must also submit a complete product list annually. This registration and listing make it possible for the FDA to inspect facilities and devices; failure to register or list has resulted in at least one criminal conviction. For example, in one case in 1994,[8] failure to properly register, concealment of adverse patient information, making product changes without FDA permission, and illegally testing products on humans resulted in criminal action against the manufacturer.

Tracking[7][Sec.821]

The FDA can impose additional tracking requirements to market clearance for some devices, most of which are implants. This happens primarily when it is thought to be necessary to track patients so that they can be contacted in the event of a recall. Generally, this activity does not qualify as research, and it is rarely seen by an IRB.

Quality Systems[7][Sec.820]

Manufacturers of devices must meet general quality standards to produce their devices. The systems must be thoroughly documented in master files. FDA inspections of registered manufacturing sites are conducted under this section. Compliance is required for the manufacture of investigational devices as well and is a part of the FDA decision about marketing.

Table 10.8.1   Routes by Which a Device Can Reach the Market

- PMA

    Traditional, Modular, or Streamlined

- Premarket Notification (510k) Substantial Equivalence

- Exempt from 510k Premarket

- Extension of Product Line

- HDE

- Reclassification

Charging[7][Sec.812.7(b)]

Device manufacturers may recover costs by charging subjects or investigators a price no larger than that necessary to recover costs of manufacture, research, development, and handling of a device. Medicare may cover these added costs through an agreement between Medicare Centers for Medicare and Medicaid Services and the FDA. The FDA provides a category: either A (experimental–risk unknown) or B (investigational–risks known enough to allow use for treatment–generally classes I or II and some class III). The category assigned is in all IDE letters. Medicare will determine the amount to be reimbursed. Although other insurers are not covered by the agreement, many follow suit.

Routes to Market[7][Sec.814]

As with drugs, before a medical device can be shipped in interstate commerce, it must be cleared for market by the FDA. Unlike drugs, devices can receive market clearance through multiple regulatory routes. Although Congress and the Cooper Committee agreed that the drug IND-to-NDA (investigational new drug to new drug application) model was appropriate for higher risk devices, it was thought to be too cumbersome and expensive for less risky devices that were often manufactured by very small companies without the resources for a long regulatory process. Thus, there are three routes to market.

Premarket Approval (PMA)

This is the device equivalent of the NDA following clinical trials to determine safety and efficacy. Clinical trials are generally required.

Substantial Equivalence[7][Sec.807E]

The 1976 medical device law, provided a shorter clearance process. A company can make a claim (now known as "510k") to the FDA, indicating that its device is "substantially equivalent" to a predicate device. If such a claim is accepted by the CDRH, the new device can join the predicate device already on the market. A device cleared by the FDA under a 510k can be *sold without demonstration of safety or efficacy or, in fact, without ever having been constructed*! The FDA will issue a determination letter within about 90 days for a 510k for a specific indication.

Exempt from 510k

The FDA also maintains a list of those devices that are exempt from 510k. These may go to market without requesting clearance. Class I devices, for instance, are exempt from the need to obtain a 510k before being sold.

Extension of a Product Line

If a company extends its product line (e.g., different sizes of a product), it is allowed to add that new form of the product to its catalog. These become part of the complete product list required in the manufacturer's annual report.

Reclassification

A brand new device (i.e., not substantially equivalent to another predicate device) is automatically in class III. The sponsor may present sufficient safety and efficacy data to request that the FDA reclassify it as a class II device.

Humanitarian Use

Similar to an orphan drug, the humanitarian use device (HUD) was added to the regulations in 1996.[7][Sec.814.100] To qualify for HUD designation, the indication must be for a disease or condition that affects fewer than 4,000 people in the United States per year. To obtain HUD designation, a humanitarian device exemption (HDE) must be submitted to the FDA and approved. A HUD designation plus an approved HDE allows marketing "notwithstanding the absence of reasonable assurance of effectiveness that would otherwise be required. . . . Although this is a product cleared for market, an HDE requires IRB approval." Humanitarian devices and device exemptions are the subject of a separate chapter in this book.

Clinical Investigation of a Medical Device

Rule: A medical device may not enter into interstate commerce until it receives FDA clearance for marketing. Interstate commerce is presumed in the case of medical devices.

Problem: How can a device be shipped across state lines for use by investigators before it is cleared?

Answer: Regulation 21 CFR 812 allows exemptions from this rule.

Modified Rule: No medical device can be shipped in interstate commerce without (1) being cleared for market (including an HDE) or (2) obtaining an exemption from the ban on interstate shipment.

Clinical data are required for submission with a PMA. Although no clinical data were required originally to substantiate a 510k claim of substantial equivalence, the FDA has increasingly requested preclearance (or postclearance) studies for safety and efficacy. Manufacturers may also perform studies for ergonomics, feasibility, preference, and acceptability and for clarity of instructions.

A common point of confusion between companies and IRBs occurs when there is no agreement (and no awareness of the lack of agreement) as to the regulatory definitions used. An institution following the Common Rule[9] would need submission of "research" to its IRB. Because the Common Rule definition of research is broader than the FDA definition of a clinical investigation, sponsors may not consider their activity to be research. For instance, under the FDA, the term *research subject* has little to do with the identifiability of samples. A test of an in vitro diagnostic kit by a laboratory may be seen as having no subjects

Table 10.8.2 Exemptions Allowing Premarket Use of a Product

- IDE
- Abbreviated IDE
- Exemption from IDE
- Nonresearch: Emergency use-one time, early expanded access

because there are no humans receiving a test article or being a control.

As recommended by the Cooper Committee, there are multiple levels of device exemptions that allow preclearance shipment. The degree of regulation for investigational devices was designed to be in proportion to their perceived risks or their circumstances.

Investigational Device Exemption (SR IDE)

Any device found to pose a significant risk of harm by the sponsor by any reviewing IRB or by the FDA must have an IDE. The IDE may be requested either before or after IRB submission; thus, IRB approval contingent on receipt of the FDA's IDE letter is not unusual. As with INDs, the FDA cannot discuss any aspect of an IDE with the IRB. (As of March 2001, there is discussion that this may change.)

Abbreviated IDE (NSR)[7[Sec. 812.2(b)]]

An abbreviated IDE is "considered to have an approved application for an IDE." Section 812.2.b lists seven sponsor requirements. The second affects the IRB: "Sponsor obtains IRB approval of the investigation after presenting the reviewing IRB with a brief explanation of why the device is not a significant risk device, and maintains such approval."[7] (Expedited review is allowed for study of a device where no IDE is required. As an abbreviated IDE is considered to be an IDE, it is presumed that full-board action is necessary.)

Exemption from an IDE[7[Sec. 812.2(c)]]

A device can be exempt from the IDE requirements. (An exemption from an exemption?) A claim that the device is exempt should be justified through reference to the exemption category being claimed. The exemption most commonly claimed is for diagnostic devices.[7[Sec. 812.2(c)(3)]] (An exemption from the IDE requirement of Part 812 is *not* an exemption from IRB review [Part 56] or informed consent [Part 50]. Studies of devices that are IDE exempt may be eligible for expedited review and, perhaps, for waiver of informed consent, but these are questions for the IRB to consider.)

Emergency Exception: Treatment Use of an Investigational Device[7[Sec.812.36]]

Very similar to an emergency use of an investigational drug, a device may be used for a serious or life-threatening condition where there is no appropriate alternative. Investigators and sponsors must comply with Parts 50 and 56,[7[Sec. 812.36(e)]] although there is little guidance concerning IRB evaluation of such an application. Most IRBs have written policies regarding emergency use of an investigational drug, which can be extended to devices.

Role of the Institutional Review Board

The use of 21 CFR 50 and 56 (or 45 CFR 46) is routine for IRBs; the application of 21 CFR 812 is considerably more difficult. These concepts and definitions are easier to understand if the three parts are separated and considered independently.

The three steps for review of a device submission are as follows:

Step 1. Is the Study Approvable? Are the Consent Form and Process Approvable?[10]

The primary purpose of any IRB is to protect the rights and welfare of the human subject. Thus, the primary IRB question remains whether the criteria for approval in the regulations and in the IRB's own written policies have been met. If the review criteria cannot be met, the study cannot be approved, and further work by the IRB (aside from assistance to the investigator) is not justified.

Occasionally, IRBs have had difficulty with the risk/benefit evaluation because of the design of the device trial. Although there are well-controlled studies of devices, a greater number of activities are more developmental in nature and are designed and run by technical instead of clinical personnel. Instead of making a drug and progressing through set stages, many device trials are done to learn more about whether the instructions are understandable, whether the ergonomics are correct, or whether the device does what it was intended to do. Therefore, the range of designs is much broader for studies of medical devices than for drugs.

The FDA may impose postapproval requirements.[7[Sec.814.80]] Often these are for continuing evaluation of the safety, effectiveness, or reliability of the device for the intended use. These may be mistaken for marketing or seeding studies rather than mandated requirements. The requirements and the reasons for them should be included with the FDA's approval letter, which the IRB may request.

Postapproval review is required for humanitarian devices. This review is particularly confusing because there is no research objective or design, no investigational device, no subjects, no study harm, or benefits. The review criteria cannot be applied as would seemingly be required. The primary reason seems to be to give notice to the institution that an HUD will be used.

HUD clearance letters contain a strong suggestion that there be further study of efficacy. The distinction between clinical treatment with an HUD and a research study should be clear to the HUD physician/investigator, the IRB, and the patient/subject.

Under 21 CFR 50 and the Common Rule, the IRB determines whether the consent process and form are appropriate. Under device regulation, however, the documents to be used to inform subjects are a part of the IDE request submitted to the FDA.[7[Sec.812.20(b)]] Many sponsors contend, incorrectly, that this means the consent materials cannot be changed by the IRB. They can be.

Step 2. Is the Regulatory Status Clear?

A drug study requires an IND; a device study requires an IDE or an exemption from the IDE. It is the applicant's responsibility—with assistance from the sponsor—to make the regulatory status of the device clear. The sponsor has access to strategic information, decisions by other IRBs, and previous FDA decisions and should be able to state clearly the intended route to market and the type of investigational exemption being sought.

The various exemptions were previously discussed; IRB actions differ depending on the type of IDE sought. Knowing the regulatory status dictates the action an IRB must take.

Significant Risk IDE

A sponsor may decide that a device poses a serious risk of harm and elect to file for an IDE. If any IRB determines that the device poses a significant risk (SR), it must be submitted to the FDA for an IDE. Making an SR decision has the potential to have a substantial impact on the sponsor. If an IDE is claimed, an IDE letter from CDRH referencing the device and the indication should be submitted before final IRB approval.

Abbreviated IDE—Nonsignificant Risk (NSR)[7][Sec.812.2(b)]

Central to an abbreviated IDE application is the need for the IRB to agree with the applicant's NSR contention. Sponsors may believe—reasonably or not—that the device does not pose a serious risk of harm to subjects. In this case, they may elect to seek an abbreviated IDE. If the claim is acceptable to the IRB and the study is approvable, the study may be approved and conducted. No report to FDA is required until the data are submitted. The IRB may, however, decide that the claim is not justified and ask for a better justification. Just as study disapproval should not occur without presenting the investigator with written reasons, the IRB should not make a final SR determination without presenting the rationale and reviewing the response.

As the difference in development time can be substantial, sponsors have a major interest in obtaining the abbreviated IDE. However, at the end of a study, the data must be presented to the FDA, and if the FDA disagrees with the NSR decision, the agency could ask for more or different data. The risk of an inappropriate decision is primarily an economic risk borne by the sponsor.

Exemption from the IDE[7][Sec.812.2(c)]

Sponsors claiming an exemption should be asked to clearly state which exemption is being claimed. The most common is for a diagnostic device. An exemption from the IDE requirement is not equivalent to an exemption from the IRB review requirement.

Step 3. Is It a Nonsignificant Risk Device?

The congressional rationale for the abbreviated IDE was that there should be a lower level of regulatory structure for devices that pose less risk. The IRB was named as an impartial body to decide what was risky enough to require submission. This triage by the IRB act would lessen the FDA workload and speed the time to approval. This provides a constant tension between IRBs, sponsors, and the FDA. If the IRB agrees with the sponsor's NSR contention, the study can proceed without any further notice to the FDA. No information (other than registering the manufacturing establishment and listing marketed devices) needs to go to the FDA. If the IRB disagrees with the contention and determines that the device is an SR device, the study may not start at that (or any other) site until the FDA has reviewed and either granted the IDE or determined that the device is, in fact, NSR.

If the sponsor believes that an abbreviated IDE is justified and it is willing to meet all seven requirements, it should provide the IRB with a statement saying that it contends that the device, as it is to be used in the context of the named protocol, poses a nonsignificant risk of harm to the subjects. The sponsor should then back up this claim. The documentation could be (1) an NSR determination made by the FDA, (2) inclusion on an FDA list of NSR devices (in their Information Sheets[11] in the section titled "Significant risk and nonsignificant risk—medical device studies"), or (3) a thorough risk analysis and a request for an IRB determination of NSR.

The NSR determination is critical to the sponsor; it is a major point on a critical path, and it can substantially alter development time. Sponsors tend to seek the speediest and least restrictive route to market, and the FDA tends to seek the most protective route. The IRB is in the middle.

Making the NSR Decision[7][Sec.812.3(m)]

The significant risk device definition has four elements each modified by the phrase "and presents a potential for serious risk to the health, safety or welfare of a subject." Grammatically, if it presents a serious risk of harm, it is an SR device; that is, an SR device is one that presents a serious risk of harm and an NSR device is one that is not found to be SR.

> 'Significant risk device' means an investigational device that:
> (1) Is intended as an implant *and* presents a potential for serious risk to the health, safety, or welfare of a subject;
> (2) Is purported or represented to be for use in supporting or sustaining human life *and* presents a potential for serious risk to the health, safety, or welfare of a subject;
> (3) Is for a use of substantial importance in diagnosing, curing, mitigating, or treating disease, or otherwise preventing impairment of human health *and* presents a potential for serious risk to the health, safety, or welfare of a subject; *or*
> (4) Otherwise presents a potential for serious risk to the health, safety, or welfare of a subject. . . ."

The first step requires a risk analysis. All of the possible and theoretical harms should be considered in terms of their potential frequency, their severity, and their permanence. The sponsor is in the best position to have the information but is not required to prepare a Report of Prior Investigations (similar to the Investigator's Brochure) except for submission of an IDE. Because a report of prior investigations is not required for submission of a 510k or for an NSR request, an IRB may need to ask for the information.

The crucial question is which of the identified risks to factor into the evaluation. Although the regulations define an SR device, the FDA guidance[12] alters the language in an important manner. It refers to a "significant risk device study." The distinction is important. Should the risks in the risk analysis be limited to one, two, or all of the following?

1. Risks from the underlying condition
2. Risks from clinical patient care
3. Risks from monitoring tests to evaluate the research results
4. Risks of the baseline device if there is one
5. Risks from the investigational form of the device
6. All of the above

The position stated in the FDA guidance is, quite logically, the more conservative view: all of the study risks must be considered. The position of the sponsor is, quite logically, the less conservative view. It is possible to have an NSR decision for study of a non-risky device (e.g., a monitor) within the context of a high-risk study.

Should It Have Been SR Rather Than NSR?

An ongoing concern is what happens if the NSR decision is "wrong." Generally, this is unknown until after the study is underway. One of three things may occur.

1. The FDA learns of the decision and disagrees. This may occur through the sponsor's submission of data; through an IRB, investigator, or sponsor audit; or in other conversation. If the IRB has made a decision in good faith, according to written policies, and with good documentation, there is little likelihood of the IRB being found to be wrong—only incorrect.

2. The same set of conditions is presented to another IRB, which determines that the device (or device study) is SR rather than NSR. In this case, the SR decision is of higher rank and the study must be submitted to the FDA. If a study hiatus might harm enrolled subjects, it is best to halt enrollment (although not follow-up or continued necessary treatment) and to call the FDA for a rapid consultation.

3. Experience suggests that there is harm. If significant new information shows up in the form of an adverse effect, the sponsor and the IRB have an obligation to reexamine the decision. The IRB may decide to change the decision from NSR to SR based on the significant new information.

In 1976 Congress and the FDA asked IRBs to perform the triage function. It was in an era in which it was unusual for IRBs to seek external consultants. IRBs were recognized as a diverse group generally without biomedical engineers or specific experts. Certainly they recognized that such a group of people would need to make these decisions with the resources and information at hand. Realistically, IRBs will do the best they can but they will reach conclusions inconsistent with those the FDA might have made. The IRB must decide whether the risks constitute a serious or significant risk to the subject. *This is a judgment left to the IRB. Each IRB must have its own written policies and procedures for making this decision.*

Conduct of an Investigational Device Study

After the IRB finds that the study is approvable (Parts 50 and 56) and that the device regulatory requirements (Part 812) have been met, the study may proceed. The postapproval requirements are, again, based on the investigational drug requirements but are slightly different.

Responsibilities of the Sponsor[7][Sec.812.40]

Instead of an FD 1572, the sponsor must obtain a signed investigator's agreement. Although the elements are dictated,[7][Sec.812.43] some of the responsibilities are different and financial disclosure is included. Because of the presence of financial information, some sponsors claim that this agreement is confidential. Because there is no section on transfer of responsibilities to a contractor, the use of contract research organizations is less common, although involvement of clinical or regulatory consultants is more common.

Responsibilities of the Investigator[7][Sec.812.100]

Investigator responsibilities are set out in the investigator's agreement rather than the FD 1572.

Adverse Device Effects[7][Sec.812.3(s),46(b),150(a)(1)]

Instead of an adverse event, devices may have an "unanticipated adverse device effect." As noted in multiple reports,[13,14] the difficulty in applying different standards makes assessment of safety issues difficult. Instead of safety reports from sponsors via the investigator, device sponsors are asked to report evaluation of "unanticipated adverse device effects" directly to the reviewing IRBs within 10 working days of their receipt of the information. If an IRB determines that the new information gained in the adverse effect reports changes their risk assessment, the IRB has the ability to reconsider its prior NSR decision and ask for FDA review.

Final Reports[7][Sec.812.150(a)(6)]

Unlike drug investigators, device investigators must submit a final report to the IRB within 3 months of termination or completion of the study.

Conclusion

Although device studies are often thought to be difficult, they are really quite similar to drug studies. When reviewing a device protocol, the IRB should ask two questions.

1. Is this study approvable using the standard IRB review criteria found in the Common Rule and in 21 CFR 50 and 56, and the institutional policies?

2. What is the regulatory status of the device?

The investigational device regulations are all contained in Title 21, Code of Federal Regulations, Part 812. Sections 812.2 and 812.3 are most important for IRB review. Unlike drugs, a device may follow one of several paths to FDA market clearance.

The SR/NSR decision is a critical factor to sponsors because it makes a considerable difference in the time and money necessary to develop the device. The IRB must have written policies and procedures for rendering the SR/NSR decision and must document each decision.

Resources

1. FDA Device Advice Page.
   http://www.fda.gov/cdrh/devadvice/index.html

References

1. 94th Congress. Report No. 94-853 by the House Committee on Interstate and Foreign Commerce (to accompany HR 11124), 29 February, 1976. Reprinted in O'Keefe DF, Spiegel RA, Murphy EG. *An Analytical Legislative History of the Medical Device Amendments of 1976: An Amendment to the Federal Food, Drug, and Cosmetic Act.* Washington, DC: Food and Drug Law Institute; 1976.

2. Museum of Questionable Medical Devices. Updated 20 January, 2001. Access date 18 April, 2001. http://www.mtn.org/quack/welcome.htm

3. U.S. Court of Appeals for the 2nd Circuit. *AMP Inc v. John W. Gardner, Secretary of HEW, and James L. Goddard, Commissioner of Food and Drugs* (389 F.2d 825). 1968. Affirmed.

4. U.S. Supreme Court. *United States v. Bacto-Unidisk* (394 US 784). 1969. Reversed.

5. 94th Congress. Medical Device Amendments of 1976. Public Law No. 94-295. 1976.

6. U.S. Food and Drug Administration. Office of Combination Products. Access date 18 August, 2005. http://www.fda.gov/oc/combination/

7. Code of Federal Regulations. Title 21, Chapter 1—Food and Drug Administration, DHHS; Subchapter H—Medical Devices; Parts 800 through 898. Updated 1 April, 1999. Access date 18 April, 2001. http://www.accessdata.fda.gov/scripts/cdrh/cfdocs/cfcfr/CFRSearch.cfm?CFRPartFrom=800&CFRPartTo=1299

8. U.S. Supreme Court. *United States v. C.R. Bard, Inc.* (848 F. Supp. 287). 1994.

9. Code of Federal Regulations. Title 21, Chapter 1—Food and Drug Administration, DHHS; Part 56—Institutional Review Boards. Updated 1 April, 1999. Access date 27 March, 2001. http://www4.law.cornell.edu/cfr/21p56.htm

10. Code of Federal Regulations. Title 21, Chapter 1—Food and Drug Administration, DHHS; Part 50—Protection of Human Subjects. Updated 1 April, 1999. Access date 18 April, 2001. http://www4.law.cornell.edu/cfr/21p50.htm

11. Food and Drug Administration. Information sheets: Guidance for institutional review boards and clinical investigators, September 1998. Access date 9 April, 2001. http://www.fda.gov/oc/oha/IRB/toc.html

12. Food and Drug Administration. Guidance sheets: Significant risk and nonsignificant risk medical device studies, September 1998. http://www.fda.gov/oc/oha/IRB/toc.html

13. National Bioethics Advisory Commission. Ethical and policy issues in research involving human participants. Report and recommendations, 20 August, 2001. Access date 31 August, 2001. http://bioethics.gov/human/overvol1.html

14. Office of Inspector General, DHHS. Protecting human research subjects: Status of recommendations (OEI-01-97-00197), April 2000. Access date 31 August, 2001. http://oig.hhs.govoei/reports/a447.pdf

CHAPTER 10-9

Humanitarian Use Devices

Robert J. Amdur

INTRODUCTION

In 1996, the Food and Drug Administration (FDA) finalized regulations regarding humanitarian use devices (HUD). The purpose of the HUD classification is to encourage the development of devices to treat or diagnose conditions that occur infrequently. When the market potential of a medical device is limited, the expense associated with extensive clinical testing is likely to discourage product development. HUD regulations are to medical devices what orphan drug laws are to medications. The HUD classification gives sponsors a mechanism for making beneficial devices available for general use without the level of testing that is required for FDA approval by other mechanisms. The process for FDA approval of a medical device is the subject of Chapter 10-8.

The HUD Classification

Information on the regulations related to HUDs may be obtained by contacting the FDA Center for Devices and Radiological Health. The specific website for HUDs is http://www.fda.gov/cdrh/ode/hdeinfo.html. All information presented in this chapter is taken from the information presented on their website on February 1, 2001.

An HUD is a device intended to benefit patients by treating or diagnosing a disease that affects fewer than 4,000 individuals in the United States per year. To be considered for HUD status, a device sponsor must complete a humanitarian device exemption (HDE) application. The HDE is similar to an FDA premarket approval application with the exception that an HDE application is not required to present evidence of effectiveness to the degree that is required for FDA approval under other conditions. Specifically, an HDE application is not required to contain the results of appropriately conducted clinical investigations. However, an HDE application must contain sufficient information for the FDA to determine that the device does not present an unreasonable risk of illness or injury and the probable benefit from its use justifies the potential risks. In considering an HDE application, the FDA is required to consider the risk/benefit profile of alternative forms of management that are currently available for the condition. The applicant must demonstrate that no comparable devices are available for the use intended for the device in question and that the applicant device could not be brought to market without the conditions of the HDE.

Conditions for Use of an HUD
An approved HDE application authorizes the applicant to market the HUD. The labeling for the HUD must state that the device is an HUD and that the effectiveness of the device has not been demonstrated. FDA regulations require that a local institutional review board (IRB) operating in compliance with FDA regulations approve the use of the HUD to treat or diagnose a medical condition as specified in the HDE application.

Longevity of an Approved HDE
An approved HDE application is valid for as long as the use of the device continues to meet the conditions of the HDE application. HDE applications do not have to be renewed. After an HDE application has been approved, there is no regular correspondence between the applicant and the FDA. The applicant is not required to inform the FDA of use of the device, the outcome of patients treated with the device, or IRB decisions regarding the device.

A Unique Assignment for the IRB

It is important for the IRB, institutional officials, the device sponsor, and local users of the HUD to understand the unique role of the IRB in this setting. This is the only situation where federal regulations require the IRB to approve and monitor an activity that is clearly not research. An approved HDE application authorizes the applicant to market the device and local physicians to use the device to treat or diagnose a medical condition. Research is not required for use of an HUD. As all IRB regulations and guidance documents are written from the point of view of research regulation, the HUD puts the IRB in a position where it must operate without the level of guidance that is the hallmark of the federal IRB system. When evaluating a request to use an HUD for medical treatment or diagnosis outside the setting of a research protocol, each IRB is free to establish its own criteria for IRB approval. Regulatory requirements and issues to consider are listed here.

1. FDA regulations require local IRB approval before use of an HUD.

2. A local IRB may defer to another IRB that has agreed to assume responsibility for reviewing the use of the HUD in the setting in question. All inter-IRB agreements must be documented in writing.

3. The holder of the HDE is responsible for ensuring that the HUD is used only at facilities that have established an IRB that operates in compliance with FDA regulations.

4. The regulations do not require the facility where the HUD is used, the local IRB, or the local user to document that an approved HDE application exists or that the device is to be used as specified in the HDE application. However, I recommend that IRB approval of the use of an HUD be contingent on IRB review of a letter or document from the device sponsor that documents the following 10 items.

   a. The generic and trade name of the device

   b. The FDA HDE number (this is a six-digit number preceded by the letter H)

   c. The date of HUD designation

   d. Indications for use of the device

   e. A description of the device

   f. Contraindications, warnings, and precautions for use of the device

   g. Adverse effects of the device on health

   h. Alternative practices and procedures

   i. Marketing history

   j. Summary of studies using the device

The HDE application contains these basic sections, and it is routine for the sponsor of an HUD to send a document with this information to local IRBs. Therefore, there should never be a situation where an IRB is pressured into approving the use of an HUD without this level of documentation.

5. Although it is not the IRB's responsibility to check HUD information directly with FDA files, the website referenced in the early part of this chapter contains a list of all approved HDEs with most of the information in the above list.

6. There is no time limit on the FDA approval of an HDE.

7. The IRB does not have to approve each individual use of an HUD. The IRB has the discretion to determine the conditions of HUD use. The IRB may approve the use of the device in general, in a specific number of patients, only under specific circumstances, etc. A local IRB may limit the use of the HUD based on any criteria that it deems appropriate.

8. The regulations require that an IRB conduct both initial and continuing review of an HUD. HUD regulations do not specify the interval of continuing review, but it is prudent to assume that this would be interpreted to be at least annually.

9. The regulations do not require informed consent to use an HUD outside the setting of a research protocol. The regulations do not discourage an IRB from requiring informed consent in any situation that it deems appropriate, and decisions of this kind on the part of local IRBs are certainly within the spirit of HUD rules.

10. The IRB should specifically ask for a statement from the local user that the HUD is not being used as part of a research project or clinical investigation designed to collect data to support an FDA premarket approval application. If the HUD is being used in research or a clinical investigation, the IRB must comply with all of the FDA regulations related to IRB review of research. The criteria for IRB approval and informed consent would be as discussed in the other chapters of this book.

Conclusion

Most IRBs have no experience reviewing the use of HUDs. The University of Florida IRB has approved the use of several different HUDs over the past year. I have discussed HUD review with IRB directors at several other institutions that have HUD experience. Most IRB members are uncomfortable approving the use of a HUD outside the setting of a research protocol. When an activity does not involve the research paradigm, the IRB is basically inventing the wheel regarding the standards for IRB approval and the endpoints for determining compliance. All of the IRB directors that I spoke with approved the use of HUDs based on the documentation listed previously here, a requirement for written informed consent stating the unproven status of the device, and a supporting opinion from a local physician who is familiar with the setting in which the device will be used.

Banking of Human Biological Materials for Research

Mark Sobel and Karen Hansen

INTRODUCTION

Institutional review boards (IRBs) face many challenges in the early 21st century, not the least of which is dealing with the role of tissue and specimen repositories in human subject research. Molecular techniques, information generated from the Human Genome Project, and advances in information technology are transforming the practice of medicine into the era of molecular medicine. The public has heightened expectations for the promise of personalized medicine as a result of the explosion of recent scientific discoveries. At the same time, the public is increasingly wary of potential invasions of privacy, including misuse of information derived from research on their tissues with consequent deleterious consequences on health, disability, and life insurance, in addition to loss of employment and social stigmatization.

The special situations and circumstances that apply to the collection, storage, and distribution of human biological materials exist above the general background of the fact that IRBs are faced with both local and national regulations for human subject research and collection of data that are not always harmonious. In the United States, there are three sets of federal regulations through which IRBs must navigate to ensure that research protocols meet minimal standards: the "Common Rule" of most agencies of the Department of Health and Human Services regulations (45 CFR Part 46), Food and Drug Administration (FDA) regulations (21 CFR Part 50), and since April 2003, HIPAA regulations (Office of Civil Rights) governing privacy.

Regulations pertaining to human subject protections apply to the use of specimens that derive from human subjects, not only in clinical trials, but also in basic research studies.

This chapter describes different types of human biological materials, ways in which they can be used in research, types of repositories, the complexity of informed consent rules as they apply to the use of human biological materials, and mechanisms to assess risk in the use of different types of human biological materials in various studies, including "genetic" research and provides some examples of how research using human biological materials has advanced the public health.

Human Biological Materials

Human biological materials range from tissue samples to blood, sputum, urine, bone marrow, and cell aspirates. Commonly used terms in protocols include "tissues" and "specimens." Although some research studies are *prospective* and are designed to use freshly obtained specimens, the vast majority of research studies using human biological materials are *retrospective* and use archived samples that were originally collected during the course of a necessary clinical procedure or collected expressly for establishment of a research tissue repository.

Archived samples may have been frozen at the time of collection or may have been preserved with fixatives that permit long-term storage for decades at room temperature. Often, samples are preserved with formalin and embedded in paraffin wax into small "paraffin blocks" that can be easily accessed. Thin tissue sections can be sliced from such blocks, permitting hundreds or even thousands of samples from a single tissue sample.

Scientists conduct research on human biological materials that have been collected and archived in laboratories of hospitals, medical centers, and repositories; however, the rights of ownership of specimens have not been clearly delineated. A recent analysis of the ownership and use of tissue specimens for research concludes that "because the benefits of medical knowledge derived from tissue research potentially accrue to all individuals and future generations (rather than a single recipient), society may justify an expansive use of these valuable resources for future studies."[1]

Types of Repositories

After tissue samples are collected, they are stored in repositories or "tissue banks." Although some specimens are stored in the frozen state, fixed tissues such as paraffin blocks and histologic slide files are stored at room temperature. Repositories vary in size from small collections under the control of one or a few investigators to departmental collections to large collections of thousands or millions of samples. Repositories should have policies to guarantee the security and confidentiality of samples and the data associated with them. Specific details and examples of operating procedures for repositories appear later in this chapter.

From a regulatory standpoint, the IRB needs to distinguish among (1) repositories of samples collected prospectively for a specific study or possible future research studies, (2) repositories of clinical samples collected during the course of routine medical procedures and that are stored purely for future clinical diagnostic and prognostic purposes, and (3) banks of clinical specimens for which there is excess tissue (beyond that needed for future clinical diagnosis) that may be accessed by researchers.

Oversight of Repositories

The authors recommend that repositories that include tissue samples that will be used in research studies (examples 1 and 2 mentioned previously here) should have policies that regulate the collection, storage, and distribution of samples that are approved by IRBs. Furthermore, IRB review and oversight would be required by OHRP if the research repository activity is federally funded.

Banks of clinical samples that are not intended for research use are generally found in the repositories of pathology departments of hospitals and medical centers. These types of specimen banks are typically not subject to OHRP regulations or IRB review unless the repository is either federally funded or institutional policy requires IRB review and oversight. However, if in a "covered entity," these types of repositories are subject to HIPAA privacy rules. Nonetheless, the College of American Pathologists recommends that pathology departments develop confidentiality, collection, and distribution policies even for repositories of samples stored solely for clinical use and that these policies should be approved by IRBs.[2]

Research Access to Stored Tissues in Repositories

Although human subject protection regulations were originally written to protect subjects from active interventions that are potentially harmful, they are also applicable to the use of human biological materials and it follows that informed consent should be obtained for the use of tissue samples in research studies. However, millions of tissue samples were archived over the past century for future research use without the type of detailed informed consent that is the current standard in the 21st century. An important consideration is that the Common Rule (45 CFR 46) definition of a human subject does not include deceased individuals; therefore, use of autopsy specimens is not considered human subject research under those regulations (however, local regulations or institutional policy may apply) nor is the use of biopsy or other specimens originally collected from living individuals considered human subject research after the individuals are deceased.

IRBs must constantly grapple with the difficulty of assessing risk in the use of subjects' tissue specimens in research studies and whether informed consent requirements can be waived in some situations. In all cases, the IRB should consider the wishes of the subject (personal autonomy) and the type of consent given for the tissue storage in the repository and whether the data associated with the sample will be secure and confidential once released from the repository. Possible risks of a breach of confidentiality for potentially identifiable tissue include loss of health insurance, denial of disability or life insurance, loss of employment, ineligibility for promotion, job demotion, and social stigmatization.

The Common Rule permits the IRB to consider waiving the informed consent in situations in which (1) there is minimal risk, (2) there is respect for the rights and personal autonomy of the individual, (3) it is impracticable to obtain consent (e.g., the samples were archived many years in the past and there is no current means of contacting the individuals), and (4) notification will be made to the individual when possible. In recognition of the potential importance of archived samples for research, the HIPAA privacy regulations that went into effect in 2003 permit the use of unidentifiable samples collected prior to April 14, 2003, without informed consent under certain circumstances. However, where applicable, IRBs should note that current FDA regulations do not permit any waivers of consent.

In assessing risk for use of stored human biological materials, the IRB should consider whether the sample is identifiable. Examples of "unidentifiable" samples are anonymous and anonymized samples. *Anonymous* samples are those that were collected without direct identifiers and involve the lowest level of risk. Although anonymous samples do not directly identify the subject, they may be associated with demographic data. *Anonymized* samples are those that were originally collected with a direct identifier and from which the identifier has been irretrievably stripped from the sample and replaced with a random alphanumeric code. Here again, demographic data may be associated with the sample. An advantage of unidentifiable samples is that their use is not considered human subject research by the Common Rule (45 CFR 46), and there is the lowest level of risk for breach of confidentiality. However, a major disadvantage is that unidentifiable samples cannot be used in long-term follow-up or prognostic studies.

There are two types of identifiable samples. *Identified* samples are those in which the identity can be readily ascertained. Examples of such identifiers include name, social security number, or hospital chart number. More commonly, *coded* or *linked* samples are used in research studies. In this case, the direct identifier is replaced with an alphanumeric code and a key to the code exists. The level of risk in the use of coded samples depends on the security of the key to the code and the policies that govern when, if ever, the code can be broken.

In general, OHRP considers private information or specimens to be identifiable when they can be linked to specific individuals by the investigator(s) either directly or indirectly through coding systems. In its most recent guidance of August 10, 2004 (www.hhs.gov/ohrp/policy/index.html#biol), the OHRP does not consider research involving only coded information or specimens to involve human subjects if the specimens were not collected specifically for the currently proposed research project through an intervention or interaction with living individuals and if the investigator(s) cannot readily ascertain the identity of the individuals to whom the coded private information or specimens pertain. For example, the key to decipher the code may have been destroyed before the research begins. Alternatively, the investigator(s) and the holder of the key (e.g., the repository gatekeeper) may enter into an agreement prohibiting the release of the key to the investigators under any circumstances or until the individuals are deceased (the regulations do not require the IRB to review and approve the agreement). Such an agreement might also require IRB-approved written policies and procedures for a repository or data management center that prohibit the release of the key or other legal requirements prohibiting the release of the key.

In assessing risk and personal autonomy factors, the IRB should consider whether the proposed study involves prospective collection of samples or is retrospective and will use archived samples:

1. Prospective collection of samples:

   a. Collection is solely for the purpose of research: The IRB should determine the safety of the method of collection and the level of pain and discomfort associated with collection and whether the informed consent clearly states the purpose of the study and explains potential risks to breach of confidentiality.

   b. In the vast majority of cases, collection will be a by-product of a necessary medical procedure (e.g., biopsy to diagnose a potential disease, blood or urine samples for clinical laboratory tests) and will not involve an additional intervention. The IRB should determine whether the informed consent permits the storage of excess tissue and clearly states the purpose for such storage and future use. The consent should also specify whether the subject can ask to have their specimen withdrawn from the repository at a later date or not. If specimens are anonymized, for example, the subject should be informed that this request is not possible because there is no link between the individual and the specimen that could allow this request for withdrawal to be met.

2. Retrospective studies of repository samples:

   a. Samples were collected for the sole purpose of research. The IRB must determine whether consent was obtained at the time of collection and the nature of that consent.

   b. Samples were collected as a by-product of a necessary medical procedure.

Another important consideration for IRB evaluation of a research study involving human biological materials is the nature of the study. A common confusion is the use of the term *genetic studies*, which in current parlance includes studies that study DNA or genetic material. However, in assessment of risk, it is critical to distinguish between germline and somatic cells. *Germline* studies have the greatest risk because germline cells represent the inherited potential of the individual and there are implications for the immediate and extended family as well as for ethnic groups. On the other hand, most research studies using human tissues are performed on *somatic cells* of diseased tissues, which may carry mutations that have been acquired during life as a result of environmental insult or injury. There is lower risk associated with somatic cell studies because there are generally no direct implications for previous or future generations.

Value and Importance of Studies Using Human Tissue Archives and Repositories

Research on human biological materials has led to critical discoveries that have improved the public health. The discipline of pathology was born in Renaissance Italy when autopsies were first performed by physicians on their deceased patients. The science of pathology, that is, the systemic study of the causes, mechanisms, and natural history of disease, was developed in the 19th century in Germany by Rudolph Virchow, who applied light microscopy to the study of diseased tissues and developed the cell theory of disease, which is the basis of modern medical research. A useful summary of examples of how archived specimens have been reused by researchers to advance the public health can be found in the *National Bioethics Advisory Commission Report on Research Involving Human Biological Materials*.[3]

Two specific examples of discoveries in the latter half of the 20th century that were based on reuse of archived human tissues that had been collected during the course of medical procedures without specific informed consent to be used for future research are the elucidation of the causes of vaginal and lung cancer. In the 1960s, Dr. Robert Scully at the Mass General Hospital noted an unusual prevalence of an unusual tumor of the vagina (clear cell adenocarcinoma). After carefully looking at the medical records of the patients, Dr. Scully noted that the cancers were appearing in the daughters of mothers who had been treated with the nonsteroidal estrogenic hormone diethylstilbestrol during their pregnancies. Dr. Scully's discovery led to the establishment of a national registry, the early detection of the cancers, and an eventual cure rate of 90%. During the same time period, Dr. Oscar Auerbach in East Orange, New Jersey noted the histopathologic changes in the lungs of autopsied smokers compared to lung cancer and provided the first evidence in human lung tissue of a link between smoking and lung cancer.

More recently, archived specimens have been used to decipher the underlying mechanisms of bronchogenic carcinoma in underground uranium workers, prion diseases, lymphomas and leukemias, and cervical cancer. The applicability of new technologies to microsamples of diseased human tissues offers the promise of new breakthroughs in understanding and managing prevalent diseases of humankind. IRBs play an important role in ensuring that studies to advance the base of biomedical knowledge that use human biological materials are conducted in an ethical manner that protects the human subjects from whom they are derived.

The IRBs Role in Review of Tissue Collection Consent Document, Repository Operations, and Subsequent Oversight of Repository

The IRB review of a tissue repository should include a review of the operating procedures of the repository (e.g., who will have access to stored samples, process to ensure individual research projects will not be conducted without prior IRB review, coding of samples). After consideration issues and several model consent forms, local IRBs may create a tissue collection consent template conforming to institutional requirements. A model consent will make it easier for an investigator when developing the IRB application and documents covering the repository function and activity. When creating the consent template, consider any of the following:

- State regulations (e.g., autopsy consent requirements)
- Federal regulations (e.g., human subject protections, FDA requirements, HIPAA)
- International regulations/guidance (e.g., International Conference on Harmonization)
- Institutional policies that may influence the content of the consent document and/or process. Institutional policy may be more stringent than regulations or other policy guidance published in the public sector.

The core elements of consent required by 45 CFR 46 help guide the development of this model consent. Experience, however, has shown that unique issues need to be evaluated by the IRB when approving repositories established for future research. Issues such as tissue ownership, privacy and confidentiality, mechanisms for withdrawing specimens from the repository, and oversight of future research involving banked specimens are critical for IRB evaluation of the repository operations and informed consent process. If a variety of potential uses are planned for the stored specimens, this needs to be clearly stated. Some organizations have used the opt-in or opt-out method in

the consent document. This method provides individuals contributing their tissue the opportunity to designate:

- Who they agree may use their tissue (e.g., nonprofit research, commercial, specific researcher)
- For what purpose the tissue may be used (e.g., lung cancer, any cancer, any disease)

Sample consent document templates are appended to this chapter.

Guidance for IRB Review of Repository Operations

OHRP developed guidance in 1996[4] that can be found at http://www.hhs.gov/ohrp/humansubjects/guidance/reposit.htm.

The IRB may wish to use this guidance when considering the management of the repository and postapproval access activity.

Additional IRB Approval Required for Each Research Project Accessing Stored Specimens in the Repository

After a repository has received IRB review and approval for banking tissues for research, each subsequent research activity involving human subject research will require an independent IRB review and approval unless the activity is considered not research involving a human subject (no identifiers). The gatekeepers of the repository will need to assure that, where applicable, access to banked specimens occurs only with IRB approval.

Depending on the nature of the study, research specimen access may require additional consent from the individual whose specimen is stored in the repository (e.g., HIV serostatus testing of identifiable specimens). Alternatively, the IRB may determine that a waiver for additional consent is appropriate. In either scenario, documentation of appropriate IRB approvals and efficient gatekeeping of specimen access and use are integral to safeguarding protections to human subjects and their tissues and the ethical advancement of research.

Other Issues

- Use of local tissue banks by commercial organizations: An institution (e.g., academic center or nonprofit) needs to advise the principal investigator overseeing the research repository (and the IRB) if the access and collaboration may include outside users, such as commercial organizations. The institution and in-house investigators may have opposing interests or contractual arrangements that prohibit any possibility of access by outside users. Alternatively, an institution may permit collaboration and access. In either scenario, this administrative issue should be clarified at the time of IRB review of the initial repository application. Furthermore, the consent document signed by individuals contributing human biological material to a research repository should address this issue of access.

- Guidance in the area of repository oversight, tissue use in research, and IRB review responsibilities is evolving. IRB administrators are encouraged to check with federal compliance agencies and professional organizations concerned with human research subject protection to keep up to date with guidance and practice.

References

1. Hakimian R, Korn D. Ownership and use of tissue specimens for research. *JAMA* 292:2500–2505, 2004.

2. Grizzle W, Grody WW, Noll WW, et al. Recommended policies for uses of human tissue in research, education, and quality control: Ad Hoc Committee on Stored Tissue, College of American Pathologists. *Arch Pathol Lab Med* 123:296–300, 1999.

3. Korn D. Contributions of the human tissue archive to the advancement of medical knowledge and the public health. *National Bioethics Advisory Commission Report on Research Involving Human Biological Materials: Ethical Issues and Policy Guidance*, Volume II. Washington, DC: United States Government Printing Office; January, 2000.

4. Office for Protection from Research Risks. Operation of human cell repositories under HHS regulations at 45 CFR 46, 19 August, 1996. http://www.hhs.gov/ohrp/humansubjects/guidance/reposit.htm

Template Consent Language for an Add-On Study Involving Biological Material
(Note: In this scenario the type of testing that is to be done on the material is known and described in the consent document. Do not use this template for consent to donate biological material for future research).

We ask your permission to test your blood or tissue for research
This study includes laboratory tests that will analyze samples of your blood or tissues. [If additional procedures, such as blood draws or biopsies, will be needed for this study then describe them here, including risks]. Blood or tissue samples will be sent to a laboratory where tests will be performed. The purpose of the tests that will be done on your blood or tissue is to determine [complete this sentence].

Will you be given the results of research tests?
The results from these tests will not be sent to you or your doctor, and will not be used in planning your care. You will not be able to find out the results of these tests even if you ask for them. These tests are only for research purposes. [If this not the case then explain the conditions under which subjects or their physicians will have access to these results. If the subject or his or her physician will have access to test results, you must explain the potential risks and implications of this disclosure. When applicable, discuss the need for genetic or psychological counseling before or after the study.]

Do you give us permission to test your blood or tissue?
Please indicate if you agree to participate by circling your response in the box below. You do not have to give permission to use your blood or tissue for research to participate in the other parts of this study. If you do not want your blood or tissue to be tested in this part of the study it will not affect your care at this institution or the ability to receive treatment as part of this study. Please ask questions if you do not understand why we are asking for your permission to use your blood or tissue for research or if you would like more information about any part of this study.

I agree to participate in the part of the study that involves testing of my blood or tissue as described above. *Please circle YES or NO.*

Yes   No

Please print and sign your name here after you circle your answer.

Your name: _____

Your signature: _____ Date: _____

Template Consent Language to Bank Biological Material for Future Research

---

We are asking you to donate your blood or tissue for future research

We are requesting your permission to donate some of your blood or tissue for future research. The blood or tissue samples that will be stored are left over from specimens that were taken, or will be taken, as part of your routine medical care [or as part of this study (if the tissue banking request is an add-on study within a primary study)]. [If additional procedures, such as blood draws or biopsies, will be done to procure the specimens that will be stored, this must be explained along with any associated risks.]

Will the blood or tissue that you donate be tested for diseases?

Some people are worried about their blood or tissue being tested for things that indicate that you have a particular disease or problem, or that a disease or problem is in the genes of your family—for example, a test for AIDS or a test for the gene for a disease called Huntington's chorea. At this time there is no plan to test your blood or tissue for things that indicate that you or your biological relatives have a serious disease or problem. [If this is not the case then describe the relevant tests and the potential implications and risks. When applicable, discuss the need for genetic or psychological counseling before or after the study.]

Will you or your doctor be given research results?

It is very important that you understand that the results from tests that are done on the blood or tissue that you donate for future research will not be given to you or your doctor, even if you ask that this be done. The results of tests that are done on the blood or tissue that you donate for future research will not be sent to your hospital medical record. These tests will be done only for research purposes. [If the subject or his or her physician will have access to research results, then describe the circumstances of this access and the potential implications and risks. When applicable, discuss the need for genetic or psychological counseling before or after the study.]

What research studies will be done on the blood or tissue that you donate?

At this time it is impossible to name all of the kinds of studies that researchers may want to use your blood or tissue for. Any research done on your blood or tissue in the future must be approved by a committee called an Institutional Review Board that is set up to determine that the research is done according to accepted standards.

Will the blood or tissue that you donate be sold in the future?

Your blood or tissue will be used only for research and will not be sold.

Will you be paid for donating blood or tissue for future research?

No. You will not be paid for the blood or tissue that you are now being asked to donate for future research. In the future it is possible that the research that is done on your blood and tissue may help to develop something that is commercially valuable—meaning something that makes a lot of money for somebody. You will not receive payment for commercial activity that results from research with your blood or tissues.

Will you be penalized if you decide not to donate blood or tissue for research?

No. You will not be penalized in any way for not donating blood or tissue for future research. If you decide not to donate blood or tissue for future research it will not affect your medical care [or your ability to participate in the treatment part of this study (if tissue storage is being requested as an add-on study within a primary study)].

Why would you donate your blood or tissue for future research?

Because research with your blood or tissue may lead to discoveries that will help people in the future.

Are there risks to donating your blood or tissue for future research?

Donating your blood or tissue for future research may have no risk. However, a serious risk that should be considered is the possibility that someone will learn things about you that you don't want them to know. It is difficult to estimate if this is a possibility in your case because we don't know exactly what studies may be done on your blood or tissue in the future. However, all reasonable efforts will be made to protect the confidentiality of information that can in any way be connected to you. As in many other kinds of research, certain authorities do have the right to review your research file. In addition to research directors, the people that may have access to your research information are representatives from the U.S. Food and Drug Administration and the Institutional Review Board. The Institutional Review Board is a committee that is set up to determine that research is done according to accepted standards.

Do you have any additional questions?

If you have questions about your rights as a research participant, please call _____

If you have questions about specimen and/or data storage, please call _____

If you have questions about your medical treatment or emergency care, please call _____

Making your choice

Please put an X in the boxes below that indicate if you want to donate your blood or tissue for future research.

❏ **Yes, I will donate my blood or tissue for future research.** *Please also check one of these boxes:*

    ❏ There are no restrictions on the kind of research that may be done with my blood or tissue.

    OR

    ❏ You may use my blood or tissue for future research as long as the only kind of research that is done is research to improve the understanding or treatment of [name specific diseases or conditions].

❏ **No, I do not want to donate my blood or tissue for future research.**

Please print and sign your name here:

Your name: _____

Your signature: _____ Date: _____

The Placebo-Controlled Clinical Trial

Robert J. Amdur and C. J. Biddle

INTRODUCTION

The use of placebo in clinical research studies is currently a topic of active debate in the medical literature.[1,2] High-profile articles appear at regular intervals that criticize the use of placebo in particular patient populations.[1,3–9] At one end of the spectrum is the argument that the current use of placebo is often unethical because alternate study designs would produce results that are of similar value to society with less risk to individual research participants. The counterargument is that current policy regarding the use of placebo is essential to protect society from the harm that would result from the widespread use of ineffective medical treatments. In view of the range of scientific and ethical issues that influence the use of placebo in clinical research, both research investigators and regulatory authorities need better guidelines to determine when placebo therapy is or is not acceptable. This chapter presents a decision algorithm to help interested members of the research community evaluate the ethics of a clinical research trial that involves concomitant placebo control. The algorithm is shown as Figure 10.11.1. The chapter presents (1) concepts and issues related to each major decision point in the algorithm and (2) case discussions to illustrate use of the algorithm in evaluating a wide range of placebo-controlled trials.

Basic Concepts

Formal definitions of placebo are referenced in a 1994 review of the placebo issue by Clark and Leaverton.[10] Basically, a placebo is any medical treatment (or component of a medical treatment) that is inactive for the condition being evaluated other than the effect that may result from a person's thinking that he or she may be receiving an active treatment. Placebo is frequently used as the control group in research studies that are designed to evaluate the efficacy of new medical treatments. The purpose of a control group in a clinical trial is to give the study the ability to distinguish between treatment-specific and treatment-nonspecific effects. The placebo effect, fluctuations in the natural history of the disease over time, and the influence of the study environment are examples of nonspecific treatment effects that may lead to false conclusions about the efficacy of a study treatment. To distribute nonspecific treatment factors equally between study groups, patients in medical trials are often assigned to a treatment group by a process called randomization, which means assignment to a treatment group by a process that involves chance.

The Use of Placebo in Place of Standard Therapy

The first step in evaluating the ethics of a placebo-controlled trial is to decide if placebo is being used in place of standard therapy. Standard therapy may be a type of active treatment (e.g., a medication with treatment-specific activity); supportive care, meaning treatment designed to alleviate symptoms but without specific activity for the underlying medical condition; or no treatment. From the ethical standpoint, the potential problem with placebo therapy is that it exposes patients to a treatment that has no specific activity for their disease. When an available therapy is considered to be beneficial, the use of placebo instead of accepted therapy may be unethical. However, when placebo is being used in addition to standard therapy, as is done in add-on and sequential treatment study

Adapted version of a contribution to *Radiation Oncology Investigations* ©2001 Wiley-Liss, Inc.[23] Used by permission of Wiley-Liss, Inc., a subsidiary of John Wiley & Sons, Inc.

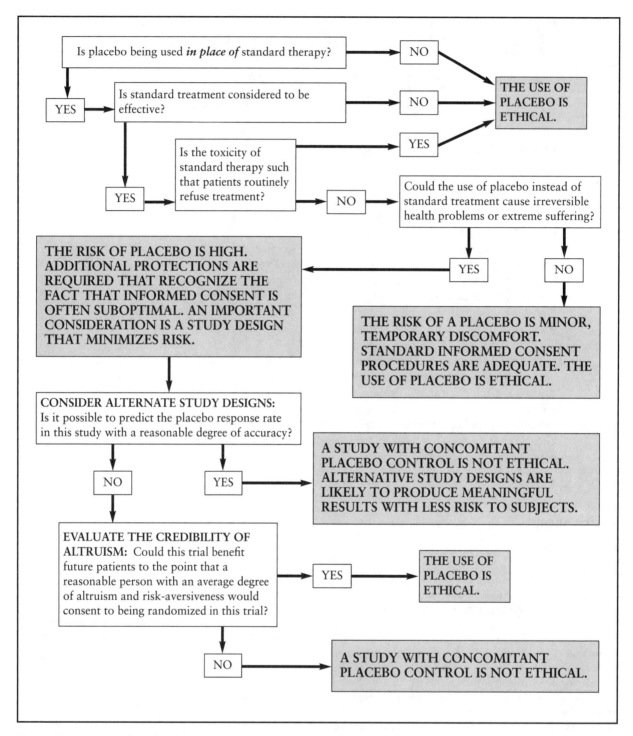

Figure 10.11.1 An algorithm for evaluating studies that use placebo control

designs,[11] there is no ethical tension related to the use of treatment without disease-specific activity.

The Efficacy of Standard Therapy

The second decision point is to determine if standard therapy is considered to be effective. With medical conditions for which there are no good treatment options, there may be legitimate controversy about the value of standard therapy. When standard therapy does not meaningfully improve length or quality of life, it is ethical to enroll informed subjects in research that uses placebo in place of standard treatment. However, when standard therapy is clearly effective in the study population, additional issues must be evaluated to determine whether it is ethical to use placebo in place of standard therapy.

Evaluating the efficacy of standard therapy may not be straightforward because controversy often exists regarding the treatment-specific activity of treatments that are commonly recommended. In the absence of overwhelming evidence, some experts will question the efficacy of treatment that is considered to be beneficial by other segments of the medical community. From the ethical standpoint, a lack of consensus within the overall medical community is less important than the opinion of the local physicians who will be asking patients to participate in research. The practice of medicine is based on the judgment of individual physicians taking care of specific patients. The evidence that a given medical treatment will or will not be effective in a specific patient is often not definitive. For this reason, the efficacy of standard therapy in any given community is best evaluated by asking local physicians how they would manage a patient who decides not to participate in research.

The Toxicity of Standard Treatment

The potential problem with the use of placebo in medical research is that subjects will be denied beneficial treatment. When evaluating the potential benefit of a medical treatment, it is important to consider both efficacy and toxicity. If the toxicity of available treatments is such that patients routinely refuse therapy that is known to have direct activity against their disease process, then it is ethical to conduct research that treats informed subjects with placebo in place of standard therapy. However, when standard treatment is both effective and well tolerated, other factors must be evaluated to determine the ethics of a placebo-controlled medical research trial.

As with treatment efficacy, there may be disagreement within the medical community about the level of toxicity of a given medical treatment in a specific patient population. Opinions about the overall effect of medical treatment are appropriately influenced to a large degree by personal values and individual experience. As discussed previously, from the ethical standpoint the important question is how the physicians who will be enrolling subjects in research view the risk/benefit profile of standard therapy. Again,

the way a physician manages patients outside the setting of a research protocol is likely to be a useful indicator of opinion about the value of alternate therapies.

Temporary Discomfort Versus Irreversible Harm

Much of the recent literature on ethical requirements for the use of placebo has emphasized the importance of making a distinction between the use of placebo in a setting that increases the risk of temporary discomfort and use of placebo in a way that increases the risk of severe morbidity or irreversible health problems.[8,9,11] This distinction is not discussed in federal research regulations or in ethical guidelines like the Nuremberg Code, Declaration of Helsinki, or *The Belmont Report*.[12] The basic concept is that protections that recognize the inherent vulnerability of medical research subjects and the limitations of the informed consent process are needed when the risk associated with placebo treatment is high.[13] In practical terms, this means that the fact that a subject enrolls in a study with a process that complies with the standard requirements for informed consent does not mean that the study is ethical.

Concern about the quality and circumstances of informed consent is not unique to research that involves placebo. An extensive body of literature now supports the view that, in many medical situations, it is not possible to obtain the type of informed consent that is considered to be a requirement for ethical research.[1,5,13,14] When the risk of research participation is high, any imperfection in the consent process has a major effect on research ethics. When the use of placebo carries a risk of irreversible and serious harm, the ethics of research will hinge on the ability of alternate study designs to provide valuable information on the study question with less risk to research subjects.[15,16[Sec.111(a)(1)]]

At the other extreme is the situation where the risk of placebo is limited to minor, temporary discomfort. In this setting, it is appropriate that research standards rely on the informed consent process to create an environment where subjects understand the main implications of their decision to participate in research and important decisions are made without coercion.[8,9,11]

Considering Alternative Study Designs

A fundamental ethical standard is that research should be designed so that the risks to subjects are minimized and reasonable in relation to anticipated benefits.[17] A major element of the placebo controversy is debate over the implications of using alternate study designs to evaluate the efficacy of new medical treatments.[1,3] This is a complex topic without definitive answers to several important questions.

The factors that influence the choice of control group in a clinical trial are discussed in detail in a recent Food and Drug Administration (FDA) guidance document.[11] The two main characteristics of a control group are the type of treatment received and the relationship of the control group to the present study population. In terms of the type of treatment received, the main options are (1) active control, meaning the control group is treated with a therapy that is known to have specific activity in the study setting, (2) placebo, and (3) no treatment.

In terms of the relationship of the control group to the present study population, the basic options are to have a control group that is chosen from the study population (concomitant control) or from an external database. Concomitant control groups are usually selected by a randomization process with blinding of subject and/or health care providers to treatment group. External control groups are usually chosen from previously conducted trials of the study medication in circumstances similar to those of the current study. A control group that is chosen from studies that were completed in the past is called a historical control group.

As a society, we want to design clinical trials to minimize the chance of a false-positive result. The scientific quality of a clinical trial refers to the aspects of the study that influence the credibility and persuasiveness of research results. The remainder of this section will summarize the main arguments that have been made to support the use of placebo control to evaluate the efficacy of medical treatments. When applicable, a point/counterpoint approach is used to explain the different schools of thought on a given subject.

Evaluating Efficacy with Concomitant Active Control

The Value of a Positive Result in a Trial with Placebo Versus Active Control

Point: Scientific quality is superior with a study design that involves concomitant placebo control because it is usually not possible to accurately determine important statistical parameters in a trial that compares a study treatment with an active control. This is especially true in medical conditions where variability in the placebo response rate is known to be high.

The fundamental question is different in a trial with active control than in a trial with placebo control. Trials that randomize subjects between study treatment and placebo use a study design that directly evaluates efficacy. Trials that use active treatment control are classified as noninferiority trials because the goal is to show that the study drug is not less effective than the control by more than a defined amount. A fundamental assumption of a noninferiority trial with active control is that noninferiority is evidence of equivalence.

A major argument against using a noninferiority (equivalence) trial to draw conclusions about treatment efficacy is that there is no accepted way to estimate some of the important statistical parameters needed to minimize the chance of a false-positive result.[11] The main problem is that a noninferiority trial requires an estimate of a parameter called the noninferiority margin, which describes

the degree of inferiority of the study medication (compared with active control) that the trial will attempt to exclude statistically. The value of the noninferiority margin is usually based on past experience in placebo-controlled trials, but clinical judgment also plays a role.

Estimating the noninferiority margin is especially difficult when there is variability in the placebo response rate between trials. For this reason, support for trials with concomitant placebo control is generally strongest in medical conditions where variability in the placebo response rate is likely to be large. There are many medical conditions for which medications that are considered to be effective cannot regularly be shown to be superior to placebo in well-designed clinical trials.[3,11,17,18]

Uncertainty in the design of a clinical trial compromises the credibility of study results. Lack of confidence in the scientific quality of an active-control trial is such that much of the scientific community, including some FDA officials, view a noninferiority trial using active control as a crude tool for evaluating the efficacy of unproven therapy in a wide range of medical conditions.[11,17] People with this point of view argue that trials with concurrent placebo control are essential to protect society from the harm that will result from approving new medical therapies based on false-positive results from noninferiority studies.[4,6,11,17]

Counterpoint: This is an example of a situation where many of the experts are mistaken. The scientific quality of results from placebo-controlled trials is overrated. The value of results from a noninferiority trial with active control is often underrated. Society would not be worse off if the FDA approval of new medical treatments were based on the results of noninferiority trials with comparison to standard therapy (concomitant active control) in many of the situations where concomitant placebo control is currently required.

Arguments that support the use of placebo control in ethically controversial situations frequently include dogmatic statements about placebo-controlled trials being the "gold standard" for evaluating the efficacy of new medical treatments.[19] These kinds of statements imply that a placebo-controlled trial is unquestionably the most accurate way to evaluate treatment efficacy. Critics argue that there is no convincing evidence to support this concept. For example, in a recent review of studies used to support FDA approval of antidepressant medications—a prime example of a situation where experts argue that the large variability in placebo response rate demands the use of placebo control—Michels[3] concluded, "We can see from the data presented that standard therapy is almost always superior to placebo and similar in effectiveness to the investigational drugs that later gained market approval. Thus, therapeutic equivalence trials would have led to the same conclusions regarding effectiveness of the investigational medications as placebo-controlled trials. So why withhold effective treatment that is likely to benefit patients?" In a 1994 article in the *New England Journal of Medicine*, Rothman and Michels[1] commented on statements about the superiority of placebo control that are frequently found in FDA documents and research textbooks: "Without justification, such statements confer on placebo control a stature that ranks it with double blinding and randomization as a hallmark of good science. . . . No scientific principle, however, requires the comparison in a trial to involve a placebo instead of, or in addition to, an active treatment."

Quality Control

Point: In a trial with placebo control, there is a built-in incentive to conduct the study as planned that is not present in a noninferiority study with active control.

A positive result in an efficacy trial with concomitant placebo control means that the outcome is better with the study treatment than with placebo. When the goal of a trial is to detect a *difference* in outcome, a built-in incentive exists for the sponsor of the trial to work hard to see that the study is conducted according to the highest level of quality. This means careful screening of subjects based on eligibility criteria, rigorous monitoring to be sure that treatment is delivered as required by the protocol, selecting and supporting subjects so that the dropout rate is as low as possible, and so forth.

In contrast to a direct efficacy trial, in a noninferiority trial with active control, a positive result is the *lack of a difference* in outcome between study groups. In this situation, the sponsor of the trial has less incentive to enforce compliance with study guidelines because study errors usually act to blur any difference that exists between treatment groups and thus increase the chance of a positive result.[11] As with the other factors mentioned in this section, concern about the value of the results of a trial that compares a study treatment with active control biases many in the research community in favor of efficacy trials with concomitant placebo control.

Counterpoint: Multiple factors determine the overall quality of the results of a clinical research trial. Although a placebo-control design may promote an environment that encourages compliance with the study protocol, other factors favor a study design that compares study treatment with active therapy.

Study Size

Point: A noninferiority trial with active control requires a larger study population than does a trial that directly evaluates efficacy with concomitant placebo control.

Study design and a variety of statistical parameters determine the number of subjects that are required for a trial to detect important differences in the activity of study therapy. Because of variability in the placebo response, the number of subjects required to minimize the possibility of a false-positive result is usually much larger for a noninferiority trial with active control compared to an efficacy study with concomitant placebo control.[11,20] A larger study population may be a negative factor for two reasons. First, the cost of a noninferiority trial may discourage researchers from evaluating new medical treatments; second, a larger study population increases the number of people who may be treated with inferior therapy.[4,11]

Although increased risk is often an argument against placebo-controlled studies, it is important to remember that the study treatment in a noninferiority trial may indeed be inferior to standard therapy.

Counterpoint: Medical progress will not be compromised by the use of active treatment control in clinical trials that evaluate the efficacy of medical treatments.

The factors that serve to decrease the value of results from trials with concomitant placebo control were discussed previously. Several aspects of these arguments suggest that larger clinical trials will meaningfully improve the quality of the treatment evaluation process. Specifically, a larger study population will increase the applicability of study results to the general population and increase the persuasiveness of study results, either positive or negative. There is also the argument that noninferiority trials ask a more important question, from the standpoint of practical value to society and stimulation of medical progress, than do comparisons of study treatment with placebo.[21]

Evaluating Efficacy with Historical Placebo Control

Historical placebo control means that efficacy is evaluated by comparing the results of a study treatment with the results from patients treated with placebo in a previously completed trial. For comparison with historical control to be meaningful, the study population and study conditions must be similar for the trial that evaluates the study treatment and the study that generated the results with placebo control.

The main problem with historical placebo control is the problem common to all studies that attempt to make conclusions based on comparison with the outcome of a group of subjects who were treated under different study conditions: namely, the difficulty in balancing the effect of important nonspecific treatment effects between the current study and the historical control group. The fact that subjects in the study and control group are treated over different time periods (often separated by years or decades) introduces the potential for differences in selection factors, placebo response rate, and study environment to affect subject outcome independent of the direct activity of the study treatment. With the exception of some well-defined situations, the FDA will not approve an application to market a new medication or medical device based on comparison with historical control.[11]

Evaluating the Credibility of Altruism

Probably the most controversial aspect of the placebo debate concerns the trade-off between the welfare of the individuals who will be the subjects of research and the welfare of people in the future who may benefit from research results.[1,5,6,8] Obviously, this tension exists in other areas of research, but the importance of the "individual-versus-society" issue to the placebo debate cannot be overemphasized. In a biomedical research study where the use of placebo increases the risk of irreversible harm, the only way to justify the use of placebo is to argue that it is ethical to increase risk to current subjects to produce information that may benefit people in the future. A major problem with this argument is that it appears to violate fundamental principles of accepted ethical guidelines. For example, the Declaration of Helsinki contains several sections that directly address the individual versus society issue.[22]

Part I (basic principles), point 5: "Every biomedical research project involving human subjects should be preceded by careful assessment of predictable risks in comparison with foreseeable benefits to the subject or to others. Concern for the interests of the subject must always prevail over the interests of science and society."

Part II, point 3: "In any medical study, every patient—including those of the control group, if any—should be assured of the best proven diagnostic and therapeutic method."

Part III (nonclinical research), point 4: "In research on man, the interest of science and society should never take precedence over considerations related to the well-being of the subject."

A *JAMA* article discusses the limitations of published ethical guidelines, including the Declaration of Helsinki.[12] Altruism may be an acceptable reason for a person to participate in research, regardless of the potential for increased risk. However, to accept the altruism argument, one must assume full and voluntary informed consent. When considering this argument, it is important to understand that an extensive body of literature now exists supporting the view that, in many medical situations, the researcher cannot obtain the type of informed consent considered to be a requirement for ethical research.[13,14] The documentation of informed consent is not credible when the nature of the study is such that reasonable people would not volunteer to participate in the research if they had a clear understanding of the implications of their decision.[1,5,13]

No definitive formula can be used to determine when a trade-off between the welfare of individual subjects and future patients is acceptable. Baruch Brody[5] has discussed a "reasonable person" standard for evaluating the ethics of clinical trials. In the context of the placebo discussion, the reasonable person standard says that a randomized, placebo-controlled trial is justified only if (1) the subjects have validly consented to being randomized and (2) a reasonable person of an average degree of altruism and risk-aversiveness might consent to being randomized. This "reasonable person" standard articulates the criteria that should be used to evaluate the ethics of placebo in the final decision point of the placebo algorithm.

Case Discussions

Use of Placebo When Standard Treatment Is Supportive Care

Proposed study: A randomized, placebo-controlled study of a new chemotherapy agent for patients with terminal cancer. Cancer has progressed despite use of all standard treatment options. Subjects are randomized between the study medication and placebo. All subjects get the best supportive care.

Discussion: There is no ethical controversy about the use of placebo in this example. Placebo does not risk denying subjects effective therapy because no treatment is known to be effective in this situation.

Use of Placebo in Addition to Active Treatment

Proposed study: A randomized, placebo-controlled trial of a new medication to relieve pain in patients with chronic pain from diabetic neuropathy. Standard therapy in this patient population is a narcotic analgesic and an antidepressant medication. The study randomizes subjects to treatment with standard therapy plus placebo or standard therapy plus the study medication.

Discussion: There is no ethical controversy about the use of placebo in this example. The use of placebo does not deny subjects effective therapy because placebo is used in addition to—not in place of—standard treatment.

Use of Placebo When Doubt Exists About the Efficacy of Standard Therapy

Proposed study: A randomized, placebo-controlled trial of an investigational gene therapy for patients with an extremely aggressive type of brain tumor called glioblastoma multiforme. The trial randomizes patients between the study treatment and placebo. Standard therapy in this patient population is either radiotherapy or supportive care. Published studies have shown that radiotherapy delays tumor progression, but patient outcome is uniformly poor. Legitimate controversy exists as to the ability of radiotherapy to meaningfully improve the length or quality of life in this setting. Some experts recommend radiotherapy as standard treatment for patients with glioblastoma multiforme, whereas other experts recommend supportive care. This trial excludes patients who have previously received radiotherapy.

Discussion: Placebo is being used in this study in place of standard therapy. If radiotherapy is considered to be effective in this setting, there may be ethical problems with using placebo in patients who have not received radiotherapy. The study may be ethical in some communities and unethical in others. To investigate local standards it is necessary to ask the local physicians who would be enrolling subjects in this trial for their opinion about the benefit of radiotherapy. If managing physicians think radiotherapy is ineffective in this setting, then the trial is without ethical controversy. However, if local physicians routinely recommend radiotherapy for patients with this tumor because they think it improves the length or quality of life, then additional issues must be evaluated to determine if placebo is ethically acceptable.

Use of Placebo When the Toxicity of Standard Therapy Is High

Proposed study: A randomized, placebo-controlled trial of a new medication for patients with multiple sclerosis (MS). The study medication is the only FDA-approved treatment that has been shown to decrease the chance of debilitating problems from MS. Only 20% of patients have a positive response to the study treatment, but in the patients who do respond, there is no question that the use of the study medication prevents or delays the progression of debilitating problems. Patients in the proposed trial will not have been treated with the study medication.

Discussion: This trial uses placebo in place of therapy that has been shown to prevent, or delay the progression of, debilitating problems. An important question to consider when evaluating the ethics of this study is the toxicity of alternative treatments. In this situation, the toxicity of the study medication is high, and many patients elect not to be treated with it. To investigate local standards, it is necessary to ask local physicians about the use of the drug in their practice. If the local physicians who would be asking patients to participate in research routinely recommend the study drug, then the study is ethical only for subjects who refuse the drug treatment with a clear understanding that it is the treatment recommended by their doctor. However, if local physicians do not recommend the study medication because they consider it to have an unfavorable risk/benefit profile, it is ethical to enroll subjects in a placebo-controlled trial without such eligibility restrictions.

Temporary Discomfort Versus Irreversible Harm

Consider two proposed studies: Study A is a randomized, placebo-controlled trial of a new medication for relief of a moderately severe tension-type headache. Study B is a randomized, placebo-controlled trial of a new antibiotic as first-line therapy for pneumonia. In both studies, placebo is used in place of standard therapy that is well tolerated and likely to be effective.

Discussion: From the ethical standpoint, the critical difference between these two studies is the nature of the risk of placebo. In Study A, the risk of placebo is temporary discomfort from a condition that is familiar to potential research subjects. The level of discomfort is not severe. The period of discomfort is temporary. In view of these factors, the standard informed consent process is sufficient ethical justification for the use of placebo. Subjects are likely to understand the implications of their decision to participate in research because they will know from past experience how it feels to have a headache for the duration of the study. The nature of this study is such that coercion is unlikely. For these reasons, additional protection from the possibility of coercion and incomplete informed consent is not necessary. The use of placebo is ethical.

In contrast to Study A, Study B involves a medical condition that will cause serious, irreversible health problems if patients are not given effective treatment within a short period of time from diagnosis. Standard therapy in this setting has a favorable risk/benefit profile and is therefore recommended by local physicians. A study with concomitant placebo control is clearly the most definitive way to evaluate efficacy of the study medication. One could argue that there are patients who would participate in this study based on altruism because an additional effective antibiotic would benefit people in the future. Altruism and informed consent would be the ethical justification for this study.

In view of the risk of irreversible, serious harm in Study B, ethical research requires a demanding standard for a study design that minimizes risk. For the sake of this discussion, let us assume that a study with concomitant placebo control is the only credible way to evaluate efficacy in this setting. Given this assumption, the final step is to evaluate the credibility of altruism (as this is the main reason that an informed subject would participate in this type of study) with the "reasonable person" standard. In the absence of coercion, it is difficult to imagine an informed person volunteering for this study. Therefore, the use of concomitant placebo control in this study is unethical.

Severe Suffering

Proposed study: A randomized, placebo-controlled trial of a new medication to prevent nausea and vomiting from chemotherapy. In the absence of effective antinausea medication, the patients in this study are expected to experience moderate nausea and vomiting for approximately three days. A variety of different medications are approved for use in this setting and are considered standard therapy by local physicians. Standard therapy is, without question, highly effective at preventing or decreasing chemotherapy-related nausea and vomiting. In this study, placebo is being used in place of standard therapy.

Discussion: This is a situation where the risk of placebo is temporary suffering with little risk of irreversible physical harm. One could argue that this study is acceptable because the risk of placebo is temporary discomfort, which is something that an informed subject should be able to accept.[9] Another view would be that, at some point, temporary suffering and irreversible harm have the same ethical implications. One could argue that severe temporary physical suffering is likely to cause long-term psychological harm. No accepted guideline or formula identifies the situation where temporary physical suffering may result in irreversible psychological harm. Personal values and individual judgment will play a major role in deciding if this study is ethical.

Considering Alternative Study Designs

Consider two examples: one with little controversy regarding the quality of a study design that does not use concomitant placebo control and one where the use of alternate study designs are currently a topic of major debate.

Proposed Study 1: The first example is that of study B as presented in the previous discussion of temporary discomfort versus irreversible harm. In the case of first-line antibiotic therapy for pneumonia, there is little variability in the placebo response rate. Specifically, in patients who would be included in this trial, it is rare for pneumonia to resolve within the timeframe of the study without effective antibiotic treatment.

Discussion: When it is possible to estimate the placebo response rate with a reasonable degree of accuracy, study designs with historical placebo control or concomitant active control are likely to yield credible results. As pneumonia is a condition that may lead to serious and permanent health problems, it is unethical to conduct a trial with concomitant placebo control in this patient population.

Proposed Study 2: The second example is that of a randomized, placebo-controlled trial of a new medication for major depression. The trial targets patients who have not been treated with approved medications that are considered standard therapy for this condition. Standard therapy, without question, has disease-specific activity in this patient population that results in meaningful benefit for many patients. The toxicity of standard medications is significant but manageable, and standard treatment is recommended by local physicians and tolerated by most patients. Major depression is a condition that causes severe suffering and irreversible health problems. From previous trials with concomitant placebo control, it is clear that variability in the placebo response rate for short-term treatment endpoints is likely to be as large as the expected effect of the study treatment.

Discussion: The use of concomitant placebo control in place of standard therapy in studies of first-line therapy for major depression is a topic of major controversy in the research community. The April 2000 issue of the journal *Archives of General Psychiatry* contains a series of articles that present both sides of this debate. The fundamental arguments presented in these articles were discussed earlier in this chapter. Basically, some experts argue that it is feasible to conduct the kind of noninferiority trials that would produce valuable and persuasive results about the efficacy of new antidepressants without the risk of placebo. The counterargument is that the quality of the results from antidepressant studies that do not use concomitant placebo control is so low that society will be harmed by the routine use of medications that are not active in this medical condition.

Credible Altruism

It is difficult to find a real-life example where a reasonable and informed person would volunteer to be randomized in a study where placebo is being used in place of standard therapy that is known to be effective for a medical condition that may cause serious, irreversible harm. This is the basis for much of the current debate regarding the use of placebo in clinical trials. The principle of credible altruism is best illustrated with a study that randomizes subjects between a major surgical procedure and symptomatic treatment.

Proposed study: A randomized trial of a major surgical procedure called radical prostatectomy for prostate cancer. This procedure has been used for many years and is considered standard therapy by local physicians. In spite of previous studies, legitimate controversy remains about the efficacy of radical prostatectomy in terms of improvement in length or quality of life. Alternative therapies are commonly used to treat prostate cancer, but none are clearly beneficial. The study under consideration randomizes patients with a curable stage of prostate cancer to either radical prostatectomy or observation (no active treatment). Both study groups will receive standard palliative therapy (treatment designed to alleviate symptoms) if cancer progresses in the future. In most of the local communities where this study would take place, observation is rarely recommended by physicians, or chosen by patients who would be eligible for this study.

Discussion: In this study, the control group does not receive potentially curative therapy. "Observation with palliative treatment as needed" is being used in place of a standard therapy that is considered to be beneficial by local physicians. The risk of treatment in the control group is severe: permanent harm (cancer progression). Although the toxicity of radical prostatectomy is significant, patients routinely choose this therapy and recommend it to other patients. Determining the effect of radical prostatectomy on length and quality of life has major implications for a large number of future prostate cancer patients. This question can only be answered by means of a large-scale clinical trial with a concomitant "symptomatic treatment" control arm. Ethical justification for this study requires that it meet the "reasonable person" standard.

In many communities, there are likely to be patients who will understand that there is legitimate controversy regarding the efficacy of radical prostatectomy, even though this is the therapy commonly recommended for their condition. In this situation, the value of study results to society may be extremely high, as the study could change the treatment recommendation for large numbers of future patients. Although the risk of the control arm of this study is high, the risk of standard therapy is significant. For these reasons, it is reasonable to conclude that a reasonable person, with an average degree of altruism and risk-aversiveness, would consent to being randomized in this trial.

References

1. Rothman KJ, Michels KB. The continuing unethical use of placebo controls [letter]. *N Engl J Med* 331:394–397, 1994.

2. Marquis D. How to resolve an ethical dilemma concerning randomized clinical trials [letter]. *N Engl J Med* 341:691–693, 1999.

3. Michels KB. The placebo problem remains [commentary]. *Arch Gen Psychiatry* 57:321–322, 2000.

4. Addington D. The use of placebos in clinical trials for acute schizophrenia. *Can J Psychiatry* 40:171–176, 1995.

5. Brody BA. When are placebo-controlled trials no longer appropriate? *Control Clin Trials* 18:602–612, 1997.

6. Freeman TB, Vawter DE, Leaverton PE, et al. Use of placebo surgery in controlled trials of a cellular-based therapy for Parkinson's disease. *N Engl J Med* 341:988–992, 1999.

7. Markman M. When regulatory requirements conflict with ethical study design: The case of oral ondansetron. *Cancer Invest* 12:654–656, 1994.

8. Stein CM, Pincus T. Placebo-controlled studies in rheumatoid arthritis: Ethical issues. *Lancet* 353:400–403, 1999.

9. Temple RJ. When are clinical trials of a given agent vs. placebo no longer appropriate or feasible? *Control Clin Trials* 18:613–620, 1997.

10. Clark PI, Leaverton PE. Scientific and ethical issues in the use of placebo controls in clinical trials. *Annu Rev Public Health* 15:19–38, 1994.

11. Food and Drug Administration. International Conference on Harmonisation: Choice of control group in clinical trials. Docket No. 99D-3082. Report number 64. September 24, 1999:51767–51780. http://www.fda.gov/OHRMS/DOCKETS/98fr/092499a.pdf.

12. Emanuel EJ, Wendler D, Grady C. What makes clinical research ethical? *JAMA* 283:2701–2711, 2000.

13. Pullman D. General provisional proxy consent to research: Redefining the role of the local research ethics board. *IRB: A Review of Human Subjects Research* 21:1–9, 1999.

14. Daugherty CK, Banik DM, Janisch L, Ratain MJ. Quantitative analysis of ethical issues in Phase 1 trials: A survey interview study of 144 advanced cancer patients. *IRB: A Review of Human Subjects Research* 22(3):6–14, 2000.

15. Ott L, Larson RF, Rexroat C, Mendenhall W. *Statistics: A Tool for the Social Sciences,* 5th ed. Boston: PWS-Kent; 1992.

16. Code of Federal Regulations. Title 45A—Department of Health and Human Services; Part 46—Protection of Human Subjects. Updated 1 October, 1997. Access date 18 April, 2001. http://www4.law.cornell.edu/cfr/45p46.htm

17. Leber P. Placebo controls. No news is good news [commentary]. *Arch Gen Psychiatry* 57:319–320, 2000.

18. Mcquay H, Moore A. Placebo mania. Placebos are essential when extent and variability of placebo response are unknown [letter]. *Br Med J* 313:1008, 1996.

19. Kahn A, Warner HA, Brown WA. Symptom reduction and suicide risk in patients treated with placebo in antidepressant clinical trials: An analysis of the Food and Drug Administration database. *Arch Gen Psychiatry* 57:311–317, 2000.

20. Leon AC. Placebo protects subjects from nonresponse: A paradox of power [commentary]. *Arch Gen Psychiatry* 57:329–330, 2000.

21. Kraemer HC. Statistical analysis to settle ethical issues? *Arch Gen Psychiatry* 57:327–328, 2000.

22. World Medical Association. Declaration of Helsinki: Ethical Principles for Medical Research Involving Human Subjects. First adopted in Helsinki, Finland, in 1964. Updated 10 July, 2000. Access date 2 September, 2001. http://www.wma.net/e/policy/17-c_e.html

23. Amdur RJ, Biddle CJ. An algorithm for evaluating the ethics of a placebo-controlled trial. *Int J Cancer (Radiat Oncol Invest)* 96:261-269, 2001.

Treatment-Withholding Studies in Psychiatry

Richard B. Ferrell

INTRODUCTION

The purpose of this chapter is to consider ethical questions raised by studies that involve withdrawal or discontinuation of current psychiatric treatment. There is overlap between the issues of treatment withdrawal and placebo control because in both of these situations there is a period of time when participants receive no active therapy. Institutional review board (IRB) management of studies involving placebo control is discussed in Chapter 10-11. This chapter focuses on the specific class of psychiatric drug studies in which active drug treatment is withheld for a period of time, which may have an important effect on the course of the illness. Washout, withdrawal, and withholding are other terms that refer to not giving active treatment. I use the word withholding to refer to all studies of this type.

Treatment withholding is not unique to psychiatric research. For patients with psychiatric illness, there is sometimes a question about the competence of the participants, but this question, although important, is also not the topic of this chapter. Psychiatric disorders are associated with a number of factors that can make ethical evaluation of treatment-withholding studies difficult. The effects of some psychiatric illnesses, such as schizophrenia, bipolar disorder, and severe depression, can be devastating, but other psychiatric illnesses can be less dangerous. Patients with the same disorder can experience a wide range of severity of symptoms, and there may be large fluctuations in the severity of a disorder in the same patient over time. With few exceptions, psychiatric drug treatments are not curative, but all carry significant risk. Another problem is a lack of exact methods to measure the effect of a given treatment in a patient. Experts do not always agree in their assessments of risks and benefits for treatment of a particular disorder. In view of this background, IRBs should expect to exercise a considerable degree of individual judgment when evaluating the ethics of a study in this category.

Ethical Guidance Documents

The Nuremberg Code, the World Medical Association Declaration of Helsinki, *The Belmont Report*, and the Code of Federal Regulations, Title 45, Part 46, of the Department of Health and Human Services are included in the reference section of this book and discussed in detail in other chapters. These guidelines all emphasize that the characteristics of ethical research are that the risks to subjects are minimized, the potential benefit of the research justifies the potential risks, and that the research is not designed with the knowledge or expectation that research participation will harm the subject. None of these guidelines specifically discusses the withholding of treatment in psychiatric research or in other fields of research.

The "Statement of Principles of Ethical Conduct for Neuropsychopharmacologic Research in Human Subjects" of the American College of Neuropsychopharmacology gives guidelines regarding ethical research design.[1] This statement discusses the importance of comparison with placebo in the evaluation of new psychiatric drugs. It does advocate careful review by the investigator and the IRB of "the use of placebo in severely ill patients, such as very disturbed and/or severely deteriorated schizophrenic patients who present gross thought disorders and hallucinations. . . ." This document does not specifically mention research in which existing treatment is to be stopped.

A Selective Literature Review

The National Alliance for the Mentally Ill (NAMI) has published standards designed to protect the welfare of psychiatric research participants.[2] Although NAMI has taken no official position on withholding treatment, prominent advocates from this organization have expressed concern about studies that do so:[3] "Many NAMI members now feel that a placebo is not acceptable, because we view schizophrenia and other psychotic disorders and affective illness as life-threatening diseases."[3] Hall and Flynn argue persuasively that studies involving withholding medication and placebo control in severe mental illness might not be ethical: "Indeed, NAMI has serious question about whether placebo-controlled studies are still necessary in this era. Researchers conducting such studies must be incredibly vigilant about these issues in their informed consent process, ongoing communication with families and patients, and follow-up to the research."[3]

Irving and Shamoo[4] and Shamoo and Keay[5] have seriously questioned the ethics of "washout" studies in schizophrenia. They assert that such studies cause unnecessary relapses in schizophrenic patients. Haas et al.[6] argued that delayed treatment of schizophrenia causes negative long-term effects. It is indeed hard to imagine how one could argue that delaying treatment could benefit a sick individual, unless one maintains that treatment is more likely to do harm than good. Nothing in my clinical experience in treating people with severe mental illness suggests to me that this is the case.

Persons with psychiatric illnesses have been stigmatized and treated with prejudice throughout history. Some would argue that informed consent is all that is needed to protect research participants and that additional protection perpetuates stigma. Others believe that people with psychiatric illness need special protection from research risk. Manschreck[7] discussed these countervailing points of view. He argued that scientific merit should not outweigh ethical concerns, and that efforts must be made to limit risks in schizophrenia studies involving placebo. Keeping the time when active treatment is not given as short as possible and having ". . . strict criteria for deciding when a patient should be withdrawn for failure to respond" are two ways of reducing risks.

One should not assume that withholding treatment could only cause harm. Cohen-Mansfield et al.[8] reported a study involving withdrawing treatment with haloperidol, thioridazine, and lorazepam from nursing home residents. This was a double-blind crossover study with a seven-week period of drug abstinence. The drugs had no clear beneficial effect.

One reason that psychiatric treatment research protocols might be controversial is that worthwhile ideals can be in conflict. Finding more effective and safer treatments for psychiatric illnesses is a worthy goal. Protecting those afflicted with such illnesses from the risk of inadequate treatment is another. Protecting people with illness and the larger public from the marketing of ineffective treatment is yet another virtuous goal. It is important to remember that advances in psychiatric treatment that resulted from clinical research have been of tremendous help to many people. Such research is extremely important for current and future patients, but the welfare of individuals who may be participants in psychiatric research is highly important also.

In recent years the ethics of clinical trials of drugs being tested as treatments for schizophrenia has been controversial. The fundamental question is whether or not it is ethical to have a period of time in a study when no drug treatment is given. Unless the study involved subjects who were not already receiving drug treatment, previous treatment would have to be stopped to achieve a drug-free state. From a scientific standpoint, it is desirable to start with subjects in a drug-free state so that therapeutic effects of previous treatment are absent, and signs and symptoms result only from the illness itself and not from previous drug treatment. The drug-free state also allows for use of a placebo study group so that there is ability to show a difference between the experimental drug treatment and placebo.[9,10]

This question of whether or not it is ethical for persons with schizophrenia to be subjects in drug studies in which they would not receive any drug with either demonstrated or possible antipsychotic effect is not finally resolved. It is very difficult to justify withholding treatment that could prevent or diminish tissue or organ injury. The more serious the illness is or the more effective existing treatment is, the harder it is to justify withholding the treatment. The argument about ethics in schizophrenia research has been fueled by the development of better therapeutic drugs, which were approved for use through clinical trials that typically included comparison of the drug to placebo. The creation of older drugs such as phenothiazines and haloperidol offered hope for improvement to sufferers from schizophrenia and their families. Newer, or "atypical" antipsychotic drugs represent a significant improvement over the older drugs, both in efficacy and in decreased unwanted effects. Yet patients, their families, clinicians, and researchers agree that better, more effective, and safer treatments, plus better understanding of the causes and pathologic effects of schizophrenia, are needed.

Currently, there are reasoned arguments on both sides of the question. Frank et al.[11] and Roberts[12] have written balanced reviews of these issues.

Quitkin argues effectively for the use of placebo in clinical trials attempting to show efficacy for potential psychotherapeutic drugs, especially antidepressant drugs.[9] He argues that if psychotherapeutic drugs are not shown to be significantly superior to placebo, then ineffective drugs may be approved for use. Subsequent treatment of large numbers of psychiatric patients with an ineffective drug would imperil the health of many people and predictably have serious negative public health consequences.

Quitkin also argues that subjects in psychiatric drug studies who might receive placebo should be closely monitored, should receive placebo for a limited time, should be withdrawn from the study if getting significantly more ill, and should receive the best possible care after the experimental treatment period.

Discontinuation studies in which some subjects are withdrawn from previous treatment and given placebo and in which the measured and expected outcome is relapse are harder to justify. Some subjects are expected to become more ill in this type of study. Such studies would appear to violate the Declaration of Helsinki and the non-maleficence principle. I should, however, point out that in psychiatric practice it is sometimes appropriate to taper and discontinue medicines of dubious efficacy for an individual patient to see whether symptoms worsen or possibly improve. This may be the only way to conclude if continuing the drug is clinically justified.

My opinion is that proscription of all drug treatment-withholding studies is not currently justified but that the IRB must critically scrutinize each such study to determine that the study is designed to maximize the safety of each participant.

Guidelines for IRB Review

Recognize the criteria that apply for IRB approval of research involving placebo are equally relevant to research involving withholding of active treatment. The IRB should use the placebo control algorithm presented in Chapter 10-11 to evaluate the ethics of trials that withhold treatment in psychiatric research. The main issues to consider are the nature of the patient's condition, the efficacy of standard therapy in the study population, and rescue plans:

1. Is the purpose of the study to learn about the natural history of the disease or to find out if a study treatment is effective?

2. Consent should be fully informed with subjects able to consult with family or friends for advice. Judicial review and use of surrogate decision makers is appropriate if subjects have decisional incapacity.

3. How effective is the treatment being withdrawn? Does it significantly alter the natural history of the disease, or greatly reduce symptoms and suffering?

4. How serious is the disease? What are its manifestations and consequences? If relapse occurs, is there likely to be permanent harm or injury? If illness recurs, is there likely to be a risk of suicide or risk of dangerous behavior toward others?

5. What is the tendency to relapse without treatment? If illness recurs, how likely is it that resumption of treatment will result in full recovery?

6. Is the period without active treatment as short as possible to answer the study question?

7. Are there possible advantages to withdrawing current treatment such as significant side effects or toxicity that might be reduced or eliminated?

8. What are the provisions in the study for timely rescue if symptoms worsen? Subjects should be removed from the study if they are getting worse. Active treatment should be resumed.

9. Close monitoring of subjects' clinical condition is essential. Hospitalization during the period of greatest risk may provide extra safety but is expensive and is an additional disruption in the life of the participant.

10. Subjects should have affordable access to effective treatment after the end of the experimental period.

Do not hesitate to ask for the opinion of an expert who is not involved in the study regarding the questions that the IRB needs to answer to make a decision about approving

the protocol. Consider making voluntary hospitalization or very careful outpatient care during the period of highest risk, a requirement for IRB approval.

Case Discussions

Example 1

A proposed study would compare two dosage schedules of an investigational antipsychotic drug for treatment of schizophrenia. Previous studies with this drug over the dose range in this study suggest a favorable risk/benefit profile. Subjects whose symptoms are not optimally treated on standard medications will have a 7-day washout period during which they receive no medication. The clinician–investigator has the option of reducing this period to 3 days, depending upon clinical judgment about the participant's condition. The study requires close monitoring of participants throughout the study with plans for immediate rescue treatment and/or hospitalization if symptoms worsen.

Withholding treatment is ethical in this study because the period without treatment is brief and flexible depending on the severity of illness. Symptom control was not optimal on standard therapy, and the study provides for close monitoring with appropriate rescue. The IRB should approve the study.

Example 2

A study would investigate treatment of attention deficit hyperactivity disorder (ADHD) in children with a new long-acting formulation of methylphenidate that is only taken once a day. An inclusion criterion is that patients are currently well controlled on the standard form of methylphenidate, which is given multiple times per day. The study requires a 2-week washout period when all subjects will be given placebo. Subjects who do well on placebo (minimal symptoms of ADHD) are excluded from the remainder of the study. Subjects who deteriorate on placebo are then randomized to treatment with the new formulation of methylphenidate or placebo for a 4-week study period.

The purpose of the washout period in this study is to identify subjects who are benefiting from methylphenidate treatment. The study is designed with a goal of producing symptomatic deterioration in a subgroup of study subjects. Consultation with several people who had experience with uncontrolled ADHD children in the classroom stressed that even a few weeks of symptom deterioration may be a serious problem for the child with ADHD and for other children in the classroom. My IRB did not approve a study similar to this.

Additional Points and Recommendations

The IRB should understand that the withdrawal of active treatment is both ethical and necessary in many research settings. To evaluate a specific study, the IRB should use the guidelines discussed in this chapter and the placebo control algorithm presented in Chapter 10-11. In my experience, most disagreements among committee members have to do with understanding the facts differently or with not enough facts being known. It is important for committee members to have as much information as possible. Prognosis is usually the greatest uncertainty and the most common source of dispute about a particular protocol.

If we knew that not treating a major illness such as schizophrenia for some period of time would result in a greater chance of neuronal injury or permanent disability or decrease the chances of successful treatment when treatment is eventually begun, then any protocol that withheld treatment would be unethical. This would be even more so if it were known that the illness was likely to cause much suffering and anguish. Although there is disagreement on this point, I do not think that it is currently ethical to withhold drug treatment from persons with schizophrenia for long time periods. This is especially true if the individual is currently receiving treatment that is improving his or her condition. This same argument might also be made for persons with severe forms of bipolar disorder, depression, anxiety disorders, and obsessive-compulsive disorder.

All psychiatric disorders cannot be lumped together. For some illnesses, the long-term consequences are clearly bad, and treatment for some illnesses is better than for others. Special attention must be paid to the risks of discontinuing treatment if the disease or disorder in question causes psychotic symptoms, produces deterioration of intellectual or social function, or is at all likely to result in dangerous behavior. If the facts are not clear, the IRB should get a consultant. For psychiatric studies involving treatment discontinuation, an actively practicing psychiatrist who regularly treats patients afflicted by the disease or disorder in question would be a good choice. A member of NAMI would also be a good choice if one were not already a member of the IRB committee. In either or both cases, a helpful consultant will have knowledge about psychiatric illness and the suffering of those afflicted. He or she should have a balanced view about the welfare of patients and the great importance of developing treatments better than those we now have.

Treatment of severe psychiatric illness is not easy. It is seldom simply a matter of correcting a "chemical imbalance" with a particular medicine. If a successful treatment is stopped and relapse occurs, restarting the medicine at a later time might not return the person to health quickly, if at all. Not only is the prognosis for repeat recovery uncertain, but also the afflicted person is suffering from symptoms and from the effects of illness on their social, emotional, family, and vocational life. Severe psychiatric illness also carries a risk of complications including other concomitant illness and suicide. For example, persons with severe depression have a higher rate of death from causes other than suicide than people who are not depressed.

It is hard to imagine that a person who has suffered from severe mental illness and who has recovered or significantly improved would want to take a substantial chance of experiencing relapse.

The IRB should be aware that future scientific advances might alter the ethical balance between currently countervailing ethical arguments. Clear and compelling evidence of nervous system damage in a psychiatric disorder that could be prevented by early treatment, or development of significantly better drug treatments than those currently available might tip the balance against psychiatric drug treatment-withholding studies.

Conclusion

It is the job of researchers to design studies that attempt to answer important research questions while, at the same time, not jeopardizing the health of those persons who volunteer to participate in the research. It is the job of IRBs to examine carefully research proposals regarding their ethical merit. Psychiatric studies that include any discontinuation of current treatment present a special challenge for IRBs. Knowledge, careful thought, and circumspect ethical judgment are necessary for making our best possible decisions.

References

1. American College of Neuropsychopharmacology. Statement of principles of ethical conduct for neuropsychopharmacologic research in human subjects. *Directory of Members* 195–208, 1996.

2. Shamoo AE, Johnson JR, Honberg R, Flynn L. National Alliance for the Mentally Ill's standards for protection of individuals with severe mental illnesses who participate as human subjects in research. In: Shamoo AE (ed.). *Ethics in Neurobiological Research with Human Subjects: The Baltimore Conference on Ethics.* Amsterdam: Gordon and Breach Publisher OPA; 1997:325–328.

3. Hall LL, Flynn L. Consumer and family concerns about research involving human subjects. In: Pincus HA, Lieberman JA, Ferris S (eds.). *Ethics in Psychiatric Research: A Resource Manual for Human Subjects Protection.* Washington, DC: American Psychiatric Association; 1999:219–238.

4. Irving DN, Shamoo AE. Washouts/relapses in patients participating in neurobiological research studies in schizophrenia. In: Shamoo AE (ed.). *Ethics in Neurobiological Research with Human Subjects: The Baltimore Conference on Ethics.* Amsterdam: Gordon and Breach Publisher OPA; 1997:119–127.

5. Shamoo AE, Keay TJ. Ethical concerns about relapse studies. *Camb Q Healthc Ethics* 5(3):373–386, 1996.

6. Haas GL, Keshavan MS, Sweeney JA. Delay to first medication in schizophrenia: Evidence for a possible negative impact of exposure to psychosis [abstract]. Proceedings of the 33rd Annual Meeting of the American College of Neuropsychopharmacology, San Juan, Puerto Rico; 1994:171.

7. Manschreck TC. Placebo studies: Lessons from psychiatric research. *Psychiatr Ann* 31(2):130–136, 2001.

8. Cohen-Mansfield J, Lipson S, Werner P, Billig N, Taylor L, Woosley R. Withdrawal of haloperidol, thioridazine, and lorazepam in the nursing home: A controlled double-blind study. *Arch Intern Med* 159(15):1733–1740, 1999.

9. Quitkin FM. Placebos, drug effects, and study design: A clinician's guide. *Am J Psychiatry* 156(6):829–836, 1999.

10. Carpenter WT. The risk of medication-free research. *Schizophrenia Bull* 23(1):11–18, 1997.

11. Frank E, Novick DM, Kupfer DJ. Beyond the question of placebo controls: Ethical issues in psychopharmacological studies. *Psychopharmacology* 171:19–26, 2003.

12. Roberts LW. Ethics and mental illness research. *Psychiatric Clin North Am* 25:525–545, 2002.

Phase I Oncology Trials

Matthew Miller

INTRODUCTION

A fundamental tension in human experimentation on patients arises from the inherent conflict between the goals of science and those of clinical care. Phase I cancer trials embody this conflict in perhaps its purest and most intense form because the subjects in these trials are terminally ill patients with advanced and incurable malignancies and the scientific goal is to effect toxicity, not cure, remission, or palliation.[1] This presents special challenges to institutional review board (IRB) review, especially in light of empirical evidence that patients overwhelmingly enroll in these trials seeking physical benefit.[2–11] Benjamin Freedman summarized the fundamental issue:

> A Phase I study of drug X is often said to be a study of X's safety and efficacy. Calling a toxicity study a study of safety seems harmless, and perhaps even reflects a laudably optimistic view of the world. Calling it a study of efficacy is, however, simply false; although to be sure, were there no hope of this drug's working it would not be tested.[1]

This chapter begins with an overview of Phase I trials, touching on the dominant dose-escalation scheme employed, historical response rates, eligibility requirements, and the special vulnerabilities of trial participants. The following section focuses on the empirical evidence that suggests most patients currently enrolled in Phase I cancer trials fail to comprehend critically important elements about the nature of the sacrifice they are being asked to make. Against this background, I explore the possibility that patient misunderstanding may be shared and reinforced by virtue of a tendency among physician–investigators to view their role as investigator as serving patients' therapeutic interests. Problematic aspects of traditional and prevailing dosing regimens are explored by contrasting them with innovative but infrequently employed designs that are in less obvious conflict with patients' expectations. Finally, suggestions are made regarding what IRB members can do to protect patients' basic right of self-determination and freedom from unwarranted harms. These suggestions focus on (1) structural elements of Phase I trials that must be disclosed clearly to patients and justified explicitly to the IRB (especially those elements that embody the conflict between the interests of science and those of personal care) and (2) accountability (beyond disclosure) for ensuring comprehending decision making by prospective patient–subjects. Throughout this chapter, I supplement findings from the empirical literature with descriptions of the difficulties I experienced navigating the tensions between research and patient care during my tenure as acting director of Phase I cancer trials at the Dana-Farber Cancer Institute in Boston.

Background

In the course of developing new anticancer compounds, agents that have demonstrated promise in cell culture and animal models must at some time be tested in human subjects. In these initial or *Phase I* human trials, compounds are administered to terminally ill cancer patients in an attempt to estimate the highest dose human beings can tolerate.[6,12–17] Evaluating a drug's anticancer effect in human cancers—a primary objective of subsequent Phase II and Phase III trials—is not a defined goal in Phase I studies.[15,17] Unlike Phase II and Phase III trials, Phase I studies do not test hypotheses (such as whether new drug X is at least Y% effective in disease Z or whether new drug X is better than old drug Y);[12] most drugs administered in Phase I trials go on to Phase II evaluation, independent

An abbreviated version of this chapter is published in *The Hastings Center Report* 30(4):34–42, 2000. Used with permission.

of an antitumor effect in Phase I. Indeed, if a partial tumor response were the basis of proceeding to Phase II trials, fewer than 5% of drugs would proceed; if a complete response were required, fewer than 0.5% would proceed.[18]

Subjects in noncancer Phase I (dose-toxicity) studies are usually healthy volunteers.[19] Because Phase I cancer trials use drugs that are selected for their ability to kill (tumor) cells and because these agents often produce their effects by causing damage to DNA, with attendant concerns about long-term carcinogenic consequences, subjects in Phase I cancer trials are never healthy volunteers.

To be considered for Phase I cancer trials, patients must have exhausted all known therapeutic options and generally have a life expectancy of at least 3 to 4 months. Typically, patients are referred by their primary oncologist to a major cancer program where a physician–investigator from the cancer center performs a physical examination, takes a medical history, and then invites eligible patients to enroll. For the duration of enrollment, a physician–investigator at the cancer center usually assumes the substantial responsibility for monitoring and caring for each patient.

Phase I dose-toxicity information is usually gathered by administering increasing doses of a new drug (or of novel combinations of known agents) to successive cohorts of three to six patients. After serious but reversible toxic effects are produced in a fixed proportion of patients (often one third of the patients in the highest dose cohort), the trial ends.[6,20–26] Examples of ill effects severe enough to be considered dose-limiting include gross hemorrhage, nausea to the point that there is no significant intake of food or fluid, and painful mouth and throat sores that make eating impossible. Unless extremely severe, irreversible toxicities are observed in Phase I trials, agents generally go on to Phase II studies, independent of whether tumor responses were observed.

Because most responses occur at 80% to 120% of the maximum tolerated dose,[6,23] subjects enrolled in the earliest cohorts have the least risk of severe toxicity but also the least likelihood of a clinical response. It has been estimated that the traditional and prevailing cohort-specific dosing strategies subject approximately 60% to 80% of patients to doses that, based on preclinical models, are thought less likely to produce a response than higher, achievable levels.[6] Thus, the predominant cohort-specific dose escalation schemes are at odds with what patients generally assume about the primacy of their interests, such as that *each* patient will receive a dose that attempts to maximize the chance for anticancer effect. Despite this significant departure from usual clinical practice, there are no formal requirements specifying that physician–investigators must share this information with patients.

Based on the long-standing rationale that the optimal therapeutic dose (of classical cytotoxic agents) is the highest safely achievable dose, the maximum tolerated dose determined from Phase I trials is usually recommended as the dose for subsequent Phase II studies.[27,28] The adoption of a therapeutic goal for Phase II trials is also reflected in patient characteristics. Patients in Phase II studies must have measurable disease (to assess response), usually have a malignancy that is thought among the most likely to respond to the agent under investigation, and often have not received extensive chemotherapy or radiotherapy in the past.[15] In contradistinction, Phase I patients need not have measurable disease and can generally have any tumor type, even types that animal models do not suggest will respond to the agent in question. Over 90% of patients eligible for Phase I trials have been extensively pretreated.[29]

Planned Toxicity and No Direct Benefit

As mentioned previously here, Phase I oncology studies are not designed to benefit the patients who participate in the trials. The nontherapeutic objective of Phase I studies is supported by empiric data. One comprehensive review of Phase I cancer trials published between 1972 and 1987 found an overall response rate among the 6,639 patients of 4.5%. There were 23 complete remissions (0.3%) and 31 toxic deaths (0.5%).[18] Of the few complete remissions, most occurred in tumor types traditionally held to be the most responsive (hematologic malignancies). When agents were classified by response rate, 9% produced an overall (i.e., partial and complete) response rate of 10% or higher and 1% produced a response rate of at least 20%. In a simulation study of 100 Phase I trials using a traditional dosing design, roughly half of all patients experienced at least mild toxicity, and approximately 20% experienced severe but reversible toxicity (grades 3 and 4 toxicity).[30] Other reviews of Phase I trials document similar response and toxicity rates.[6,20,31–34] As mentioned, patients in Phase I trials survive, on average, 6 months from the date of enrollment.[35] Among the few who achieve a complete response, half relapse within 6 months; partial responses last approximately three months.[28] It is also unknown whether the few patient–subjects who responded actually lived any longer or better as a result.[4]

The predominant structure of Phase I trials embodies peculiarly contrasting tensions at opposing ends of the dosing spectrum: at one extreme, requiring that at least one patient suffer severe (but reversible) toxicity,[12] and at the other, subjecting 60% to 80% of patients to doses that, based on preclinical models, are a priori expected to prove less likely to produce a response than higher achievable levels.[6] Given a remission rate of under 1% and a comparable rate of death due to drug toxicity,[18] few would claim any aggregate survival advantage for participants. In fact, consent documents state that Phase I cancer trials are primarily toxicity studies and that response is neither intended nor expected.[6] Yet, when asked, patients enrolled in these trials overwhelmingly cite hope of physical benefit (rarely altruism) as their primary motivation for enrolling.[3–5,9,11]

Therapeutic Misconceptions of Subjects

This section explores the empirical evidence suggesting that Phase I cancer patients agree to participate in these trials largely in hope of physical benefit and generally assume that the structure of the trial itself serves their personal therapeutic goal. These beliefs reflect a profound trust patients have in the doctor–patient relationship and an underlying assumption about the immutability of this trusting relationship even in the face of the demands of science. This misunderstanding, whereby patients do not fully recognize the way that science sometimes deprives them of care chosen solely out of concern for their well being (what Fried[36] calls the right of "personal care"), has been called the "therapeutic misconception."[37] After reviewing evidence that suggests Phase I cancer patients are particularly susceptible to the therapeutic misconception, I explored the possibility that physician–investigators share elements of the therapeutic misconception. Finally, I argue that this shared misconception has moral consequences for these trials, resulting in mutually reinforcing behaviors that are inimical to attaining truly informed consent.

Empirical studies of patient comprehension in Phase I cancer trials consistently suggest that patients participating in Phase I oncology trials are primarily motivated by the hope that they will derive physical benefit. Making a contribution to generalizable knowledge or to future patients appears to play an inconsequential and greatly subordinate role.[2-11] Although cancer patients participating in Phase I trials appear to have adequate knowledge of the risks of the investigational agents,[3] seldom do they understand that the purpose of Phase I studies is not to produce a tumor response or to palliate human suffering, but rather to establish a relationship between dose and toxicity.[2-6]

In 1995, a prominent team of ethicists and oncologists at the University of Chicago published one of the first empirical studies to explore the motivations and perceptions of cancer patients enrolled in Phase I trials.[3] Thirty consecutive cancer patients enrolled in Phase I trials were surveyed. Although 93% of patients said that they understood most of the information given them, only 33% were able to state that the purpose of the trial in which they were subjects was to determine toxicities, tolerability, or the safest dose of the administered agents. Fewer than one third said that the option of no treatment was discussed. Eighty-five percent decided to participate for reasons of possible therapeutic benefit, 11% because of advice or trust in a physician, and 4% because of family pressure. No one identified altruism as the primary motivation for participating. Of note, patients who were unable to state the purpose of Phase I trials were more likely to believe that they would derive benefit from the study. These findings are consistent with previous expectations: 94% of Phase I investigators and 85% of IRB chairs believe that patients enroll in these trials for physical benefit, not for altruistic reasons.[38]

Other studies reveal similar deficiencies in what terminally ill patients generally comprehend about clinical trials.[2,4,7-10,39] These studies consistently find that patients enroll in research primarily motivated by a hope for improving their condition and that, frequently, therapeutic misconceptions are wedded to despair.[39] One comparative study of patient understanding in clinical trials found that the therapeutic misconception is particularly strong among Phase I cancer trial subjects.[11] In this study, 127 subjects enrolled in four types of research protocols (three groups of ill subjects—Phase I and Phase II cancer patients, Phase III HIV-positive symptom-free patients—and one group of healthy volunteers). All Phase I subjects stated that their study's goal (as distinct from their hopes) was related both to treatment and research; a majority considered that cure or remission was a benefit of participating. Patients held these beliefs despite the written consent document, which states that the purpose of their trial was "to determine the side effects of Ormaplatin in patients with cancer and to determine the highest safe dose that can be used in future patients." Eighty percent of Phase II subjects and 60% of Phase III subjects described their study as both research and treatment. Ninety-one percent of the healthy volunteers responded that they believed their study was mostly research versus 35% of Phase III subjects and 8% of Phase II subjects. Significantly more subjects in the diagnosed groups than healthy volunteers reported that the consent document itself had no effect on their decision to participate in the study. In addition, responses were inversely related to health status: the greatest percentage of subjects reporting no effect were enrolled in the Phase I study (50%), followed by Phase II (42%), Phase III (23%), and healthy volunteers (17%). The two factors reported most frequently by both Phase I and Phase II subjects for deciding to participate in a research study were (1) "hope for control of disease" and (2) "present medical condition." In contrast, healthier Phase III subjects reported "NIH reputation" and "hope others benefit" most frequently. Healthy volunteers reported "hope others benefit" and "payment for participation in the study."

A particularly innovative study of the perceptions of patient–subjects enrolled in Phase I trials assessed the feasibility of a clinical trial design that uses an interactive informed-consent process in which patient–subjects can choose to become directly involved in decisions of dose escalation.[4] Subjects were patients with advanced cancer who were eligible to participate in a Phase I trial. These subjects underwent a three-step informed-consent process that used cohort-specific consent and allowed them the option to choose their own doses of the chemotherapeutic agents under study within predetermined limits. The agents in this Phase I study were known drugs, but the combination of the two drugs was novel. (In this way, the trial differed from the more problematic nature of trials that use untried agents.) Participants in this study were surveyed, and the survey results were compared with a similar survey of a matched control population of subjects who participated in other concurrently active, conventional Phase I trials at the same institution. Almost all the subjects in both the cohort-specific and the matched control groups claimed that they understood all or most of what was told to them. Respondents felt that having been given cohort-specific information and the option to choose a dose within predetermined ranges made them feel better informed. Nevertheless, there were no statistically significant improvements in objective measures of the informed consent process in this group.

Therapeutic Misconceptions of Physicians

My experience as acting director of Phase I trials at the Dana-Farber Cancer Institute is consistent with the empirical literature. I found that patients in Phase I cancer trials agree to participate almost exclusively in hopes of physical benefit. Moreover, before our first meeting, almost every patient assumed that the imperatives of ordinary patient-centered care would prevail over any protocol constraints. They were wrong.

When patients came to see me, they did not appreciate critical aspects of Phase I trial design—aspects that were absolutely necessary for them to grasp if they were to have anything approaching an adequate understanding of the nature of the sacrifice they were being asked to consider. For example, patient–subjects did not have the faintest expectation that the drug on which their hopes were pinned would be administered at doses that depended on contingencies unrelated to maximizing the likelihood of antitumor effect. They did not expect that the dosing structure was designed around parameters of toxicity, not effectiveness. They did not expect that the fixed dose they would receive depended on, for example, what day of the week they enrolled relative to others. In addition, few had been told by their primary oncologist that these trials historically have a partial response rate of less than 5% and a complete response rate equal to that of acute toxic death (0.5%). Few understood that these trials aim to induce grade 3 or grade 4 toxicity in at least one subject or that the trial would end as soon as that endpoint was reached. None had imagined possible the reality that moved one leading figure in modern oncology to write this: "It is reasonably certain that if the full reality of subtherapeutic dosing were getting through to patients and families, very few would volunteer for Phase I studies."[6]

The direction our conversation took and, it turned out, the likelihood patients would enroll depended largely on whether, and the extent to which, we discussed the particular ways in which the protocol offered opposed customary assumptions about medical practice and physician loyalty. Yet, because terminally ill patients rarely if ever initiate such a discussion, no conversation was more tempting or easier to avoid.

Telling patients that they are unlikely to respond favorably is an inference drawn from historical data and reflects, apart from any research agenda, the limitations of medicine's capabilities in the face of advanced malignancy. It is a conversation familiar to anyone who has cared for sick patients and is peculiar neither to oncology nor to the Phase I setting. Telling a patient that his or her chance of responding will not necessarily be maximized is, however, less familiar and more difficult because this limitation is imposed by a particular methodology. In the one case, there is no need, per se, to redefine the doctor–patient relationship in ways that distinguish research from usual patient care; in the other, the distinction is inescapable.

One strategy to avoid discussing the way a patient's interests yield before those of protocol is to conflate the limitations inherent in medicine's capabilities with those that are imposed by protocol. My reluctance to distinguish between medicine's limitations and those imposed by protocol stemmed, in part, from an impulse to protect my patients. I was reluctant to further debilitate a patient's hope. However, I was also reluctant to acknowledge (to myself and to my patients) the extent to which my clinical authority was undercut by protocol and to examine the extent to which I had already been complicit in maintaining the status quo.

Another way to avoid making clear the therapy versus research distinction is to adopt a sweeping and undifferentiated concept of the uncertainty inherent in the proposed trial. To say, for example, one never knows when the next breakthrough drug will come along is to allow a vague conceptualization of uncertainty to devour the morally relevant little we do know, such as the fact that no one has ever been cured in a Phase I trial. Even the essential premise of the underlying design could be overshadowed—for what does the monotonicity of dose-response have to do with the advent of the miraculous? Cohort-specific dose escalation is, in fact, rarely a part of the consent form. So rare that even though more than a decade has passed since the late Benjamin Freedman argued persuasively that it is morally necessary to include a specific and clear explanation of the cohort-specific nature of the dosing design, few institutions have adopted his suggestion.[40]

In addition to unwitting strategies of avoidance, physician–investigators, by virtue of being physicians, tend to reinforce expectations patients have about the primacy of their individual therapeutic interests.[39,41–43] Katz has written:[41]

> Investigators who appear before patient–subjects as physicians in white coats create confusion. Patients come to hospitals with the trusting expectation that their doctor will care for them. They will view an invitation to participate in research as a professional recommendation that is intended to serve their individual interests.

What, after all, is a patient supposed to assume about a clinical trial proposed as an untried but promising new "therapy" or "treatment?" Add to this that the invitation is extended in a hospital clinic by a doctor who has just finished performing a history and physical examination—an act that is powerfully symbolic and intimate, one customarily the privilege and almost exclusive province of the personal physician. Unless explicitly and particularly addressed, why would a dying patient ever think that the dose she or he would be given is based on contingencies unrelated to maximizing the response?

There are many ways in which the language physicians use when speaking about these trials may reinforce the tendency among patients to distort those elements of experimental investigation that threaten to undermine hope of clinical benefit.[2,41,43,44] For example, speaking of these trials as offering experimental "therapy" or using consent forms that refer to investigational interventions as novel "treatments" lends misleading credibility to the proposed project as one designed to promote patients' interests. Even factually accurate information in a particular juxtaposition can mislead. Saying to a patient on the one hand that the probability of remission is slight and on the other that one never knows when a miracle drug will come along gives equal rhetorical weight to clinical success and failure. More importantly, it is a formulation of the trial that omits specific reference to potential harms, to how the needs of science trump those of medicine, to the absence of intrapatient (individualized) dose escalation, and to the uncertainty that even the rare responder benefits at all.

It took far longer for me to appreciate that these same words and surroundings performed a similar function for me, preserving the illusion that what I was engaged in was an extension of usual clinical practice. This, in turn, made it easier for me to assume that my patient's interests were not in conflict with those of protocol, nor with my own interests for career advancement. Viewing these trials as an extension of medical practice makes it harder for physicians (and therefore for our patients) to identify the troubling ways in which patients' interests yield to those of protocol or the additional responsibilities of disclosure in human experimentation.

Physicians, it seems to me, do not adopt the oxymoronic language of "therapeutic research" in order to deceive subjects into thinking that they are patients. Rather, we do so unwittingly and in order that we may continue to see ourselves as compassionate physicians even as we perform duties in service of dispassionate science. It is not that we disingenuously hide from patients information we deem relevant; rather, it is that we are so adept at hiding it from ourselves. It is an accommodation that allows us to take comfort in our own good intentions. Unfortunately, it also makes it easier to characterize these trials wrongly, if inadvertently, as serving patients' interests.

Little empirical attention has been paid to the possibility that physicians, too, are susceptible to the therapeutic misconception. A few empirical findings indirectly hint at such a misconception among physicians. In one study of 144 patients enrolled in Phase I, Phase II, and Phase III trials at three cancer centers, virtually all of the 68 oncologists thought that their patients would benefit from the investigational agents being tested. Moreover, 43% of physicians said they had "no doubts at all about benefits of treatment" despite a statement in the consent form that benefit could not be assured.[45]

In another study of exclusively Phase I cancer patients, 18 oncologists who had primary responsibility for enrolling and caring for Phase I patients were asked to estimate the likelihood of risks and benefit. Overall, physicians tended to overestimate both the likelihood of severe and fatal toxicity and the likelihood of anticancer effect. For example, approximately half of these physicians thought that the frequency of fatal toxicity was at least 5% (historically it is 0.5%) and that the chance of antitumor response (partial plus complete) was 15% (historically it is approximately 5%). These data may be superficially seen as consistent with physicians presenting to patients relatively more bias of ill effects than of benefits by virtue of the greater exaggeration of the likelihood of ill effects (10-fold) than of likely benefits (3-fold). To me, however, the exaggerations of response (and toxicity) indicate that physician-investigators are thinking about untried agents the way that they would view a tried and powerfully successful agent if it were administered at the maximum tolerated dose to each patient. These exaggerated estimates may represent ignorance, itself a worrisome finding as the physicians in this study were the ones to invite patients to participate. Yet physicians generally are quite skillful at knowing the response rates for given agents in specific diseases. Such wildly exaggerated projections, anchored as they appear to be to estimates of response and toxicity rates for proven chemotherapeutics in advanced disease, suggest another possibility: that these projections reflect a heuristic that physician-investigators adopt to avoid acknowledging to themselves the trade-off they are asking patient-subjects to make. In any event, these physician-investigators are attributing to untried agents a degree of effectiveness that, whatever else it betrays, makes it easier for them to see themselves as caring physicians rather than dispassionate researchers. To the extent that both patient-subjects and physician-investigators share the perspective that these trials provide dying patients with a venue in which to pursue their best chance for clinical benefit, their perspectives will be mutually reinforcing. For patients, the belief that their interests come first reflects a profound trust that patients have in the doctor-patient relationship. For physicians, it reflects the socializing force of clinical training steeped in the longstanding Hippocratic tradition of beneficence. As Katz has written:

> It is that belief, that trust, which physician-investigators must vigorously challenge so that patient-subjects appreciate that in research, unlike therapy, the research question comes first. This takes time and is difficult to convey. It can be conveyed to patient-subjects only if physician-investigators are willing to challenge the misperceptions that many patients bring to the invitation.[41]

This challenge is a difficult one because physicians, too, may have deep-seated, not fully recognized needs that these trials serve. Which is to say that the challenge is difficult because it is not strictly a matter of volition, but one of self-discovery and acknowledgment of complicity, however well intended. To meet this challenge successfully requires that physician-investigators repudiate intention-based definitions of what constitutes therapy. It asks that we acknowledge fundamental and irreducible conflicts between the role of researcher and that of clinician, an acknowledgment that conflicts with our identity as caregiver before all else. Ironically, if physician-investigators did not care so deeply about the well-being of their patients, they would be less susceptible to this therapeutic misconception. In my experience, physician-investigators are susceptible precisely because they care and because they are drawn to search for new, more effective treatments out of a deep frustration with medicine's present capabilities and out of a painful awareness of their patients' suffering.

Alternatives to the Standard Phase I Dosing Strategy

IRB members and researchers should recognize that there are methodologically acceptable alternatives to the dosing schedules currently used in Phase I studies. This section examines one such alternative—intrapatient dose escalation—and contrasts it with the dominant cohort-specific dosing schemes described earlier in the background section of this chapter. Intrapatient dose escalation is chosen as an example of innovative dosing strategies because it is precisely the proscription of individualized (i.e., within-patient) dose adjustments that most clearly demonstrated to my patients how research interests trump their medical interests. These trials are also of interest because the rarity with which they are employed throughout the United States illustrates a cultural refractoriness to change that stems from deep-seated but dimly acknowledged needs of patients, physicians, and the medical community as a whole. After reviewing the mechanics of intrapatient dose escalation, I discuss why the reasons most commonly offered in rejecting this dosing scheme do not hold up to scrutiny.

Intrapatient dose escalation is a dosing scheme that allows patients to be given successively higher doses of an experimental drug (within certain safety parameters) if the initial dose administered proves to be well tolerated but unable to shrink the tumor. Intrapatient dose escalation is based on the rationale that typical anticancer agents have the best chance of killing cancer cells when administered at the highest safely achievable dose. For more than 10 years, trial strategies (such as, and in addition to, intrapatient dose escalation) have been proposed that avoid consigning the bulk of patients to doses that animal data suggest do not maximize the chance for response.[6,12,16,21,30,33,46-55] Yet, fewer than 15% of Phase I cancer trials in the United States employ these innovative approaches.[20,28]

The initial interdiction of intrapatient dose escalation in Phase I trials occurred in the early 1960s, after clinical studies with nitrosoureas that resulted in delayed toxicity.[6,56] Although the movement away from intrapatient dose escalation is linked historically to the misfortune with nitrosoureas, there is no scientific justification for the persistence of this avoidance. In reviewing the National Cancer Institute's Phase I database, an expert panel concluded that cumulative toxicity does not appear to be a valid reason to prohibit intrapatient dose escalation:[28] Where intrapatient dose escalation was used, there was no evidence that it had a negative impact on the trial or on individual patients. In fact, comparing conventional dosing schemes with these innovative designs[6,30,49] suggests that innovative individualized approaches (e.g., intrapatient dose escalation) effectively reduce the number of patients treated at doses substantially less than that recommended for Phase II trials and speed the completion of the trials.

Changing the dosing strategy does not, unfortunately, change the nature of a patient's incurable disease. It is unlikely, therefore, that any foreseeable technical modification (including intrapatient dose escalation) will greatly improve clinically meaningful Phase I trial response rates.

Nevertheless, dosing schemes that attempt to maximize the response that each patient can expect, small as that chance may remain, bring into closer alignment what patients expect from their doctors and what protocol allows doctors to provide. Because of this, a critical impediment to open dialogue between doctor and patient is, if not removed, made less formidable. Similarly, if eligibility for Phase I trials resembled eligibility for Phase II trials, where tumor types that appear most likely to respond to the agent under investigation are the tumor types admitted, patients enrolled would at least be given a drug that has a specific anticancer rationale for their particular disease.

There are, however, dangers in an overly zealous attachment to making technical changes if such attachments serve to divert attention from the more fundamental issue of using persons as the means for other's ends. Perhaps intrapatient dose escalation (and like modifications) will unintentionally reinforce patients' and physicians' expectations that Phase I trials are therapy when, in fact, the gain under this regimen may be so slight as to be indistinguishable from that under more traditional approaches. If so, the specter of clinical benefit might obscure questions about what else is risked, who is most likely to benefit, and how the trial itself is still configured in service of science, not medicine. In addition, if these structural modifications encourage physicians to see these trials as enterprises that are therapeutic, the standards of disclosure in purely therapeutic doctor–patient encounters risk becoming, and thereby lowering, the standards for these trials. The admonition inherent in these critiques does not excuse inaction that would maintain a clearly suboptimal status quo. Rather, it warns us to be alert to the likely influence of proposed changes, to the conflicts of interest that remain, and to the particular susceptibility of some patients to choose harm.

Among some of my oncology colleagues not directly involved in Phase I trials, these initial human trials were viewed as ethically untenable, and consequently, they rarely, if ever, referred patients for Phase I trials. Among physicians involved in Phase I studies, some stated that they prefer innovative designs but that costs and the level of sophistication required to coordinate and conduct such trials were impediments to employing them more commonly. Many, however, offered explanations that sustained current practice.

The most common explanations put forward by defenders of current practice fit into one of four groups. First, intrapatient dose escalation is not a workable Phase I strategy because it vitiates determination of the agents' acute and chronic toxicities. Although I accepted this explanation as creditable when I first heard it, after further investigation, it became clear that this view is not supported by the literature.[6,28,30,49] Second, newer anticancer agents were unlike the old chemotoxic drugs in that tumor response is not assumed to be roughly proportionate to drug dosage and that, therefore, the problem of predictably undertreating so many patients was soon to be a concern of the past. Although some of the newer agents, such as angiogenesis inhibitors, have anticancer effects at nontoxic levels, arguments regarding noncytotoxic agents do not apply to most of today's Phase I cancer trials. Third, because of our profound ignorance about these new agents, any dose can be considered (equally) potentially therapeutic. Although we are indeed profoundly ignorant about these agents, the little we do know from preclinical models is not generally being used in designing and implementing dosing strategies in most of today's trials.[6,20,28,57] Fourth, someone would have already made these changes if they were technically possible. Indeed, this last explanation was what I assumed when I first agreed to become a member of the Phase I clinical team.

What is striking about these explanations (offered by deeply committed and thoughtful professionals) is the way that the perception of technical necessity (to use traditional design) served to abruptly arrest attempts to think through the ethical imperatives in human experimentation. This perception may serve an important function within the Phase I community (or within the broader oncology community), an adverting rationalization that distracts ethical inquiry, looks to a monolithic notion of uncertainty as a way to avoid discussing the morally relevant little we do know, and maintains the status quo. Indeed, the status quo may be resistant to change because of the deeply embedded cultural and psychological function these trials, in their long-standing incarnation, serve. One of these deeply embedded functions may be as an instrument of affect management, as the magic card that referring physicians, physician–investigators, and patients can play together to keep in abeyance difficult and uncomfortable discussions that loom when therapeutic options have been exhausted. Referring physicians can rationalize putting off these difficult matters because the physician–investigator is offering one last hope. Physician–investigators, in a compromised state to speak about the lack of therapeutic options because they have not had the chance to earn the trust of a new recruit, can focus instead on the possibility of benefit to both society and patients, and patients, perhaps in the most compromised position of all to raise difficult questions about their fears and about possible conflicts of interest, can acquiesce in this avoidance and misunderstanding as a way of preserving a desperate hope.

Recommendations for IRB Review

With all of these misperceptions, is anything approaching truly informed decision making possible? As others have noted, many investigators have maintained that truly informed consent is a more difficult problem in clinical research than in usual clinical practice because patient–subjects are even less capable of understanding the additional scientific complexities that a clinical trial seeks to resolve.[41] These investigators are right that it is more difficult to achieve truly informed decision making in clinical research than in clinical practice, but for the wrong reasons. It is not the recondite nature of scientific complexities that stymies understanding. Indeed, morally relevant information is too readily obscured by an over-

whelming amount of unnecessary scientific minutiae. Rather, it is that physician–investigators are susceptible to unwittingly obscure the distinction between their roles as physician and as investigator.

As has been noted, given how little we know about the way fear and illness, being thought incompetent, and being kept ignorant limit a patient's capacity for reflective thought, it would be irresponsible to reach any conclusive judgments about what patients can and cannot understand.[41] This does not, of course, excuse trading on patients' desperate hopes. Perhaps Phase I cancer trials will accrue far more slowly if informed and uncoerced consent is even partially achieved, but that is a price that IRBs are obliged to insist on in the name of protecting potential subjects' rights to self-determination and the inviolability of their bodies. To this end, what can IRBs do? At the very least, IRBs can insist on clarity with regard to two critical aspects of Phase I trials: (1) the dosing strategy proposed and (2) how investigators plan to assure that participating subjects understand the nature of the sacrifice they are being asked to make. What follows are some specific suggestions.

Require Investigators to Explain and Justify the Dose Schedule

IRBs should require that investigators explicitly justify to the committee whatever dosing schemes they propose to use. Investigators should be required to explain why a drug that showed promise in an animal model of a particular cancer (e.g., breast cancer) is to be administered to subjects with cancers unrelated to the animal model in question (e.g., brain tumors). IRBs should reject the use of traditional schemata if the justification rests on any of the fallacious rationalizations laid out in the previous section.

Determine Whether the Study Agent Is Being Evaluated Simultaneously in Other Centers

IRBs should require that investigators report whether the agent proposed for study is being simultaneously studied in other Phase I centers and, if so, in what way information already known about the agent is going to be incorporated into the current proposal. Phase I research studies that seek to repeat other Phase I trials or are contemporaneous with other trials of the same agent must justify the rationale for repetition and must demonstrate, in the case of contemporaneous trials, how the centers will coordinate their dosing strategies based on daily exchange of shared data. As Katz[41] has written, we must not seek truth when it is already known or progress when it is already a reality.

Reject Justifications for a Phase I Protocol That Are Based on Adjunctive Elements Unrelated to the Research Question

Arguments that the general quality of the medical care that they receive will be higher if they participate in a research study should never offset ethical compromises in research design. Subjects should not participate in a Phase I trial because they benefit from "close follow-up" or have access to "free medical care."

Make Clear the Distinction Between Research and Patient Care

IRBs should reject in all written forms and should discourage, in the consenting dialogue itself, the use of oxymoronic language that serves to blur the distinction between the enterprise of research and the activity of patient-centered care. As Annas[43] has written: "Research is research, designed to test a hypothesis and performed based on the rules of the protocol; treatment is something else, designed to benefit a patient, and subject to change whenever change is seen in the patient's best interest. Confusing research with treatment confuses both the researcher and subject and permits self-interested self-deception by both of them." Examples of words that are likely to compromise the informed consent process include "experimental therapy" and "novel treatment."

Require a Cohort-Specific Consent Document

If cohort-specific escalation is employed, so too should a cohort-specific consenting process and cohort-specific consent form be used. This is based on the broadly agreed-on notion that subjects of research are entitled to relevant information about purpose and consequent design of the study.[19] Benjamin Freedman has provided a template for such a cohort-specific consent form and for the way the invitation ought to be extended.[40] Freedman's template attempts to explain clearly the structure of the study and where a particular patient–subject fits into that structure—specifically, into which cohort he or she would be enrolled. It attempts to make clear how an individual's dose is cohort specific. To this I would add the explicit statement that the dose administered is not chosen to maximize the chance of antitumor effect and that, in this way, it differs from alternatives such as second- or third-line chemotherapy. The invitation to participate must, as Freedman urges, make clear to patients that individuals enrolled in the earliest group are least likely to experience severe toxicity (but may nonetheless) and are also least likely to get a dose that is potent against their cancer. His template notes that it is often, but not always, true that the higher the dose, the more powerful are the effects against cancer, but also the more likely to produce unacceptable reactions. Finally, patients are to be explicitly told that if they agree to enroll, they will be assigned to the *nth* group of subjects and told as well what is known about the responses and toxicities experienced by subjects previously enrolled.

Require a Commitment to Eliminating Misconceptions About Risks and Benefits

The principle of respect for persons requires that potential subjects understand the important implications of their decision to participate in research. This principle emphasizes the need to clarify the goals of Phase I trials to the people who are being asked to participate in them. Specifically, potential subjects should be told that Phase I trials are designed to determine toxicity, that severe toxicity is a planned event for a subset of subjects, and that direct benefit is both not intended and extremely unlikely.

As others have cautioned, this fact must not be disguised by drafting a protocol as a combined Phase I/Phase II trial and calling it one of effectiveness and safety on the basis that the endpoint of the second, Phase II component.[40] The President's Commission's comments on Phase I cancer trials emphasize that it is "important that patients who are asked to participate in tests of new anticancer drugs not be misled about the likelihood (or remoteness) of any therapeutic benefit they might derive." In accordance with this emphasis, patients should be told that historically only one of 20 subjects has a partial response and that the complete response rate is roughly equal to that of fatal toxicity, 0.5%. Furthermore, patients should also be told that even if their cancer responds to the experimental agent, no one has ever been cured in a Phase I trial, and that any response is expected to be temporary, with most cancers recurring within 3 to 6 months. Patients must also be told that although it is possible that response correlates with physical benefit, it is also possible that even the few patient–subjects whose disease responds may not actually derive any benefit either in terms of prolonging life or in improving the quality of life. The recommended standard wording for the consent document in all Phase I studies is presented in Figure 10.13.1.

Evaluate the Quality of Informed Consent

Telling patients what they need to know is not enough. Institutions and researchers must be held accountable not merely for a signature on a consent form but for some minimal level of patient comprehension. Mandating that specific steps are taken is one approach to improving the consent process. There is, however, a drawback to an overly specified series of required steps: It introduces rigidity and diverts attention from creative approaches to achieving informed decision making. An approach that may prove more effective (especially once fundamental

---

Purpose: The purpose of this study is to find the highest dose of _____ that people can tolerate without getting extremely ill.

Risks: In this study, the dose of _____ will be increased until people get extremely sick. It is impossible to predict the side effects that you will experience.

Benefits: This study is not being done to treat your cancer. Based on prior experience, the chance that you will feel better or live longer as a result of participating in this study is almost zero. This study is being done in the hope that it will provide information that will improve the treatment of people in the future.

Figure 10.13.1 Recommended standard wording for consent document in Phase I oncology studies

inputs are identified) is to make physicians and institutions accountable not merely for incorporating a limited number of prespecified actions (important as these requirements are), but also for achieving some minimal threshold of patient understanding. Creative efforts will be stimulated, offering the best hope of amelioration, precisely because attention to the consenting process is demanded by the challenge to bring about the desired end: adequate patient comprehension.

IRBs ideally should insist on an objective assessment of patient understanding, with a special emphasis on the requirement that patients understand the ways in which their therapeutic interests are possibly opposed by the structure of the trial. The assessment of comprehending consent cannot rest on the signature of the consent form or the good intentions of the informing physician–investigator. To this end, IRBs should require the use (or development) of a validated instrument that assesses patient comprehension, such as the MacArthur Competence Assessment Tool for Clinical Research (MacCAT-CR)[58] or others in the literature.[59] In demanding higher standards of informed consent in clinical research compared with clinical practice, it should be remembered that respect for the subject's right to self-determination requires that he or she know the decision to participate entails making a gift for the sake of others. It is not an act of enlightened self-interest, not a quid pro quo, for these untried agents offer no more objective likelihood of effective anticancer effect than do existing agents that have been deemed unlikely to avail.

It is worth noting that research suggests that informed, uncoerced, voluntary, and understanding decision making may not be a quixotic goal. Researchers have demonstrated that patients can be taught to recognize that research sometimes conflicts with the goals of ordinary treatment.[60] A technique that proved particularly helpful was to have a third party supplement what investigators disclose to subjects with a "preconsent disclosure." This discussion was led by a third party, distinct from the Phase I team, who was trained to teach potential subjects about critical methodological aspects of the protocol, especially those that might conflict with the principle of personal, individualized care. The authors of this study concluded that there is no reason to think that subjects will refuse to hear clear-cut efforts to dispel the therapeutic misconception. In my experience, patients could recognize that the requirements of Phase I trials were those of science, not of medicine, but only if and when we discussed the way the particular protocol offered undermined fundamental assumptions they held about the doctor–patient relationship. This, however, very often discouraged participation: patients wanted to be given a dose adjusted according to their own needs, as in intrapatient dose escalation schemes, or at least one predicted to have maximal anticancer effect.

References

1. Freedman B. The ethical analysis of clinical trials: New lessons for and from cancer research. In: Vanderpool HY (ed.). *The Ethics of Research Involving Human Subjects: Facing the 21st Century.* Frederick, MD: University Publishing Group; 1996:319–338.
2. Miller M. Phase I cancer trials: A collusion of misunderstanding. *Hastings Cent Rep* 30(4):34–43, 2000.
3. Daugherty C, Ratain MJ, Grochowski E, et al. Perceptions of cancer patients and their physicians involved in Phase I trials [published erratum appears in *J Clin Oncol* 1995 Sep;13(9):2476]. *J Clin Oncol* 13(5):1062–1072, 1995.
4. Daugherty CK, Ratain MJ, Minami H, et al. Study of cohort-specific consent and patient control in Phase I cancer trials. *J Clin Oncol* 16(7):2305–2312, 1998.
5. Daugherty CK. Informed consent, the cancer patient, and Phase I clinical trials. *Cancer Treat Res* 102(1):77–89, 2000.
6. Frei E. Clinical trials of antitumor agents: Experimental design and timeline considerations. *Cancer J* 3(3):127–136, 1997.
7. Tomamichel M, Sessa C, Herzig S, et al. Informed consent for Phase I studies: Evaluation of quantity and quality of information provided to patients. *Ann Oncol* 6(4):363–369, 1995.
8. Yoder LH, O'Rourke TJ, Etnyre A, Spears DT, Brown TD. Expectations and experiences of patients with cancer participating in Phase I clinical trials. *Oncol Nurs Forum* 24(5):891–896, 1997.
9. Rodenhuis S, Van Den Heuvel WJ, Annyas AA, Koops HS, Sleijfer DT, Mulder NH. Patient motivation and informed consent in a Phase I study of an anticancer agent. *Eur J Cancer Clin Oncol* 20(4):457–462, 1984.
10. Willems Y, Sessa C. Informing patients about Phase I trials—How should it be done? *Acta Oncol* 28(1):106–107, 1989.
11. Schaeffer MH, Krantz DS, Wichman A, Masur H, Reed E, Vinicky JK. The impact of disease severity on the informed consent process in clinical research. *Am J Med* 100(3):261–268, 1996.
12. Ratain MJ, Mick R, Schilsky RL, Siegler M. Statistical and ethical issues in the design and conduct of Phase I and II clinical trials of new anticancer agents. *J Natl Cancer Inst* 85(20):1637–1643, 1993.
13. Storer B, DeMets D. Current Phase I/II designs: Are they adequate? *J Clin Res Drug Dev* 1:121–130, 1987.
14. Gordon NH, Wilson JK. Using toxicity grades in the design and analysis of cancer Phase I clinical trials. *Stat Med* 11(16):2063–2075, 1992.
15. Fisher B. Clinical trials for the evaluation of cancer therapy. *Cancer* 54(11 Suppl):2609–2617, 1984.
16. Hawkins MJ. Early cancer clinical trials: Safety, numbers, and consent (editorial comment). *J Natl Cancer Inst* 85(20):1618–1619, 1993.
17. Freedman B. A response to a purported ethical difficulty with randomized clinical trials involving cancer patients. *J Clin Ethics* 3(3):231–234, 1992.
18. Decoster G, Stein G, Holdener EE. Responses and toxic deaths in Phase I clinical trials. *Ann Oncol* 1(3):175–181, 1990.
19. Levine RJ. *Ethics and Regulation of Clinical Research,* 2nd ed. Baltimore, MD: Urban and Schwarzenberg; 1986.
20. Dent SF, Eisenhauer EA. Phase I trial design: Are new methodologies being put into practice? *Ann Oncol* 7(6):561–566, 1996.

21. Gatsonis C, Greenhouse JB. Bayesian methods for Phase I clinical trials. *Stat Med* 11(10):1377–1389, 1992.

22. Storer BE. Design and analysis of Phase I clinical trials. *Biometrics* 45(3):925–937, 1989.

23. Van Hoff D, Kuh J, Clark G. Design and conduct of Phase I trials. In: Buyse M, Staquet M, Sylvester R (eds.). *Cancer Clinical Trials: Methods and Practice.* Oxford: Oxford University Press; 1984.

24. EORTC New Drug Development Committee, Rozencweig M, Staquet M, Hansen H, et al. EORTC guidelines for Phase I trials with single agents in adults. *Eur J Cancer Clin Oncol* 21(9):1005–1007, 1985.

25. Geller NL. Design of Phase I and II clinical trials in cancer: A statistician's view. *Cancer Invest* 2(6):483–491, 1984.

26. Carter SK, Selawry O, Slavik M. Phase I clinical trials. *Natl Cancer Inst Monogr* 45:75–80, 1977.

27. *Cancer: Principles and Practice of Oncology,* 5th ed. Philadelphia: Lippincott-Raven; 1997.

28. Von Hoff DD. Is response in Phase I trials a useful predictor for the future clinical activity of a new agent [abstract]? *Ann Oncol* 7(Suppl 1):14, 1996.

29. Decoster G, Cavalli F. Design of Phase I and II clinical trials in cancer: A statistician's view. *Cancer Invest* 5(6):649–650, 1987.

30. Mick R, Ratain MJ. Model-guided determination of maximum tolerated dose in Phase I clinical trials: Evidence for increased precision. *J Natl Cancer Inst* 85(3):217–223, 1993.

31. Von Hoff DD, Turner J. Response rates, duration of response, and dose response effects in Phase I studies of antineoplastics. *Invest New Drugs* 9(1):115–122, 1991.

32. Estey E, Hoth D, Wittes R, Marsoni S, Simon R, Leyland-Jones B. Therapeutic response in Phase I trials of antineoplastic agents. *Cancer Treat Rep* 70(9):1105–1115, 1986.

33. Penta JS, Rosner GL, Trump DL. Choice of starting dose and escalation for Phase I studies of antitumor agents. *Cancer Chemother Pharmacol* 31(3):247–250, 1992.

34. Smith TL, Lee JJ, Kantarjian HM, Legha SS, Raber MN. Design and results of Phase I cancer clinical trials: Three-year experience at M.D. Anderson Cancer Center. *J Clin Oncol* 14(1):287–295, 1996.

35. Janisch L, Mick R, Schilsky RL, et al. Prognostic factors for survival in patients treated in Phase I clinical trials. *Cancer* 74(7):1965–1973, 1994.

36. Fried C. *Medical Experimentation: Personal Integrity and Social Policy.* New York: American Elsevier; 1974.

37. Appelbaum PS, Roth LH, Lidz C. The therapeutic misconception: Informed consent in psychiatric research. *Int J Law Psychiatry* 5(3–4):319–329, 1982.

38. Kodish E, Stocking C, Ratain MJ, Kohrman A, Siegler M. Ethical issues in Phase I oncology research: A comparison of investigators and institutional review board chairpersons. *J Clin Oncol* 10(11):1810–1816, 1992.

39. Kass NE, Sugarman J, Faden R, Schoch-Spana M. Trust, the fragile foundation of contemporary biomedical research. *Hastings Cent Rep* 26(5):25–29, 1996.

40. Freedman B. Cohort-specific consent: An honest approach to Phase I clinical cancer studies. *IRB: A Review of Human Subjects Research* 12(1):5–7, 1990.

41. Katz J. Human experimentation and human rights. *St Louis Univ Law J* 38:7–54, 1993.

42. Katz JM. "Ethics and clinical research" revisited: A tribute to Henry K. Beecher. *Hastings Cent Rep* 23(5):31–39, 1993.

43. Annas GJ. Questing for grails: Duplicity, betrayal, and self-deception in postmodern medical research. *J Contemp Health Law Policy* 12(2):297–324, 1996.

44. Katz J. Informed consent—must it remain a fairy tale? *J Contemp Health Law Policy* 10:69–91, 1994.

45. Penman DT, Holland JC, Bahna GF, et al. Informed consent for investigational chemotherapy: Patients' and physicians' perceptions. *J Clin Oncol* 2(7):849–855, 1984.

46. O'Quigley J. Sequential design and analysis of dose finding studies in patients with life threatening disease. *Fundam Clin Pharmacol* 4(Suppl 2):81s–91s, 1990.

47. O'Quigley J, Pepe M, Fisher L. Continual reassessment method: A practical design for Phase I clinical trials in cancer. *Biometrics* 46(1):33–48, 1990.

48. O'Quigley J, Chevret S. Methods for dose finding studies in cancer clinical trials: A review and results of a Monte Carlo study. *Stat Med* 10(11):1647–1664, 1991.

49. O'Quigley J. Estimating the probability of toxicity at the recommended dose following a Phase I clinical trial in cancer [published erratum appears in *Biometrics* 1994 March;50(1):322]. *Biometrics* 48(3):853–862, 1992.

50. Piantadosi S, Liu G. Improved designs for dose escalation studies using pharmacokinetic measurements. *Stat Med* 15(15):1605–1618, 1996.

51. Mick R, Lane N, Daugherty C, Ratain MJ. Physician-determined patient risk of toxic effects: Impact on enrollment and decision making in Phase I cancer trials. *J Natl Cancer Inst* 86(22):1685–1693, 1994.

52. Moller S. An extension of the continual reassessment methods using a preliminary up-and-down design in a dose finding study in cancer patients, in order to investigate a greater range of doses. *Stat Med* 14(9–10):911–922, 1995.

53. Eichhorn BH, Zacks S. Sequential search for an optimal dosage. *J Am Stat Assoc* 68(343):594–598, 1973.

54. Goodman SN, Zahurak ML, Piantadosi S. Some practical improvements in the continual reassessment method for Phase I studies. *Stat Med* 14(11):1149–1161, 1995.

55. Faries D. Practical modifications of the continual reassessment method for Phase I cancer clinical trials. *J Biopharm Stat* 4(2):147–164, 1994.

56. Hansen HH, Selawry OS, Muggia FM, Walker MD. Clinical studies with 1-(2-chloroethyl)-3-cyclohexyl-1-nitrosourea (NSC 79037). *Cancer Res* 31(3):223–227, 1971.

57. Eisenhauer EA. Phase I and II trials of novel anti-cancer agents: Endpoints, efficacy and existentialism. *Ann Oncol* 9(10):1047–1052, 1998.

58. Applebaum PS, Grisso T. The MacArthur Treatment Competence Study: Mental illness and competence to consent to treatment. *Law Hum Behav* 19:105–126, 1995.

59. Joffe S, Cook EF, Cleary PD, Clark JW, Weeks JC. Quality of informed consent: A new measure of understanding among research subjects. *J Natl Cancer Inst* 93(2):139–147, 2001.

60. Appelbaum PS, Roth LH, Lidz CW, Benson P, Winslade W. False hopes and best data: Consent to research and the therapeutic misconception. *Hastings Cent Rep* 17(2):20–24, 1987.

Research Involving Genetic Testing

Eric C. Larsen

INTRODUCTION

The rapid pace of genetic research creates unique challenges to the institutional review board (IRB) review process. The dramatic progress in our understanding of the genetic basis of health and disease raises a number of key regulatory issues.[1-5] This chapter focuses on the issues that are important to consider when the IRB reviews genetic research studies.

When discussing genetic research, it is important to understand the difference between the study of *constitutional* (also called *host*) genes, meaning the genes common to all normal tissues in the body, and the study of genetic material from the pathologic tissue of humans, such as malignancies. Research on constitutional genes is likely to involve sensitive information about research participants and demand careful IRB review. An example of this type of research is the determination of the expression of certain genes that result in the subsequent development of a serious medical illness. The information collected in such a study clearly has potential for psychological and financial harm to research participants. In contrast, genetic research involving pathologic human tissue rarely poses risk to participants because genetic abnormalities in this setting are usually not representative of the subject's underlying genetic makeup. An example of genetic research with pathologic tissue is the study of the relationship between gene expression in tumor tissue with clinical outcome. This type of research poses almost no risk (and no direct benefit) to the participant.

Genetic research typically presents risks of social and psychologic harm to participants rather than risks of physical harm. Several areas in genetic research pose challenges to the IRB process, including selection of participants, confidentiality, disclosure of information, storage of data and samples, and participant withdrawal.

Selection of Participants

Certain genetic research studies involve the investigations of individuals within a certain family pedigree or a certain social or ethnic group. The design of these studies may place undue influence on an individual's decision to participate in the study. An example of this is the analysis of the types of mutations of the von Willebrand gene in large kindred affected by severe clinical bleeding. There will be an attempt to include all family members because the more complete the pedigree is the more useful the resulting information will be. Family members who are not interested in participating will likely experience pressure to participate in order to enhance the quality of the study. At this point, the decision not to participate affects more than just the individual. The federal regulations provide little guidance in this situation: "Selection of subjects is equitable."[6(Sec.111(a)(3))] "An investigator shall seek such consent only under circumstances that provide the prospective subject or the representative sufficient opportunity to consider whether or not to participate and that minimize the possibility of coercion or undue influence."[6(Sec.116)] The IRB review of pedigree studies must take into account the potential coercion of family members and be aware of alternative recruitment strategies.

Confidentiality and Privacy

Privacy and confidentiality issues are perhaps the most challenging regulatory aspects of genetic research. Because of the sensitive nature of the information that may be generated from genetic research studies, it is critical that investigators establish a method to secure information in a highly confidential manner. Studies that have the potential to ultimately predict the likelihood of subsequent serious illness could place participants at high risk for psychological and social harm. This type of sensitive information could adversely affect an individual's future insurability and employability as well as have significant impact on his or her psychological well-being. For example, consider the study of the expression of a particular gene that places individuals at a very high risk of developing colon cancer at a young age. Personal knowledge of this finding presents a psychologic burden on the individual, and disclosure of this information could affect one's ability to obtain medical insurance and/or employment. The regulation[6][Sec.111(a)(6)] states, "When appropriate, the research plan makes adequate provisions to protect the privacy of subjects and to maintain the confidentiality of data." Whereas confidentiality of research data is important in all studies, it is particularly crucial in genetic research studies because of the sensitivity of the data. Thus, IRB review must be scrupulous in assuring that privacy and confidentiality are always maintained.

Disclosure of Information

As genetic research may yield information of the most private nature, the IRB and potential research subject must understand exactly who will have access to study information and under what circumstances. This issue of disclosing research results to the subject should be explicitly addressed in the protocol application and consent document. This topic is the subject of Chapter 6-9. Investigators and IRBs have to weigh the risks and benefits of giving a subject access to research results. There are many different scenarios to consider. Something that may be overlooked is the possibility that the disclosure of unanticipated or incidental information may harm the subject. A common example of an incidental finding in genetic research that may have serious consequences is the finding that family members are not biologically related. During the informed consent process, potential participants should always be given the opportunity not to receive information, if they so desire.

An additional important consideration is the potential need for genetic counseling. There are situations in which genetic counseling is appropriate for participants involved in genetic research studies. It is impossible to define clearly the situations for which counseling is indicated, but IRBs should consider the potential benefits of genetic counseling to participants in these studies.

Secure Storage of Data and Tissue Samples

Genetic studies often involve the use of tissue or cell banks that may involve the long-term storage of biological materials.[7,8] In some studies, the precise nature of subsequent experiments on banked samples is not clear and/or not disclosed to the participant at the time of banking. Because the results of these studies may pose harm to individuals as

outlined previously here, it is crucial that participants be fully informed about their subsequent knowledge of research results. For example, a study banks tissue on participants as an optional part of the study; in the future, these samples are screened for the expression of a gene that predicts for alcoholism. Clearly, the results of this subsequent study, which is conceived and carried out long after the actual collection of samples, carries substantial social and financial risk to the participants. Whenever possible, genetic test results should be stored in a secure manner. When participants are informed, there is really no way to make genetic samples completely anonymous. During the informed consent process, it is critical that participants understand both the inherent risk of this type of research and, if it is the case, that they will not be informed of the results of subsequent studies performed on their tissue. IRB management of studies that involve the storage of tissue for future research is the subject of Chapter 10-10.

Participant Withdrawal

Ethical research requires that subjects have the right to withdraw from research participation at any point in the study. In genetic research, there is the potential for continuation of individual risk after withdrawal from the study when there is long-term storage of tissue. For this reason, it is important to determine whether the research plan provides for the destruction of all stored data and tissue if the subject wants this to be done. If the research plan does not provide for tissue or data destruction, the study may still be ethical as long as participants understand this limitation.

IRB Evaluation of Genetic Research Studies

A critical first step in the IRB review process of genetic studies is the determination of the predictive value of the study results. This determination should be made through an interactive dialogue between the IRB and the investigator. If there is reasonable scientific evidence that the expression of certain genetic markers within a study accurately predicts for a particular disease or condition, then participants are at risk, and the IRB must know the answers to a detailed list of questions before a determination can be made. Alternatively, if there is no clear evidence that a particular marker has predictive value, then there is virtually no risk to participants. At Dartmouth, questions about genetic testing are included as an attachment to the general IRB application package. The text of the attachment follows and may be found at: http://www.dartmouth.edu/~cphs/tosubmit/forms/ within the CPHS Study Plan. When a study involves genetic testing, the principal investigator is first asked to make a determination about the predictive value of the genetic tests that will be done as part of the project. An investigator who thinks that the genetic testing is clinically useful in predicting the development of disease (answer "b" in the first section) is required to go on to the second part of the attachment, which is a detailed list of questions related to the risk of research participation. This list of questions is adapted from the OHRP *IRB Guidebook*.[3(Chap.5H)] The third section of the attachment guides both the investigator and IRB in identifying the information that must be included in the consent document when research involves tests for markers that clearly predict the development of disease.

Attachment C of the CPHS Study Plan

Genetic Research
For research studies involving genetic testing the CPHS has developed two basic categories to assist in the determination of further review. The researcher should determine if the research falls into category (a) or (b) as described below.

If the research falls into category (a) indicate by circling below and add comments as appropriate to this project. If the research falls into category (b) please respond to questions that follow.

(a) The study is looking for an association between a genetic marker and a specific disease or condition, but at this point it is not clear if the genetic marker has predictive value. *The uncertainty regarding the predictive value of the genetic marker is such that studies in this category will not involve participant counseling.*

Comment:

(b) The study is based on the premise that a link between a genetic marker and a specific disease or condition is such that the marker *is* clinically useful in predicting the development of that specific disease or condition. *Respond to the questions in* Human Genetic Research Questions for CPHS Review, *which follow.*

Human Genetic Research Questions for CPHS Review
For studies involving genetic testing, the PI must respond to the following items (if an item is not applicable to the study, please state NA).

1. Are clear guidelines established for disclosure of information, including interim or inconclusive research results to the participants?
2. Will participants be told about what information (and its meaning) they may receive at what point in the research?
3. Will family members be protected against disclosure of medical or other personal information about themselves to other family members?
4. Will they be given the option not to receive information about themselves?
5. Will limits on such protections be clearly communicated to participants, including obtaining advance consent to such disclosures (e.g., when family members will be warned about health risks)?
6. Will the possible psychological and social risks of genetic research be adequately considered in the consent process?
7. Will appropriate counseling be provided, both as part of the consent process and when communicating test or other research results to participants?
8. Will participants be informed about the possibility of important incidental findings such as paternity, disease, or conditions other than the one(s) under the study?
9. Will the data be protected from disclosure to third parties, such as employers and insurance companies?
10. Will the participant be told about the potential consequences of a third party, such as an employer or insurance company, becoming aware of the study findings?
11. Will the data be stored in a secure manner?
12. Will the data be coded so as to protect the identity of subjects?
13. Is a request for a certificate of confidentiality appropriate?
14. Does the investigator plan to disclose research findings to subjects' physicians for clinical use?
15. Are such plans appropriate?
16. Will the possibility of such disclosures be discussed with and consented to by prospective participants?
17. Will vulnerable populations (e.g., children, persons with impaired mental capacities) be adequately protected?
18. Under what circumstances can a research participant serve to grant permission to involve a minor or an incapacitated adult in a study?
19. Have adequate provisions been made for protecting against misuse of tissue samples (e.g., confidentiality, obtaining consent for any used not within the original purpose of this study)?
20. What agreements with participants are necessary to use stored materials for new studies or for clinical diagnoses?
21. Have adequate provisions been made for the treatment of data and tissue samples in the event of subject withdrawal from the study?
22. Do the investigator's publication plans threaten the privacy or confidentiality of participants?
23. Has adequate consideration been given to ways in which participants' privacy and confidentiality can be protected (e.g., providing for consent to publication of identifying information)?
24. If research may involve family members:
    a. Has the appropriateness of various strategies for recruiting participants been considered?
    b. Will information be obtained via clinical medical records of family members?
    c. If so, should consent be obtained prior to use of the data, or is the permission of participant sufficient?

Information for Consent Document
Participants should be informed of the following:
- The kind of information with which they will be provided (e.g., only information the investigator feels is significant and reliable, or no genetic information will be provided) and at what point in the study they will receive that information
- They may find out things about themselves or their family that they did not really want to know, or that they may be uncomfortable knowing
- Information about themselves may be learned by others in their family
- Whether or not information they learn or information generated about them during the study could compromise their insurability
- Actions they may take as a result of their participation may expose them to risks (e.g., submitting insurance claim forms for reimbursement of costs for genetic counseling or procedures not covered by the protocol)

- What assurance can be given to protect confidentiality and what lack of assurance can be given
- The rights they retain and the rights they must give up regarding control over what can be done with tissue they donate (e.g., blood samples)
- Consequences of withdrawal from the study
- Costs associated with participation (e.g., the cost of genetic and/or psychological counseling, if those costs will not be covered by the investigator or the institution).

References

1. Allen HJ. Genetic protocols review by institutional review boards at National Cancer Institute-designated Cancer Centers. *Genetic Testing* 2(4):329–335, 1998.

2. American Society of Human Genetics. Statement on informed consent for genetic research. *Am J Hum Genet* 59(2):471–474, 1996.

3. Penslar RL, Porter JP, Office for Human Research Protections. *Institutional Review Board Guidebook*, 2nd ed. Updated 6 February, 2001. Access date 29 March, 2001. http://ohrp.osophs.dhhs.gov/irbirb_guidebook.htm

4. Reilly PR, Boshar MF, Holtzman SH. Ethical issues in genetic research: Disclosure and informed consent. *Nat Genet* 15(4):16–20, 1997.

5. Weir RF, Horton JR. Genetic research, adolescents, and informed consent. *Theor Med* 16(4):347–373, 1995.

6. Code of Federal Regulations. Title 45A—Department of Health and Human Services; Part 46—Protection of Human Subjects. Updated 1 October, 1997. Access date 18 April, 2001. http:www4.law.cornell.edu/cfr/45p46.htm

7. Clayton EW, Steinberg KK, Khoury MJ, et al. Informed consent for genetic research on stored tissue samples. *JAMA* 274(22):1786–1792, 1995.

8. Knoppers BM, Laberge CM. Research and stored tissues: Persons as sources, samples as persons. *JAMA* 274(2):1806–1807, 1995.

International Research

David A. Borasky

INTRODUCTION

It is currently not unusual for institutional review boards (IRBs) to review research proposed for international settings. Much of the new research is in less-developed countries, where investigators have limited experience with U.S.-sponsored studies, potential research participants are unfamiliar with concepts such as informed consent, and institutions have not established strong human subjects protection programs. In addition, some studies, such as the placebo-controlled HIV prevention trials in sub-Saharan Africa, sparked a firestorm of criticism both within the research community and among IRBs. As a result, international research is the focus of a great deal of scrutiny. IRBs must be continuously vigilant when reviewing research intended for international settings.

Because of these heightened sensitivities, mechanisms for the protection of international research subjects have been strengthened. The Declaration of Helsinki was revised in 2000, and the National Bioethics Advisory Commission in April 2001 completed a report on issues in international research.[1] A copy of the Declaration of Helsinki[2] is included in Part 11 of this book. More recently, the Office for Human Research Protections (OHRP) has revised the assurance process, replacing the single-project assurance with a federalwide assurance (FWA) that allows foreign research institutions to rely on procedural standards other than 45 CFR 46.[3] This chapter is intended to guide IRBs through the process of reviewing international research, beginning before IRB review and following through the review process to the end of the study.

Before IRB Review

For an IRB that has received its first international research proposal, there can be feelings of trepidation on the part of the staff and membership. Before the first reviewer receives the proposal, several questions should be answered up front. Taking correct steps in the beginning will save time and effort in the long run. The following questions will help steer the IRB in the right direction.

Does Your Institution Hold a Multiple-Project Assurance or FWA?

If the answer is yes, then the proposed research site(s) will most likely need to file an FWA application. Instructions and templates are available on the OHRP Registration and Assurance Filing web page.[3]

Does a U.S. Department or Agency Fund the Research?

If the answer is yes, then it is probable that the institution will need to file a FWA. Check with the funding officer for the project and/or contact the OHRP assurance manager for your geographic region. Assurance coordinator assignments are listed on the OHRP web page.[3]

Is Your IRB Qualified to Review the Proposal?

This question is particularly important if your IRB will be the only one reviewing the proposal. A FWA requires an institution to name a designated IRB. The OHRP expects the designated IRB to have knowledge of the local research context.[4] This is important because the local research environment and the characteristics of the subjects being enrolled can vary greatly. The level of local knowledge required by the OHRP is based in part on the degree of risk presented by the research. For example, if the research involves minimal risk to subjects, the IRB should demonstrate that it has obtained necessary information about the local research context through written materials or discussions with appropriate consultants. As the level of risk increases, the steps an IRB must take to demonstrate local knowledge also increase. Additional steps might include adding a consultant to the IRB who is familiar with the research location or sending IRB members on regular visits to the research site.

Local IRBs

In many cases, it is required that a local IRB review the proposal. This may be due to policies of the host institution or local regulations or a requirement of OHRP or the research sponsor. In more experienced institutions, there will be an established review system in place, but if you are working with an independent investigator or a smaller institution, you may have to search for an appropriate local IRB. (The term *IRB* is not widely used outside of the United States. In foreign countries, the IRB may be known as the ethics committee, the research ethics committee, the ethical review committee, etc.) If you are having trouble finding a local IRB, you might look at nearby universities or research centers, government agencies such as the local ministry of health, or U.S. agencies with international experience (such as OHRP). Be aware that the infrastructure for ethical review can vary greatly, and the quality of review may vary as well.

Reviewing the Proposal

When reviewing the proposal, the IRB must be aware of local conditions and situations that may affect the design and implementation of the research. For example, local regulations governing research with minors can vary from country to country, just as they can vary by state in the United States. Also, local social and political conditions may distort the way informed consent documents are viewed by foreign participants, and a request for a subject's signature may be viewed with suspicion. Also, offering monetary compensation or access to health care may be coercive in certain research settings. The IRB should be prepared to bring in a consultant if sufficient knowledge of the local context is lacking. In addition, the IRB must be sure that all of its questions are satisfactorily answered before granting approval. Finally, the IRB is encouraged to review informed consent document translations for accuracy. The original approved English version and the back-translation should be compared, and major discrepancies should be addressed.

Monitoring Approved Research

After research is approved, IRBs that are responsible for international projects need effective mechanisms for ongoing review of research. IRB administrators should work closely with their own research staff to assure reliable access to collaborating investigators in the field. Regular correspondence between the field investigator and the IRB should be maintained. Because many foreign IRBs do not have continuing review requirements, foreign investigators should be informed of this requirement and any other related responsibilities. In addition, adverse event reporting requirements should be made clear so that IRBs receive required information in a timely manner. Any problems encountered with a foreign investigator should be reported to the study sponsor, relevant regulatory bodies, and when applicable, all reviewing IRBs for the project.

Conclusion

Reviewing international research is a challenge for any IRB. Problems that are considered routine for domestic IRBs can become much more complicated when encountered in an international setting. One example is the new education and training requirement for investigators and

research staff, which may be difficult to implement in less-developed countries where access to online resources is limited or where English is not the primary language. IRBs should move forward with caution and should take advantage of resources such as ARENA and the IRB Forum (formerly MCWIRB) when looking for answers to difficult questions.

References

1. National Bioethics Advisory Commission. Ethical and policy issues in international research: Clinical trials in developing countries. Updated 18 April, 2001. Access date 3 September, 2001. http:bioethics.gov/clinical/Vol1.pdf

2. World Medical Association. *Declaration of Helsinki: Ethical Principles for Medical Research Involving Human Subjects.* First adopted in Helsinki, Finland, in 1964. Updated 10 July, 2000. Access date 2 September, 2001. http://www.wma.net/e/policy/17-c_e.html

3. Office for Human Research Protections. Procedures for registering institutional review boards and filing federal-wide assurances of protection for human subjects (FWAs). Updated 22 August, 2001. Access date 3 September, 2001. http://ohrp.osophs.dhhs.gov/polasur.htm

4. Office for Protection from Research Risks. Knowledge of local research context. Updated 27 August, 1998. Access date 3 September, 2001. http://ohrp.osophs.dhhs.gov/humansubjects/guidance/local.htm

Example

1. Please describe the rationale for conducting research at an international site:

   Site location(s):
   Host site principal investigator (PI) name(s):
   Name of ethics committee:
   FWA No. (if applicable):
   Contact information (e-mail):

The IRB relies on communication with the host sites (PI and ethics committee) to ensure the research protocol addresses local issues. The following items should be completed via communication/collaboration with the host PI and/or local ethics committee:

a. Local standards for health care (describe):
b. Is the research responsive to the health needs of the host site?
c. Are the risks acceptable in the social context of the host country?
d. How will the research team ensure informed consent is obtained (describe process):
e. If compensation is being offered, is it appropriate for the setting?
f. Are there sufficient resources available to conduct the research (e.g., will research staff have appropriate training)?
g. Are there sufficient resources to monitor the research?
h. What provisions, if any, are there to continue if the health care intervention proves effective?
i. Will the results of the research be used at the host site?

Alternative Medicine Research

Timothy Callahan

INTRODUCTION

In this chapter, I briefly survey the terrain of complementary and alternative medicine, indicating some areas of contemporary discussion and disagreement as to what constitutes the parameters of the field. As complementary and alternative medical practices become more popular in the United States and are being used by an increasing percentage of the population, they are coming under greater scrutiny. The American public is demanding unfettered access to insurance reimbursement for therapies whose safety and effectiveness may be as yet unknown. Evaluation of these practices has begun to move from collections of anecdotes and testimonials to established methods of scientific inquiry, including controlled research studies involving the use of human subjects. As more medical professionals begin to practice in an "integrative" fashion, there is an increased need for focused research on alternative therapies and modalities.

With the establishment of the National Center for Complementary and Alternative Medicine (NCCAM) at the National Institutes of Health in 1998,[1] the federal government is supporting examination of alternative medical practices through an increased budget for competitive research proposals. From a research budget of $2 million in 1992 under the Office of Alternative Medicine to an FY2004 budget of $ 117.7 million under NCCAM, efforts have grown exponentially in the past decade. These efforts are being used to investigate various practices that Americans are seeking out and using in record numbers. According to a widely publicized 1998 study, as many as 42% of Americans currently use one or more medical practices labeled as "alternative" by the medical establishment.[2] As more research institutions compete for available funds, their institutional review boards (IRBs) will have to consider the safety of these interventions, modalities, and practices along with risks and benefits to subjects and society. This task is complicated by a relative lack of information available to IRBs about many alternative treatment modalities and substances. I do not attempt to provide definitive answers to questions of safety regarding particular interventions, such as acupuncture or bodywork, or ingestible substances, such as herbs or vitamins. However, I will attempt to provide a framework for IRB members to approach their task of evaluating complementary and alternative medical research proposals.

The Present Scope of Complementary and Alternative Medicine

The field of complementary and alternative medicine, often referred to as CAM, is a somewhat nebulous area of medicine. Medical practices labeled "alternative" are generally those that are not accepted or practiced by adherents of the allopathic model currently dominant in Western medicine. Many such alternative modalities have been practiced for centuries, such as traditional Chinese medicine (China, Japan, Korea), Ayurvedic medicine (India, Sri Lanka, Nepal), and Tibetan medicine (Tibet). Alternative medical practices generally do not fit into the standard Western biomedical model. Many practices are labeled as folk medicine, unproven, controversial, fraudulent, quackery, unscientific, and questionable by conventional medical practitioners.[3]

There is considerable disagreement in the literature as to what practices comprise the field of CAM. Some have noted that "alternative medicine is defined as consisting of medical interventions not taught widely at U.S. medical schools or generally available at U.S. hospitals."[4] Others have claimed, "There is no alternative medicine. There is only scientifically proven, evidence-based medicine supported by solid data or unproven medicine, for which scientific evidence is lacking."[5] No widespread agreement exists as to what actually constitutes the area of alternative medicine. Clearly, numerous practices and modalities ranging from acupuncture, massage, yoga, and chiropractic to distance healing, biofeedback, and therapeutic touch have practitioners and adherents worldwide. Nevertheless, these practices are not embraced or even accepted by the dominant Western medical orthodoxy. Although CAM practitioners practice a wide range of healing modalities that encompass incredible diversity, most practitioners do hold some common beliefs. These include the belief that the human body possesses innate healing powers; that religious and spiritual values are important determinants of health; and that physical, mental, emotional, and psychosocial aspects of an individual must be considered in the context of the whole individual and his or her particular condition or illness.[3]

Current Research Projects

Current NCCAM-supported research projects include investigation of acupuncture in the treatment of osteoarthritis, back pain, depression, fibromyalgia, and irritable bowel syndrome. Also funded are investigations of the role of biofeedback in the treatment of hypertension, chromium and glucose tolerance, ginkgo and vascular function, and echinacea in fighting colds. There are also numerous other funded centers dedicated to investigation of a broad variety of alternative interventions into specific populations such as women, children, older persons, and HIV-positive individuals. Individual investigators with a wide variety of backgrounds and levels of experience perform most federally funded CAM research at conventional medical institutions, although some funding has been awarded to colleges and universities specializing in CAM.

CAM Research and the IRB Process

Although CAM research presents the opportunity for IRB members to review many new and perhaps unfamiliar conceptual issues in medical research, the IRB process itself does not have to be modified to meet the demands of reviewing proposals intending to use human subjects in studies of various CAM therapies. At Bastyr University, the largest accredited, science-based, natural medicine university in the country, our IRB has had the opportunity to review a wide variety of CAM proposals. Our review process adheres to the regulations established in 45 CFR 46 and is thus the same as at any medical research institution that receives federal funding. The IRB is constituted according to the regulatory guidelines and meets regularly to consider full proposals, renewals, and reports on expedited reviews.

We have, however, added a few more steps to make the human subjects review process more robust and meaningful in the context of our institution. For example, we have instituted a research seminar in which prospective principal investigators have an opportunity to present their research ideas to the community in a collegial fashion. They can get feedback, form collaborations, and generate discussion of possible future research agendas. In addition, we have instituted a scientific review committee that is charged with evaluating the scientific merit of proposals before they are sent out to granting agencies. Research proposals are generated both in response to NCCAM funding cycles as well as industry-sponsored research agendas, and we found that the IRB required additional support and expertise in evaluating the scientific merit of proposed research. These two stages of research seminar presentation and focused scientific merit review support the work of the IRB as the committee strives to determine the risks and benefits of participation for potential subjects.

Review of Proposals Involving Substances Not Controlled by the Food and Drug Administration

Many substances commonly used in complementary and alternative medicine, such as herbs and other botanicals, vitamins, minerals, and amino acids, are not regulated by the Food and Drug Administration (FDA). They are considered to be dietary supplements, as determined by the 1990 Nutrition Labeling and Education Act and further defined by the 1994 Dietary Supplement Health and Education Act. Under these acts, herbal and other dietary supplement manufacturers cannot make specific health claims regarding the ability of the supplement to treat or cure a specific disease in most cases. However, the product label may indicate "the supplement's effects on 'structure or function' of the body or the 'well-being' achieved by consuming the dietary ingredient."[6] Manufacturers must be able to substantiate the truth of any such statements and specifically state that the FDA has not evaluated any such claims. However, specific health claims may be made on product labels in certain cases, if previously approved by the FDA, as is the case with the claim that the use of calcium may reduce the risk of osteoporosis.

IRB committees that are more familiar with evaluating the use of investigational new drug applications in studies sponsored by pharmaceutical companies may be unsure how to approach the evaluation of products that are not required to undergo comprehensive testing by the FDA. Package inserts are not necessarily available for most herbs and nutritional supplements. IRB members at conventional research institutions may have had no experience with evaluating homeopathic medicines or ultrahigh dilutions of FDA-approved drugs such as interleukin-2.

Steps Preceding Evaluation

In the absence of recognized expertise on the IRB, the committee should perhaps take a few preliminary steps before evaluating any such proposals. First, it should make sure that the investigator has done the appropriate background research to ascertain whether the study substance in question is indeed subject to FDA regulation. If it is, FDA procedures should be followed. If it is not, the investigator should be asked to provide available evidence of use of that substance in humans and/or animals in previous research studies. If there is no available evidence for the safety of an herbal product, for example, perhaps the committee should look carefully at the scale of the trial. This is to determine whether a pilot study may be more appropriate to investigate the substance in question. In the case of Chinese herbal medicines, they are usually purchased in bulk from a Chinese herbal dispensary, and the IRB may rightly have concerns about the purity, consistency, and potency of the herbs. The investigator should be responsible for providing evidence regarding methods of cultivating and processing the herbs in question. It may be helpful to consult with a pharmacologist and/or pharmacist to obtain the needed expertise if the IRB has questions about potential drug–herb interactions.

Perhaps a research forum could be organized to provide the scientific community, including the IRB, with relevant background information to familiarize the community with the proposed new area of research. If a separate scientific review committee is utilized to support the work of the IRB, that group may wish to hear from experts in the field of study under consideration. If the IRB approaches unfamiliar areas of proposed research with an openness to learning about different or perhaps unfamiliar medical paradigms, they may find their human subjects review experience to be more rewarding than frustrating. There are several good references available on complementary and alternative medicine that can help to educate and inform IRB members.[7–12]

Conclusion

Complementary and alternative medicine practices have become quite popular with the American public in the past decade. Some practitioners have begun to move toward an integrative model whereby CAM practices that have been shown to be efficacious are being adopted into mainstream medicine. As more research is initiated on CAM therapies at major medical institutions, IRB members face new challenges in evaluating the risks and benefits of proposed research studies. In the absence of FDA jurisdiction over many of the substances used in CAM therapies, IRB members need to become educated about the nature of the proposed interventions. They will also need to work closely with principal investigators to gain the appropriate information required to make an informed judgment about the potential impact on human subjects of participation in the proposed study. This is part of the ongoing effort to protect human subjects of research from harm.

References

1. National Institutes of Health. National Center for Complementary and Alternative Medicine. Updated 7 June, 2004. Access date 11 June, 2004. http://nccam.nih.gov/

2. Eisenberg DM, Davis RB, Ettner SL, et al. Trends in alternative medicine use in the United States, 1990–1997: Results of a follow-up national survey. *JAMA* 280(18):1569–1575, 1998.

3. Patel V. Understanding the integration of alternative modalities into an emerging healthcare model in the United States. In: Humber JM, Almeder RF (eds.). *Alternative Medicine and Ethics*. Totowa, NJ: Humana Press; 1998:46–48.

4. Eisenberg DM, Kessler RC, Foster C, Norlock FE, Calkins DR, Delbanco TL. Unconventional medicine in the United States: Prevalence, costs, and patterns of use. *N Engl J Med* 328(4):246–252, 1993.

5. Fontanarosa PB, Lundberg GD. Alternative medicine meets science. *JAMA* 280(18):1618–1619, 1998.

6. Food and Drug Administration. The Dietary Supplement Health and Education Act of 1994. Updated 27 November, 2000. Access date 23 Aug, 2005. http://www.cfsan.fda.gov/~dms/dietsupp.html

7. Murray M, Pizzorno J. *Encyclopedia of Natural Medicine*. Rocklin, CA: Prima Publishing; 1990.

8. Collinge W. *The American Holistic Health Association Complete Guide to Alternative Medicine*. New York: Warner Books; 1996.

9. Humber JM, Almeder RF (eds.). *Alternative Medicine and Ethics*. Totowa, NJ: Humana Press; 1998.

10. Spencer J (ed.). *Complementary Medicine: An Integrated Approach*. St. Louis: Mosby Year Books; 1999.

11. Spencer JW, Jacobs JJ. *Complementary/Alternative Medicine: An Evidence-Based Approach*. St. Louis: Mosby; 1999.

12. Cohen MH. *Complementary and Alternative Medicine: Legal Boundaries and Regulatory Perspectives*. Baltimore: Johns Hopkins University Press; 1998.

PART 11

Reference Material and Contact Information*

*Compiled by Elizabeth Bankert with assistance from the office of Public Responsibility in Medicine and Research (PRIM&R) and Applied Research Ethics National Association (ARENA)

Ethical Codes

The Nuremberg Code
Web site: http://ohrp.osophs.dhhs.gov/irb/irb_appendices.htm
Note: Full text attached

The Belmont Report
Ethical Principles and Guidelines for the Protection of Human Subjects of Research
The National Commission for the Protection of Human Subjects of Biomedical and Behavioral Research. April 18, 1979
Web site: http://ohrp.osophs.dhhs.gov/humansubjects/guidance/belmont.htm
Note: Full text attached

The World Medical Association Declaration of Helsinki
Web site: http://www.wma.net/e/policy/17-c_e.html

Council For International Organizations of Medical Sciences (CIOMS)
Web site: http://www.cioms.ch

The Nuremberg Code

[From Trials of War Criminals before the Nuremberg Military Tribunals under Control Council Law No. 10. Vol. 2, Nuremberg, October 1946–April 1949. Washington D.C.: U.S. G.P.O., 1949–1953. pp. 181-182.]

Permissible Medical Experiments

The great weight of the evidence before us is to the effect that certain types of medical experiments on human beings, when kept within reasonably well-defined bounds, conform to the ethics of the medical profession generally. The protagonists of the practice of human experimentation justify their views on the basis that such experiments yield results for the good of society that are unprocurable by other methods or means of study. All agree, however, that certain basic principles must be observed in order to satisfy moral, ethical and legal concepts:

1. The voluntary consent of the human subject is absolutely essential.

   This means that the person involved should have legal capacity to give consent; should be so situated as to be able to exercise free power of choice, without the intervention of any element of force, fraud, deceit, duress, over-reaching, or other ulterior form of constraint or coercion; and should have sufficient knowledge and comprehension of the elements of the subject matter involved as to enable him to make an understanding and enlightened decision. This latter element requires that before the acceptance of an affirmative decision by the experimental subject there should be made known to him the nature, duration, and purpose of the experiment; the method and means by which it is to be conducted; all inconveniences and hazards reasonably to be expected; and the effects upon his health or person which may possibly come from his participation in the experiment. The duty and responsibility for ascertaining the quality of the consent rests upon each individual who initiates, directs or engages in the experiment. It is a personal duty and responsibility which may not be delegated to another with impunity.

2. The experiment should be such as to yield fruitful results for the good of society, unprocurable by other methods or means of study, and not random and unnecessary in nature.

3. The experiment should be so designed and based on the results of animal experimentation and a knowledge of the natural history of the disease or other problem under study that the anticipated results will justify the performance of the experiment.

4. The experiment should be so conducted as to avoid all unnecessary physical and mental suffering and injury.

5. No experiment should be conducted where there is an a priori reason to believe that death or disabling injury will occur; except, perhaps, in those experiments where the experimental physicians also serve as subjects.

6. The degree of risk to be taken should never exceed that determined by the humanitarian importance of the problem to be solved by the experiment.

7. Proper preparations should be made and adequate facilities provided to protect the experimental subject against even remote possibilities of injury, disability, or death.

8. The experiment should be conducted only by scientifically qualified persons. The highest degree of skill and care should be required through all stages of the experiment of those who conduct or engage in the experiment.

9. During the course of the experiment the human subject should be at liberty to bring the experiment to an end if he has reached the physical or mental state where continuation of the experiment seems to him to be impossible.

10. During the course of the experiment the scientist in charge must be prepared to terminate the experiment at any stage, if he has probably cause to believe, in the exercise of the good faith, superior skill and careful judgment required of him that a continuation of the experiment is likely to result in injury, disability, or death to the experimental subject.

Of the ten principles which have been enumerated our judicial concern, of course, is with those requirements which are purely legal in nature—or which at least are so clearly related to matters legal that they assist us in determining criminal culpability and punishment. To go beyond that point would lead us into a field that would be beyond our sphere of competence. However, the point need not be labored. We find from the evidence that in the medical experiments which have been proved, these ten principles were much more frequently honored in their breach than in their observance. Many of the concentration camp inmates who were the victims of these atrocities were citizens of countries other than the German Reich. They were non-German nationals, including Jews and "asocial persons", both prisoners of war and civilians, who had been imprisoned and forced to submit to these tortures and barbarities without so much as a semblance of trial. In every single instance appearing in the record, subjects were used who did not consent to the experiments; indeed, as to some of the experiments, it is not even contended by the defendants that the subjects occupied the status of volunteers. In no case was the experimental subject at liberty of his own free choice to withdraw from any experiment. In many cases experiments were performed by unqualified persons; were conducted at random for no adequate scientific reason, and under revolting physical conditions. All of the experiments were conducted with unnecessary suffering and injury and but very little, if any, precautions were taken to protect or safeguard the human subjects from the possibilities of injury, disability, or death. In every one of the experiments the subjects experienced extreme pain or torture, and in most of them they suffered permanent injury, mutilation, or death, either as a direct result of the experiments or because of lack of adequate follow-up care.

Obviously all of these experiments involving brutalities, tortures, disabling injury, and death were performed in complete disregard of international conventions, the laws and customs of war, the general principles of criminal law as derived from the criminal laws of all civilized nations, and Control Council Law No. 10. Manifestly human experiments under such conditions are contrary to "the principles of the law of nations as they result from the usages established among civilized peoples, from the laws of humanity, and from the dictates of public conscience."

The Belmont Report

**OFFICE OF THE SECRETARY
ETHICAL PRINCIPLES AND GUIDELINES
FOR THE PROTECTION OF HUMAN
SUBJECTS OF RESEARCH
THE NATIONAL COMMISSION FOR THE PROTECTION
OF HUMAN SUBJECTS
OF BIOMEDICAL AND BEHAVIORAL RESEARCH
APRIL 18, 1979**

AGENCY: Department of Health, Education, and Welfare.

SUMMARY: On July 12, 1974, the National Research Act (Pub. L. 93-348) was signed into law, there-by creating the National Commission for the Protection of Human Subjects of Biomedical and Behavioral Research. One of the charges to the Commission was to identify the basic ethical principles that should underlie the conduct of biomedical and behavioral research involving human subjects. To develop guidelines that should be followed to assure that such research is conducted in accordance with those principles. In carrying out the above, the Commission was directed to consider: (i) the boundaries between biomedical and behavioral research and the accepted and routine practice of medicine, (ii) the role of assessment of the risk-benefit criteria in the determination of the appropriateness of research involving human subjects, (iii) appropriate guidelines for the selection of human subjects for participation in such research and (iv) the nature and definition of informed consent in various research settings.

The Belmont Report attempts to summarize the basic ethical principles identified by the Commission in the course of its deliberations. It is the outgrowth of an intensive four-day period of discussions that were held in February 1976 at the Smithsonian Institution's Belmont Conference Center supplemented by the monthly deliberations of the Commission that were held over a period of nearly four years. It is a statement of basic ethical principles and guidelines that should assist in resolving the ethical problems that surround the conduct of research with human subjects. By publishing the Report in the Federal Register, and providing reprints upon request, the Secretary intends that it may be made readily available to scientists, members of Institutional Review Boards, and Federal employees. The two-volume Appendix, containing the lengthy reports of experts and specialists who assisted the Commission in fulfilling this part of its charge, is available as DHEW Publication No. (OS) 78-0013 and No. (OS) 78-0014, for sale by the Superintendent of Documents, U.S. Government Printing Office, Washington, D.C. 20402.

Unlike most other reports of the Commission, the Belmont Report does not make specific recommendations for administrative action by the Secretary of Health, Education, and Welfare. Rather, the Commission recommended that the Belmont Report be adopted in its entirety, as a statement of the Department's policy. The Department requests public comment on this recommendation.

National Commission for the Protection of Human Subjects of Biomedical
and Behavioral Research

Members of the Commission

Kenneth John Ryan, M.D., Chairman, Chief of Staff, Boston Hospital for Women
Joseph V. Brady, Ph.D., Professor of Behavioral Biology, Johns Hopkins University

Robert E. Cooke, M.D., President, Medical College of Pennsylvania
Dorothy I. Height, President, National Council of Negro Women, Inc.
Albert R. Jonsen, Ph.D., Associate Professor of Bioethics,
University of California at San Francisco
Patricia King, J.D., Associate Professor of Law, Georgetown University Law Center
Karen Lebacqz, Ph.D., Associate Professor of Christian Ethics, Pacific School of Religion
***David W. Louisell, J.D., Professor of Law, University of California at Berkeley
Donald W. Seldin, M.D., Professor and Chairman, Department of Internal Medicine,
University of Texas at Dallas
***Eliot Stellar, Ph.D., Provost of the University and Professor of Physiological Psychology,
University of Pennsylvania
***Robert H. Turtle, LL.B., Attorney, VomBaur, Coburn, Simmons & Turtle, Washington,
D.C.
***Deceased.

Table of Contents

Ethical Principles and Guidelines for Research Involving Human Subjects

Scientific research has produced substantial social benefits. It has also posed some troubling ethical questions. Public attention was drawn to these questions by reported abuses of human subjects in biomedical experiments, especially during the Second World War. During the Nuremberg War Crime Trials, the Nuremberg code was drafted as a set of standards for judging physicians and scientists who had conducted biomedical experiments on concentration camp prisoners. This code became the prototype of many later codes (1) intended to assure that research involving human subjects would be carried out in an ethical manner.

The codes consist of rules, some general, others specific, that guide the investigators or the reviewers of research in their work. Such rules often are inadequate to cover complex situations; at times they come into conflict, and they are frequently difficult to interpret or apply. Broader ethical principles will provide a basis on which specific rules may be formulated, criticized and interpreted.

Three principles, or general prescriptive judgments, that are relevant to research involving human subjects are identified in this statement. Other principles may also be relevant. These three are comprehensive, however, and are stated at a level of generalization that should assist scientists, subjects, reviewers and interested citizens to understand the ethical issues inherent in research involving human subjects. These principles cannot always be applied so as to resolve beyond dispute particular ethical problems. The objective is to provide an analytical framework that will guide the resolution of ethical problems arising from research involving human subjects.

This statement consists of a distinction between research and practice, a discussion of the three basic ethical principles, and remarks about the application of these principles.

Part A: Boundaries Between Practice & Research

It is important to distinguish between biomedical and behavioral research on the one hand, and the practice of accepted therapy on the other, in order to know what activities ought to undergo review for the protection of human subjects of research. The distinction between research and practice is blurred partly because both often occur together (as in research designed to evaluate a therapy) and partly because notable departures from standard practice are often called "experimental" when the terms "experimental" and "research" are not carefully defined. For the most part, the term "practice" refers to interventions that are designed solely to enhance the well-being of an individual patient or client and that have a reasonable expectation of success. The purpose of medical or behavioral practice is to provide diagnosis, preventive treatment or therapy to particular individuals. (2) By contrast, the term "research" designates an activity designed to test an hypothesis, permit conclusions to be drawn, and thereby to develop or contribute to generalizable knowledge (expressed, for example, in theories, principles, and statements of relationships). Research is usually described in a formal protocol that sets forth an objective and a set of procedures designed to reach that objective.

When a clinician departs in a significant way from standard or accepted practice, the innovation does not, in and of itself, constitute research. The fact that a procedure is "experimental," in the sense of new, untested or different, does not automatically place it in the category of research. Radically new procedures of this description should, however, be made the object of formal research at an early stage in order to determine whether they are safe and effective. Thus, it is the responsibility of medical practice committees, for example, to insist that a major innovation be incorporated into a formal research project.(3)

Research and practice may be carried on together when research is designed to evaluate the safety and efficacy of a therapy. This need not cause any confusion regarding whether or not the activity requires review; the general rule is that if there is any element of research in an activity, that activity should undergo review for the protection of human subjects.

Part B: Basic Ethical Principles
The expression "basic ethical principles" refers to those general judgments that serve as a basic justification for the many particular ethical prescriptions and evaluations of human actions. Three basic principles, among those generally accepted in our cultural tradition, are particularly relevant to the ethics of research involving human subjects: the principles of respect of persons, beneficence and justice.

1. Respect for Persons.—
Respect for persons incorporates at least two ethical convictions: first, that individuals should be treated as autonomous agents, and second, that persons with diminished autonomy are entitled to protection. The principle of respect for persons thus divides into two separate moral requirements: the requirement to acknowledge autonomy and the requirement to protect those with diminished autonomy.

An autonomous person is an individual capable of deliberation about personal goals and of acting under the direction of such deliberation. To respect autonomy is to give weight to autonomous persons' considered opinions and choices while refraining from obstructing their actions unless they are clearly detrimental to others. To show lack of respect for an autonomous agent is to repudiate that person's considered judgments, to deny an individual the freedom to act on those considered judgments, or to withhold information necessary to make a considered judgment, when there are no compelling reasons to do so.

However, not every human being is capable of self-determination. The capacity for self-determination matures during an individual's life, and some individuals lose this capacity wholly or in part because of illness, mental disability, or circumstances that severely restrict liberty. Respect for the immature and the incapacitated may require protecting them as they mature or while they are incapacitated.

Some persons are in need of extensive protection, even to the point of excluding them from activities which may harm them; other persons require little protection beyond making sure they undertake activities freely and with awareness of possible adverse consequence. The extent of protection afforded should depend upon the risk of harm and the likelihood of benefit. The judgment that any individual lacks autonomy should be periodically reevaluated and will vary in different situations.

In most cases of research involving human subjects, respect for persons demands that subjects enter the research voluntarily and with adequate information. In some situations, however, application of the principle is not obvious. The involvement of prisoners as subjects of research provides an instructive example. On the one hand, it would seem that the principle of respect for persons requires that prisoners not be deprived of the opportunity to volunteer for research. On the other hand, under prison conditions they may be subtly coerced or unduly influenced to engage in research activities for which they would not otherwise volunteer. Respect for persons would then dictate prisoners be protected. Whether to allow prisoners to "volunteer" or to "protect" them presents a dilemma. Respecting persons, in most hard cases, is often a matter of balancing competing claims urged by the principle of respect itself.

2. Beneficence.—
Persons are treated in an ethical manner not only by respecting their decisions and protecting them from harm, but also by making efforts to secure their well-being. Such treatment falls under the principle of beneficence. The term "beneficence" is often understood to cover acts of kindness or charity that go beyond strict obligation. In this document, beneficence is understood in a stronger sense, as an obligation. Two general rules have been formulated as complementary expressions of beneficent actions in this sense: (1) do not harm and (2) maximize possible benefits and minimize possible harms.

The Hippocratic maxim "do no harm" has long been a fundamental principle of medical ethics. Claude Bernard extended it to the realm of research, saying that one should not injure one person regardless of the benefits that might come to others. However, even avoiding harm requires learning what is harmful; and, in the process of obtaining this information, persons may be exposed to risk of harm. Further, the Hippocratic Oath requires physicians to benefit their patients "according to their best judgment." Learning what will in fact benefit may require exposing persons to risk. The problem posed by these imperatives is to decide when it is justifiable to seek certain benefits despite the risks involved, and when the benefits should be foregone because of the risks.

The obligations of beneficence affect both individual investigators and society at large, because they extend both to particular research projects and to the entire enterprise of research. In the case of particular projects, investigators and members of their institutions are obliged to give forethought to the maximization of benefits and the reduction of risk that might occur from the research investigation. In the case of scientific research in general, members of the larger society are obliged to recognize the longer term benefits and risks that may result from the improvement of knowledge and from the development of novel medical, psychotherapeutic, and social procedures.

The principle of beneficence often occupies a well-defined justifying role in many areas of research involving human subjects. An example is found in research involving children. Effective ways of treating childhood diseases and fostering healthy development are benefits that serve to justify research involving children—even when individual research subjects are not direct beneficiaries. Research also makes it possible to avoid the harm that may result from the application of previously accepted routine practices that on closer investigation turn out to be dangerous. But the role of the principle of beneficence is not always so unambiguous. A difficult ethical problem remains, for example, about research that presents more than minimal risk without immediate prospect of direct benefit to the children involved. Some have argued that such research is inadmissible, while others have pointed out that this limit would rule out much research promising great benefit to children in the future. Here again, as with all hard cases, the different claims covered by the principle of beneficence may come into conflict and force difficult choices.

3. Justice.—

Who ought to receive the benefits of research and bear its burdens? This is a question of justice, in the sense of "fairness in distribution" or "what is deserved." An injustice occurs when some benefit to which a person is entitled is denied without good reason or a burden is imposed unduly. Another way of conceiving the principle of justice is that equals ought to be treated equally. However, this statement requires explication. Who is equal and unequal? What considerations justify departure from equal distribution? Almost all commentators allow that distinctions based on experience, age, deprivation, competence, merit and position do sometimes constitute criteria justifying differential treatment for certain purposes. It is necessary, then, to explain in what respects people should be treated equally. There are several widely accepted formulations of just ways to distribute burdens and benefits. Each formulation mentions some relevant property on the basis of which burdens and benefits should be distributed. These formulations are (1) to each person an equal share; (2) to each person according to individual need; (3) to each person according to individual effort; (4) to each person according to societal contribution; and (5) to each person according to merit.

Questions of justice have long been associated with social practices such as punishment, taxation, and political representation. Until recently these questions have not generally been associated with scientific research. However, they are foreshadowed even in the earliest reflections on the ethics of research involving human subjects. For example, during the 19th and early 20th centuries the burdens of serving as research subjects fell largely upon poor ward patients, while the benefits of improved medical care flowed primarily to private patients. Subsequently, the exploitation of unwilling prisoners as research subjects in Nazi concentration camps was condemned as a particularly flagrant injustice. In this country, in the 1940's, the Tuskegee syphilis study used disadvantaged, rural black men to study the untreated course of a disease that is by no means confined to that population. These subjects were deprived of demonstrably effective treatment in order not to interrupt the project, long after such treatment became generally available.

Against this historical background, it can be seen how conceptions of justice are relevant to research involving human subjects. For example, the selection of research subjects needs to be scrutinized in order to determine whether some classes (e.g., welfare patients, particular racial and ethnic minorities, or persons confined to institutions) are being systematically selected simply because of their easy availability, to their compromised position, or their manipulability, rather than for reasons directly related to the problem being studied. Finally, whenever research supported by public funds leads to the development of therapeutic devices and procedures, justice demands that these not provide advantages only to those who can afford them and that such research should not unduly involve persons from groups unlikely to be among the beneficiaries of subsequent applications of the research.

Part C: Applications

C. Applications

Applications of the general principles to the conduct of research leads to consideration of the following requirements: informed consent, risk/benefit assessment, and the selection of subjects of research.

1. Informed Consent.—

Respect for persons requires that subjects, to the degree that they are capable, be given the opportunity to choose what shall or shall not happen to them. This opportunity is provided when adequate standards for informed consent are satisfied.

While the importance of informed consent is unquestioned, controversy prevails over the nature and possibility of an informed consent. Nonetheless, there is widespread agreement that the consent process can be analyzed as containing three elements: information, comprehension, and voluntariness.

Information

Most codes of research establish specific items for disclosure intended to assure that subjects are given sufficient information. These items generally include: the research procedure, their purposes, risks and anticipated benefits, alternative procedures (where therapy is involved), and a statement offering the subject the opportunity to ask questions and to withdraw at any time from the research. Additional items have been proposed, including how subjects are selected, the person responsible for the research, etc.

However, a simple listing of items does not answer the question of what the standard should be for judging how much and what sort of information should be provided. One standard frequently invoked in medical practice, namely the information commonly provided by practitioners in the field or in the locale, is inadequate since research takes place precisely when a common understanding does not exist. Another standard, currently popular in malpractice law, requires the practitioner to reveal the information that reasonable persons would wish to know in order to make a decision regarding their care. This, too, seems insufficient since the research subject, being in essence a volunteer, may wish to know considerably more about risks gratuitously undertaken than do patients who deliver themselves into the hand of a clinician for needed care. It may be that a standard of "the reasonable volunteer" should be proposed: the extent and nature of information should be such that persons, knowing that the procedure is neither necessary for their care nor perhaps fully understood, can decide whether they wish to participate in the furthering of knowledge. Even when some direct benefit to them is anticipated, the subjects should understand clearly the range of risk and the voluntary nature of participation.

A special problem of consent arises where informing subjects of some pertinent aspect of the research is likely to impair the validity of the research. In many cases, it is sufficient to indicate to subjects that they are being invited to participate in research of which some features will not be revealed until the research is concluded. In all cases of research involving incomplete disclosure, such research is justified only if it is clear that (1) incomplete disclosure is truly necessary to accomplish the goals of the research, (2) there are no undisclosed risks to subjects that are more than minimal, and (3) there is an adequate plan for debriefing subjects, when appropriate, and for dissemination of research results to them. Information about risks should never be withheld for eliciting the cooperation of subjects, and truthful answers should always be given to direct questions about the research. Care should be taken to distinguish cases in which disclosure would destroy or invalidate the research from cases in which disclosure would simply inconvenience the investigator.

Comprehension
The manner and context in which information is conveyed is as important as the information itself. For example, presenting information in a disorganized and rapid fashion, allowing too little time for consideration or curtailing opportunities for questioning, all may adversely affect a subject's ability to make an informed choice.

Because the subject's ability to understand is a function of intelligence, rationality, maturity, and language, it is necessary to adapt the presentation of the information to the subject's capacities. Investigators are responsible for ascertaining that the subject has comprehended the information. While there is always an obligation to ascertain that the information about risk to subjects is complete and adequately comprehended, when the risks are more serious, that obligation increases. On occasion, it may be suitable to give some oral or written tests of comprehension.

Special provision may need to be made when comprehension is severely limited—for example, by conditions of immaturity or mental disability. Each class of subjects that one might consider as incompetent (e.g., infants and young children, mentally disabled patients, the terminally ill, and the comatose) should be considered on its own terms. Even for these persons, however, respect requires giving them the opportunity to choose to the extent that they are able, whether to participate in research. The objections of these subjects to involvement should be honored, unless the research entails providing them a therapy unavailable elsewhere. Respect for persons also requires seeking the permission of other parties in order to protect the subjects from harm. Such persons are thus respected both by acknowledging their own wishes and by the use of third parties to protect them from harm.

The third parties chosen should be those who are most likely to understand the incompetent subject's situation and to act in that person's best interest. The person authorized to act on behalf of the subject should be given an opportunity to observe the research as it proceeds in order to be able to withdraw the subject from the research, if such action appears in the subject's best interest.

Voluntariness
An agreement to participate in research constitutes a valid consent only if voluntarily given. This element of informed consent requires conditions free of coercion and undue influence. Coercion occurs when an overt threat of harm is intentionally presented by one person to another in order to obtain compliance. Undue influence, by contrast, occurs through an offer of an excessive, unwarranted, inappropriate, or improper reward or other overture in order to obtain compliance. Also, inducements that would ordinarily be acceptable may become undue influences if the subject is especially vulnerable.

Unjustifiable pressures usually occur when persons in positions of authority or commanding influence—especially where possible sanctions are involved—urge a course of action for a subject. A continuum of such influencing factors exists, however, and it is impossible to state precisely where justifiable persuasion ends and undue influence begins. But undue influence would include actions such as manipulating a person's choice through the controlling influence of a close relative and threatening to withdraw health services to which an individual would otherwise be entitled.

2. Assessment of Risks and Benefits.—
The assessment of risks and benefits requires a careful array of relevant data, including, in some cases, alternative ways of obtaining the benefits sought in the research. Thus, the assessment presents both an opportunity and a responsibility to gather systematic and comprehensive information about proposed research. For the investigator, it is a means to examine whether the proposed research is properly designed. For a review committee, it is a method for determining whether the risks that will be presented to subjects are justified. For prospective subjects, the assessment will assist the determination whether or not to participate.

The Nature and Scope of Risks and Benefits
The requirement that research be justified on the basis of a favorable risk/benefit assessment bears a close relation to the principle of beneficence, just as the moral requirement that informed consent be obtained is derived primarily from the principle of respect for persons. The term "risk" refers to a possibility that harm may occur. However, when expressions such as "small risk" or "high risk" are used, they usually refer (often ambiguously) both to the chance

(probability) of experiencing a harm and the severity (magnitude) of the envisioned harm.

The term "benefit" is used in the research context to refer to something of positive value related to health or welfare. Unlike "risk," "benefit" is not a term that expresses probabilities. Risk is properly contrasted to probability of benefits, and benefits are properly contrasted with harms rather than risks of harm. Accordingly, so-called risk/benefit assessments are concerned with the probabilities and magnitudes of possible harm and anticipated benefits. Many kinds of possible harms and benefits need to be taken into account. There are, for example, risks of psychological harm, physical harm, legal harm, social harm, and economic harm, and the corresponding benefits. While the most likely types of harms to research subjects are those of psychological or physical pain or injury, other possible kinds should not be overlooked.

Risks and benefits of research may affect the individual subjects, the families of the individual subjects, and society at large (or special groups of subjects in society). Previous codes and Federal regulations have required that risks to subjects be outweighed by the sum of both the anticipated benefit to the subject, if any, and the anticipated benefit to society in the form of knowledge to be gained from the research. In balancing these different elements, the risks and benefits affecting the immediate research subject will normally carry special weight. On the other hand, interests other than those of the subject may on occasion be sufficient by themselves to justify the risks involved in the research, so long as the subjects' rights have been protected. Beneficence thus requires that we protect against risk of harm to subjects and that we be concerned about the loss of the substantial benefits that might be gained from research.

The Systematic Assessment of Risks and Benefits
It is commonly said that benefits and risks must be "balanced" and shown to be "in a favorable ratio." The metaphorical character of these terms draws attention to the difficulty of making precise judgments. Only on rare occasions will quantitative techniques be available for the scrutiny of research protocols. However, the idea of systematic, nonarbitrary analysis of risks and benefits should be emulated insofar as possible. This ideal requires those making decisions about the justifiability of research to be thorough in the accumulation and assessment of information about all aspects of the research, and to consider alternatives systematically. This procedure renders the assessment of research more rigorous and precise, while making communication between review board members and investigators less subject to misinterpretation, misinformation, and conflicting judgments. Thus, there should first be a determination of the validity of the presuppositions of the research; then the nature, probability, and magnitude of risk should be distinguished with as much clarity as possible. The method of ascertaining risks should be explicit, especially where there is no alternative to the use of such vague categories as small or slight risk. It should also be determined whether an investigator's estimates of

the probability of harm or benefits are reasonable, as judged by known facts or other available studies.

Finally, assessment of the justifiability of research should reflect at least the following considerations: (i) Brutal or inhumane treatment of human subjects is never morally justified. (ii) Risks should be reduced to those necessary to achieve the research objective. It should be determined whether it is in fact necessary to use human subjects at all. Risk perhaps can never entirely be eliminated, but it can often be reduced by careful attention to alternative procedures. (iii) When research involves significant risk of serious impairment, review committees should be extraordinarily insistent on the justification of the risk (looking at the likelihood of benefit to the subject—or, in some rare cases, to the manifest voluntariness of the participation). (iv) When vulnerable populations are involved in research, the appropriateness of involving them should itself be demonstrated. A number of variables go into such judgments, including the nature and degree of risk, the condition of the particular population involved, and the nature and level of the anticipated benefits. (v) Relevant risks and benefits must be thoroughly arrayed in documents and procedures used in the informed consent process.

3. Selection of Subjects.—
Just as the principle of respect for persons finds expression in the requirements for consent, and the principle of beneficence in risk/benefit assessment, the principle of justice gives rise to moral requirements that there be fair procedures and outcomes in the selection of research subjects.

Justice is relevant to the selection of subjects of research at two levels: the social and the individual. Individual justice in the selection of subjects would require that researchers exhibit fairness: thus, they should not offer potentially beneficial research only to some patients who are in their favor or select only "undesirable" persons for risky research. Social justice requires that distinction be drawn between classes of subjects that ought, and ought not, to participate in any particular kind of research, based on the ability of members of that class to bear burdens and on the appropriateness of placing further burdens on already burdened persons. Thus, it can be considered a matter of social justice that there is an order of preference in the selection of classes of subjects (e.g., adults before children) and that some classes of potential subjects (e.g., the institutionalized mentally infirm or prisoners) that may be involved as research subjects, if at all, only on certain conditions.

Injustice may appear in the selection of subjects, even if individual subjects are selected fairly by investigators and treated fairly in the course of research. Injustice arises from social, racial, sexual, and cultural biases institutionalized in society. Thus, even if individual researchers are treating their research subjects fairly, and the IRBs are taking care to assure that subjects are selected fairly within a particular institution, unjust social patterns may nevertheless appear in the overall distribution of the burdens and benefits of research. Although individual institutions or investigators may not be able to resolve a problem that is pervasive in their social setting, they can consider distributive justice in selecting research subjects.

Some populations, especially institutionalized ones, are already burdened in many ways by their infirmities and environments. When research is proposed that involves risks and does not include a therapeutic component, other less burdened classes of persons should be called upon first to accept these risks of research, except where the research is directly related to the specific conditions of the class involved. Also, even though public funds for research may often flow in the same directions as public funds for health care, it seems unfair that populations dependent on public health care constitute a pool of preferred research subjects, especially when more advantaged populations are likely to be the recipients of the benefits.

One special instance of injustice results from the involvement of vulnerable subjects. Certain groups, such as racial minorities, the economically disadvantaged, the very sick, and the institutionalized, may continually be sought as research subjects, owing to their ready availability in settings where research is conducted. Given their dependent status and their frequently compromised capacity for free consent, they should be protected against the danger of being involved in research solely for administrative convenience, or because they are easy to manipulate as a result of their illness or socioeconomic condition.

(1) Since 1945, various codes for the proper and responsible conduct of human experimentation in medical research have been adopted by different organizations. The best known codes are the Nuremberg Code of 1947, the Helsinki Declaration of 1964 (revised in 1975), and the 1971 Guidelines (codified into Federal Regulations in 1974) issued by the U.S. Department of Health, Education, and Welfare Codes for the conduct of social and behavioral research have also been adopted, the best known being that of the American Psychological Association, published in 1973.

(2) Although practice usually involves interventions designed solely to enhance the well-being of a particular individual, interventions are sometimes applied to one individual for the enhancement of the well-being of another (e.g., blood donation, skin grafts, organ transplants) or an intervention may have the dual purpose of enhancing the well-being of a particular individual, and, at the same time, providing some benefit to others (e.g., vaccination, which protects both the person who is vaccinated and society generally). The fact that some forms of practice have elements other than immediate benefit to the individual receiving an intervention, however, should not confuse the general distinction between research and practice. Even when a procedure applied in practice may benefit some other person, it remains an intervention designed to enhance the well-being of a particular individual or groups of individuals; thus, it is practice and need not be reviewed as research.

(3) Because the problems related to social experimentation may differ substantially from those of biomedical and behavioral research, the Commission specifically declines to make any policy determination regarding such research at this time. Rather, the Commission believes that the problem ought to be addressed by one of its successor bodies.

National Institutes of Health, Bethesda, Maryland 20892

Selected U.S. Government Regulations

Department of Health and Human Services

Office for Human Research Protections (OHRP)
Web site: http://ohrp.osophs.dhhs.gov/

Protection of Human Subjects
45 Code of Federal Regulations Part 46
Web site: http://ohrp.osophs.dhhs.gov/humansubjects/guidance/45cfr46.htm
Note: Full text attached

Revised Expedited Review Criteria (1998)
Web site: http://ohrp.osophs.dhhs.gov/humansubjects/guidance/expedited98.htm
Note: Full text attached

Food and Drug Administration (FDA)
Web site: http://www.fda.gov/

Protection of Human Subjects
21 Code of Federal Regulations Part 50
Web site: http://www.access.gpo.gov/nara/cfr/waisidx_00/21cfr50_00.html
Note: Full text attached

Institutional Review Boards
21 Code of Federal Regulations Part 56
Web site: http://www.access.gpo.gov/nara/cfr/waisidx_00/21cfr56_00.html
Includes:
Appendix A: A List of Selected FDA Regulations Relating to the Protection of Human Subjects
Appendix B: Significant Differences in FDA and HHS Regulations for Protection of Human Subjects
Note: Full text attached

Financial Disclosure by Clinical Investigators
21 Code of Federal Regulations Part 54
Web site: http://www.access.gpo.gov/nara/cfr/waisidx_00/21cfr54_00.html

Biologic Products: General
21 Code of Federal Regulations Part 600
Web site: http://www.access.gpo.gov/nara/cfr/waisidx_00/21cfr600_00.html

Investigational New Drug Application
21 Code of Federal Regulations Part 312
Web site: http://www.access.gpo.gov/nara/cfr/waisidx_00/21cfr312_00.html

Investigational Device Exemptions
21 Code of Federal Regulations Part 812
Web site: http://www.access.gpo.gov/nara/cfr/waisidx_00/21cfr812_00.html

Health Insurance Portability and Accountability Act (HIPAA)
Web site: http://aspe.hhs.gov/admnsimp/

Code of Federal Regulations: Title 45, Part 46

CODE OF FEDERAL REGULATIONS: TITLE 45, PUBLIC WELFARE
PARTMENT OF HEALTH AND HUMAN SERVICES
NATIONAL INSTITUTES OF HEALTH
OFFICE FOR PROTECTION FROM RESEARCH RISKS

PART 46
PROTECTION OF HUMAN SUBJECTS

* * *

Revised June 18, 1991
Effective August 19, 1991

* * *

Authority: 5 U.S.C. 301; Sec. 474(a), 88 Stat. 352 (42 U.S.C. 2891-3(a))

Note: As revised, Subpart A of the DHHS regulations incorporates the Common Rule (Federal Policy) for the Protection of Human Subjects (56 FR 28003). Subpart D of the HHS regulations has been amended at Section 46.401(b) to reference the revised Subpart A

The Common Rule (Federal Policy) is also codified at:

7 CFR Part 1c	Department of Agriculture
10 CFR Part 745	Department of Energy
14 CFR Part 1230	National Aeronautics and Space Administration
15 CFR Part 27	Department of Commerce
16 CFR Part 1028	Consumer Product Safety Commission
22 CFR Part 225	International Development Cooperation Agency, Agency for International Development
24 CFR Part 60	Department of Housing and Urban Development
28 CFR Part 46	Department of Justice
32 CFR Part 219	Department of Defense
34 CFR Part 97	Department of Education
38 CFR Part 16	Department of Veterans Affairs
40 CFR Part 26	Environmental Protection Agency
45 CFR Part 690	National Science Foundation
49 CFR Part 11	Department of Transportation

Title 45
Code of Federal Regulations

Part 46
Protection of Human Subjects

* * *

Revised June 18, 1991
Effective August 19, 1991

* * *

Subpart A

Federal Policy for the Protection of Human Subjects (Basic DHHS Policy for Protection of Human Research Subjects)
Source: 56 FR 28003, June 18, 1991.

§46.101 To what does this policy apply?

(a) Except as provided in paragraph (b) of this section, this policy applies to all research involving human subjects conducted, supported or otherwise subject to regulation by any federal department or agency which takes appropriate administrative action to make the policy applicable to such research. This includes research conducted by federal civilian employees or military personnel, except that each department or agency head may adopt such procedural modifications as may be appropriate from an administrative standpoint. It also includes research conducted, supported, or otherwise subject to regulation by the federal government outside the United States.

(1) Research that is conducted or supported by a federal department or agency, whether or not it is regulated as defined in §46.102(e), must comply with all sections of this policy.

(2) Research that is neither conducted nor supported by a federal department or agency but is subject to regulation as defined in §46.102(e) must be reviewed and approved, in compliance with §46.101, §46.102, and §46.107 through §46.117 of this policy, by an institutional review board (IRB) that operates in accordance with the pertinent requirements of this policy.

(b) Unless otherwise required by department or agency heads, research activities in which the only involvement of human subjects will be in one or more of the following categories are exempt from this policy:

(1) Research conducted in established or commonly accepted educational settings, involving normal educational practices, such as (i) research on regular and special education instructional strategies, or (ii) research on the effectiveness of or the comparison among instructional techniques, curricula, or classroom management methods.

(2) Research involving the use of educational tests (cognitive, diagnostic, aptitude, achievement), survey procedures, interview procedures or observation of public behavior, unless:

(i) information obtained is recorded in such a manner that human subjects can be identified, directly or through identifiers linked to the subjects; and

(ii) any disclosure of the human subjects' responses outside the research could reasonably place the subjects at risk of criminal or civil liability or be damaging to the subjects' financial standing, employability, or reputation.

(3) Research involving the use of educational tests (cognitive, diagnostic, aptitude, achievement), survey procedures, interview procedures, or observation of public behavior that is not exempt under paragraph (b)(2) of this section, if:

(i) the human subjects are elected or appointed public officials or candidates for public office; or

(ii) Federal statute(s) require(s) without exception that the confidentiality of the personally identifiable information will be maintained throughout the research and thereafter.

(4) Research involving the collection or study of existing data, documents, records, pathological specimens, or diagnostic specimens, if these sources are publicly available or if the information is recorded by the investigator in such a manner that subjects cannot be identified, directly or through identifiers linked to the subjects.

(5) Research and demonstration projects which are conducted by or subject to the approval of department or agency heads, and which are designed to study, evaluate, or otherwise examine:

(i) Public benefit or service programs; (ii) procedures for obtaining benefits or services under those programs; (iii) possible changes in or alternatives to those programs or procedures; or (iv) possible changes in methods or levels of payment for benefits or services under those programs.

(6) Taste and food quality evaluation and consumer acceptance studies, (i) if wholesome foods without additives are consumed or (ii) if a food is consumed that contains a food ingredient at or below the level and for a use found to be safe, or agricultural chemical or environmental contaminant at or below the level found to be safe, by the Food and Drug Administration or approved by the Environmental Protection Agency or the Food Safety and Inspection Service of the U.S. Department of Agriculture.

(c) Department or agency heads retain final judgment as to whether a particular activity is covered by this policy.

(d) Department or agency heads may require that specific research activities or classes of research activities conducted, supported, or otherwise subject to regulation by the department or agency but not otherwise covered by this policy, comply with some or all of the requirements of this policy.

(e) Compliance with this policy requires compliance with pertinent federal laws or regulations which provide additional protections for human subjects.

(f) This policy does not affect any state or local laws or regulations which may otherwise be applicable and which provide additional protections for human subjects.

(g) This policy does not affect any foreign laws or regulations which may otherwise be applicable and which provide additional protections to human subjects of research.

(h) When research covered by this policy takes place in foreign countries, procedures normally followed in the foreign countries to protect human subjects may differ from those set forth in this policy. [An example is a foreign institution which complies with guidelines consistent with the World Medical Assembly Declaration (Declaration of Helsinki amended 1989) issued either by sovereign states or by an organization whose function for the protection of human research subjects is internationally recognized.] In these circumstances, if a department or agency head determines that the procedures prescribed by the institution afford protections that are at least equivalent to those provided in this policy, the department or agency head may approve the substitution of the foreign procedures in lieu of the procedural requirements provided in this policy. Except when otherwise required by statute, Executive Order, or the department or agency head, notices of these actions as they occur will be published in the Federal Register or will be otherwise published as provided in department or agency procedures.

(i) Unless otherwise required by law, department or agency heads may waive the applicability of some or all of the provisions of this policy to specific research activities or classes or research activities otherwise covered by this policy. Except when otherwise required by statute or Executive Order, the department or agency head shall forward advance notices of these actions to the Office for Protection from Research Risks, National Institutes of Health, Department of Health and Human Services (DHHS), and shall also publish them in the Federal Register or in such other manner as provided in department or agency procedures.[1]

Institutions with DHHS-approved assurances on file will abide by provisions of title 45 CFR part 46 subparts A-D. Some of the other departments and agencies have incorporated all provisions of title 45 CFR part 46 into their policies and procedures as well. However, the exemptions at 45 CFR 46.101(b) do not apply to research involving prisoners, fetuses, pregnant women, or human in vitro fertilization, subparts B and C. The exemption at 45 CFR 46.101(b)(2), for research involving survey or interview procedures or observation of public behavior, does not apply to research with children, subpart D, except for research involving observations of public behavior when the investigator(s) do not participate in the activities being observed.

§46.102 Definitions

(a) Department or agency head means the head of any federal department or agency and any other officer or employee of any department or agency to whom authority has been delegated.

(b) Institution means any public or private entity or agency (including federal, state, and other agencies).

(c) Legally authorized representative means an individual or judicial or other body authorized under applicable law to consent on behalf of a prospective subject to the subject's participation in the procedure(s) involved in the research.

(d) Research means a systematic investigation, including research development, testing and evaluation, designed to develop or contribute to generalizable knowledge. Activities which meet this definition constitute research for purposes of this policy, whether or not they are conducted or supported under a program which is considered research for other purposes. For example, some demonstration and service programs may include research activities.

(e) Research subject to regulation, and similar terms are intended to encompass those research activities for which a federal department or agency has specific responsibility for regulating as a research activity, (for example, Investigational New Drug requirements administered by the Food and Drug Administration). It does not include research activities which are incidentally regulated by a federal department or agency solely as part of the department's or agency's broader responsibility to regulate certain types of activities whether research or non-research in nature (for example, Wage and Hour requirements administered by the Department of Labor).

(f) Human subject means a living individual about whom an investigator (whether professional or student) conducting research obtains

(1) Data through intervention or interaction with the individual, or

(2) Identifiable private information.

Intervention includes both physical procedures by which data are gathered (for example, venipuncture) and manipulations of the subject or the subject's environment that are performed for research purposes. Interaction includes communication or interpersonal contact between investigator and subject. Private information includes information about behavior that occurs in a context in which an individual can reasonably expect that no observation or recording is taking place, and information which has been provided for specific purposes by an individual and which the individual can reasonably expect will not be made public (for example, a medical record). Private information must be individually identifiable (i.e., the identity of the subject is or may readily be ascertained by the investigator or associated with the information) in order for obtaining the information to constitute research involving human subjects.

(g) IRB means an institutional review board established in accord with and for the purposes expressed in this policy.

(h) IRB approval means the determination of the IRB that the research has been reviewed and may be conducted at an institution within the constraints set forth by the IRB and by other institutional and federal requirements.

(i) Minimal risk means that the probability and magnitude of harm or discomfort anticipated in the research are not greater in and of themselves than those ordinarily encountered in daily life or during the performance of routine physical or psychological examinations or tests.

(j) Certification means the official notification by the institution to the supporting department or agency, in accordance with the requirements of this policy, that a research project or activity involving human subjects has been reviewed and approved by an IRB in accordance with an approved assurance.

§46.103 Assuring compliance with this policy—research conducted or supported by any federal department or agency

(a) Each institution engaged in research which is covered by this policy and which is conducted or supported by a federal department or agency shall provide written assurance satisfactory to the department or agency head that it will comply with the requirements set forth in this policy. In lieu of requiring submission of an assurance, individual department or agency heads shall accept the existence of a current assurance, appropriate for the research in question, on file with the Office for Protection from Research Risks, National Institutes Health, DHHS, and approved for federal wide use by that office. When the existence of an DHHS-approved assurance is accepted in lieu of requiring submission of an assurance, reports (except certification) required by this policy to be made to department and agency heads shall also be made to the Office for Protection from Research Risks, National Institutes of Health, DHHS.

(b) Departments and agencies will conduct or support research covered by this policy only if the institution has an assurance approved as provided in this section, and only if the institution has certified to the department or agency head that the research has been reviewed and approved by an IRB provided for in the assurance, and will be subject to continuing review by the IRB. Assurances applicable to federally supported or conducted research shall at a minimum include:

(1) A statement of principles governing the institution in the discharge of its responsibilities for protecting the rights and welfare of human subjects of research conducted at or sponsored by the institution, regardless of whether the research is subject to federal regulation. This may include an appropriate existing code, declaration, or statement of ethical principles, or a statement formulated by the institution itself. This requirement does not preempt provisions of this policy applicable to department- or agency-supported or regulated research and need not be applicable to any research exempted or waived under §46.101 (b) or (i).

(2) Designation of one or more IRBs established in accordance with the requirements of this policy, and for which provisions are made for meeting space and sufficient staff to support the IRB's review and record keeping duties.

(3) A list of IRB members identified by name; earned degrees; representative capacity; indications of experience such as board certifications, licenses, etc., sufficient to describe each member's chief anticipated contributions to IRB deliberations; and any employment or other relationship between each member and the institution; for example: full-time employee, part-time employee, member of governing panel or board, stockholder, paid or unpaid consultant. Changes in IRB membership shall be reported to the department or agency head, unless in accord with §46.103(a) of this policy, the existence of a DHHS-approved assurance is accepted. In this case, change in IRB membership shall be reported to the

Office for Protection from Research Risks, National Institutes of Health, DHHS.

(4) Written procedures which the IRB will follow (i) for conducting its initial and continuing review of research and for reporting its findings and actions to the investigator and the institution; (ii) for determining which projects require review more often than annually and which projects need verification from sources other than the investigators that no material changes have occurred since previous IRB review; and (iii) for ensuring prompt reporting to the IRB of proposed changes in a research activity, and for ensuring that such changes in approved research, during the period for which IRB approval has already been given, may not be initiated without IRB review and approval except when necessary to eliminate apparent immediate hazards to the subject.

(5) Written procedures for ensuring prompt reporting to the IRB, appropriate institutional officials, and the department or agency head of (i) any unanticipated problems involving risks to subjects or others or any serious or continuing noncompliance with this policy or the requirements or determinations of the IRB; and (ii) any suspension or termination of IRB approval.

(c) The assurance shall be executed by an individual authorized to act for the institution and to assume on behalf of the institution the obligations imposed by this policy and shall be filed in such form and manner as the department or agency head prescribes.

(d) The department or agency head will evaluate all assurances submitted in accordance with this policy through such officers and employees of the department or agency and such experts or consultants engaged for this purpose as the department or agency head determines to be appropriate. The department or agency head's evaluation will take into consideration the adequacy of the proposed IRB in light of the anticipated scope of the institution's research activities and the types of subject populations likely to be involved, the appropriateness of the proposed initial and continuing review procedures in light of the probable risks, and the size and complexity of the institution.

(e) On the basis of this evaluation, the department or agency head may approve or disapprove the assurance, or enter into negotiations to develop an approvable one. The department or agency head may limit the period during which any particular approved assurance or class of approved assurances shall remain effective or otherwise condition or restrict approval.

(f) Certification is required when the research is supported by a federal department or agency and not otherwise exempted or waived under §46.101 (b) or (i). An institution with an approved assurance shall certify that each application or proposal for research covered by the assurance and by §46.103 of this policy has been reviewed and approved by the IRB. Such certification must be submitted with the application or proposal or by such later date as may be prescribed by the department or agency to which the application or proposal is submitted. Under no condition shall research covered by §46.103 of the policy be supported prior to receipt of the certification that the research has been reviewed and approved by the IRB. Institutions without an approved assurance covering the research shall certify within 30 days after receipt of a request for such a certification from the department or agency, that the application or proposal has been approved by the IRB. If the certification is not submitted within these time limits, the application or proposal may be returned to the institution.

(Approved by the Office of Management and Budget under Control Number 9999-0020.)

§§46.104—46.106 [Reserved]

§46.107 IRB membership

(a) Each IRB shall have at least five members, with varying backgrounds to promote complete and adequate review of research activities commonly conducted by the institution. The IRB shall be sufficiently qualified through the experience and expertise of its members, and the diversity of the members, including consideration of race, gender, and cultural backgrounds and sensitivity to such issues as community attitudes, to promote respect for its advice and counsel in safeguarding the rights and welfare of human subjects. In addition to possessing the professional competence necessary to review specific research activities, the IRB shall be able to ascertain the acceptability of proposed research in terms of institutional commitments and regulations, applicable law, and standards of professional conduct and practice. The IRB shall therefore include persons knowledgeable in these areas. If an IRB regularly reviews research that involves a vulnerable category of subjects, such as children, prisoners, pregnant women, or handicapped or mentally disabled persons, consideration shall be given to the inclusion of one or more individuals who are knowledgeable about and experienced in working with these subjects.

(b) Every nondiscriminatory effort will be made to ensure that no IRB consists entirely of men or entirely of women, including the institution's consideration of qualified persons of both sexes, so long as no selection is made to the IRB on the basis of gender. No IRB may consist entirely of members of one profession.

(c) Each IRB shall include at least one member whose primary concerns are in scientific areas and at least one member whose primary concerns are in nonscientific areas.

(d) Each IRB shall include at least one member who is not otherwise affiliated with the institution and who is not part of the immediate family of a person who is affiliated with the institution.

(e) No IRB may have a member participate in the IRB's initial or continuing review of any project in which the member has a conflicting interest, except to provide information requested by the IRB.

(f) An IRB may, in its discretion, invite individuals with competence in special areas to assist in the review of issues which require expertise beyond or in addition to that available on the IRB. These individuals may not vote with the IRB.

§46.108 IRB functions and operations

In order to fulfill the requirements of this policy each IRB shall:

(a) Follow written procedures in the same detail as described in §46.103(b)(4) and to the extent required by §46.103(b)(5).

(b) Except when an expedited review procedure is used (see §46.110), review proposed research at convened meetings at which a majority of the members of the IRB are present, including at least one member whose primary concerns are in nonscientific areas. In order for the research to be approved, it shall receive the approval of a majority of those members present at the meeting

§46.109 IRB review of research

(a) An IRB shall review and have authority to approve, require modifications in (to secure approval), or disapprove all research activities covered by this policy.

(b) An IRB shall require that information given to subjects as part of informed consent is in accordance with §46.116. The IRB may require that information, in addition to that specifically mentioned in §46.116, be given to the subjects when in the IRB's judgment the information would meaningfully add to the protection of the rights and welfare of subjects.

(c) An IRB shall require documentation of informed consent or may waive documentation in accordance with §46.117.

(d) An IRB shall notify investigators and the institution in writing of its decision to approve or disapprove the proposed research activity, or of modifications required to secure IRB approval of the research activity. If the IRB decides to disapprove a research activity, it shall include in its written notification a statement of the reasons for its decision and give the investigator an opportunity to respond in person or in writing.

(e) An IRB shall conduct continuing review of research covered by this policy at intervals appropriate to the degree of risk, but not less than once per year, and shall have authority to observe or have a third party observe the consent process and the research.

(Approved by the Office of Management and Budget under Control Number 9999-0020.)

§46.110 Expedited review procedures for certain kinds of research involving no more than minimal risk, and for minor changes in approved research

(a) The Secretary, HHS, has established, and published as a Notice in the Federal Register, a list of categories of research that may be reviewed by the IRB through an expedited review procedure. The list will be amended, as appropriate, after consultation with other departments and agencies, through periodic republication by the Secretary, HHS, in the Federal Register. A copy of the list is available from the Office for Protection from Research Risks, National Institutes of Health, DHHS, Bethesda, Maryland 20892.

(b) An IRB may use the expedited review procedure to review either or both of the following:

(1) Some or all of the research appearing on the list and found by the reviewer(s) to involve no more than minimal risk,

(2) Minor changes in previously approved research during the period (of one year or less) for which approval is authorized.

Under an expedited review procedure, the review may be carried out by the IRB chairperson or by one or more experienced reviewers designated by the chairperson from among members of the IRB. In reviewing the research, the reviewers may exercise all of the authorities of the IRB except that the reviewers may not disapprove the research. A research activity may be disapproved only after review in accordance with the non-expedited procedure set forth in §46.108(b).

(c) Each IRB which uses an expedited review procedure shall adopt a method for keeping all members advised of research proposals which have been approved under the procedure.

(d) The department or agency head may restrict, suspend, terminate, or choose not to authorize an institution's or IRB's use of the expedited review procedure.

§46.111 Criteria for IRB approval of research

(a) In order to approve research covered by this policy the IRB shall determine that all of the following requirements are satisfied:

(1) Risks to subjects are minimized: (i) By using procedures which are consistent with sound research design and which do not unnecessarily expose subjects to risk, and (ii) whenever appropriate, by using procedures already being performed on the subjects for diagnostic or treatment purposes.

(2) Risks to subjects are reasonable in relation to anticipated benefits, if any, to subjects, and the importance of the knowledge that may reasonably be expected to result. In evaluating risks and benefits, the IRB should consider only those risks and benefits that may result from the research (as distinguished from risks and benefits of therapies subjects would receive even if not participating in the research). The IRB should not consider possible long-range effects of applying knowledge gained in the research (for example, the possible effects of the research on public policy) as among those research risks that fall within the purview of its responsibility.

(3) Selection of subjects is equitable. In making this assessment the IRB should take into account the purposes of the research and the setting in which the research will be conducted and should be particularly cognizant of the special problems of research involving vulnerable populations, such as children, prisoners, pregnant women, mentally disabled persons, or economically or educationally disadvantaged persons.

(4) Informed consent will be sought from each prospective subject or the subject's legally authorized representative, in accordance with, and to the extent required by §46.116.

(5) Informed consent will be appropriately documented, in accordance with, and to the extent required by §46.117.

(6) When appropriate, the research plan makes adequate provision for monitoring the data collected to ensure the safety of subjects.

(7) When appropriate, there are adequate provisions to protect the privacy of subjects and to maintain the confidentiality of data.

(b) When some or all of the subjects are likely to be vulnerable to coercion or undue influence, such as children, prisoners, pregnant women, mentally disabled persons, or economically or educationally disadvantaged persons, additional safeguards have been included in the study to protect the rights and welfare of these subjects.

§46.112 Review by institution

Research covered by this policy that has been approved by an IRB may be subject to further appropriate review and approval or disapproval by officials of the institution. However, those officials may not approve the research if it has not been approved by an IRB.

§46.113 Suspension or termination of IRB approval of research

An IRB shall have authority to suspend or terminate approval of research that is not being conducted in accordance with the IRB's requirements or that has been associated with unexpected serious harm to subjects. Any suspension or termination or approval shall include a statement of the reasons for the IRB's action and shall be reported promptly to the investigator, appropriate institutional officials, and the department or agency head.

(Approved by the Office of Management and Budget under Control Number 9999-0020.)

§46.114 Cooperative research

Cooperative research projects are those projects covered by this policy which involve more than one institution. In the conduct of cooperative research projects, each institution is responsible for safeguarding the rights and welfare of human subjects and for complying with this policy. With the approval of the department or agency head, an institution participating in a cooperative project may enter into a joint review arrangement, rely upon the review of another qualified IRB, or make similar arrangements for avoiding duplication of effort.

§46.115 IRB records

(a) An institution, or when appropriate an IRB, shall prepare and maintain adequate documentation of IRB activities, including the following:

(1) Copies of all research proposals reviewed, scientific evaluations, if any, that accompany the proposals, approved sample consent documents, progress reports submitted by investigators, and reports of injuries to subjects.

(2) Minutes of IRB meetings which shall be in sufficient detail to show attendance at the meetings; actions taken by the IRB; the vote on these actions including the number of members voting for, against, and abstaining; the basis for requiring changes in or disapproving research; and a written summary of the discussion of controverted issues and their resolution.

(3) Records of continuing review activities.

(4) Copies of all correspondence between the IRB and the investigators.

(5) A list of IRB members in the same detail as described in §46.103(b)(3).

(6) Written procedures for the IRB in the same detail as described in §46.103(b)(4) and §46.103(b)(5).

(7) Statements of significant new findings provided to subjects, as required by §46.116(b)(5).

(b) The records required by this policy shall be retained for at least 3 years, and records relating to research which is conducted shall be retained for at least 3 years after completion of the research. All records shall be accessible for inspection and copying by authorized representatives of the department or agency at reasonable times and in a reasonable manner.

(Approved by the Office of Management and Budget under Control Number 9999-0020.)

§46.116 General requirements for informed consent

Except as provided elsewhere in this policy, no investigator may involve a human being as a subject in research covered by this policy unless the investigator has obtained the legally effective informed consent of the subject or the subject's legally authorized representative. An investigator shall seek such consent only under circumstances that provide the prospective subject or the representative sufficient opportunity to consider whether or not to participate and that minimize the possibility of coercion or undue influence. The information that is given to the subject or the representative shall be in language understandable to the subject or the representative. No informed consent, whether oral or written, may include any exculpatory language through which the subject or the representative is made to waive or appear to waive any of the subject's legal rights, or releases or appears to release the investigator, the sponsor, the institution or its agents from liability for negligence.

(a) Basic elements of informed consent. Except as provided in paragraph (c) or (d) of this section, in seeking informed consent the following information shall be provided to each subject:

(1) A statement that the study involves research, an explanation of the purposes of the research and the expected duration of the subject's participation, a description of the procedures to be followed, and identification of any procedures which are experimental;

(2) A description of any reasonably foreseeable risks or discomforts to the subject;

(3) A description of any benefits to the subject or to others which may reasonably be expected from the research;

(4) A disclosure of appropriate alternative procedures or courses of treatment, if any, that might be advantageous to the subject;

(5) A statement describing the extent, if any, to which confidentiality of records identifying the subject will be maintained;

(6) For research involving more than minimal risk, an explanation as to whether any compensation and an explanation as to whether any medical treatments are available if injury occurs and, if so, what they consist of, or where further information may be obtained;

(7) An explanation of whom to contact for answers to pertinent questions about the research and research subjects' rights, and whom to contact in the event of a research-related injury to the subject; and

(8) A statement that participation is voluntary, refusal to participate will involve no penalty or loss of benefits to which the subject is otherwise entitled, and the subject may discontinue participation at any time without penalty or loss of benefits to which the subject is otherwise entitled.

(b) Additional elements of informed consent. When appropriate, one or more of the following elements of information shall also be provided to each subject:

(1) A statement that the particular treatment or procedure may involve risks to the subject (or to the embryo or fetus, if the subject is or may become pregnant) which are currently unforeseeable;

(2) Anticipated circumstances under which the subject's participation may be terminated by the investigator without regard to the subject's consent;

(3) Any additional costs to the subject that may result from participation in the research;

(4) The consequences of a subject's decision to withdraw from the research and procedures for orderly termination of participation by the subject;

(5) A statement that significant new findings developed during the course of the research which may relate to the subject's willingness to continue participation will be provided to the subject; and

(6) The approximate number of subjects involved in the study.

(c) An IRB may approve a consent procedure which does not include, or which alters, some or all of the elements of informed consent set forth above, or waive the requirement to obtain informed consent provided the IRB finds and documents that:

(1) The research or demonstration project is to be conducted by or subject to the approval of state or local government officials and is designed to study, evaluate, or otherwise examine: (i) public benefit or service programs; (ii) procedures for obtaining benefits or services under those programs; (iii) possible changes in or alternatives to those programs or procedures; or (iv) possible changes in methods or levels of payment for benefits or services under those programs; and

(2) The research could not practicably be carried out without the waiver or alteration.

(d) An IRB may approve a consent procedure which does not include, or which alters, some or all of the elements of informed consent set forth in this section, or waive the requirements to obtain informed consent provided the IRB finds and documents that:

(1) The research involves no more than minimal risk to the subjects;

(2) The waiver or alteration will not adversely affect the rights and welfare of the subjects;

(3) The research could not practicably be carried out without the waiver or alteration; and

(4) Whenever appropriate, the subjects will be provided with additional pertinent information after participation.

(e) The informed consent requirements in this policy are not intended to preempt any applicable federal, state, or local laws which require additional information to be disclosed in order for informed consent to be legally effective.

(f) Nothing in this policy is intended to limit the authority of a physician to provide emergency medical care, to the extent the physician is permitted to do so under applicable federal, state, or local law.

(Approved by the Office of Management and Budget under Control Number 9999-0020.)

§46.117 Documentation of informed consent

(a) Except as provided in paragraph (c) of this section, informed consent shall be documented by the use of a written consent form approved by the IRB and signed by the subject or the subject's legally authorized representative. A copy shall be given to the person signing the form.

(b) Except as provided in paragraph (c) of this section, the consent form may be either of the following:

(1) A written consent document that embodies the elements of informed consent required by §46.116. This form may be read to the subject or the subject's legally authorized representative, but in any event, the investigator shall give either the subject or the representative adequate opportunity to read it before it is signed; or

(2) A short form written consent document stating that the elements of informed consent required by §46.116 have been presented orally to the subject or the subject's legally authorized representative. When this method is used, there shall be a witness to the oral presentation. Also, the IRB shall approve a written summary of what is to be said to the subject or the representative. Only the short form itself is to be signed by the subject or the representative. However, the witness shall sign both the short form and a copy of the summary, and the person actually obtaining consent shall sign a copy of the summary. A copy of the summary shall be given to the subject or the representative, in addition to a copy of the short form.

(c) IRB may waive the requirement for the investigator to obtain a signed consent form for some or all subjects if it finds either:

(1) That the only record linking the subject and the research would be the consent document and the principal risk would be potential harm resulting from a breach of confidentiality. Each subject will be asked whether the subject wants documentation linking the subject with the research, and the subject's wishes will govern; or

(2) That the research presents no more than minimal risk of harm to subjects and involves no procedures for which written consent is normally required outside of the research context.

In cases in which the documentation requirement is waived, the IRB may require the investigator to provide subjects with a written statement regarding the research. (Approved by the Office of Management and Budget under Control Number 9999-0020.)

§46.118 Applications and proposals lacking definite plans for involvement of human subjects

Certain types of applications for grants, cooperative agreements, or contracts are submitted to departments or agencies with the knowledge that subjects may be involved within the period of support, but definite plans would not normally be set forth in the application or proposal. These include activities such as institutional type grants when selection of specific projects is the institution's responsibility; research training grants in which the activities involving subjects remain to be selected; and projects in which human subjects' involvement will depend upon completion of instruments, prior animal studies, or purification of compounds. These applications need not be reviewed by an IRB before an award may be made. However, except for research exempted or waived under §46.101 (b) or (i), no human subjects may be involved in

any project supported by these awards until the project has been reviewed and approved by the IRB, as provided in this policy, and certification submitted, by the institution, to the department or agency.

§46.119 Research undertaken without the intention of involving human subjects

In the event research is undertaken without the intention of involving human subjects, but it is later proposed to involve human subjects in the research, the research shall first be reviewed and approved by an IRB, as provided in this policy, a certification submitted, by the institution, to the department or agency, and final approval given to the proposed change by the department or agency.

§46.120 Evaluation and disposition of applications and proposals for research to be conducted or supported by a federal department or agency.

(a) The department or agency head will evaluate all applications and proposals involving human subjects submitted to the department or agency through such officers and employees of the department or agency and such experts and consultants as the department or agency head determines to be appropriate. This evaluation will take into consideration the risks to the subjects, the adequacy of protection against these risks, the potential benefits of the research to the subjects and others, and the importance of the knowledge gained or to be gained.

(b) On the basis of this evaluation, the department or agency head may approve or disapprove the application or proposal, or enter into negotiations to develop an approvable one.

§46.121 [Reserved]

§46.122 Use of federal funds

Federal funds administered by a department or agency may not be expended for research involving human subjects unless the requirements of this policy have been satisfied.

§46.123 Early termination of research support: Evaluation of applications and proposals

(a) The department or agency head may require that department or agency support for any project be terminated or suspended in the manner prescribed in applicable program requirements, when the department or agency head finds an institution has materially failed to comply with the terms of this policy.

(b) In making decisions about supporting or approving applications or proposals covered by this policy the department or agency head may take into account, in addition to all other eligibility requirements and program criteria, factors such as whether the applicant has been subject to a termination or suspension under paragraph (a) of this section and whether the applicant or the person or persons who would direct or has/have directed the scientific and technical aspects of an activity has/have, in the judgment of the department or agency head, materially failed to discharge responsibility for the protection of the rights and welfare of human subjects (whether or not the research was subject to federal regulation).

§46.124 Conditions

With respect to any research project or any class of research projects the department or agency head may impose additional conditions prior to or at the time of approval when in the judgment of the department or agency head additional conditions are necessary for the protection of human subjects.

Subpart B
Additional DHHS Protections Pertaining to Research, Development, and Related Activities Involving Fetuses, Pregnant Women, and Human In Vitro Fertilization

Source: 40 FR 33528, Aug. 8, 1975; 43 FR 1758, January 11, 1978;
43 FR 51559, November 3, 1978.

§46.201 Applicability

(a) The regulations in this subpart are applicable to all Department of Health and Human Services grants and contracts supporting research, development, and related activities involving: (1) the fetus, (2) pregnant women, and (3) human in vitro fertilization.

(b) Nothing in this subpart shall be construed as indicating that compliance with the procedures set forth herein will in any way render inapplicable pertinent State or local laws bearing upon activities covered by this subpart.

(c) The requirements of this subpart are in addition to those imposed under the other subparts of this part.

§46.202 Purpose

It is the purpose of this subpart to provide additional safeguards in reviewing activities to which this subpart is applicable to assure that they conform to appropriate ethical standards and relate to important societal needs.

§46.203 Definitions

As used in this subpart:

(a) Secretary means the Secretary of Health and Human Services and any other officer or employee of the Department of Health and Human Services (DHHS) to whom authority has been delegated.

(b) Pregnancy encompasses the period of time from confirmation of implantation (through any of the presumptive signs of pregnancy, such as missed menses, or by a medically acceptable pregnancy test), until expulsion or extraction of the fetus.

(c) Fetus means the product of conception from the time of implantation (as evidenced by any of the presumptive signs of pregnancy, such as missed menses, or a medically acceptable pregnancy test), until a determination is made, following expulsion or extraction of the fetus, that it is viable.

(d) Viable as it pertains to the fetus means being able, after either spontaneous or induced delivery, to survive (given the benefit of available medical therapy) to the point of independently maintaining heart beat and respiration. The Secretary may from time to time, taking into account medical advances, publish in the Federal Register guidelines to assist in determining whether a fetus is viable for purposes of this subpart. If a fetus is viable after delivery, it is a premature infant.

(e) Nonviable fetus means a fetus ex utero which, although living, is not viable.

(f) Dead fetus means a fetus ex utero which exhibits neither heartbeat, spontaneous respiratory activity, spontaneous movement of voluntary muscles, nor pulsation of the umbilical cord (if still attached).

(g) In vitro fertilization means any fertilization of human ova which occurs outside the body of a female, either through admixture of donor human sperm and ova or by any other means.

§46.204 Ethical Advisory Boards

(a) One or more Ethical Advisory Boards shall be established by the Secretary. Members of these board(s) shall be so selected that the board(s) will be competent to deal with medical, legal, social, ethical, and related issues and may include, for example, research scientists, physicians, psychologists, sociologists, educators, lawyers, and ethicists, as well as representatives of the general public. No board member may be a regular, full-time employee of the Department of Health and Human Services.

(b) At the request of the Secretary, the Ethical Advisory Board shall render advice consistent with the policies and requirements of this part as to ethical issues, involving activities covered by this subpart, raised by individual applications or proposals. In addition, upon request by the Secretary, the Board shall render advice as to classes of applications or proposals and general policies, guidelines, and procedures.

(c) A Board may establish, with the approval of the Secretary, classes of applications or proposals which: (1) Must be submitted to the Board, or (2) Need not be submitted to the Board. Where the Board so establishes a class of applications or proposals which must be submitted, no application or proposal within the class may be funded by the department or any component thereof until the application or proposal has been reviewed by the Board and the Board has rendered advice as to its acceptability from an ethical standpoint.

(d) [Nullified under Public Law 103-43, June 10, 1993]

§46.205 Additional duties of the Institutional Review Boards in connection with activities involving fetuses, pregnant women, or human in vitro fertilization

(a) In addition to the responsibilities prescribed for Institutional Review Boards under Subpart A of this part, the applicant's or offeror's Board shall, with respect to activities covered by this subpart, carry out the following additional duties:

(1) Determine that all aspects of the activity meet the requirements of this subpart;

(2) Determine that adequate consideration has been given to the manner in which potential subjects will be selected, and adequate provision has been made by the applicant or offeror for monitoring the actual informed consent process (e.g., through such mechanisms, when appropriate, as participation by the Institutional Review Board or subject advocates in: (i) Overseeing the actual process by which individual consents required by this subpart are secured either by approving induction of each individual into the

activity or verifying, perhaps through sampling, that approved procedures for induction of individuals into the activity are being followed, and (ii) monitoring the progress of the activity and intervening as necessary through such steps as visits to the activity site and continuing evaluation to determine if any unanticipated risks have arisen);

(3) Carry out such other responsibilities as may be assigned by the Secretary.

(b) No award may be issued until the applicant or offeror has certified to the Secretary that the Institutional Review Board has made the determinations required under paragraph (a) of this section and the Secretary has approved these determinations, as provided in §46.120 of Subpart A of this part.

(c) Applicants or offerors seeking support for activities covered by this subpart must provide for the designation of an Institutional Review Board, subject to approval by the Secretary, where no such Board has been established under Subpart A of this part.

§46.206 General limitations

(a) No activity to which this subpart is applicable may be undertaken unless:

(1) Appropriate studies on animals and nonpregnant individuals have been completed;

(2) Except where the purpose of the activity is to meet the health needs of the mother or the particular fetus, the risk to the fetus is minimal and, in all cases, is the least possible risk for achieving the objectives of the activity;

(3) Individuals engaged in the activity will have no part in: (i) Any decisions as to the timing, method, and procedures used to terminate the pregnancy, and (ii) determining the viability of the fetus at the termination of the pregnancy; and

(4) No procedural changes which may cause greater than minimal risk to the fetus or the pregnant woman will be introduced into the procedure for terminating the pregnancy solely in the interest of the activity.

(b) No inducements, monetary or otherwise, may be offered to terminate pregnancy for purposes of the activity. Source: 40 FR 33528, Aug. 8, 1975, as amended at 40 FR 51638, Nov. 6, 1975.

§46.207 Activities directed toward pregnant women as subjects

(a) No pregnant woman may be involved as a subject in an activity covered by this subpart unless: (1) The purpose of the activity is to meet the health needs of the mother and the fetus will be placed at risk only to the minimum extent necessary to meet such needs, or (2) the risk to the fetus is minimal.

(b) An activity permitted under paragraph (a) of this section may be conducted only if the mother and father are legally competent and have given their informed consent after having been fully informed regarding possible impact on the fetus, except that the father's informed consent need not be secured if: (1) The purpose of the activity is to meet the health needs of the mother; (2) his identity or whereabouts cannot reasonably be ascertained; (3) he is not reasonably available; or (4) the pregnancy resulted from rape.

§46.208 Activities directed toward fetuses in utero as subjects

(a) No fetus in utero may be involved as a subject in any activity covered by this subpart unless: (1) The purpose of the activity is to meet the health needs of the particular fetus and the fetus will be placed at risk only to the minimum extent necessary to meet such needs, or (2) the risk to the fetus imposed by the research is minimal and the purpose of the activity is the development of important biomedical knowledge which cannot be obtained by other means.

(b) An activity permitted under paragraph (a) of this section may be conducted only if the mother and father are legally competent and have given their informed consent, except that the father's consent need not be secured if: (1) His identity or whereabouts cannot reasonably be ascertained, (2) he is not reasonably available, or (3) the pregnancy resulted from rape.

§46.209 Activities directed toward fetuses ex utero, including nonviable fetuses, as subjects

(a) Until it has been ascertained whether or not a fetus ex utero is viable, a fetus ex utero may not be involved as a subject in an activity covered by this subpart unless:

(1) There will be no added risk to the fetus resulting from the activity, and the purpose of the activity is the development of important biomedical knowledge which cannot be obtained by other means, or

(2) The purpose of the activity is to enhance the possibility of survival of the particular fetus to the point of viability.

(b) No nonviable fetus may be involved as a subject in an activity covered by this subpart unless:

(1) Vital functions of the fetus will not be artificially maintained,

(2) Experimental activities which of themselves would terminate the heartbeat or respiration of the fetus will not be employed, and

(3) The purpose of the activity is the development of important biomedical knowledge which cannot be obtained by other means.

(c) In the event the fetus ex utero is found to be viable, it may be included as a subject in the activity only to the extent permitted by and in accordance with the requirements of other subparts of this part.

(d) An activity permitted under paragraph (a) or (b) of this section may be conducted only if the mother and father are legally competent and have given their informed consent, except that the father's informed consent need not be secured if: (1) His identity or whereabouts cannot reasonably be ascertained, (2) he is not reasonably available, or (3) the pregnancy resulted from rape.

§46.210 Activities involving the dead fetus, fetal material, or the placenta

Activities involving the dead fetus, mascerated fetal material, or cells, tissue, or organs excised from a dead fetus shall be conducted only in accordance with any applicable State or local laws regarding such activities.

§46.211 Modification or waiver of specific requirements

Upon the request of an applicant or offeror (with the approval of its Institutional Review Board), the Secretary may modify or waive specific requirements of this subpart, with the approval of the Ethical Advisory Board after such opportunity for public comment as the Ethical Advisory Board considers appropriate in the particular instance. In making such decisions, the Secretary will consider whether the risks to the subject are so outweighed by the sum of the benefit to the subject and the importance of the knowledge to be gained as to warrant such modification or waiver and that such benefits cannot be gained except through a modification or waiver. Any such modifications or waivers will be published as notices in the Federal Register.

Subpart C

Additional DHHS Protections Pertaining to Biomedical and Behavioral Research Involving Prisoners as Subjects

Source: 43 FR 53655, Nov. 16, 1978.

§46.301 Applicability

(a) The regulations in this subpart are applicable to all biomedical and behavioral research conducted or supported by the Department of Health and Human Services involving prisoners as subjects.

(b) Nothing in this subpart shall be construed as indicating that compliance with the procedures set forth herein will authorize research involving prisoners as subjects, to the extent such research is limited or barred by applicable State or local law.

(c) The requirements of this subpart are in addition to those imposed under the other subparts of this part.

§46.302 Purpose

Inasmuch as prisoners may be under constraints because of their incarceration which could affect their ability to make a truly voluntary and uncoerced decision whether or not to participate as subjects in research, it is the purpose of this subpart to provide additional safeguards for the protection of prisoners involved in activities to which this subpart is applicable.

§46.303 Definitions

As used in this subpart:

(a) Secretary means the Secretary of Health and Human Services and any other officer or employee of the Department of Health and Human Services to whom authority has been delegated.

(b) DHHS means the Department of Health and Human Services.

(c) Prisoner means any individual involuntarily confined or detained in a penal institution. The term is intended to encompass individuals sentenced to such an institution under a criminal or civil statute, individuals detained in other facilities by virtue of statutes or commitment procedures which provide alternatives to criminal prosecution or incarceration in a penal institution, and individuals detained pending arraignment, trial, or sentencing.

(d) Minimal risk is the probability and magnitude of physical or psychological harm that is normally encountered in the daily lives, or in the routine medical, dental, or psychological examination of healthy persons.

§46.304 Composition of Institutional Review Boards where prisoners are involved

In addition to satisfying the requirements in §46.107 of this part, an Institutional Review Board, carrying out responsibilities under this part with respect to research covered by this subpart, shall also meet the following specific requirements:

(a) A majority of the Board (exclusive of prisoner members) shall have no association with the prison(s) involved, apart from their membership on the Board.

(b) At least one member of the Board shall be a prisoner, or a prisoner representative with appropriate background and experience to serve in that capacity, except that where a particular research project is reviewed by more than one Board only one Board need satisfy this requirement.

§46.305 Additional duties of the Institutional Review Boards where prisoners are involved

(a) In addition to all other responsibilities prescribed for Institutional Review Boards under this part, the Board shall review research covered by this subpart and approve such research only if it finds that:

(1) The research under review represents one of the categories of research permissible under §46.306(a)(2);

(2) Any possible advantages accruing to the prisoner through his or her participation in the research, when compared to the general living conditions, medical care, quality of food, amenities and opportunity for earnings in the prison, are not of such a magnitude that his or her ability to weigh the risks of the research against the value of such advantages in the limited choice environment of the prison is impaired;

(3) The risks involved in the research are commensurate with risks that would be accepted by nonprisoner volunteers;

(4) Procedures for the selection of subjects within the prison are fair to all prisoners and immune from arbitrary intervention by prison authorities or prisoners. Unless the principal investigator provides to the Board justification in writing for following some other procedures, control subjects must be selected randomly from the group of available prisoners who meet the characteristics needed for that particular research project;

(5) The information is presented in language which is understandable to the subject population;

(6) Adequate assurance exists that parole boards will not take into account a prisoner's participation in the research in making decisions regarding parole, and each prisoner is clearly informed in advance that participation in the research will have no effect on his or her parole; and

(7) Where the Board finds there may be a need for follow-up examination or care of participants after the end of their participation, adequate provision has been made for such examination or care, taking into account the varying lengths of individual prisoners' sentences, and for informing participants of this fact.

(b) The Board shall carry out such other duties as may be assigned by the Secretary.

(c) The institution shall certify to the Secretary, in such form and manner as the Secretary may require, that the duties of the Board under this section have been fulfilled.

§46.306 Permitted research involving prisoners

(a) Biomedical or behavioral research conducted or supported by DHHS may involve prisoners as subjects only if:

(1) The institution responsible for the conduct of the research has certified to the Secretary that the Institutional Review Board has approved the research under §46.305 of this subpart; and

(2) In the judgment of the Secretary the proposed research involves solely the following:

(i) Study of the possible causes, effects, and processes of incarceration, and of criminal behavior, provided that the study presents no more than minimal risk and no more than inconvenience to the subjects;

(ii) Study of prisons as institutional structures or of prisoners as incarcerated persons, provided that the study presents no more than minimal risk and no more than inconvenience to the subjects;

(iii) Research on conditions particularly affecting prisoners as a class (for example, vaccine trials and other research on hepatitis which is much more prevalent in prisons than elsewhere; and research on social and psychological problems such as alcoholism, drug addiction, and sexual assaults) provided that the study may proceed only after the Secretary has consulted with appropriate experts including experts in penology, medicine, and ethics, and published notice, in the Federal Register, of his intent to approve such research; or

(iv) Research on practices, both innovative and accepted, which have the intent and reasonable probability of improving the health or well-being of the subject. In cases in which those studies require the assignment of prisoners in a manner consistent with protocols approved by the IRB to control groups which may not benefit from the research, the study may proceed only after the Secretary has consulted with appropriate experts, including experts in penology, medicine, and ethics, and published notice, in the Federal Register, of the intent to approve such research.

(b) Except as provided in paragraph (a) of this section, biomedical or behavioral research conducted or supported by DHHS shall not involve prisoners as subjects.

Subpart D

Additional DHHS Protections for Children Involved as Subjects in Research

Source: 48 FR 9818, March 8, 1983; 56 FR 28032, June 18, 1991.

§46.401 To what do these regulations apply?

(a) This subpart applies to all research involving children as subjects, conducted or supported by the Department of Health and Human Services.

(1) This includes research conducted by Department employees, except that each head of an Operating Division of the Department may adopt such nonsubstantive, procedural modifications as may be appropriate from an administrative standpoint.

(2) It also includes research conducted or supported by the Department of Health and Human Services outside the United States, but in appropriate circumstances, the Secretary may, under paragraph (i) of §46.101 of Subpart A, waive the applicability of some or all of the requirements of these regulations for research of this type.

(b) Exemptions at §46.101(b)(1) and (b)(3) through (b)(6) are applicable to this subpart. The exemption at §46.101(b)(2) regarding educational tests is also applicable to this subpart. However, the exemption at §46.101(b)(2) for research involving survey or interview procedures or observations of public behavior does not apply to research covered by this subpart, except for research involving observation of public behavior when the investigator(s) do not participate in the activities being observed.

(c) The exceptions, additions, and provisions for waiver as they appear in paragraphs (c) through (i) of §46.101 of Subpart A are applicable to this subpart.

§46.402 Definitions

The definitions in §46.102 of Subpart A shall be applicable to this subpart as well. In addition, as used in this subpart:

(a) Children are persons who have not attained the legal age for consent to treatments or procedures involved in the research, under the applicable law of the jurisdiction in which the research will be conducted.

(b) Assent means a child's affirmative agreement to participate in research. Mere failure to object should not, absent affirmative agreement, be construed as assent.

(c) Permission means the agreement of parent(s) or guardian to the participation of their child or ward in research.

(d) Parent means a child's biological or adoptive parent.

(e) Guardian means an individual who is authorized under applicable State or local law to consent on behalf of a child to general medical care.

§46.403 IRB duties

In addition to other responsibilities assigned to IRBs under this part, each IRB shall review research covered by this subpart and approve only research which satisfies the conditions of all applicable sections of this subpart.

§46.404 Research not involving greater than minimal risk

DHHS will conduct or fund research in which the IRB finds that no greater than minimal risk to children is presented, only if the IRB finds that adequate provisions are made for soliciting the assent of the children and the permission of their parents or guardians, as set forth in §46.408.

§46.405 Research involving greater than minimal risk but presenting the prospect of direct benefit to the individual subjects

DHHS will conduct or fund research in which the IRB finds that more than minimal risk to children is presented by an intervention or procedure that holds out the prospect of direct benefit for the individual subject, or by a monitoring procedure that is likely to contribute to the subject's well-being, only if the IRB finds that:

(a) The risk is justified by the anticipated benefit to the subjects;

(b) The relation of the anticipated benefit to the risk is at least as favorable to the subjects as that presented by available alternative approaches; and

(c) Adequate provisions are made for soliciting the assent of the children and permission of their parents or guardians, as set forth in §46.408.

§46.406 Research involving greater than minimal risk and no prospect of direct benefit to individual subjects, but likely to yield generalizable knowledge about the subject's disorder or condition

DHHS will conduct or fund research in which the IRB finds that more than minimal risk to children is presented by an intervention or procedure that does not hold out the prospect of direct benefit for the individual subject, or by a monitoring procedure which is not likely to contribute to the well-being of the subject, only if the IRB finds that:

(a) The risk represents a minor increase over minimal risk;

(b) The intervention or procedure presents experiences to subjects that are reasonably commensurate with those inherent in their actual or expected medical, dental, psychological, social, or educational situations;

(c) The intervention or procedure is likely to yield generalizable knowledge about the subjects' disorder or condition which is of vital importance for the understanding or amelioration of the subjects' disorder or condition; and

(d) Adequate provisions are made for soliciting assent of the children and permission of their parents or guardians, as set forth in §46.408.

§46.407 Research not otherwise approvable which presents an opportunity to understand, prevent, or alleviate a serious problem affecting the health or welfare of children

DHHS will conduct or fund research that the IRB does not believe meets the requirements of §46.404, §46.405, or §46.406 only if:

(a) The IRB finds that the research presents a reasonable opportunity to further the understanding, prevention, or alleviation of a serious problem affecting the health or welfare of children; and

(b) The Secretary, after consultation with a panel of experts in pertinent disciplines (for example: science, medicine, education, ethics, law) and following opportunity for public review and comment, has determined either:

(1) That the research in fact satisfies the conditions of §46.404, §46.405, or §46.406, as applicable, or

(2) the following:

(i) The research presents a reasonable opportunity to further the understanding, prevention, or alleviation of a serious problem affecting the health or welfare of children;

(ii) The research will be conducted in accordance with sound ethical principles;

(iii) Adequate provisions are made for soliciting the assent of children and the permission of their parents or guardians, as set forth in §46.408.

§46.408 Requirements for permission by parents or guardians and for assent by children

(a) In addition to the determinations required under other applicable sections of this subpart, the IRB shall determine that adequate provisions are made for soliciting the assent of the children, when in the judgment of the IRB the children are capable of providing assent. In determining whether children are capable of assenting, the IRB shall take into account the ages, maturity, and psychological state of the children involved. This judgment may be made for all children to be involved in research under a particular protocol, or for each child, as the IRB deems appropriate. If the IRB determines that the capability of some or all of the children is so limited that they cannot reasonably be consulted or that the intervention or procedure involved in the research holds out a prospect of direct benefit that is important to the health or well-being of the children and is available only in the context of the research, the assent of the children is not a necessary condition for proceeding with the research. Even where the IRB determines that the subjects are capable of assenting, the IRB may still waive the assent requirement under circumstances in which consent may be waived in accord with §46.116 of Subpart A.

(b) In addition to the determinations required under other applicable sections of this subpart, the IRB shall determine, in accordance with and to the extent that consent is required by §46.116 of Subpart A, that adequate provisions are made for soliciting the permission of each child's parents or guardian. Where parental permission is to be obtained, the IRB may find that the permission of one parent is sufficient for research to be conducted under §46.404 or §46.405. Where research is covered by §46.406 and §46.407 and permission is to be obtained from parents, both parents must give their permission unless one parent is deceased, unknown, incompetent, or not reasonably available, or when only one parent has legal responsibility for the care and custody of the child.

(c) In addition to the provisions for waiver contained in §46.116 of Subpart A, if the IRB determines that a research protocol is designed for conditions or for a subject population for which parental or guardian permission is not a reasonable requirement to protect the subjects (for example, neglected or abused children), it may waive the consent requirements in Subpart A of this part and paragraph (b) of this section, provided an appropriate mechanism for protecting the children who will participate as subjects in the research is substituted, and provided further that the waiver is not inconsistent with Federal, State, or local law. The choice of an appropriate mechanism would depend upon the nature and purpose of the activities described in the protocol, the risk and anticipated benefit to the research subjects, and their age, maturity, status, and condition.

(d) Permission by parents or guardians shall be documented in accordance with and to the extent required by §46.117 of Subpart A.

(e) When the IRB determines that assent is required, it shall also determine whether and how assent must be documented.

§46.409 Wards

(a) Children who are wards of the State or any other agency, institution, or entity can be included in research approved under §46.406 or §46.407 only if such research is:

(1) Related to their status as wards; or

(2) Conducted in schools, camps, hospitals, institutions, or similar settings in which the majority of children involved as subjects are not wards.

(b) If the research is approved under paragraph (a) of this section, the IRB shall require appointment of an advocate for each child who is a ward, in addition to any other individual acting on behalf of the child as guardian or in loco parentis. One individual may serve as advocate for more than one child. The advocate shall be an individual who has the background and experience to act in, and agrees to act in, the best interests of the child for the duration of the child's participation in the research and who is not associated in any way (except in the role as advocate or member of the IRB) with the research, the investigator(s), or the guardian organization.

CHAPTER 11-2B

Code of Federal Regulations: Title 21, Part 50

21 CFR Part 50—Protection of Human Subjects—Food and Drug Administration

Subpart A—General Provisions
50.1 Scope
50.3 Definitions

Subpart B—Informed Consent of Human Subjects
50.20 General requirements for informed consent
50.23 Exception from general requirements
50.24 Exception from informed consent requirements for emergency research
50.25 Elements of informed consent
50.27 Documentation of informed consent
[Source: 45 FR 36390, May 30, 1980, unless otherwise noted.]

Subpart A—General Provisions

§ 50.1 Scope

(a) This part applies to all clinical investigations regulated by the Food and Drug Administration under sections 505(i) and 520(g) of the Federal Food, Drug, and Cosmetic Act, as well as clinical investigations that support applications for research or marketing permits for products by the Food and Drug Administration, including food and color additives, drugs for human use, medical devices for human use, biological products for human use, and electronic products. Additional specific obligations and commitments of, and standards of conduct for, persons who sponsor or monitor clinical investigations involving particular test articles may also be found in other parts (e.g., 21 CFR parts 312 and 812). Compliance with these parts is intended to protect the rights and safety of subjects involved in investigations filed with the Food and Drug Administration pursuant to sections 406, 409, 502, 503, 505, 506, 507, 510, 513-516, 518, 520, 706, and 801 of the Federal Food, Drug and Cosmetic Act and sections 351 and 354-360F of the Public Health Service Act.

(b) References in this part to regulatory sections of the Code of Federal Regulations are to chapter I of title 21, unless otherwise noted.

[45 FR 36390, May 30, 1980; 46 FR 8979, Jan. 27, 1981]

§ 50.3 Definitions
As used in this part:

(a) Act means the Federal Food, Drug, and Cosmetic Act, as amended (secs. 201-902, 52 Stat. 1040 et seq. as amended (21 U.S.C. 321-392)).

(b) Application for research or marketing permit includes:

(1) A color additive petition, described in part 71.

(2) A food additive petition, described in parts 171 and 571.

(3) Data and information about a substance submitted as part of the procedures for establishing that the substance is generally recognized as safe for use that results or may reasonably be expected to result, directly or indirectly, in its becoming a component or otherwise affecting the characteristics of any food, described in §§ 170.30 and 570.30.

(4) Data and information about a food additive submitted as part of the procedures for food additives permitted to be used on an interim basis pending additional study, described in § 180.1.

(5) Data and information about a substance submitted as part of the procedures for establishing a tolerance for unavoidable contaminants in food and food-packaging materials described in section 406 of the act.

(6) An investigational new drug application described in part 312 of this chapter.

(7) A new drug application described in' part 314.

(8) Data and information about the bio-availability or bio-equivalence of drugs for human use submitted as part of the procedures for issuing, amending, or repealing a bio-equivalence requirement, described in part 320.

(9) Data and information about an over-the-counter drug for human use submitted as part of the procedures for classifying these drugs as generally recognized as safe and effective and not misbranded, described in part 330.

(10) Data and information about a prescription drug for human use submitted as part of the procedures for classifying these drugs as generally recognized as safe and effective and not misbranded, described in this chapter.

(11) Data and information about an antibiotic drug submitted as part of the procedures for issuing, amending or repealing regulations for these drugs, described in § 314.300 of this chapter.

(12) An application for a biological product license, described in part 601.

(13) Data and information about a biological product submitted as part of the procedures for determining that licensed biological products are safe and effective and not misbranded, described in part 601.

(14) Data and information about an in vitro diagnostic product submitted as part of the procedures for establishing, amending, or repealing a standard for these products, described in part 809.

(15) An Application for an Investigational Device Exemption, described in part 812.

(16) Data and information about a medical device submitted as part of the procedures for classifying these devices, described in section 513.

(17) Data and information about a medical device submitted as part of the procedures for establishing, amending, or repealing a standard for these devices, described in section 514.

(18) An application for premarket approval of a medical device, described in section 515.

(19) A product development protocol for a medical device, described in section 515.

(20) Data and information about an electronic product submitted as part of the procedures for establishing, amending or repealing a standard for these products, described in section 358 of the Public Health Service Act.

(21) Data and information about an electronic product submitted as part of the procedures for obtaining a variance from any electronic product performance standard, as described in § 1010.4.

(22) Data and information about an electronic product submitted as part of the procedures for granting amending, or extending an exemption from a radiation safety performance standard, as described in § 1010.5.

(c) Clinical investigation means any experiment that involves a test article and one or more human subjects and that either is subject to requirements for prior submission to the Food and Drug Administration under section 505(i), or 520(g) of the act, or is not subject to requirements for prior submission to the Food and Drug Administration under these sections of the act, but the results of which are intended to be submitted later to, or held for inspection by, the Food and Drug Administration as part of an application for a research or marketing permit. The term does not include experiments that are subject to the provisions of part 58 of this chapter, regarding nonclinical laboratory studies.

(d) Investigator means an individual who actually conducts a clinical investigation, i.e., under whose immediate direction the test article is administered or dispensed to or used involving, a subject, or, in the event of an investigation conducted by a team of individuals, is the responsible leader of that team.

(e) Sponsor means a person who initiates a clinical investigation, but who does not actually conduct the investigation, i.e., the test article is administered or dispensed to or used involving, a subject under the immediate direction of another individual. A person other than an individual (e.g., corporation or agency) that uses one or more of its own employees to conduct a clinical investigation it has initiated is considered to be a sponsor (not a sponsor-investigator) and the employees are considered to be investigators.

(f) Sponsor-investigator means an individual who both initiates and actually conducts, alone or with others a clinical investigation, i.e., under whose immediate direction the test article is administered or dispensed to, or used involving, a subject. The term does not include any person other than an individual, e.g., corporation or agency.

(g) Human subject means an individual who is or becomes a participant in research, either as a recipient of the test article as a control. A subject may be either a healthy human or a patient.

(h) Institution means any public or private entity or Agency (including Federal, State, and other agencies). The word facility as used in section 520(g) of the act is deemed to be synonymous with the term institution for purposes of this part.

(i) Institutional review board (IRB) means any board, committee, or other group formally designated by an institution to review biomedical research involving humans as subjects, to approve the initiation of and conduct periodic review of such research. The term has the same meaning as the phrase institutional review committee as used in section 520(g) of the act.

(j) Test article means any drug (including a biological product for human use), medical device for human use, human food additive, color additive, electronic product, or any other article subject to regulation under the act or under sections 351 and 354-360F of the Public Health Service Act (42 U.S.C. 262 and 263b-263n).

(k) Minimal risk means that the probability and magnitude of harm or discomfort anticipated in the research are not greater in and of themselves than those ordinarily encountered in daily life or during the performance of routine physical or psychological examinations or tests.

(l) Legally authorized representative means an individual or judicial or other body authorized under applicable law to consent on behalf of a prospective subject to the subject's participation in the procedure(s) involved in the research.

(m) Family member means any one of the following legally competent persons: Spouse; parents; children (including adopted children); brothers and sisters; and any individual related by blood or affinity whose close association with the subject is the equivalent of a family relationship.

[45 FR 36390, May 30, 1980, as amended at 46 FR 8950 Jan. 27,1981; 54 FR 9038, Mar. 3, 1989; 56 FR 28028, June 18, 1991; 61 FR 51497, Oct. 2, 1996; 62 FR 39440, July 23, 1997]

Subpart B—Informed Consent of Human Subjects
Source: 46 FR 8951, Jan. 27, 1981, unless otherwise noted.

Sec. 50.20 General requirements for informed consent

Except as provided in Secs. 50.23 and 50.24, no investigator may involve a human being as a subject in research covered by these regulations unless the investigator has obtained the legally effective informed consent of the subject or the subject's legally authorized representative. An investigator shall seek such consent only under circumstances that provide the prospective subject or the representative sufficient opportunity to consider whether or not to participate and that minimize the possibility of coercion or undue influence. The information that is given to the subject or the representative shall be in language understandable to the subject or the representative. No informed consent, whether oral or written, may include any exculpatory language through which the subject or the representative is made to waive or appear to waive any of the subject's legal rights, or releases or appears to release the investigator, the sponsor, the institution, or its agents from liability for negligence.

[46 FR 8951, Jan. 27, 1981, as amended at 64 FR 10942, Mar. 8, 1999]

Sec. 50.23 Exception from general requirements

(a) The obtaining of informed consent shall be deemed feasible unless, before use of the test article (except as provided in paragraph (b) of this section), both the investigator and a physician who is not otherwise participating in the clinical investigation certify in writing all of the following:

(1) The human subject is confronted by a life-threatening situation necessitating the use of the test article.

(2) Informed consent cannot be obtained from the subject because of an inability to communicate with, or obtain legally effective consent from, the subject.

(3) Time is not sufficient to obtain consent from the subject's legal representative.

(4) There is available no alternative method of approved or generally recognized therapy that provides an equal or greater likelihood of saving the life of the subject.

(b) If immediate use of the test article is, in the investigator's opinion, required to preserve the life of the subject, and time is not sufficient to obtain the independent determination required in paragraph (a) of this section in advance of using the test article, the determinations of the clinical investigator shall be made and, within 5 working days after the use of the article, be reviewed and evaluated in writing by a physician who is not participating in the clinical investigation.

(c) The documentation required in paragraph (a) or (b) of this section shall be submitted to the IRB within 5 working days after the use of the test article.

(d)(1) Under 10 U.S.C. 1107(f) the President may waive the prior consent requirement for the administration of an investigational new drug to a member of the armed forces in connection with the member's participation in a particular military operation. The statute specifies that only the President may waive informed consent in this connection and the President may grant such a waiver only if the President determines in writing that obtaining consent: Is not feasible; is contrary to the best interests of the military member; or is not in the interests of national security. The statute further provides that in making a determination to waive prior informed consent on the ground that it is not feasible or the ground that it is contrary to the best interests of the military members involved, the President shall apply the standards and criteria that are set forth in the relevant FDA regulations for a waiver of the prior informed consent requirements of section 505(i)(4) of the Federal Food, Drug, and Cosmetic Act (21 U.S.C. 355(i)(4)). Before such a determination may be made that obtaining informed consent from military personnel prior to the use of an investigational drug (including an antibiotic or biological product) in a specific protocol under an investigational new drug application (IND) sponsored by the Department of Defense (DOD) and limited to specific military personnel involved in a particular military operation is not feasible or is contrary to the best interests of the military members involved the Secretary of Defense must first request such a determination from the President, and certify and document to the President that the following standards and criteria contained in paragraphs (d)(1) through (d)(4) of this section have been met.

(i) The extent and strength of evidence of the safety and effectiveness of the investigational new drug in relation to the medical risk that could be encountered during the military operation supports the drug's administration under an IND.

(ii) The military operation presents a substantial risk that military personnel may be subject to a chemical, biological, nuclear, or other exposure likely to produce death or serious or life-threatening injury or illness.

(iii) There is no available satisfactory alternative therapeutic or preventive treatment in relation to the intended use of the investigational new drug.

(iv) Conditioning use of the investigational new drug on the voluntary participation of each member could significantly risk the safety and health of any individual member who would decline its use, the safety of other military personnel, and the accomplishment of the military mission.

(v) A duly constituted institutional review board (IRB) established and operated in accordance with the requirements of paragraphs (d)(2) and (d)(3) of this section, responsible for review of the study, has reviewed and approved the investigational new drug protocol and the administration of the investigational new drug without informed consent. DOD's request is to include the documentation required by 56.115(a)(2) of this chapter.

(vi) DOD has explained:

(A) The context in which the investigational drug will be administered, e.g., the setting or whether it will be self-administered or it will be administered by a health professional;

(B) The nature of the disease or condition for which the preventive or therapeutic treatment is intended; and

(C) To the extent there are existing data or information available, information on conditions that could alter the effects of the investigational drug.

(vii) DOD's record keeping system is capable of tracking and will be used to track the proposed treatment from supplier to the individual recipient.

(viii) Each member involved in the military operation will be given, prior to the administration of the investigational new drug, a specific written information sheet (including information required by 10 U.S.C. 1107(d)) concerning the investigational new drug, the risks and benefits of its use, potential side effects, and other pertinent information about the appropriate use of the product.

(ix) Medical records of members involved in the military operation will accurately document the receipt by members of the notification required by paragraph (d)(1)(viii) of this section.

(x) Medical records of members involved in the military operation will accurately document the receipt by members of any investigational new drugs in accordance with FDA regulations including part 312 of this chapter.

(xi) DOD will provide adequate follow-up to assess whether there are beneficial or adverse health consequences that result from the use of the investigational product.

(xii) DOD is pursuing drug development, including a time line, and marketing approval with due diligence.

(xiii) FDA has concluded that the investigational new drug protocol may proceed subject to a decision by the President on the informed consent waiver request.

(xiv) DOD will provide training to the appropriate medical personnel and potential recipients on the specific investigational new drug to be administered prior to its use.

(xv) DOD has stated and justified the time period for which the waiver is needed, not to exceed one year, unless separately renewed under these standards and criteria.

(xvi) DOD shall have a continuing obligation to report to the FDA and to the President any changed circumstances relating to these standards and criteria (including the time period referred to in paragraph (d)(1)(xv) of this section) or that otherwise might affect the determination to use an investigational new drug without informed consent.

(xvii) DOD is to provide public notice as soon as practicable and consistent with classification requirements through notice in the Federal Register describing each waiver of informed consent determination, a summary of the most updated scientific information on the products used, and other pertinent information.

(xviii) Use of the investigational drug without informed consent otherwise conforms with applicable law.

(xix) The duly constituted institutional review board, described in paragraph (d)(1)(v) of this section, must include at least 3 nonaffiliated members who shall not be employees or officers of the Federal Government (other than for purposes of membership on the IRB) and shall be required to obtain any necessary security clearances. This IRB shall review the proposed IND protocol at a convened meeting at which a majority of the members are present including at least one member whose primary concerns are in nonscientific areas and, if feasible, including a majority of the nonaffiliated members. The information required by Sec. 56.115(a)(2) of this chapter is to be provided to the Secretary of Defense for further review.

(3) The duly constituted institutional review board, described in paragraph (d)(1)(v) of this section, must review and approve:

(i) The required information sheet;

(ii) The adequacy of the plan to disseminate information, including distribution of the information sheet to potential recipients, on the investigational product (e.g., in forms other than written);

(iii) The adequacy of the information and plans for its dissemination to health care providers including

potential side effects, contraindications, potential interactions, and other pertinent considerations; and

(iv) An informed consent form as required by part 50 of this chapter, in those circumstances in which DOD determines that informed consent may be obtained from some or all personnel involved.

(4) DOD is to submit to FDA summaries of institutional review board meetings at which the proposed protocol has been reviewed.

(5) Nothing in these criteria or standards is intended to preempt or limit FDA's and DOD's authority or obligations under applicable statutes and regulations.

[46 FR 8951, Jan. 27, 1981, as amended at 55 FR 52817, Dec. 21, 1990; 64 FR 399, Jan. 5, 1999; 64 FR 54188, Oct. 5, 1999]

Sec. 50.24 Exception from informed consent requirements for emergency research

(a) The IRB responsible for the review, approval, and continuing review of the clinical investigation described in this section may approve that investigation without requiring that informed consent of all research subjects be obtained if the IRB (with the concurrence of a licensed physician who is a member of or consultant to the IRB and who is not otherwise participating in the clinical investigation) finds and documents each of the following:

(1) The human subjects are in a life-threatening situation, available treatments are unproven or unsatisfactory, and the collection of valid scientific evidence, which may include evidence obtained through randomized placebo-controlled investigations, is necessary to determine the safety and effectiveness of particular interventions.

(2) Obtaining informed consent is not feasible because:

(i) The subjects will not be able to give their informed consent as a result of their medical condition;

(ii) The intervention under investigation must be administered before consent from the subjects' legally authorized representatives is feasible; and

(iii) There is no reasonable way to identify prospectively the individuals likely to become eligible for participation in the clinical investigation.

(3) Participation in the research holds out the prospect of direct benefit to the subjects because:

(i) Subjects are facing a life-threatening situation that necessitates intervention;

(ii) Appropriate animal and other preclinical studies have been conducted, and the information derived from those studies and related evidence support the potential for the intervention to provide a direct benefit to the individual subjects; and

(iii) Risks associated with the investigation are reasonable in relation to what is known about the medical condition of the potential class of subjects, the risks and benefits of standard therapy, if any, and what is known about the risks and benefits of the proposed intervention or activity.

(4) The clinical investigation could not practicably be carried out without the waiver.

(5) The proposed investigational plan defines the length of the potential therapeutic window based on scientific evidence, and the investigator has committed to attempting to contact a legally authorized representative for each subject within that window of time and, if feasible, to asking the legally authorized representative contacted for consent within that window rather than proceeding without consent. The investigator will summarize efforts made to contact legally authorized representatives and make this information available to the IRB at the time of continuing review.

(6) The IRB has reviewed and approved informed consent procedures and an informed consent document consistent with Sec. 50.25. These procedures and the informed consent document are to be used with subjects or their legally authorized representatives in situations where use of such procedures and documents is feasible. The IRB has reviewed and approved procedures and information to be used when providing an opportunity for a family member to object to a subject's participation in the clinical investigation consistent with paragraph (a)(7)(v) of this section.

(7) Additional protections of the rights and welfare of the subjects will be provided, including, at least:

(i)   Consultation (including, where appropriate, consultation carried out by the IRB) with representatives of the communities in which the clinical investigation will be conducted and from which the subjects be drawn;

(ii)   Public disclosure to the communities in which the clinical investigation will be conducted and from which the subjects will be drawn, prior to initiation of the clinical investigation, of plans for the investigation and its risks and expected benefits;

(iii)   Public disclosure of sufficient information following completion of the clinical investigation to apprise the community and researchers of the study, including the demographic characteristics of the research population, and its results;

(iv)   Establishment of an independent data monitoring committee to exercise oversight of the clinical investigation; and

(v)   If obtaining informed consent is not feasible and a legally authorized representative is not reasonably available, the investigator has committed, if feasible, to attempting to contact within the therapeutic window the subject's family member who is not a legally authorized representative, and asking whether he or she objects to the subject's participation in the clinical investigation. The investigator summarize efforts made to contact family members and make this information available to the IRB at the time of continuing review.

(b)The IRB is responsible for ensuring that procedures are in place to inform, at the earliest feasible opportunity, each subject, or if the subject remains incapacitated, a legally authorized representative of the subject, or if such a representative is not reasonably available, a family member, of the subject's inclusion in the clinical investigation, the details of the investigation and other information contained in the informed consent document. The IRB shall also ensure that there is a procedure to inform the subject, or if the subject remains incapacitated, a legally authorized

representative of the subject, or if such a representative is not reasonably available, a family member, that he or she may discontinue the subject's participation at any time without penalty or loss of benefits to which the subject is otherwise entitled. If a legally authorized representative or family member is told about the clinical investigation and the subject's condition improves, the subject is also to be informed as soon as feasible. If a subject is into a clinical investigation with waived consent and the subject dies before a legally authorized representative or family member can be contacted, information about the clinical investigation is to be provided to the subject's legally authorized representative or family member, if feasible.

(c) The IRB determinations required by paragraph (a) of this section and the documentation required by paragraph (e) of this section are to be retained by the IRB for at least 3 years after completion of the clinical investigation, and the records shall be accessible for inspection and copying by FDA in accordance with Sec. 56.115(b) of this chapter.

(d) Protocols involving an exception to the informed consent requirement under this section must be performed under a separate investigational new drug application (IND) or investigational device exemption (IDE) that clearly identifies such protocols as protocols that may include subjects who are unable to consent. The submission of those protocols in a separate IND/IDE is required even if an IND for the same drug product or an IDE for the same device already exists. Applications for investigations under this section may not be submitted as amendments under Secs. 312.30 or 812.35 of this chapter.

(e) If an IRB determines that it cannot approve a clinical investigation because the investigation does not meet the criteria in the exception provided under paragraph (a) of this section or because of other relevant ethical concerns, the IRB must document its findings and provide these findings promptly in writing to the clinical investigator and to the sponsor of the clinical investigation. The sponsor of the clinical investigation must promptly disclose this information to FDA and to the sponsor's clinical investigators who are participating or are asked to participate in this or a substantially equivalent clinical investigation of the sponsor, and to other IRB's that have been, or are, asked to review this or a substantially equivalent investigation by that sponsor.

[61 FR 51528, Oct. 2, 1996]

Sec. 50.25 Elements of informed consent

(a) Basic elements of informed consent. In seeking informed consent, the following information shall be provided to each subject:

(1) A statement that the study involves research, an explanation of the purposes of the research and the expected duration of the subject's participation, a description of the procedures to be followed, and identification of any procedures which are experimental.

(2) A description of any reasonably foreseeable risks or discomforts to the subject.

(3) A description of any benefits to the subject or to others which may reasonably be expected from the research.

(4) A disclosure of appropriate alternative procedures or courses of treatment, if any, that might be advantageous to the subject.

(5) A statement describing the extent, if any, to which confidentiality of records identifying the subject will be maintained and that notes the possibility that the Food and Drug Administration may inspect the records.

(6) For research involving more than minimal risk, an explanation as to whether any compensation and an explanation as to whether any medical treatments are available if injury occurs and, if so, what they consist of, or where further information may be obtained.

(7) An explanation of whom to contact for answers to pertinent questions about the research and research subjects' rights, and whom to contact in the event of a research-related injury to the subject.

(8) A statement that participation is voluntary, that refusal to participate will involve no penalty or loss of benefits to which the subject is otherwise entitled, and that the subject may discontinue participation at any time without penalty or loss of benefits to which the subject is otherwise entitled.

(b) Additional elements of informed consent. When appropriate, one or more of the following elements of information shall also be provided to each subject:

(1) A statement that the particular treatment or procedure may involve risks to the subject (or to the embryo or fetus, if the subject is or may become pregnant) which are currently unforeseeable.

(2) Anticipated circumstances under which the subject's participation may be terminated by the investigator without regard to the subject's consent.

(3) Any additional costs to the subject that may result from participation in the research.

(4) The consequences of a subject's decision to withdraw from the research and procedures for orderly termination of participation by the subject.

(5) A statement that significant new findings developed during the course of the research which may relate to the subject's willingness to continue participation will be provided to the subject.

(6) The approximate number of subjects involved in the study.

(c) The informed consent requirements in these regulations are not intended to preempt any applicable Federal, State, or local laws which require additional information to be disclosed for informed consent to be legally effective.

(d) Nothing in these regulations is intended to limit the authority of a physician to provide emergency medical care to the extent the physician is permitted to do so under applicable Federal, State, or local law.

Sec. 50.27 Documentation of informed consent

(a) Except as provided in Sec. 56.109(c), informed consent shall be documented by the use of a written consent form approved by the IRB and signed and dated by the subject or the subject's legally authorized representative at the time of consent. A copy shall be given to the person signing the form.

(b) Except as provided in Sec. 56.109(c), the consent form may be either of the following:

(1) A written consent document that embodies the elements of informed consent required by Sec. 50.25. This form may be read to the subject or the subject's legally authorized representative, but, in any event, the investigator shall give either the subject or the representative adequate opportunity to read it before it is signed.

(2) A short form written consent document stating that the elements of informed consent required by Sec. 50.25 have been presented orally to the subject or the subject's legally authorized representative. When this method is used, there shall be a witness to the oral presentation. Also, the IRB shall approve a written summary of what is to be said to the subject or the representative. Only the short form itself is to be signed by the subject or the representative. However, the witness shall sign both the short form and a copy of the summary, and the person actually obtaining the consent shall sign a copy of the summary. A copy of the summary shall be given to the subject or the representative in addition to a copy of the short form.

[46 FR 8951, Jan. 27, 1981, as amended at 61 FR 57280, Nov. 5, 1996]
[61FR 51497, October 2, 1996]

Code of Federal Regulations: Title 21, Part 56

21 CFR Part 56—Institutional Review Boards—Food and Drug Administration

Subpart A—General Provisions

Subpart B—Organization and personnel

Subpart C—IRB Functions and operations

Subpart D—Records and Reports

Subpart E—Administrative Action for Noncompliance

[Source: 46 FR 8975, Jan 27, 1981, unless otherwise noted.]

Subpart A—General Provisions

§ 56.101 Scope

(a) This part contains the general standards for the composition operation, and responsibility of an Institutional Review Board (IRB) that reviews clinical investigations regulated by the Food and Drug Administration under sections 505(i) and 520(g) of the act, as well as clinical that support applications for research or marketing permits for products regulated by the Food and Drug Administration including food and color additives, drugs for human use medical devices for human use, biological products for human use, and electronic products. Compliance with this part is intended to protect the rights and welfare of human subjects involved in such investigations.

(b) References in this part to regulatory sections of the Code of Federal Regulations are to chapter I of title 21, unless otherwise noted.

§ 56.102 Definitions

As used in this part:

(a) Act means the Federal Food, Drug, and Cosmetic Act, as amended (secs. 201-902, 52 Stat. 1040 et seq., as amended (21 U.S.C. 321-392)).

(b) Application for research or marketing permit includes:

(1) A color additive petition, described in part 71.

(2) Data and information regarding a substance submitted as part of the procedures for establishing that a substance is generally recognized as safe for a use which results or may reasonably be expected to result, directly or indirectly, in its becoming a component or otherwise affecting the characteristics of any food, described in § 170.35.

(3) A food additive petition, described in part 171.

(4) Data and information regarding a food additive submitted as part of the procedures regarding food additives permitted to be used on an interim basis pending additional study, described in § 180.1.

(5) Data and information regarding a substance submitted as part of the procedures for establishing a tolerance for unavoidable contaminants in food and food-packaging materials described in section 406 of the act.

(6) An investigational new drug application, described in part 312 of this chapter.

(7) A new drug application, described in part 314.

(8) Data and information regarding the bioavailability or bioequivalence of drugs for human use submitted as part of the procedures for issuing, amending, or repealing a bioequivalence requirement, described in part 320.

(9) Data and information regarding an over-the-counter drug for human use submitted as part of the procedures for classifying such drugs as generally recognized as safe and effective and not misbranded, described in part 330.

(10) An application for a biological product license, described in part 601.

(11) Data and information regarding a biological product submitted as part of the procedures for determining that licensed biological products are safe and effective and not misbranded, as described in part 601.

(12) An Application for an Investigational Device Exemption, described in parts 812 and 813.

(13) Data and information regarding a medical device for human use submitted as part of the procedures for classifying such devices, described in part 860.

(14) Data and information regarding a medical device for human use submitted as part of the procedures for establishing, amending, or repealing a standard for such device, described in part 861.

(15) An application for premarket approval of a medical device for human use, described in section 515 of the act.

(16) A product development protocol for a medical device for human use, described in section 515 of the act.

(17) Data and information regarding an electronic product submitted as part of the procedures for establishing, amending, or repealing a standard for such products, described in section 358 of the Public Health Service Act.

(18) Data and information regarding an electronic product submitted as part of the procedures for obtaining a variance from any electronic product performance standard, as described in § 1010.4.

(19) Data and information regarding an electronic product submitted as part of the procedures for granting, amending, or extending an exemption from a radiation safety performance standard as described in § 1010.5.

(20) Data and information regarding an electronic product submitted as part of the procedures for obtaining an exemption from notification of a radiation safety defect or failure of compliance with a radiation safety performance standard, described in subpart D of part 1003.

(c) Clinical investigation means any experiment that involves a test article and one or more human subjects, and that either must meet the requirements for prior submission to the Food and Drug Administration under section 505(i), or 520(g) of the act, or need not meet the requirements for prior submission to the Food and Drug Administration under these sections of the act, but the results of which are intended to be later submitted to, or held for inspection by, the Food and Drug Administration as part of an application for a research or marketing permit. The term does not include experiments that must meet the provisions of part 58, regarding nonclinical laboratory studies. The terms research, clinical research, clinical study, study, and clinical investigation are deemed to be synonymous for purposes of this part.

(d) Emergency use means the use of a test article on a human subject in a life-threatening situation in which no standard acceptable treatment is available, and in which there is not sufficient time to obtain IRB approval.

(e) Human subject means an individual who is or becomes a participant in research, either as a recipient of the test article or as a control. A subject may be either a healthy individual or a patient.

(f) Institution means any public or private entity or Agency (including Federal, State, and other agencies). The term facility as used in section 520(g) of the act is deemed to be synonymous with the term institution for purposes of this part.

(g) Institutional Review Board (IRB) means any board committee, or other group formally designated by an institution to review, to approve the initiation of, and to conduct periodic review of, biomedical research involving human subjects. The primary purpose of such review is to assure the protection of the rights and welfare of the human subjects. The term has the same meaning as the phrase institutional review committee as used in section 520(g) of the act.

(h) Investigator means an individual who actually conducts a clinical investigation (i.e., under whose immediate direction the test article is administered or dispensed to or used involving, a subject) or, in the event of an investigation conducted by a team of individuals, is the responsible leader of that team.

(i) Minimal risk means that the probability and magnitude of harm or discomfort anticipated in the research are not greater in and of themselves than those ordinarily encountered in daily life or during the performance of routine physical or psychological examinations or tests.

(j) Sponsor means a person or other entity that initiates a clinical investigation, but that does not actually conduct the investigation, i.e., the test article is administered or dispensed to, or used involving, a subject under the immediate direction of another individual. A person other than an individual (e.g., a corporation or agency) that uses one or more of its own employees to conduct an investigation that it has initiated is considered to be a sponsor (not a sponsor-investigator) and the employees are considered to be investigators.

(k) Sponsor-investigator means an individual who both initiates and actually conducts, alone or with others a clinical investigation, i.e., under whose immediate direction the test article is administered or dispensed to, or used involving, a subject. The term does not include any person other than an individual, e.g., it does not include a corporation or agency. The obligations of a sponsor-investigator under this part include both those of a sponsor and those of an investigator.

(l) Test article means any drug for human use, biological product for human use, medical device for human use, human food additive, color additive, electronic product, or any other article subject to regulation under the act or under sections 351 or 354-360F of the Public Health Service Act.

(m) IRB approval means the determination of the IRB that the clinical investigation has been reviewed and may be conducted at an institution within the constraints set forth by the IRB and by other institutional and Federal requirements.

[46 FR 8975, Jan. 27, 1981, as amended at 54 FR 9038 Mar. 3, 1989; 56 FR 28028, June 18, 1991; 64 FR 399, Jan. 5, 1999; 64 FR 56448, Oct. 20, 1999; 65 FR 52302, Aug. 29, 2000]

§ 56.103 Circumstances in which IRB review is required

(a) Except as provided in §§ 56.104 and 56.105, any clinical investigation which must meet the requirements for prior submission (as required in parts 312, 812, and 813) to the Food and Drug Administration shall not be initiated unless that investigation has been reviewed and approved by, and remains subject to continuing review by, an IRB meeting the requirements of this part.

(b) Except as provided in §§ 56.104 and 56.105, the Food and Drug Administration may decide not to consider in support of an application for research or marketing permit any data or information that has been derived from a clinical investigation that has not been approved by, and that was not subject to initial and continuing review by, an IRB meeting the requirements of this part. The determination that a clinical investigation may not be considered in support of an application for a research or marketing permit does not, however, relieve the applicant for such a permit of any obligation under any other applicable regulations to submit the results of the investigation to the Food and Drug Administration.

(c) Compliance with these regulations will in no way render inapplicable pertinent Federal, State, or local laws or regulations.

[46 FR 8975, Jan. 27, 1981; 46 FR 14340, Feb. 27, 1981]

§ 56.104 Exemptions from IRB requirement

The following categories of clinical investigations are exempt from the requirements of this part for IRB review:

(a) Any investigation which commenced before July 27, 1981 and was subject to requirements for IRB review under FDA regulations before that date, provided that the investigation remains subject to review of an IRB which meets the FDA requirements in effect before July 27, 1981.

(b) Any investigation commenced before July 27, 1981 and was not otherwise subject to requirements for IRB review under Food and Drug Administration regulations before that date.

(c) Emergency use of a test article, provided that such emergency use is reported to the IRB within 5 working days. Any subsequent use of the test article at the institution is subject to IRB review.

(d) Taste and food quality evaluations and consumer acceptance studies, if wholesome foods without additives are consumed or if a food is consumed that contains a food ingredient at or below the level and for a use found to be safe, or agricultural, chemical, or environmental contaminant at or below the level found to be safe, by the Food and Drug Administration or approved by the Environmental Protection Agency or the Food Safety and Inspection Service of the U.S. Department of Agriculture.

[46 FR 8975, Jan. 27 1981, as amended at 56 FR 28028, June 18, 1991]

§ 56.105 Waiver of IRB requirement

On the application of a sponsor or sponsor-investigator, the Food and Drug Administration may waive any of the requirements contained in these regulations including the requirements for IRB review, for specific research activities or for classes of research activities otherwise covered by these regulations.

Subpart B—Organization and Personnel

§ 56.107 IRB membership

(a) Each IRB shall have at least five members, with varying backgrounds to promote complete and adequate review of research activities commonly conducted by the institution. The IRB shall be sufficiently qualified through the experience and expertise of its members and the diversity of the members, including consideration of race, gender, cultural backgrounds, and sensitivity to such issues as community attitudes, to promote respect for its advice and counsel in safeguarding the rights and welfare of human subjects. In addition to possessing the professional competence necessary to review the specific research activities, the IRB shall be able to ascertain the acceptability of proposed research in terms of institutional commitments and regulations applicable law, and standards of professional conduct and practice. The IRB shall therefore include persons knowledgeable in these areas. If an IRB regularly reviews research that involves a vulnerable category of subjects, such as children, prisoners, pregnant women, or handicapped or mentally disabled persons, consideration shall be given to the inclusion of one or more individuals who are knowledgeable about and experienced in working with those subjects.

(b) Every nondiscriminatory effort will be made to ensure that no IRB consists entirely of men or entirely of women, including the institution's consideration of qualified persons of both sexes, so long as no selection is made to the IRB on the basis of gender. No IRB may consist entirely of members of one profession.

(c) Each IRB shall include at least one member whose primary concerns are in the scientific area and at least one member whose primary concerns are in nonscientific areas.

(d) Each IRB shall include at least one member who is not otherwise affiliated with the institution and who is not part of the immediate family of a person who is affiliated with the institution.

(e) No IRB may have a member participate in the IRB's initial or continuing review of any project in which the member has a conflicting interest, except to provide information requested by the IRB.

(f) An IRB may, in its discretion, invite individuals with competence in special areas to assist in the review of complex issues which require expertise beyond or in addition to that available on the IRB. These individuals may not vote with the IRB.

[46 FR 8975, Jan 27, 1981, as amended at 56 FR 28028, June 18, 1991; 56 FR 29756 June 28, 1991]

Subpart C—IRB Functions and Operations

§ 56.108 IRB functions and operations

In order to fulfill the requirements of these regulations, each IRB shall:

(a) Follow written procedures: (1) For conducting its initial and continuing review of research and for reporting its findings and actions to the investigator and the institution; (2) for determining which projects require review more often than annually and which projects need verification from sources other than the investigator that no material changes have occurred since previous IRB review; (3) for ensuring prompt reporting to the IRB of changes in research activity; and (4) for ensuring that changes in approved research, during the period for which

IRB approval has already been given may not be initiated without IRB review and approval except where necessary to eliminate apparent immediate hazards to the human subjects.

(b) Follow written procedures for ensuring prompt reporting to the IRB, appropriate institutional officials, and the Food and Drug Administration of: (1) Any unanticipated problems involving risks to human subjects or others; (2) any instance of serious or continuing noncompliance with these or the requirements or determinations of the IRB; or (3) any suspension or termination of IRB approval.

(c) Except when an expedited review procedure is used (see § 56.110), review proposed research at convened meetings at which a majority of the members of the IRB are present including at least one member whose primary concerns are in nonscientific areas. In order for the research to be approved it shall receive the approval of a majority of those members present at the meeting.

[46 FR 8975, Jan. 27, 1981, as amended at 56 FR 28028, June 18, 1991]

§ 56.109 IRB review of research

(a) An IRB shall review and have authority to approve, require modifications in (to secure approval), or disapprove all research activities covered by these regulations.

(b) An IRB shall require that information given to subjects as part of informed consent is in accordance with § 50.25. The IRB may require that information in addition to that specifically mentioned in § 50.25, be given to the subjects when in the IRB's judgment the information would meaningfully add to the protection of the rights and welfare of subjects.

(c) An IRB shall require documentation of informed consent in accordance with Sec. 50.27 of this chapter, except as follows:

  (1) The IRB may, for some or all subjects, waive the requirement that the subject, or the subject's legally authorized representative, sign a written consent form if it finds that the research presents no more than minimal risk of harm to subjects and involves no procedures for which written consent is normally required outside the research context; or

  (2) The IRB may, for some or all, find that the requirements in Sec. 50.24 of this chapter for an exception from informed consent for emergency research are met.

(d) In cases where the documentation requirement is waived under paragraph (c)(1) of this section, the IRB may require the investigator to provide subjects with a written statement regarding the research.

(e) An IRB shall notify investigators and the institution in writing of its decision to approve or disapprove the proposed research activity, or of modifications required to secure IRB approval of the research activity. If the IRB decides to disapprove a research activity, it shall include in its written notification a statement of the reasons for its decision and give the investigator an opportunity to respond in person or in writing. For investigations involving an exception to informed consent under Sec. 50.24 of this chapter, an IRB shall promptly notify in writing the investigator and the sponsor of the research when an IRB determines that it cannot approve the research because it does not meet the criteria in the exception provided under Sec. 50.24(a) of this chapter or because of other relevant ethical concerns. The written notification shall include a statement of the reasons for the IRB's determination.

(f) An IRB shall conduct continuing review of research covered by these regulations at intervals appropriate to the degree of risk, but not less than once per year, and shall have authority to observe or have a third party observe the consent process and the research.

(g) An IRB shall provide in writing to the sponsor of research involving an exception to informed consent under Sec. 50.24 of this chapter a copy of information that has been publicly disclosed under Sec. 50.24(a)(7)(ii) and (a)(7)(iii) of this chapter. The IRB shall provide this information to the sponsor promptly so that the sponsor is aware that such disclosure has occurred. Upon receipt, the sponsor shall provide copies of the information disclosed to FDA.

[46 FR 8975, Jan. 27, 1981, as amended at 56 FR 28028, June 18, 1991, and at 61 FR 51497, Oct. 2, 1996]

§ 56.110 Expedited review procedures for certain kinds of research involving no more than minimal risk, and for minor changes in approved research

(a) The Food and Drug Administration has established, and published in the Federal Register, a list of categories of research that may be reviewed by the IRB through an expedited review procedure. The list will be amended, as appropriate through periodic republication in the Federal Register.

(b) An IRB may use the expedited review procedure to review either or both of the following: (1) Some or all of the research appearing on the list and found by the reviewer(s) to involve no more than minimal risk, (2) minor changes in previously approved research during the period (of 1 year or less) for which approval is authorized. Under an expedited review procedure the review may be carried out by the IRB chairperson or by one or more experienced reviewers designated by the IRB chairperson from among the members of the IRB. In reviewing the research, the reviewers may exercise all of the authorities of the IRB except that the reviewers may not disapprove the research. A research activity may be disapproved only after review in accordance with the non-expedited review procedure set forth in § 56.108(c).

(c) Each IRB which uses an expedited review procedure shall adopt a method for keeping all members advised of research proposals which have been approved under the procedure.

(d) The Food and Drug Administration may restrict, suspend, or terminate an institution's or IRB's use of the expedited review procedure when necessary to protect the rights or welfare of subjects.

[46 FR 8975, Jan. 27, 1981, as amended at 56 FR 28029, June 18, 1991]

§ 56.111 Criteria for IRB approval of research

(a) In order to approve research covered by these regulations the IRB shall determine that all of the following requirements are satisfied:

(1) Risks to subjects are minimized: (i) By using procedures which are consistent with sound research design and which do not unnecessarily expose subjects to risk, and (ii) whenever appropriate, by using procedures already being performed on the subjects for diagnostic or treatment purposes.

(2) Risks to subjects are reasonable in relation to anticipated benefits, if any, to subjects and the importance of the knowledge that may be expected to result. In evaluating risks and benefits, the IRB should consider only those risks and benefits that may result from the research (as distinguished from risks and benefits therapies that subjects would receive even if not participating in the research). The IRB should not consider possible long-range effects of applying knowledge gained in the research (for example, the possible effects of the research on public policy) as among those research risks that fall within the purview of its responsibility.

(3) Selection of subjects is equitable. In making this assessment the IRB should take into account the purposes of the research and the setting in which the research will be conducted and should be particularly cognizant of the special problems of research involving vulnerable populations, such as children, prisoners, pregnant women, handicapped, or mentally disabled persons, or economically or educationally disadvantaged persons.

(4) Informed consent will be sought from each prospective subject or the subject's legally authorized representative, in accordance with and to the extent required by part 50.

(5) Informed consent will be appropriately documented, in accordance with and to the extent required by § 50.27.

(6) Where appropriate, the research plan makes adequate provision for monitoring the data collected to ensure the safety of subjects.

(7) Where appropriate, there are adequate provisions to protect the privacy of subjects and to maintain the confidentiality of data.

(b) When some or all of the subjects, such as children, prisoners, pregnant women, handicapped, or mentally disabled persons, or economically or educationally disadvantaged persons, are likely to be vulnerable to coercion or undue influence additional safeguards have been included in the study to protect the rights and welfare of these subjects.
[46 FR 8975, Jan. 27, 1981, as amended at 56 FR 28029, June 18, 1991]

§ 56.112 Review by institution

Research covered by these regulations that has been approved by an IRB may be subject to further appropriate review and approval or disapproval by officials of the institution. However, those officials may not approve the research if it has not been approved by an IRB.

§ 56.113 Suspension or termination of IRB approval of research

An IRB shall have authority to suspend or terminate approval of research that is not being conducted in accordance with the IRB's requirements or that has been associated with unexpected serious harm to subjects. Any suspension or termination of approval shall include a statement of the reasons for the IRB's action and shall be reported promptly to the investigator appropriate institutional officials, and the Food and Drug Administration.

§ 56.114 Cooperative research

In complying with these regulations, institutions involved in multi-institutional studies may use joint review, reliance upon the review of another qualified IRB, or similar arrangements aimed at avoidance of duplication of effort.

Subpart D—Records and Reports

§ 56.115 IRB records

(a) An institution, or where appropriate an IRB, shall prepare and maintain adequate documentation of IRB activities including the following:

(1) Copies of all research proposals reviewed, scientific evaluations, if any, that accompany the proposals, approved sample consent documents progress reports submitted by investigators, and reports of injuries to subjects.

(2) Minutes of IRB meetings which shall be in sufficient detail to show attendance at the meetings; actions taken by the IRB; the vote on these actions including the number of members voting for, against and abstaining; the basis for requiring changes in or disapproving research; and a written summary of the discussion of controverted issues and their resolution.

(3) Records of continuing review activities.

(4) Copies of all correspondence between the IRB and the investigators.

(5) A list of IRB members identified by name; earned degrees; representative capacity; indications of experience such as board certifications licenses, etc., sufficient to describe each member's chief anticipated contributions to IRB deliberations; and any employment or other relationship between each member and the institution; for example: full-time employee, part-time employee, a member of governing panel or board, stockholder, paid or unpaid consultant.

(6) Written procedures for the IRB as required by § 56.108(a) and (b).

(7) Statements of significant new findings provided to subjects, as required by § 50.25.

(b) The records required by this regulation shall be retained for at least 3 years after completion of the research, and the records shall be accessible for inspection and copying by authorized representatives of the Food and Drug Administration at reasonable times and in a reasonable manner.

(c) The Food and Drug Administration may refuse to consider a clinical investigation in support of an application for a research or marketing permit if the institution or the IRB that reviewed the investigation refuses to allow an inspection under this section.
(Information collection requirements in this section were approved by the Office of Management and Budget (OMB) and assigned OMB control number 0910-0130)
[46 FR 8975, Jan. 27, 1981, as amended at 56 FR 28029, June 18, 1991]

Subpart E—Administrative Actions for Noncompliance

§ 56.120 Lesser administrative actions

(a) If apparent noncompliance with these regulations in the operation of an IRB is observed by an FDA investigator during an inspection, the inspector will present an oral or written summary of observations to an appropriate representative of the IRB. The Food and Drug Administration may subsequently send a letter describing the noncompliance to the IRB and to the parent institution. The agency will require that the IRB or the parent institution respond to this letter within a time period specified by FDA and describe the corrective actions that will be taken by the IRB, the institution, or both to achieve compliance with these regulations.

(b) On the basis of the IRB's or the institution's response FDA may schedule a reinspection to confirm the adequacy of corrective actions. In addition, until the IRB or the parent institution takes appropriate corrective action, the agency may:

(1) Withhold approval of new studies subject to the requirements of this part that are conducted at the institution or reviewed by the IRB;

(2) Direct that no new subjects be added to ongoing studies subject to this part;

(3) Terminate ongoing studies subject to this part when doing so would not endanger the subjects; or

(4) When the apparent noncompliance creates a significant threat to the rights and welfare of human subjects notify relevant State and Federal regulatory agencies and other parties with a direct interest in the agency's action of the deficiencies in the operation of the IRB.

(c) The parent institution is presumed to be responsible for the operation of an IRB, and the Food and Drug Administration will ordinarily direct any administrative action under this subpart against the institution. However, depending on the evidence of responsibility for deficiencies, determined during the investigation, the Food and Drug Administration may restrict its administrative actions to the IRB or to a component of the parent institution determined to be responsible for formal designation of the IRB.

§ 56.121 Disqualification of an IRB or an institution

(a) Whenever the IRB or the institution has failed to take adequate steps to correct the noncompliance stated in the letter sent by the agency under § 56.120(a), and the Commissioner of Food and Drugs determines that this noncompliance may justify the disqualification of the IRB or of the parent, the Commissioner will institute proceedings in accordance with the requirements for a regulatory hearing set forth in part 16.

(b) The Commissioner may disqualify an IRB or the parent if the Commissioner determines that:

(1) The IRB has refused or repeatedly failed to comply with any of the regulations set forth in this part, and;

(2) The noncompliance adversely affects the rights or welfare of the human subjects in a clinical investigation.

(c) If the Commissioner determines that disqualification is appropriate, the Commissioner will issue an order that explains the basis for the determination and that prescribes any actions to be taken with regard to ongoing clinical research conducted under the review of the IRB. The Food and Drug Administration will send notice of the disqualification to the IRB and the parent institution. Other parties with a direct interest, such as sponsors and clinical investigators, may also be sent a notice of the disqualification. In addition, the agency may elect to publish a notice of its action in the Federal Register.

(d) The Food and Drug Administration will not approve an application for a research permit for a clinical investigation that is to be under the review of a disqualified IRB or that is to be conducted at a disqualified institution, and it may refuse to consider in support of a marketing permit the data from a clinical investigation that was reviewed by a disqualified IRB as conducted at a disqualified institution unless the IRB or the parent institution is reinstated as provided in § 56.123.

§ 56.122 Public disclosure of information regarding revocation

A determination that the Food and Drug Administration has disqualified an institution and the administrative record regarding that determination are disclosable to the public under part 20.

§ 56.123 Reinstatement of an IRB or an institution

An IRB or an institution may be reinstated if the Commissioner determines upon an evaluation of a written submission from the IRB or institution that explains the corrective action that the institution or IRB plans to take, that the IRB or institution has provided adequate assurance that it will operate in compliance with the standards set forth in this part. Notification of reinstatement shall be provided to all persons notified under § 56.121(c).

§ 56.124 Actions alternative or additional to disqualification

Disqualification of an IRB or of an institution is independent of, and neither in lieu of nor a precondition to, other proceedings or actions authorized by the act. The Food and Drug Administration may at any time, through the Department of Justice institute any appropriate judicial proceedings (civil or criminal) and any other appropriate regulatory action, in addition to or in lieu of, and before, at the time of, or after, disqualification. The Agency may also refer pertinent matters to another Federal, State, or local government Agency for any action that Agency determines to be appropriate.

Appendix A: List of Selected FDA Regulations Relating to the Protection of Human Subjects

This list contains Food and Drug Administration (FDA) regulations that specifically relate to the protection of human subjects in clinical investigations. The citations selected below are only a few of the FDA regulations (contained in nine volumes) that apply to clinical investigations and govern the development and approval of drugs, biologics, and devices. The regulations are contained in Title 21 of the Code of Federal Regulations (CFR), which can be purchased from the Superintendent of Documents, Attn: New Orders, P.O. Box 371954,

Pittsburgh, PA 15250-7954; (202-512-1800, fax: 202-512-2233)

I. FDA HUMAN SUBJECT PROTECTIONS
Part 50—Protection of Human Subjects (Informed Consent)
Part 56—Institutional Review Boards

II. SUBSTANCES AND ARTICLES REGULATED BY FDA

Foods
Part 71—Color Additives
Part 171—Food Additive Petitions
Part 180—Food Additives (Interim)

Drugs
Part 312—Investigational New Drug Application
Part 314—New Drug Applications
Part 320—Bioavailability and Bioequivalence Requirements
Part 330—Over-the-Counter Human Drugs Part 361.1—Radioactive Drugs for Certain Research Uses

Biologics
Part 312—Investigational New Drug Application
Part 601—Licensing
Part 630—Additional Standards for Viral Vaccines Medical Devices
Part 812—Investigational Device Exemptions
Part 814—Premarket Approval of Medical Devices

Radiological Health
Part 361.1—Radioactive Drugs for Certain Research Uses
Part 1010—Performance Standards for Electronic Products

III. RELATED FDA PROCEDURES
Part 10—General Agency Administrative Procedures
Part 16—Regulatory Hearings before the FDA
Part 20—Public Information

IV. STATUTES PROVIDING AUTHORITY FOR REGULATIONS LISTED ABOVE:
Biological Control Act of 1902/Virus, Serum and Toxin Act of 1902
Food, Drug and Cosmetic Act of 1938 (as amended)
Public Health Service Act of 1944 (as amended)
Food Additive Amendments of 1958
Color Additives Amendment of 1960
New Drug Amendments of 1962
Radiation Control for Public Health and Safety Act of 1968
National Research Act of 1974
Medical Device Amendments of 1976
Safe Medical Devices Act of 1990
Device Amendments of 1992
FDA Modernization Act of 1997

Appendix B: Significant Differences in FDA and HHS Regulations for Protection of Human Subjects

The Department of Health and Human Services (HHS) regulations [45 CFR part 46] apply to research involving human subjects conducted by the HHS or funded in whole or in part by the HHS. The Food and Drug Administration (FDA) regulations [21 CFR parts 50 and 56] apply to research involving products regulated by the FDA. Federal support is not necessary for the FDA regulations to be applicable. When research involving products regulated by the FDA is funded, supported or conducted by FDA and/or HHS, both the HHS and FDA regulations apply.

IRB Regulations

§ 56.102 (FDA)	FDA definitions are included for terms
§ 46.102 (HHS)	specific to the type of research covered by the FDA regulations (test article, application for research or marketing permit, clinical investigation). A definition for emergency use is provided in the FDA regulations.
§ 56.104 (FDA)	FDA provides exemption from the prospective
§ 46.116 (HHS)	IRB review requirement for "emergency use" of test article in specific situations. HHS regulations state that they are not intended to limit the provision of emergency medical care.
§ 56.105 (FDA)	FDA provides for sponsors and sponsor-investigators to request a waiver of IRB review requirements (but not informed consent requirements).
§ 46.101 (HHS)	HHS exempts certain categories of research and provides for a Secretarial waiver.
§ 56.109 (FDA)	Unlike HHS, FDA does not provide that an IRB
§ 46.109 (HHS)	may waive the requirement for signed consent
§ 46.117(c)(HHS)	when the principal risk is a breach of confidentiality because FDA does not regulate studies which would fall into that category of research. (Both regulations allow for IRB waiver of documentation of informed consent in instances of minimal risk.)
§ 56.110 (FDA)	The FDA list of investigations eligible for
§ 46.110 (HHS)	expedited review (published in the Federal Register) does not include the studies described in category 9

	of the HHS list because these types of studies are not regulated by FDA
§ 56.114 (FDA)	FDA does not discuss administrative matters
§ 46.114 (HHS)	dealing with grants and contracts because they are irrelevant to the scope of the Agency's regulation. (Both regulations make allowances for review of multi-institutional studies.)
§ 56.115 (FDA)	FDA has neither an assurance mechanism nor
§ 46.115 (HHS)	files of IRB membership. Therefore, FDA does not require the IRB or institution to report changes in membership whereas HHS does require such notification.
§ 56.115(c) (FDA)	FDA may refuse to consider a study in support of a research or marketing permit if the IRB or the institution refuses to allow FDA to inspect IRB records. HHS has no such provision because it does not issue research or marketing permits.
§ 56.120—	FDA regulations provide sanctions for
§ 56.124 (FDA)	non-compliance with regulations.

Informed Consent Regulations

§ 50.23 (FDA)	FDA, but not HHS, provides for an exception from the informed consent requirements in emergency situations. The provision is based on the Medical Device Amendments of 1976, but may be used in investigations involving drugs, devices, and other FDA regulated products in situations described in § 50.23.
§ 46.116(c)&(d)	HHS provides for waiving or altering elements (HHS) of informed consent under certain conditions. FDA has no such provision because the types of studies which would qualify for such waivers are either not regulated by FDA or are covered by the emergency treatment provisions (§ 50.23).
§ 50.25(a)(5) (FDA)	FDA explicitly requires that subjects be
§ 46.116(a) (5) (HHS)	informed that FDA may inspect the records of the study because FDA may occasionally examine a subject's medical records when they pertain to the study. While HHS has the right to inspect records of studies it funds, it does not impose that same informed consent requirement.
§ 50.27(a)	FDA explicitly requires that consent forms be dated as well as signed by the subject or the subject's legally authorized representative. The HHS regulations do not explicitly require consent forms to be dated.

IRB Expedited Review Criteria

Dept. of Health and Human Services, National Institutes of Health, Office for Protection from Research Risks

Categories of Research That May Be Reviewed by the Institutional Review Board (IRB) through an Expedited Review Procedure*
63 FR 60364-60367, November 9, 1998

Applicability

(A) Research activities that (1) present no more than minimal risk to human subjects, and (2) involve only procedures listed in one or more of the following categories, may be reviewed by the IRB through the expedited review procedure authorized by 45 CFR 46.110 and 21 CFR 56.110. The activities listed should not be deemed to be of minimal risk simply because they are included on this list. Inclusion on this list merely means that the activity is eligible for review through the expedited review procedure when the specific circumstances of the proposed research involve no more than minimal risk to human subjects.

(B) The categories in this list apply regardless of the age of subjects, except as noted.

(C) The expedited review procedure may not be used where identification of the subjects and/or their responses would reasonably place them at risk of criminal or civil liability. Nor may it be damaging to the subjects financial standing, employability, insurability, reputation, or be stigmatizing. Unless reasonable and appropriate protections will be implemented so that risks related to invasion of privacy and breach of confidentiality are no greater than minimal.

(D) The expedited review procedure may not be used for classified research involving human subjects.

(E) IRBs are reminded that the standard requirements for informed consent (or its waiver, alteration, or exception) apply regardless of the type of review—expedited or convened—utilized by the IRB.

(F) Categories one (1) through seven (7) pertain to both initial and continuing IRB review.

Research Categories

(1) Clinical studies of drugs and medical devices only when condition (a) or (b) is met.

    (a) Research on drugs for which an investigational new drug application (21 CFR Part 312) is not required. (Note: Research on marketed drugs that significantly increases the risks or decreases the acceptability of the risks associated with the use of the product is not eligible for expedited review.)

    (b) Research on medical devices for which (i) an investigational device exemption application (21 CFR Part 812) is not required; or (ii) the medical device is cleared/approved for marketing and the medical device is being used in accordance with its cleared/approved labeling.

(2) Collection of blood samples by finger stick, heel stick, ear stick, or venipuncture as follows:

    (a) from healthy, nonpregnant adults who weigh at least 110 pounds. For these subjects, the amounts drawn may not exceed 550 ml in an 8 week period and collection may not occur more frequently than 2 times per week; or

    (b) from other adults and children**, considering the age, weight, and health of the subjects, the collection procedure, the amount of blood to be collected, and the frequency with which it will be collected. For these subjects, the amount drawn may not exceed the lesser of 50 ml or 3 ml per kg in an 8 week period and collection may not occur more frequently than 2 times per week.

(3) Prospective collection of biological specimens for research purposes by noninvasive means.

Examples:

(a) hair and nail clippings in a nondisfiguring manner; (b) deciduous teeth at time of exfoliation or if routine patient care indicates a need for extraction; (c) permanent teeth if routine patient care indicates a need for extraction; (d) excreta and external secretions (including sweat); (e) uncannulated saliva collected either in an unstimulated fashion or stimulated by chewing gumbase orwax or by applying a dilute citric solution to the tongue; (f) placenta removed at delivery; (g) amniotic fluid obtained at the time of rupture of the membrane prior to or during labor; (h) supra-and subgingival dental plaque and calculus, provided the collection procedure is not more invasive than routine prophylactic scaling of the teeth and the process is accomplished in accordance with accepted prophylactic techniques; (i) mucosal and skin cells collected by buccal scraping or swab, skin swab, or mouth washings; (j) sputum collected after saline mist nebulization.

(4) Collection of data through noninvasive procedures (not involving general anesthesia or sedation) routinely employed in clinical practice, excluding procedures involving x-rays or microwaves. Where medical devices are employed, they must be cleared/approved for marketing. (Studies intended to evaluate the safety and effectiveness of the medical device are not generally eligible for expedited review, including studies of cleared medical devices for new indications.)

Examples:

(a) physical sensors that are applied either to the surface of the body or at a distance and do not involve input of significant amounts of energy into the subject or an invasion of the subjects privacy; (b) weighing or testing sensory acuity; (c) magnetic resonance imaging; (d) electrocardiography, electroencephalography, thermography, detection of naturally occurring radioactivity, electroretinography, ultrasound, diagnostic infrared imaging, doppler blood flow, and echocardiography; (e) moderate exercise, muscular strength testing, body composition assessment, and flexibility testing where appropriate given the age, weight, and health of the individual.

(5) Research involving materials (data, documents, records, or specimens) that have been collected, or will be collected solely for nonresearch purposes (such as medical treatment or diagnosis). (NOTE: Some research in this category may be exempt from the HHS regulations for the protection of human subjects. 45 CFR 46.101(b)(4). This listing refers only to research that is not exempt.)

(6) Collection of data from voice, video, digital, or image recordings made for research purposes.

(7) Research on individual or group characteristics or behavior (including, but not limited to, research on perception, cognition, motivation, identity, language, communication, cultural beliefs or practices, and social behavior) or research employing survey, interview, oral history, focus group, program evaluation, human factors evaluation, or quality assurance methodologies. (NOTE: Some research in this category may be exempt from the HHS regulations for the protection of human subjects. 45 CFR 46.101(b)(2) and (b)(3). This listing refers only to research that is not exempt.)

(8) Continuing review of research previously approved by the convened IRB as follows:

(a) where (i) the research is permanently closed to the enrollment of new subjects; (ii) all subjects have completed all research-related interventions; and (iii) the research remains active only for long-term follow-up of subjects; or

(b) where no subjects have been enrolled and no additional risks have been identified; or

(c) where the remaining research activities are limited to data analysis.

(9) Continuing review of research, not conducted under an investigational new drug application or investigational device exemption where categories two (2) through eight (8) do not apply but the IRB has determined and documented at a convened meeting that the research involves no greater than minimal risk and no additional risks have been identified.

* An expedited review procedure consists of a review of research involving human subjects by the IRB chairperson or by one or more experienced reviewers designated by the chairperson from among members of the IRB in accordance with the requirements set forth in 45 CFR 46.110.

**Children are defined in the HHS regulations as "persons who have not attained the legal age for consent to treatments or procedures involved in the research, under the applicable law of the jurisdiction in which the research will be conducted." 45 CFR 46.402(a).

Guidelines and Resources

U.S. Government Guidance and Resources

Office for Human Research Protections (OHRP): Dear Colleague Letters
Web site: http://ohrp.osophs.dhhs.gov/dearcoll.htm

Office for Human Research Protections (OHRP): Guidance Topics by Subject
Web site: http://ohrp.osophs.dhhs.gov/g-topics.htm

OHRP Compliance Activities: Common Findings and Guidance
Web site: http://ohrp.osophs.gov/compovr.htm

FDA Information Sheets (1998 edition)
Guidance for Institutional Review Boards and Clinical Investigators
Web site: http://www.fda.gov/oc/oha/IRB/toc.html

FDA Clinical Trials/ Human Subjects Protection
Information for Health Professionals
Web site: http://www.fda.gov/oc/oha/default.htm#clinical

National Bioethics Advisory Commission
Web site: http://bioethics.gov/nbac.html

Office of Research Integrity
Web site: http://ori.dhhs.gov/

Health Care Financing Administration (HCFA)
Medicare Coverage Policy—Clinical Trials
Web site: http://www.hcfa.gov/coverage/8d2.htm

Bioethics Resources on the Web—National Institutes of Health
Web site: http://www.nih.gov/sigs/bioethics/

National Human Genome Research Institute
Ethical, Legal and Social Implications of Human Genetics Research
Web site: http://www.nhgri.nih.gov/ELSI/

National Reference Center for Bioethics Literature—Kennedy Institute
Web site: http://www.georgetown.edu/research/nrcbl/

Office of Biotechnology Activities—NIH
Web site: http://www.nih.gov/od/oba/index.htm

International Guidelines

International Committee on Harmonisation (ICH)
Good Clinical Practice Guidelines
Web site: www.ifpma.org/ich5e.html

Council for International Organizations of Medical Sciences (CIOMS)
International Ethical Guidelines for Biomedical Research
Web site: http://www.who.int/ina-ngo/ngo/ngo011.htm

Canadian Institutes of Health Research
Web site: http://www.nserc.ca/programs/ethics.htm

National Council on Ethics in Human Research—Canada
Web site: http://www.ncehr-cnerh.org/english/mstr_frm.html

Danish Council on Ethics
Web site:
http://www.etiskraad.dk/english/about_the_council.html

French National Consultative Committee on Ethics
Web site: http://www.ccne-ethique.org/

National Committee for Medical Research Ethics—Norway
Web site: http://www.etikkom.no/E/index.htm

Periodicals, IRB Forum, and Selected Organizations

Periodicals and IRB Forum

ARENA Newsletter
Applied Research Ethics in Medicine and Research
http://140.239.168.132/arena.html

Bulletin of Medical Ethics
Dr. Richard Nicholson, Editor
Email: bulletin_of_medical_ethics@compuserve.com

The Hastings Center
Web site: http://www.thehastingscenter.org/

Hastings Center Report
Web site:
    http://www.thehastingscenter.org/publications.htm

IRB: A Review of Human Subjects Research
Web site:
    http://www.thehastingscenter.org/publications.htm

Human Research Report
Web site: http://www.humansubjects.com/

Kennedy Institute of Ethics Journal
Web site:
    http://muse.jhu.edu/journals/kennedy_institute_of_
    ethics_journal/

The IRB Forum (previously MCWIRB)
Web site: http://www.irbforum.org/
The IRB Forum promotes the discussion of ethical,
    regulatory, and policy concerns with human subjects
    research.

Research Practitioner
Web site:
    http://www.researchpractice.com/rp_about.shtml

Selected Organizations

American Medical Association (AMA)
Web site: http://www.ama-assn.org

American Psychiatric Association
Web site: http://www.psych.org/

American Psychological Association
Web site: http://www.apa.org/

**American Society of Law, Medicine, and Ethics
    (ASLME)**
Web site: http://www.aslme.org/

Applied Research Ethics National Association (ARENA)
Web site: http://140.239.168.132/arena.html

Association of American Medical Colleges (AAMC)
Web site: http://www.aamc.org

Association of Clinical Research Professionals (ACRP)
Web site: http://www.acrpnet.org/

Center for Clinical Research Practice (CCRP)
Web site: http://www.ccrp.com/index.shtlm

CenterWatch Clinical Trials
http://www.centerwatch.com

Drug Information Association (DIA)
Web site: http://www.diahome.org

National Association of IRB Managers (NIAM)
Web site: http://www.naim.org

**National Council of University Research Administrators
    (NCURA)**
Web site: http://www.ncura.edu

Oral History Association (OHA)
Web site: http://omega.dickinson.edu/organizations/oha

**Public Responsibility in Medicine and Research
    (PRIM&R)**
Web site: http://www.primr.org

World Medical Association (WMA)
Web site: http://www.wma.net

Index